CURRENT THERAPY IN NEUROLOGIC DISEASE

CURRENT THERAPY SERIES

CURRENT THERAPY IN NEUROLOGIC DISEASE

FOURTH EDITION

RICHARD T. JOHNSON, M.D.

Professor and Director of Neurology
Professor of Microbiology and Neuroscience
The Johns Hopkins University School of Medicine
Neurologist-in-Chief
The Johns Hopkins Hospital
Baltimore, Maryland

JOHN W. GRIFFIN, M.D.

Professor of Neurology and Neuroscience
The Johns Hopkins University School of Medicine
Baltimore, Maryland

B.C. Decker
An Imprint of Mosby–Year Book, Inc.

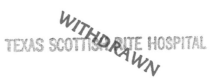

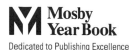

Executive Editor: Susan M. Gay
Senior Managing Editor: Lynne Gery
Project Supervisor: Victoria Hoenigke

FOURTH EDITION

Printed in the United States of America

Mosby–Year Book, Inc.
11830 Westline Industrial Drive
St. Louis, Missouri 63146

NOTICE: The authors and publisher have made every effort to ensure that the patient care recommended
herein, including choice of drugs and drug dosages, is in accord with the accepted standards and practice at
the time of publication. However, since research and regulation constantly change clinical standards, the
reader is urged to check the product information sheet included in the package of each drug, which includes
recommended doses, warnings, and contraindications. This is particularly important with new or infrequently
used drugs.

ISBN 0-8016-7730-0

MICHAEL P. ALEXANDER, M.D.

Associate Professor of Neurology, Boston University School of Medicine, Boston; Aphasia Program Director, Braintree Hospital, Braintree, Massachusetts

ROBERT R. ALLEN, M.D.

Neurology Pain Fellow, University of California, San Francisco, School of Medicine, San Francisco, California

JOHN ARYANPUR, M.D.

Assistant Professor of Neurosurgery, The Johns Hopkins University School of Medicine, Baltimore, Maryland

J. RICHARD BARINGER, M.D.

Professor and Chair, Department of Neurology, University of Utah School of Medicine; Staff Physician, Veterans Affairs Medical Center, Salt Lake City, Utah

ALLAN J. BELZBERG, M.D., FRCSC

Assistant Professor of Neurosurgery, The Johns Hopkins University School of Medicine; Attending Neurosurgeon, The Johns Hopkins Hospital, Baltimore, Maryland

GREGORY KENT BERGEY, M.D.

Associate Professor of Neurology, University of Maryland School of Medicine; Director, Maryland Epilepsy Center, University of Maryland Medical Center, Baltimore, Maryland

LEWIS S. BLEVINS, Jr., M.D.

Senior Clinical Fellow, Department of Internal Medicine, The Johns Hopkins University School of Medicine, Baltimore, Maryland

H. ROBERT BRASHEAR, M.D.

Associate Professor of Neurology and of Behavioral Medicine and Psychiatry, University of Virginia School of Medicine, Charlottesville, Virginia

MITCHELL F. BRIN, M.D.

Assistant Professor of Neurology, Columbia University College of Physicians and Surgeons, New York, New York

WILLIAM D. BROWN, M.D.

Department of Neurology, University of Southern California School of Medicine; Fellow, Child Neurology, Children's Hospital of Los Angeles, Los Angeles, California

THOMAS M. BRUSHART, M.D.

Assistant Professor of Orthopaedics and Neurology, The Johns Hopkins University School of Medicine; Attending Surgeon, Raymond M. Curtis Hand Center, Baltimore, Maryland

JAMES N. CAMPBELL, M.D.

Professor of Neurosurgery, The Johns Hopkins University School of Medicine, Baltimore, Maryland

RICHARD J. CASELLI, M.D.

Assistant Professor, Mayo Medical School, Rochester, Minnesota; Consultant in Neurology, Mayo Clinic Scottsdale, Scottsdale, Arizona

KENNETH L. CASEY, M.D.

Professor of Neurology and Physiology, University of Michigan Medical School; Chief, Neurology Service, Veterans Affairs Medical Center, Ann Arbor, Michigan

VINAY CHAUDHRY, M.B., B.S., M.R.C.P. (UK)

Assistant Professor of Neurology, The Johns Hopkins University School of Medicine; Co-Director, EMG Laboratory, The Johns Hopkins Hospital, Baltimore, Maryland

LORA L. CLAWSON, R.N., B.S.N.

ALS Research Coordinator, The Johns Hopkins Hospital, Baltimore, Maryland

MONROE COLE, M.D.

Associate Professor of Neurology, Case Western Reserve University School of Medicine; Neurologist, MetroHealth Medical Center, Cleveland, Ohio

JAMES J. CORBETT, M.D.

Professor and Chairman of Neurology, and Professor of Ophthalmology, University of Mississippi School of Medicine, Jackson, Mississippi

DAVID R. CORNBLATH, M.D.

Associate Professor of Neurology, The Johns Hopkins University School of Medicine, Baltimore, Maryland

ANDREA M. CORSE, M.D.

Senior Neuromuscular Fellow, The Johns Hopkins University School of Medicine, Baltimore, Maryland

PATRICIA K. COYLE, M.D.

Associate Professor of Neurology, State University of New York at Stony Brook Health Sciences Center School of Medicine; Director, Multiple Sclerosis Comprehensive Care Center, The University Hospital, Stony Brook, New York

THOMAS O. CRAWFORD, M.D.

Assistant Professor of Neurology, The Johns Hopkins University School of Medicine, Baltimore, Maryland

MARTHA BRIDGE DENCKLA, M.D.

Professor of Neurology and Pediatrics, The Johns Hopkins University School of Medicine; Director, Developmental Cognitive Neurology, Kennedy Krieger Institute, Baltimore, Maryland

MICHAEL N. DIRINGER, M.D.

Assistant Professor of Neurology and Neurological Surgery, Washington University School of Medicine; Director, Neurology/Neurosurgery Intensive Care Unit, Barnes Hospital, St. Louis, Missouri

W. EDWIN DODSON, M.D.

Professor of Pediatrics and Neurology, and Associate Dean, Washington University School of Medicine; Staff, Division of Pediatric Neurology, St. Louis Children's Hospital, St. Louis, Missouri

JAMES O. DONALDSON, M.D.

Professor of Neurology, University of Connecticut School of Medicine, Farmington, Connecticut

DANIEL B. DRACHMAN, M.D.

Professor of Neurology and Neuroscience, The Johns Hopkins University School of Medicine, Baltimore, Maryland

THOMAS B. DUCKER, M.D.

Associate Professor of Neurosurgery, The Johns Hopkins University School of Medicine, Baltimore, Maryland

CHRISTOPHER J. EARLEY, M.D., Ph.D.

Assistant Professor of Neurology, The Johns Hopkins University School of Medicine, Baltimore, Maryland

JOHN S. ELSTON, B.Sc, M.D., F.R.C.S.

Consultant Ophthalmic Surgeon, The Eye Hospital, Radcliffe Infirmary, Oxford, England

JANET R. FARHIE, M.D.

Psychiatrist, Sinai Hospital of Baltimore, Baltimore, Maryland

THOMAS E. FEASBY, M.D.

Professor and Head of Clinical Neurosciences, The University of Calgary Faculty of Medicine; Director, Department of Clinical Neurosciences, Foothills Hospital, Calgary, Alberta, Canada

EVA L. FELDMAN, M.D., Ph.D.

Assistant Professor of Neurology, University of Michigan Medical School; Medical Doctor, University of Michigan Medical Center, Ann Arbor, Michigan

GERALD M. FENICHEL, M.D.

Professor of Neurology and Pediatrics, and Chairman, Department of Neurology, Vanderbilt University School of Medicine; Neurologist-in-Chief, Vanderbilt University Medical Center and Vanderbilt's Children's Hospital, Nashville, Tennessee

ALEXANDRA FLOWERS, M.D.

Junior Faculty Associate and Fellow, Department of Neuro-Oncology, University of Texas M. D. Anderson Cancer Center, Houston, Texas

SUSAN E. FOLSTEIN, M.D.

Professor of Psychiatry and Pediatrics, The Johns Hopkins University School of Medicine; Director, Divisions of Psychiatric Genetics and Child and Adolescent Psychiatry, The Johns Hopkins Medical Institutions, Baltimore, Maryland

JOHN M. FREEMAN, M.D.

Professor of Neurology and Pediatrics, and Lederer Professor of Pediatric Epilepsy, The Johns Hopkins Medical Institutions, Baltimore, Maryland

MIRIAM L. FREIMER, M.D.

Assistant Professor of Neurology, The Ohio State University College of Medicine, Columbus, Ohio

JOSEPH H. FRIEDMAN, M.D.

Associate Professor of Clinical Neurosciences, Brown University School of Medicine; Director, Brown University Parkinson's Disease and Movement Disorder Unit, and Chief, Division of Neurology, Roger Williams Medical Center, Providence, Rhode Island

EDWIN B. GEORGE, M.D., Ph.D.

Instructor of Neurology, The Johns Hopkins University School of Medicine, Baltimore, Maryland

MARK R. GILBERT, M.D.

Assistant Professor of Neurology and Medicine, University of Pittsburgh School of Medicine; Co-Director, Neuro-Oncology Program, The Pittsburgh Cancer Institute, Pittsburgh, Pennsylvania

JONATHAN D. GLASS, M.D.

Assistant Professor of Neurology and Pathology, The Johns Hopkins University School of Medicine; Attending Neurologist, The Johns Hopkins Hospital, Baltimore, Maryland

LYNN M. GRATTAN, Ph.D.

Assistant Professor of Neurology, University of Maryland School of Medicine; Director, Neuropsychological Diagnostic and Research Laboratory, Baltimore, Maryland

JOHN E. GREENLEE, M.D.

Chief, Neurology Service, Veterans Affairs Medical Center; Professor and Vice-Chairman, Department of Neurology, University of Utah School of Medicine, Salt Lake City, Utah

JOHN W. GRIFFIN, M.D.

Professor of Neurology and Neuroscience, The Johns Hopkins University School of Medicine, Baltimore, Maryland

STUART A. GROSSMAN, M.D.

Associate Professor of Oncology, Medicine, and Neurosurgery, The Johns Hopkins University School of Medicine; Director of Neuro-Oncology, The Johns Hopkins Oncology Center, Baltimore, Maryland

MICHAEL L. GRUBER, M.D.

Assistant Professor of Neurology, Harvard Medical School; Attending Neurologist, Massachusetts General Hospital, Boston, Massachusetts

RONALD G. HALLER, M.D.

Associate Professor of Neurology and Internal Medicine, University of Texas Southwestern Medical Center; Chief, Neurology Service, Veterans Affairs Medical Center, Dallas, Texas

DANIEL F. HANLEY, M.D.

Associate Professor of Anesthesiology and Critical Care Medicine, Neurology, and Neurosurgery, The Johns Hopkins University School of Medicine; Director, Neurosciences Critical Care Unit, The Johns Hopkins Hospital, Baltimore, Maryland

MARY W. HAWKE, M.D.

Assistant Professor, Division of Cardiology, University of Maryland School of Medicine; Director of Transesophageal Echo and Director of Graphics, University Hospital, Baltimore, Maryland

THIRAVAT HEMACHUDHA, M.D.

Professor of Neurology, Department of Medicine, Chulalongkorn University; Director, World Health Organization Collaborating Center for Research in Rabies Pathogenesis and Prevention, Science Division, Queen Saovabha Memorial Institute, Thai Red Cross Society, Bangkok, Thailand

SUSAN J. HERDMAN, Ph.D.

Associate Professor of Otolaryngology–Head and Neck Surgery, The Johns Hopkins University School of Medicine, Baltimore, Maryland

FRED H. HOCHBERG, M.D.

Associate Professor of Neurology, Harvard Medical School; Attending Neurologist, Massachusetts General Hospital, Boston, Massachusetts

GENE G. HUNDER, M.D.

Professor of Medicine, Mayo Medical School; Consultant, Internal Medicine/Rheumatology, and Chair, Division of Rheumatology, Mayo Clinic, Rochester, Minnesota

OREST HURKO, M.D.

Associate Professor of Neurology and Medicine, Center for Medical Genetics, The Johns Hopkins Hospital, Baltimore, Maryland

REBECCA N. ICHORD, M.D.

Clinical Instructor of Pediatric Neurology, The Johns Hopkins University School of Medicine, Baltimore, Maryland

DONALD R. JOHNS, M.D.

Assistant Professor of Neurology, The Johns Hopkins University School of Medicine, Baltimore, Maryland

RICHARD T. JOHNSON, M.D.

Profesor and Director of Neurology, and Professor of Microbiology and Neuroscience, The Johns Hopkins University School of Medicine; Neurologist-in-Chief, The Johns Hopkins Hospital, Baltimore, Maryland

MICHAEL J. KAMINSKY, M.D.

Assistant Professor of Psychiatry and Behavioral Sciences and of Emergency Medicine and Trauma, The Johns Hopkins University School of Medicine; Clinical Director, Ambulatory Services, Department of Psychiatry and Behavioral Sciences, and Director, Psychiatric Emergency Services, The Johns Hopkins Hospital, Baltimore, Maryland

GEORGE KARPATI, M.D., FRCPC

Isaac Walton Killam Professor of Neurology, Montreal Neurological Institute, McGill University Faculty of Medicine; Senior Neurologist, Montreal Neurological Hospital, Montreal, Quebec, Canada

STEPHEN L. KINSMAN, M.D.

Instructor of Neurology, The Johns Hopkins University School of Medicine; Director, Birth Defects Clinic, Kennedy Krieger Institute, Baltimore, Maryland

JOHN T. KISSEL, M.D.

Associate Professor of Neurology, Division of Neuromuscular Disease, The Ohio State University College of Medicine, Columbus, Ohio

STEVEN J. KITTNER, M.D., M.P.H.

Assistant Professor of Neurology, University of Maryland School of Medicine, Baltimore, Maryland

JAMES P. KNOCHEL, M.D.

Clinical Professor of Internal Medicine, University of Texas Southwestern Medical Center; Chairman, Department of Internal Medicine, Presbyterian Hospital, Dallas, Texas

GREGORY L. KRAUSS, M.D.

Instructor of Neurology, The Johns Hopkins University School of Medicine, Baltimore, Maryland

ALLAN KRUMHOLZ, M.D.

Professor of Neurology, University of Maryland School of Medicine, Baltimore, Maryland

RALPH W. KUNCL, M.D., Ph.D.

Associate Professor of Neurology, and Co-Director, Neuromuscular Clinical Laboratory, The Johns Hopkins University School of Medicine, Baltimore, Maryland

ROGER KURLAN, M.D.

Associate Professor of Neurology, University of Rochester School of Medicine and Dentistry; Attending Neurologist, Strong Memorial Hospital, Rochester, New York

R. JOHN LEIGH, M.D.

Professor of Neurology, Case Western Reserve University School of Medicine; Staff Neurologist, Cleveland Veterans Affairs Medical Center, Cleveland, Ohio

GLENN J. LESSER, M.D.

Senior Clinical Fellow in Medical Oncology, Johns Hopkins Oncology Center, Baltimore, Maryland

JOHN LINDENBAUM, M.D.

Professor of Medicine and Associate Chairman, Department of Medicine, Columbia University College of Physicians and Surgeons; Associate Director of Medical Service and Attending Physician, The Presbyterian Hospital in the City of New York, and Attending Physician, Harlem Hospital Center, New York, New York

PHILLIP A. LOW, M.D.

Professor of Neurology, Mayo Medical School; Chairman, Division of Clinical Neurophysiology, Department of Neurology, Mayo Clinic, Rochester, Minnesota

J. DOUGLAS MANN, M.D.

Associate Professor of Neurology and Medicine, University of North Carolina School of Medicine, Chapel Hill, North Carolina

DOUGLAS E. MATTOX, M.D.

Professor of Otolaryngology–Head and Neck Surgery, The Johns Hopkins University School of Medicine, Baltimore, Maryland

RICHARD MAYEUX, M.D.

Gertrude H. Sergievsky Professor of Neurology and Psychiatry, Columbia University College of Physicians and Surgeons; Director, Gertrude H. Sergievsky Center, New York, New York

JUSTIN C. McARTHUR, M.B., B.S., M.P.H.

Associate Professor of Neurology and Epidemiology, The Johns Hopkins University School of Medicine, Baltimore, Maryland

UNA D. McCANN, M.D.

Chief, Sleep Laboratory, Section on Anxiety and Affective Disorders, Biological Psychiatry Branch, National Institute of Mental Health, National Institutes of Health, and Assistant Professor of Psychiatry, Uniformed Services University of the Health Sciences; Senior Staff Researcher and Medical Staff Member, Warren G. Magnusen Clinical Center, National Institutes of Health, Bethesda, Maryland

KATHLEEN M. McEVOY, M.D., Ph.D.

Assistant Professor of Neurology, Mayo Medical School; Consultant in Neurology, Mayo Clinic and Foundation, Rochester, Minnesota

JERRY R. MENDELL, M.D.

Professor of Neurology and Pathology, Division of Neuromuscular Disease, and Chairman, Department of Neurology, The Ohio State University College of Medicine; Chairman, Columbus, Ohio

CONSTANCE J. MEYD, M.D., M.S.

Assistant Professor of Neurology, The Johns Hopkins University School of Medicine; Director, Neurovascular Center, Francis Scott Key Medical Center, Baltimore, Maryland

WENDY G. MITCHELL, M.D.

Associate Professor of Neurology and Pediatrics, University of Southern California School of Medicine; Attending Child Neurologist, Children's Hospital Los Angeles, Los Angeles, California

THOMAS MOENCH, M.D.

Assistant Professor of Medicine and Neurology, The Johns Hopkins University School of Medicine, Baltimore, Maryland

JOEL C. MORGENLANDER, M.D.

Assistant Professor of Medicine (Neurology), Duke University Medical Center, Durham, North Carolina

HOWARD MOSES, M.D., M.S.

Assistant Professor of Neurology, The Johns Hopkins University School of Medicine; Neurologist, The Johns Hopkins Hospital, Baltimore, and Chief, Division of Neurology, Greater Baltimore Medical Center, Towson, Maryland

KEVIN D. MULLEN, M.B., F.R.C.P.I

Assistant Professor of Medicine, Case Western Reserve University School of Medicine; Consultant Gastroenterologist, MetroHealth Medical Center, Cleveland, Ohio

SAKKUBAI NAIDU, M.D.

Associate Professor of Neurology and Pediatrics, The Johns Hopkins University School of Medicine; Director, Clinical Neurogenetics Unit, Kennedy Krieger Institute, Baltimore, Maryland

JOHN K. NIPARKO, M.D.

Associate Professor of Otolaryngology–Head and Neck Surgery, The Johns Hopkins University School of Medicine, Baltimore, Maryland

RICHARD B. NORTH, M.D.

Associate Professor of Neurosurgery, The Johns Hopkins University School of Medicine, Baltimore, Maryland

STEPHEN M. OPPENHEIMER, M.B., M.R.C.P., FRCPC, F.A.C.T.

Director, Cerebrovascular Program, and Assistant Professor of Neurology and of Medicine (Cardiology), The Johns Hopkins University School of Medicine; Physician, The Johns Hopkins Hospital, Baltimore, Maryland

ROGER J. PACKER, M.D.

Professor of Neurology and Pediatrics, The George Washington University School of Medicine, Washington, D.C., and Clinical Professor of Neurosurgery, University of Virginia School of Medicine, Charlottesville, Virginia; Chairman, Department of Neurology, Children's National Medical Center, Washington, D.C.

MARCO PAPPAGALLO, M.D.

Senior Clinical and Research Fellow, Pain Treatment Center, Departments of Neurology and Neurosurgery, The Johns Hopkins Hospital, Baltimore, Maryland

SYDNEY J. PEERLESS, M.D., FRCSC

Professor of Neurological Surgery, University of Miami School of Medicine; Director, Cerebrovascular Unit, and Neurosurgical Staff, Jackson Memorial Hospital, Miami, Florida

HENRY A. PETERS, M.D.

Professor of Neurology, Psychiatry, and Rehabilitation, University of Wisconsin Medical School; Co-Director, Muscular Dystrophy Clinic, and Director, Parkinson's Disease Clinic, University of Wisconsin Hospital and Clinics, Madison, Wisconsin

CAROL E. PEYSER, M.D.

Assistant Professor of Psychiatry, The Johns Hopkins University School of Medicine; Clinical Director, Baltimore Huntington's Disease Project, The Johns Hopkins Medical Institutions, Baltimore, Maryland

NABIH M. RAMADAN, M.D.

Director, Cerebrovascular Diseases Laboratory, Center for Stroke Research, and Staff Neurologist, Department of Neurology, Henry Ford Hospital and Health Sciences Center, Detroit, Michigan

STEPHEN G. REICH, M.D.

Assistant Professor of Neurology, and Co-Director, Parkinson's Disease Center, The Johns Hopkins University School of Medicine, Baltimore, Maryland

GEORGE A. RICAURTE, M.D., Ph.D.

Assistant Professor, Department of Neurology, Francis Scott Key Medical Center, Baltimore, Maryland

RAYMOND P. ROOS, M.D.

Professor of Neurology, University of Chicago Pritzker School of Medicine, Chicago, Illinois

JEFFREY D. ROTHSTEIN, M.D., Ph.D.

Assistant Professor of Neurology, The Johns Hopkins University School of Medicine, Baltimore, Maryland

HELENE RUBEIZ, M.D.

Fellow, Clinical Neurophysiology, University of Chicago Hospital, Chicago, Illinois

RICHARD A. RUDICK, M.D.

Director, Mellen Center for Multiple Sclerosis Treatment and Research, Cleveland Clinic Foundation, Cleveland, Ohio

JOHN DEAN RYBOCK, M.D.

Assistant Professor of Neurosurgery, The Johns Hopkins University School of Medicine, Baltimore, Maryland

NED SACKTOR, M.D.

Instructor of Neurology, and Aaron Diamond Foundation Research Fellow, Gertrude H. Sergievsky Center, Department of Neurology, Neurological Institute of New York, New York, New York

MERLE A. SANDE, M.D.

Professor and Vice Chairman of Medicine, University of California, San Francisco, School of Medicine; Chief, Medical Services, San Francisco General Hospital, San Francisco, California

ROBERT N. SAWYER, Jr., M.D.

Assistant Clinical Professor of Neurology, Case Western Reserve University School of Medicine; Staff, Departments of Neurology and Surgery, MetroHealth Medical Center, Cleveland, Ohio

ALAN R. SEAY, M.D.

Associate Professor of Neurology and Pediatrics, University of Colorado School of Medicine; Head, Division of Child Neurology, The Children's Hospital, Denver, Colorado

WILLIAM R. SHAPIRO, M.D.

Chairman, Division of Neurology, Barrow Neurological Institute, St. Joseph's Hospital and Medical Center, Phoenix, Arizona

ZACHARY SIMMONS, M.D.

Assistant Professor of Neurology, The Pennsylvania State University College of Medicine; Director, EMG Laboratory, The Milton S. Hershey Medical Center, Hershey, Pennsylvania

CARLOS SINGER, M.D.

Assistant Professor of Neurology, and Director, Botulinum Toxin Treatment Clinic, University of Miami School of Medicine, Miami, Florida

PHILLIP R. SLAVNEY, M.D.

Professor of Psychiatry, The Johns Hopkins University School of Medicine; Attending Psychiatrist, The Johns Hopkins Hospital, Baltimore, Maryland

O. CARTER SNEAD III, M.D.

Professor and Vice Chairman, Department of Neurology, and Professor of Pediatrics and of Molecular Pharmacology and Toxicology, University of Southern California School of Medicine; Chief, Division of Neurology, Children's Hospital Los Angeles, Los Angeles, California

S. ROBERT SNODGRASS, M.D.

Professor of Neurology and Pediatrics, University of Mississippi School of Medicine; Chief, Pediatric Neurology, University of Mississippi Medical Center, Jackson, Mississippi

BARNEY J. STERN, M.D.

Associate Professor of Neurology, The Johns Hopkins University School of Medicine; Director, Division of Neurology, Sinai Hospital, Baltimore, Maryland

MATTHEW B. STERN, M.D.

Associate Professor of Neurology, University of Pennsylvania School of Medicine; Director, Parkinson's Disease and Movement Disorder Center, Graduate Hospital, Philadelphia, Pennsylvania

DAVID A. STUMPF, M.D., Ph.D.

Benjamin and Virginia T. Boshes Professor and Chairman, Department of Neurology, and Professor of Pediatrics, Northwestern University Medical School; Chairman of Neurology, Northwestern Memorial Hospital, Northwestern Medical Faculty Foundation; and Attending Neurologist, Northwestern Memorial Hospital, Children's Memorial Hospital, Rehabilitation Institute of Chicago, and Evanston Hospital, Chicago, Illinois

JERRY W. SWANSON, M.D.

Associate Professor of Neurology, Mayo Medical School; Consultant in Neurology, Mayo Clinic, Rochester, Minnesota

THOMAS K. TATEMICHI, M.D.

Assistant Professor of Neurology, and Director, Stroke and Aging Research Project, Columbia University College of Physicians and Surgeons, New York, New York

MARTIN G. TÄUBER, M.D.

Assistant Professor of Medicine, University of California, San Francisco, School of Medicine; Attending Physician in Medicine and Infectious Diseases, San Francisco General Hospital, San Francisco, California

LEON J. THAL, M.D.

Professor of Neurosciences, University of California, San Diego, School of Medicine; Chief, Neurology Service, Veterans Affairs Medical Center, San Diego, California

J. DAVID THOMPSON, M.D.

Assistant Professor of Orthopaedic Surgery, The Johns Hopkins University School of Medicine, Baltimore, Maryland

DAVID M. TREIMAN, M.D.

Professor of Neurology, University of California, Los Angeles, School of Medicine; Co-Director, DVA Southwest Regional Epilepsy Center, DVA Medical Center, West Los Angeles, California

JAY H. TUREEN, M.D.

Associate Clinical Professor of Pediatrics, University of California, San Francisco, School of Medicine, San Francisco, California

RONALD J. TUSA, M.D., Ph.D.

Associate Professor of Neurology and Otolaryngology, The Johns Hopkins University School of Medicine, Baltimore, Maryland

WILLIAM R. TYOR, M.D.

Assistant Professor of Neurology and of Microbiology and Immunology, Medical University of South Carolina, Charleston, South Carolina

GARY S. WAND, M.D.

Associate Professor of Medicine, The Johns Hopkins University School of Medicine; Director, Neuroendocrine Clinic, The Johns Hopkins Hospital, Baltimore, Maryland

WILLIAM J. WEINER, M.D.

Director of Movement Disorders Center, and Professor of Neurology, University of Miami School of Medicine; National Parkinson Foundation Clinical Research Scholar, National Parkinson Foundation, Miami, Florida

K.M.A. WELCH, M.D.

William T. Gossett Chair of Neurology, Henry Ford Hospital and Health Sciences Center, Detroit, Michigan

HENRY WILDE, M.D., F.A.C.P.

Professor of Medicine, Chulalongkorn University; Attending Staff, Chulalongkorn University Hospital, Bangkok General Hospital, Bangkok, Thailand, and Bartlett Memorial Hospital, Juneau, Alaska; Senior Consultant Physician, World Health Organization Collaborating Center for Research in Rabies Pathogenesis and Prevention, Queen Saovabha Memorial Institute, Bangkok, Thailand

SHIRLEY H. WRAY, M.D., Ph.D., F.R.C.P.

Associate Professor of Neurology, Harvard Medical School; Director, Unit for Neurovisual Disorders, and Staff Neurologist, Massachusetts General Hospital, Boston, Massachusetts

WISE YOUNG, Ph.D., M.D.

Professor of Neurosurgery, Physiology, and Biophysics, Department of Neurosurgery, and Director, Neurosurgery Research, New York University Medical Center, and Bellevue Hospital, New York, New York

W. K. ALFRED YUNG, M.D.

Professor of Neurology, University of Texas Medical School at Houston; Neurologist and Professor of Neurology, Department of Neuro-Oncology, University of Texas M.D. Anderson Cancer Center, Houston, Texas

SETH M. ZEIDMAN, M.D.

Senior Resident, Department of Neurosurgery, The Johns Hopkins Hospital, Baltimore, and Senior Resident and Clinical Associate, Surgical Neurology Branch, National Institutes of Health, Bethesda, Maryland

PREFACE

In this fourth edition, John Griffin joins *Current Therapy in Neurologic Disease* as co-editor. His expertise has enhanced the coverage of neuromuscular diseases, as evidenced by the expanded discussion of these diseases in this edition. Neuromuscular diseases, which represent one third of neurologic referrals, deserve and have received greater emphasis.

The goal of *Current Therapy in Neurologic Disease* has not changed. It has been designed to supplement textbooks that emphasize etiology, pathophysiology, and diagnosis. We wish to present clear-cut therapeutic solutions, which are often hard to find in clinical texts, journals, or even texts of pharmacology. This book was designed to fill a gap. We asked experienced clinicians with specialized expertise in treating specific diseases to state simply and straightforwardly how they treat a particular ailment. These collections of "second opinions" have been well received.

As before, we have changed authors in each edition. Some differing approaches presented in this edition are the result of differences of opinion, but others genuinely reflect new information that has become available over the past three years. This is particularly notable in the treatments of cerebrovascular disease and brain tumors, which have been more critically evaluated; the new approach to Parkinson's disease; the use of IgG in the Guillain-Barré syndrome and other immune-mediated diseases; the wider and better defined use of botulinum toxin; and even a quick validated treatment for benign, postural vertigo.

We asked each author also to present a few selected references and, when available, patient resources. Drug doses have been checked, but the reader should scrutinize product information sheets for dosage changes or contraindications, particularly in new and infrequently used drugs.

We wish to express our sincere appreciation to the authors who shared their expertise and experience with us. We also thank Laura Neuberger and Sheila Garrity for their editorial assistance.

Richard T. Johnson
John W. Griffin

CONTENTS

DISORDERS OF CONSCIOUSNESS AND EQUILIBRIUM

THE UNCONSCIOUS PATIENT

R. JOHN LEIGH, M.D.
ROBERT N. SAWYER, Jr., M.D.

Impairment of consciousness is a manifestation of many serious diseases. It may be complete (coma, unarousable psychological unresponsiveness) or partial (stupor, behavioral unresponsiveness from which the patient can be aroused only by vigorous and repeated stimulation). In this chapter we include the entire spectrum of disturbances of consciousness, which may reflect impaired function of the brain stem reticular formation, of the cerebral hemispheres, or both. Because therapy depends so much on the underlying disorder, accurate diagnosis is important. Nevertheless, time is of the essence, and it is often necessary to institute certain emergency treatments that may not be specific but are so potentially beneficial for certain conditions—and so otherwise innocuous—that they cannot be withheld. Therefore, our strategy is this: (1) to carry out initial evaluation and emergency measures; (2) to perform a focused general and neurologic examination with the goal of determining the cause; (3) to implement tests and treatments on the basis of this examination; and (4) to re-examine the patient to evaluate the effectiveness of these measures and estimate prognosis.

INITIAL EVALUATION AND EMERGENCY MEASURES

The first measure is to assess airway patency and breathing. Patients unable to protect their airway should be intubated. The cervical spine should be protected until injury is ruled out (radiologic assessment may be necessary). If the patient is breathing spontaneously, the respiratory rate and pattern are noted; patients with very irregular or ataxic respiration often progress to respiratory arrest and should be intubated. It is much better to intubate early under controlled conditions than to intubate as an emergency. Airway obstruction, respiratory or circulatory failure, and cardiac dysrhythmia or arrest are treated according to the guidelines published by the American Heart Association (*Advanced Cardiac Life Support*). The patient is undressed and examined carefully for signs of trauma. Measures are taken to correct extremes of body temperature, and the patient's eyes are protected. If the patient is agitated, sedative drugs are withheld until the cause is better understood, in favor of reassurance or limb restraints. Arterial and venous blood should be sent to the laboratory for studies (Table 1). A Foley catheter is placed to obtain urine for urinalysis, culture, and toxicology. Electrocardiography and portable chest radiography are ordered.

Thiamine is given, 100 mg IV. If immediate analysis of blood glucose (fingerstick method) indicates hypoglycemia, or if such rapid analysis is not available, 25 g of IV glucose is given (50 ml of 50 percent solution). Although glucose is not indicated for diabetic coma or after cerebral infarction, the risks are outweighed by the greater danger of not treating hypoglycemia.

If infection is likely, antibiotics are given. If bacterial meningitis is suspected, lumbar puncture should be considered, although if there is reason to suspect an intracranial mass lesion, computed tomography (CT) should be performed before lumbar puncture. In any case, antibiotics should be administered immediately: ceftriaxone sodium (Rocephin), 2 g IV or IM to patients aged 12 or older (100 mg per kilogram IV for younger patients). For about 2 hours after starting antibiotics, cerebrospinal fluid may still be cultured to grow the offending organism.

Patients who show signs of cerebral herniation or are suspected of having raised intracranial pressure should undergo endotracheal intubation (if they have not already) and hyperventilation to a $Paco_2$ of 20 to 25 mm Hg. In addition, 25 to 75 g of 20 percent mannitol solution IV can be given to reduce brain water content. Placement of a Foley catheter permits monitoring of urine output and the effect of mannitol. Arrangements are made for prompt CT of such patients.

In the case of status epilepticus, administer IV lorazepam, 0.2 mg per kilogram at the rate of 0.5 mg per minute, or diazepam, 3 to 10 mg. This should be followed immediately by the phenytoin, 18 mg per kilogram IV at 50 mg per minute while the patient is monitored for hypotension and arrhythmias. Electroencephalography should be performed in patients with unexplained coma,

Table 1 Laboratory Studies to Evaluate the Unconscious Patient

Immediate
  Arterial blood gas with carboxyhemoglobin
  Glucose
  Electrolytes, including magnesium and calcium
  Creatinine, blood urea nitrogen
  Prothrombin, partial thromboplastin time
  Complete blood count with differential, platelets,
    erythrocyte sedimentation rate
  Osmolality
  Electrocardiography
  Chest radiography
  Computed tomography of head
  Cerebrospinal fluid (see text)
Deferred
  Toxicology screen (blood and urine)
  Liver function tests
  Ammonia
  Blood cultures
  Urinalysis
  Thyroid and adrenal functions

to look for nonmotor status epilepsy. Additional measures for treatment of status epilepticus are discussed in the chapter *Status Epilepticus.*

If drug intoxication is likely, depending on available information, the physician should consider administering specific antidotes: for narcotic overdose, naloxone, 0.4 to 2 mg IV at 2 to 3 minute intervals for patients older than 5 years and 0.01 mg per kilogram IV for those younger than 5 years. For benzodiazepine overdose, the treatment is flumenazil, 0.2 mg IV, followed by another 0.3 mg IV if not effective, followed by further 0.5 mg IV doses to a cumulative dose of 3 mg. Flumenazil can produce seizures in patients who use benzodiazepines long term or who have taken a massive overdose of a tricyclic antidepressant. Physostigmine, 1 mg IV, may be given to patients who are intoxicated with anticholinergic agents such as some of the tricyclic antidepressants. Before a suspected toxin is removed from the stomach via a nasogastric tube, adequate airway protection must be ensured with a cuffed endotracheal tube.

EXAMINATION OF THE UNCONSCIOUS PATIENT

The goal of the history and examination is to determine the cause of unconsciousness and, in particular, to establish whether it is due to a supratentorial mass lesion, a subtentorial mass or destructive lesion, a metabolic, toxic, or infective encephalopathy, or psychogenic unresponsiveness. Treatment of each of these respective categories of disease requires specific measures.

Relatives, friends, paramedics, or police are questioned to quickly ascertain the history of illness. When information is lacking, a colleague should try to telephone the patient's family or physician. Key items of the history include time of onset of coma, and whether it was abrupt or gradual, history of headache, depression, focal weakness, vertigo, and injury. Previous medical and psychiatric illnesses and current medications are also determined.

A general examination should be directed toward identifying signs of trauma, drug abuse, and severe systemic disease. Next, the level of consciousness is assessed by observing the patient's verbal, motor, and eye-opening responses (Table 2). The physician should always start by asking the patient to open and move the eyes and limbs, and, if no tube interferes, to tell where he or she is (use the patient's first name). In this way, certain patients who appear to be unconscious but are not (e.g., those who are "locked in" or paralyzed but conscious) may be identified and spared discomfort. If there are no responses, noxious stimuli are next applied; the safest of these are compression of the nail beds and pressure over the supraorbital notch. Systematic written notes of the responses are made (Table 2), as they help not only with diagnosis but with estimation of prognosis (see below). Interpretation of the motor responses focuses on movements at the elbows, which are coded as flexion or extension. In lighter states of unconsciousness, the patient may flex the elbow to withdraw or reach out to remove the examiner's hand (localizing response). Abnormal flexor and extensor responses are characterized by lack of localization of the noxious stimulus and by adduction of the shoulder. The tensor of fascia lata muscle (lateral thigh) contracts during a triple flexor response of the lower limbs but not during a withdrawal response.

Next, the optic fundi and brain stem reflexes are examined. With the ophthalmoscope the examiner looks for papilledema and subhyaloid hemorrhage. The retina may bear stigmata of hypertensive or diabetic retinopathy or show retinal infarctions (reflecting septicemia or IV drug abuse). The resting size and shape of the pupils are noted and the responses to light tested using a bright flashlight. Pinpoint pupils suggest narcotic overdose or a pontine lesion. A unilateral dilated pupil (which may or may not respond to light) suggests herniation of the uncus of the temporal lobe, arterial berry aneurysm at the carotid–posterior communicating junction, or the effects of medications that dilate the pupil.

The ocular motor examination is often valuable for determining the cause of coma. First the resting position of the eyes is observed. Sustained, conjugate, horizontal deviation of the eyes may reflect a unilateral lesion of the cerebral hemispheres, in which case the eyes are usually directed toward the side of the lesion and away from hemiparesis. A vestibular stimulus can usually drive the eyes across the midline. If the conjugate deviation is due to a lesion of the brain stem, especially the pons, the eyes are directed away from the side of the lesion and toward the hemiparesis; the eyes usually do not respond to vestibular stimuli. Intermittent deviation of the eyes and head turning are usually due to seizure activity. Tonic downward deviation of the eyes, often accompanied by convergence, occurs with thalamic hemorrhage or with lesions affecting the dorsal midbrain. Tonic upward

Table 2 Neurologic Examination of the Comatose Patient

Verbal responses	Corneal responses
Oriented speech	Present
Confused conversation	Absent
Inappropriate speech	
Incomprehensible speech	Respiratory pattern
No speech	Regular
	Periodic
Eye opening	Ataxic
Spontaneous	
Response to verbal stimuli	Motor responses
Response to noxious stimuli	Obeying commands
None	Localizing
	Withdrawal
Pupillary reactions	Abnormal flexion
Present	Abnormal extension
Absent	None
Spontaneous eye movements	Deep tendon reflexes
Orienting	Normal
Roving conjugate	Increased
Roving disconjugate	Absent
Miscellaneous abnormal	
movements	Skeletal muscle tone
None	Normal
	Paratonic
Eye movements with head rotation	Flexor
(oculocephalic responses)	Extensor
Normal	Flaccid
Full	
Minimal	
None	
Eye movement with caloric	
stimulation (oculovestibular	
responses)	
Normal	
Tonic conjugate	
Minimal or dysconjugate	
None	

Adapted from Plum F, Posner JB. The Diagnosis of Stupor and Coma. 3rd ed. Philadelphia: FA Davis, 1980; with permission.

deviation of the eyes follows hypoxic-ischemic insult and may be encountered as a component of oculogyric crisis induced by certain drugs, especially phenothiazines. Deviations of the visual axes in coma may be due to oculomotor, trochlear, or abducens nerve palsy, skew deviation, or a phoria that is normally compensated for by fusional mechanisms. Complete oculomotor nerve palsy causes pupillary dilatation, ptosis, and deviation of the eye down and out. Vertical tropias are usually due to skew deviation or trochlear nerve palsy; the latter is common following head trauma. Bilateral abducens nerve palsy occurs when increased intracranial pressure compromises the nerves as they bend over the petroclinoid ligament. Spontaneous eye movements that occur include slow roving movements that are similar to the eye movements of light sleep; these imply that brain stem gaze mechanisms are intact. Classic ocular bobbing consists of intermittent, usually conjugate, rapid downward movement of the eyes followed by a slower return to the original position. It is usually a sign of destructive pontine lesions. A number of variants of ocular bobbing have been described, but they are less reliable for localization. Ping-pong gaze consists of slow, horizontal, conjugate deviations of the eyes alternating every few seconds; it is usually a sign of bilateral infarction of the cerebral hemispheres.

Reflex eye movements may be elicited in unconscious patients either by head rotation (the doll's head-eye or oculocephalic maneuver) or by caloric stimulation (the oculovestibular test); both stimuli test the vestibulo-ocular reflex. Head rotations should not be used in unconscious patients unless it is certain that no neck injury or abnormality is present. Both horizontal and vertical rotations should be performed. Before caloric stimulation, we always check to see that the tympanic membrane is intact and unobstructed. A large quantity (at least 100 ml) of ice water may be needed. In testing reflex eye movements in unresponsive patients, it is important to note the magnitude of the response, whether the ocular deviation is conjugate, and any quick phases of nystagmus, particularly during caloric stimulation. Impaired abduction suggests sixth nerve palsy; impaired adduction implies either internuclear ophthalmoplegia or third nerve palsy. Occasionally, metabolic coma or drug intoxication may mimic such deficits. Vertical responses may be impaired with disease of the midbrain or bilateral lesions of the medial longitudinal fasciculus. Pontine lesions may abolish the reflex eye movements in the horizontal plane but spare the vertical responses. When reflex eye movements are present in an unresponsive patient, the brain stem is likely to be structurally intact. When reflex eye movements are abnormal or absent, the cause may be structural disease, profound metabolic coma, or drug intoxication (any of a variety of medications). Quick phases of nystagmus are usually absent in acutely unconscious patients, and their presence without a tonic deviation of the eyes should raise the possibility of feigned coma. Patients who survive coma but are left in a persistent vegetative state, with severe damage to the cerebral hemispheres but preservation of the brain stem, regain nystagmus with caloric or rotational stimulation, as well as spontaneous eye opening.

The corneal reflex and the gag reflex are also tested. The response to tracheal suctioning of patients who are intubated should be noted. Absence of these brain stem reflexes suggests a subtentorial lesion.

SPECIFIC TREATMENT MEASURES

An expanding supratentorial mass may initially produce focal neurologic deficits, but it also impairs consciousness by compressing the diencephalon or brain stem. Progressive rostrocaudal deterioration may be observed, reflecting transtentorial herniation that may be central or uncal (herniation of the temporal lobe with compression of the oculomotor nerve, midbrain, and posterior cerebral artery against the tentorial edge). The first imperative is to treat intracranial hypertension using hyperventilation and mannitol (see above) and, for tumor-associated edema, corticosteroids. Prompt CT is necessary. Careful attention should be given to electrolyte balance and blood gases. If the patient's condition is deteriorating rapidly, emergency placement of burr holes may be indicated. Patients who develop fixed, dilated, or irregular (oval) pupils are likely to have suffered hemorrhagic infarction of the midbrain.

Subtentorial lesions include destructive processes of the brain stem and mass lesions that compress the brain stem. Sometimes complaints of headache, vertigo, vomiting, or diplopia are reported before the patient loses consciousness. Brain stem dysfunction is usually evident from abnormalities of the eye movements, pupillary responses, and other brain stem reflexes. Although destructive lesions of the brain stem are not treatable, cerebellar mass lesions (including hemorrhage and infarction) are amenable to surgical decompression, which may be life saving. Intracranial hypertension is treated (see above) while CT is rapidly performed. If progressive basilar occlusion is suspected and CT shows no blood, heparinization may be indicated.

Metabolic-toxic-infective encephalopathy is usually characterized by more gradual onset of coma and by the absence of lateralizing signs. In addition, tremor, asterixis, myoclonus, and respiratory disturbance are common. The preservation of pupillary reflexes and a full range of reflexive eye movements helps support the diagnosis. Firm diagnosis, however, rests on laboratory evidence of metabolic, toxic, or infective cause, and normal CT findings. (Remember that, for example, subdural hematoma and hepatic coma may coexist.) Effective treatment consists of correction of an underlying metabolic disorder, elimination or specific antidote for a toxin, or administration of appropriate antibiotics.

Patients who are psychogenically unresponsive often show signs that are inconsistent with true coma: eyelids are held tightly closed; pupils are usually reactive; caloric stimulation induces nystagmus with quick phases; motor tone is normal or inconsistent; tendon reflexes are physiologic. Such patients should usually be admitted so that they may receive psychiatric help.

EVALUATION OF EFFECTIVENESS OF TREATMENT AND ESTIMATION OF PROGNOSIS

After emergency measures are instituted and the patient examined, the success of treatment should be re-evaluated. In particular it is worthwhile to ask these questions:

1. What are the current vital signs and temperature?
2. Is there adequate oxygenation?
3. What is the circulatory status?
4. What is the intracranial pressure?
5. Are there seizures (subclinical status)?
6. Is infection being treated?
7. What is the acid-base and electrolyte status?
8. Have appropriate specific antidotes been given?
9. Is agitation controlled adequately?
10. Are the corneas protected? (Corneal ulcers occur within 4 to 6 hours when they are not protected.)

Part of the treatment of coma is to render a prediction about the final outcome of events, as many therapeutic decisions are based on prognosis. This cannot be done immediately, but, by serially noting certain important clinical signs (see Table 2), some estimation of likely outcome eventually is possible. It is important to note, however, that drug intoxication or hypothermia can confound such attempts. In cases of medical, and especially hypoxic-ischemic coma, Levy and colleagues found that pupillary light reactions, spontaneous and reflex eye movements, eye opening, and motor responses were all useful for predicting eventual outcome when evaluated 1, 3, and 7 days after the onset of coma. These studies reinforce the importance of a focused neurologic examination for evaluating the prognosis of unconscious patients. Unfortunately, unless coma is the result of sedative overdose, the prognosis is usually poor.

SUGGESTED READING

Levy DE, Bates D, Caronna JJ, et al. Prognosis in nontraumatic coma. Ann Intern Med 1981;94:293–301.
Levy DE, Caronna JJ, Singer BH, et al. Predicting outcome from hypoxic-ischemic coma. JAMA 1985;253:1420–1426.
Plum F, Posner JB. The diagnosis of stupor and coma. 3rd ed. Philadelphia: FA Davis, 1980.

SYNCOPE

JERRY W. SWANSON, M.D.

Syncope comes from the Greek word *synkopē,* which means pause or cessation, and refers to a brief loss of consciousness. Syncope results from a diffuse decrease in cerebral perfusion. It must be distinguished from other mechanisms of loss of consciousness, such as seizures and concussion. Syncope is a common presenting symptom, and estimates are that it accounts for 3 percent of visits to emergency departments and 6 percent of medical admissions to general hospitals. Despite extensive evaluation, no specific cause for syncope is found in up to 50 percent of patients.

Syncope can be classified as cardiovascular, noncardiovascular, or of uncertain origin (Table 1). Syncope as an isolated symptom is almost never secondary to disease of the brain.

HISTORY

As with all transient events, the history is usually the most valuable information for the diagnosis of episodic loss of consciousness. By definition, patients are not aware during the entirety of an attack, and additional information about the attack must be gathered from observers. Features such as precipitating factors, posture, rapidity of onset, head and neck position, presence

Table 1 Classification of Syncopal Disorders

Cardiovascular
  Reflex
    Vasovagal (vasodepressor)
    Vasovagal (situational)
      Micturition
      Cough (tussive)
      Defecation
      Deglutition (swallow)
      Vagoglossopharyngeal (glossopharyngeal) neuralgia
      Other types of situational syncope
    Orthostatic
      Hyperadrenergic (e.g., blood loss)
      Hypoadrenergic
        Progressive autonomic failure
        Secondary autonomic insufficiency (e.g., neurologic
          disorders or medications)
    Carotid sinus syncope
      Cardioinhibitory
      Vasodepressor
      Mixed
    Cardiac
      Mechanical (obstructive)
      Electrical (dysrhythmia)
Noncardiovascular
  Cerebrovascular
  Hyperventilation
  Psychogenic
Syncope of uncertain origin

and duration of antecedent and associated symptoms, duration of loss of consciousness, rate of recovery, and sequelae should be sought. Tonic or clonic motor activity may accompany prolonged cerebral hypoperfusion and hence is not always symptomatic of seizures. A careful review of the medical history is important when seeking predisposing factors. A history of medications is essential. Medications that may predispose to syncope include prazosin, captopril, nitroglycerin, antiarrhythmia agents, phenothiazines, tricyclic antidepressants, methyldopa, beta-adrenergic receptor blockers, and digoxin.

PHYSICAL EXAMINATION

Blood pressure and heart rate should be measured when the patient is lying supine and standing. Blood pressure should be measured in both arms. Bruits should be sought over the carotid and subclavian vessels as well as over the cranium. During cardiac auscultation, evidence of cardiac murmurs and abnormalities of the heart sounds should be sought. Heart sounds may reveal evidence of aortic stenosis, idiopathic hypertrophic subaortic stenosis, pulmonary hypertension, mitral valve prolapse, atrial myxoma, or pericarditis. Carotid sinus compression, if it is to be performed, should be done only if intravenous access and electrocardiographic monitoring have been established and atropine is available. The presence of carotid occlusive disease is a relative contraindication to carotid sinus compression because of the increased risk of ipsilateral cerebral hemisphere ischemia. Hyperventilation during the examination may reproduce symptoms when this is the underlying mechanism of syncope. Finally, a neurologic examination helps support or exclude a neurologic disorder that has syncope as one feature.

CARDIOVASCULAR SYNCOPE

Cardiovascular syncope has been subdivided into reflex and cardiac syncope.

Reflex Syncope

Reflex syncope occurs principally because of underfilling on the right side of the heart. It most commonly is related to pooling of peripheral blood and usually occurs when the individual is standing (or, occasionally, sitting).

Vasovagal (Vasodepressor) Syncope

Vasovagal syncope is the most common type of classifiable syncope. It most often is seen in young, healthy people, although it can be observed in older people. There are usually premonitory symptoms and signs, such as weakness, apprehension, epigastric discomfort, nausea, pallor, diaphoresis, and blurred vision. Vasovagal syncope can also be situational and can be

5

classified with respect to its precipitant (see below). Patients with a typical history of vasovagal syncope do not need investigation. Individuals who recognize the precipitating circumstances should try to avoid them.

Vasovagal (Situational) Syncope

Micturition Syncope. Micturition syncope occurs predominantly in men. It is typically associated with rapid emptying of the bladder, which causes reflex vasodilatation and decreased cerebral perfusion that may be magnified by the effects of Valsalva's maneuver during urination. Most affected persons have ingested alcohol and have been recumbent prior to the episode. If the history is characteristic, treatment consists of advising male patients to sit when urinating, particularly at night.

Cough (Tussive) Syncope. Tussive syncope is quite uncommon and usually occurs in association with chronic obstructive pulmonary disease in persons who have a prolonged or a violent episode of coughing. The mechanism appears to be vagally mediated hypotension or bradycardia precipitated by coughing and magnified by a decrease in venous return caused by the increase in intrathoracic pressure. The loss of consciousness is usually brief. Treatment is aimed at the underlying pulmonary disorder.

Defecation Syncope. Defecation syncope has been thought to be related to a reflex mechanism such as prolonged Valsalva's maneuver. It can usually be treated by avoiding prolonged straining during defecation.

Deglutition (Swallow) Syncope. Swallowing is a rarely observed precipitant of syncope. Like other forms of reflex syncope, it is mediated by the vasovagal reflex. It usually is seen with esophageal disease, cardiac disease, or both. Endoscopy is necessary to exclude esophageal disease. An attempt to precipitate syncope during cardiac monitoring can also be informative with respect to the associated cardiac arrhythmias, which are of several types. If esophageal disease is present, it is treated when possible. Atropine may be effective in abolishing the episodes. Occasionally, placement of a cardiac pacemaker may be necessary.

Vagoglossopharyngeal (Glossopharyngeal) Neuralgia–Induced Syncope. Vagoglossopharyngeal neuralgia is characterized by paroxysmal pain in the throat or the ear and can be associated with bradycardia and even asystole. Syncope in association with this disorder has been reported in fewer than 50 cases. Treatment of the arrhythmia often requires placement of a cardiac pacemaker, at least temporarily. Although vagoglossopharyngeal neuralgia may respond to carbamazepine, often surgical sectioning of the glossopharyngeal nerve and upper roots of the vagus nerve is necessary for treatment. This procedure relieves both the pain of the disorder and the associated syncope.

Orthostatic Syncope

Orthostatic hypotension with resultant syncope is a commonly observed problem in neurologic practice. Orthostatic hypotension is particularly common in the elderly and often becomes symptomatic in those receiving cardiovascular or psychotropic drugs.

Progressive autonomic failure, multiple-system atrophy, neuropathies with autonomic involvement, tabes dorsalis, and spinal cord lesions of various types are neurologic conditions associated with orthostatic hypotension. The diagnosis of these conditions depends on the associated neurologic symptoms and signs. Usually, the treatment of orthostatic hypotension in these conditions is primarily symptomatic and the results are often unsatisfactory.

Elevation of the head of the bed approximately 15 degrees for sleep is advised. Patients are instructed to rise slowly from a seated or recumbent position. An elasticized body garment (leotard) can be worn to decrease venous pooling of blood in the lower limbs.

A high-salt diet (≥ 150 mEq per day) is usually advised. Fludrocortisone (9-alpha-fluorohydrocortisone) is administered, if needed, in doses of 0.1 to 1.0 mg per day. In patients with cardiac disease, the volume expansion must be monitored carefully to avoid precipitation of congestive heart failure.

Indomethacin in doses of 25 to 50 mg three times per day has been of some help to some patients. For some individuals, methylphenidate may be utilized, either alone or with a small dose of monoamine oxidase inhibitor, and the blood pressure is observed closely. Midodrine, a peripheral alpha-adrenergic receptor agonist that produces vasoconstriction of arterioles and venous capacitance vessels, has been shown to be effective in treating orthostatic hypotension in some patients. It is not yet available for general use.

Further discussion of orthostatic hypotension related to autonomic failure is in the chapter *Neurogenic Orthostatic Hypotension*.

Carotid Sinus Syncope

Carotid sinus syncope has been categorized into two main types. The cardioinhibitory type is associated with the block of the sinus node and the atrioventricular node. This can sometimes be effectively treated with atropine sulfate in doses of 0.5 mg three or four times daily. Effective treatment may require placement of a transvenous pacemaker. The vasodepressor type of carotid sinus hypersensitivity predominates, but hypotension can be associated with bradycardia. Treatment of this type of carotid sinus syncope is often unsatisfactory; treatment with ephedrine and dihydroergotamine and denervation of the carotid sinus may have limited success. A cardiac pacemaker may be needed. A mixed type of carotid sinus syndrome, with both cardioinhibitory and vasodepressor responses, can also occur.

Cardiac Syncope

Cardiac syncope results from insufficient output of the left side of the heart and usually indicates underlying cardiac disease. It can be attributed to mechanical (obstructive) causes or dysrhythmia. It may be characterized by an abrupt onset without premonitory signs, although sometimes it is preceded by dyspnea, palpitations, or angina. Obstructive causes can usually be suspected on the basis of the cardiac history and clinical examination. However, cardiac dysrhythmias may be episodic and difficult to document when the patient is asymptomatic. Treatment is aimed at the specific cardiac disorder and should be directed by a physician who is expert in the treatment of these disorders.

NONCARDIOVASCULAR SYNCOPE

Cerebrovascular Syncope

Cerebrovascular disease is a very infrequent cause of syncope. It has been seen in the presence of high-grade stenosis or occlusion of the large cervicocephalic arteries. Specifically, it has occasionally been seen with stenoses in the vertebrobasilar system as well as with bilateral carotid disease. Usually, a careful history reveals focal central nervous system ischemic symptoms that point to the diagnosis. Treatment depends on the underlying anatomic abnormality demonstrated at angiography.

Recurrent syncope associated with positional head changes such as hyperextension and lateral rotation can be related to mechanical compression of vertebral arteries due to a cervical rib or cervical spondylosis. Again, documentation requires visualization of the cervical cephalic arteries with angiography. Surgical removal of the mechanical obstruction may be indicated.

The subclavian steal syndrome is due to occlusive disease proximal to the vertebral artery, with associated reversal of flow in the vertebral artery. Its most commonly described presentation is weakness of the left arm during exercise, but it has been reported to be associated sometimes with focal brain-stem ischemia and syncope. The presence of a physiologic subclavian steal documented by either noninvasive testing or angiography is a common finding and in most cases no symptoms can be attributed to it. If recurrent syncope can be convincingly shown to be symptomatic of a subclavian steal, surgical treatment of the obstructing lesion can be considered.

Takayasu's arteritis (pulseless disease) is a vasculitic disorder that affects the aorta and its large branches. It most commonly affects women, who experience the onset of symptoms at a young age. It is suspected on the basis of systemic and central nervous system ischemic symptoms associated with a decrease of peripheral pulses. Syncope can be associated with the disorder. Treatment is directed at the underlying vasculitis process, which usually responds to corticosteroid therapy.

Hyperventilation Syndrome

Hyperventilation is usually accompanied by light-headedness, paresthesias of the face and distal limbs, blurred vision, and dry mouth. There also may be a sensation of chest tightness and anxiety. Occasionally, hyperventilation may result in syncope. When this diagnosis is suspected, having the patient hyperventilate for 3 to 5 minutes usually reproduces the symptoms.

Treatment with rebreathing in a paper bag is effective in terminating an attack. This, coupled with an explanation of the mechanism of the symptoms, may suffice to reassure the patient. If an underlying anxiety disorder or other psychiatric disorder is suspected, psychiatric consultation is appropriate.

Psychogenic Unresponsiveness

A history typical of syncope is not common in patients with psychiatric disorders. More common presentations are pseudoseizures and fugue states. Confirmation of the diagnosis typically requires a history provided by an accurate observer. Sometimes, to be certain of the diagnosis, an episode must be observed by a physician; electroencephalographic and electrocardiographic monitoring may be helpful as well. Evaluation and management by a psychiatrist are helpful once the diagnosis has been established.

SYNCOPE OF UNCERTAIN ORIGIN

After the initial history and examination are performed, approximately 50 percent of patients have no obvious cause for their syncope. In these situations, standard hematologic studies, chemistry studies, and an electrocardiogram are performed. If results of these routine studies are normal; if there has been only a single, isolated event; and if the patient is not thought to be at high risk for cardiac syncope, further investigations are difficult to justify. If the events recur, an electroencephalogram during waking and sleep and 24 hour electrocardiographic monitoring should be done. If, after these studies a cardiac disorder is still a possibility, a cardiologic opinion is obtained and invasive electrophysiologic studies are considered. Electrophysiologic studies are probably warranted if there have been frequent, recurrent events or if the patient is judged to be at high risk for cardiac syncope. In the view of some the usefulness of these studies is still controversial.

SUGGESTED READING

Kapoor WN. Evaluation and outcome of patients with syncope. Medicine (Baltimore) 1990; 69:160–175.

Manolis AS, Linzer M, Salem D, Estes NAM III. Syncope: Current diagnostic evaluation and management. Ann Intern Med 1990; 112:850–863.

Thomas JE, Schirger A, Fealey RD, Sheps SG. Orthostatic hypotension. Mayo Clin Proc 1981; 56:117–125.

Yanagihara T, Klass DW, Piepgras DG, Houser OW. Brief loss of consciousness in bilateral carotid occlusive disease. Arch Neurol 1989; 46:858–861.

VERTIGO AND DYSEQUILIBRIUM

RONALD J. TUSA, M.D., Ph.D.
SUSAN J. HERDMAN, Ph.D.

Dizziness is a very common symptom, especially in elderly persons. Out of a group of 1,000 patients seen in a housestaff outpatient clinic, dizziness was the third most common complaint. It affects more than 50 percent of the elderly population and is the most common reason for visiting a physician after age 75 years. The fear of sudden dizziness can cause persons to be withdrawn and may lead to agoraphobia. The fear of falling adversely affects the sense of independence and the quality of life.

CLASSIFICATION

Dizziness is an imprecise term used to describe a variety of symptoms, including vertigo, unsteadiness, lightheadedness, and giddiness, each of which has a different pathophysiologic mechanism. *Vertigo* is the illusion of movement (rotation, translation, or tilt) caused by an imbalance of tonic vestibular signals. *Dysequilibrium,* an imbalance or unsteadiness while standing or walking, is caused by loss of vestibulospinal, proprioceptive, visual, or motor function. A number of *psychological disorders* frequently elicit complaints of dizziness (usually floating, swimming, giddiness, rocking, falling, spinning inside the head). These include anxiety disorders (including panic attacks, agoraphobia, obsessive-compulsive disorder), somatoform disorders (including conversion disorder), and depression. *Presyncope* or lightheadedness is caused by decreased blood flow to the brain.

The most common reason for failure of treatment of dizziness is misdiagnosis and use of the wrong treatment. Antivert and other related drugs are not the treatment of choice for the majority of patients with dizziness. In this chapter we emphasize key features to facilitate correct diagnosis and describe the most helpful forms of therapy.

COMMON PATIENT PRESENTATION

Most patients with dizziness complain of either spells of dizziness or chronic dysequilibrium. In our outpatient neuro-otology clinic the most common causes of spells of dizziness are migraine (prevalence 38 percent), benign paroxysmal positional vertigo (25 percent), psychological disorders (10 percent), Meniere's disease (9 percent), and transient ischemic attack (7 percent). The most common causes of chronic dysequilibrium are peripheral or central neurologic disorders (including cerebrovascular accident, 34 percent), psychological disorders (28 percent), and uncompensated peripheral vestibular defects (24 percent).

SPELLS OF DIZZINESS

When confronted with a patient with spells of dizziness, it is very helpful to determine the average duration of the spell. Table 1 lists the duration, method of diagnosis, and management of the more common causes of spells.

Benign Paroxysmal Positional Vertigo

Patients with benign paroxysmal positional vertigo (BPPV) usually complain of vertigo that lasts less than 1 minute. It usually occurs in the morning, when they get up or turn over in bed. It may also occur when they lie down in bed or move the head back (sitting in a dentist or beauty parlor chair, taking a shower, looking up to a high shelf). After a bad attack, they frequently complain of dysequilibrium that lasts for several hours.

BPPV is usually idiopathic, but it can also follow head trauma, labyrinthitis, or ischemia in the distribution of the anterior vestibular artery, which arises from anterior inferior cerebellar artery via the labyrinthine artery. The pathophysiologic mechanism for BPPV is believed to be debris that is either free floating in the long arm of the posterior semicircular canal (SCC, canalithiasis) or debris attached to the cupula of this canal (cupulolithiasis). Both conditions inappropriately cause the afferents from the posterior SCC to continue to discharge after the head stops moving backward. The debris is most likely calcium particles that have broken free from the macula of the utricle, which is superior to the posterior SCC when the head is erect.

The diagnosis of BPPV is secured by eliciting a torsional-upbeat nystagmus associated with vertigo dur-

---

Table 1 Spells of Dizziness

Seconds to 1 minute
  Benign paroxysmal positional vertigo
    DX: Positive Hallpike-Dix maneuver
    RX: Epley's, Semont's, or Brandt's maneuver

Minutes to 1 hour
  Transient ischemic attacks
    DX: Cerebrovascular and cardiac studies
    RX: Reduce risk factors, antiplatelet medications
  Migraine
    DX: International Headache Society (IHS) criteria for migraine
    RX: Reduce risk factors, antiserotonin medication
  Panic attacks
    DX: DSM-III R criteria
    RX: Imipramine and psychiatric intervention

Hours to days
  Meniere's syndrome
    DX: Fluctuating hearing loss, low-frequency sensorineural
      hearing loss (SNHL)
    RX: Low salt, no caffeine, Diamox, surgery

ing the Hallpike-Dix (Barany's) maneuver when the affected ear is inferior. The nystagmus usually has a latency of 3 to 20 seconds, exhibits fatigue in less than 1 minute, and habituates with repeated maneuvers.

BPPV is best treated by a maneuver that moves the debris out of the posterior SCC. We use two single treatment approaches, a modified Epley's maneuver and Semont's maneuver. We found total remission or significant improvement in BPPV in 90 percent of patients treated with either of these maneuvers in a randomized study of 60 patients. In the modified Epley's maneuver, a Hallpike-Dix manuever is performed toward the side of the affected ear and the head is kept down for 4 minutes (Fig. 1B). Then, the head is slowly rotated toward the unaffected side over the course of 1 minute and kept in the new position 4 minutes (Fig. 1C). Keeping the head deviated toward the unaffected side, the patient slowly sits up (Fig. 1D). This series of maneuvers is designed to move free-floating material in the posterior SCC (arrows in Fig. 1) away from the cupula and into the common crus of the labyrinth. To make certain the debris does not move back toward the cupula, the patient is fitted with a soft collar and told not to bend over or look up or down for 2 days. In addition, they sleep sitting up during this period. For the

subsequent 5 days they are allowed to lie down, but only on the unaffected side. After 7 days the patient is reevaluated to make certain the maneuver worked. It is unclear what happens to the debris after the treatment; presumably, it either adheres to the wall of one of the canals or otoliths, or dissolves. In Semont's maneuver, the patient sits sideways on a table (Fig. 2A). The patient is then rapidly moved onto one side with the affected canal down (Fig. 2B). Prior to this movement the head is turned 45 degrees toward the unaffected side, such that the movement is parallel to the plane of the affected posterior canal. After 4 minutes, the patient is rapidly moved through the initial sitting position to the opposite side while the head is still positioned 45 degrees toward the unaffected side (movement is always parallel to the affected posterior canal) (Fig. 2C). The patient holds this position for 4 minutes and then moves slowly to a sitting position. The patient is then placed in a soft collar and given the same instructions described for modified Epley's maneuver. This series of maneuvers is designed to treat BPPV by dislodging material from the cupula and moving it away from the cupula. If the initial treatment (Epley's or Semont's) does not work, the patient is treated again but with the other technique.

For patients who cannot tolerate sleeping upright

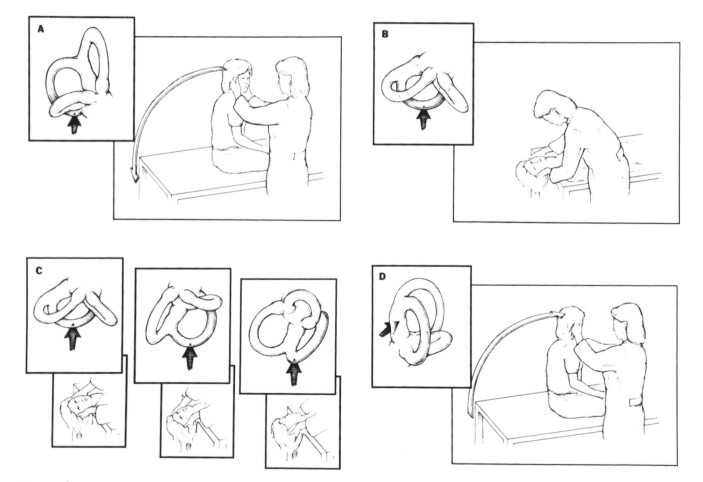

Figure 1 Modified Epley's maneuver for treatment of BPPV. Filled arrows indicate location of free-floating debris in the posterior SCC. See text for description.

for 2 days we use a third maneuver described by Brandt and Daroff. The patient sits on a table sideways then rapidly lies down on one side and waits until the vertigo has resolved or 30 seconds. The patient then rapidly sits up and waits for the same period of time. The movement is then repeated in the opposite direction. This "set" is repeated 10 to 20 times and performed three times a week. Unlike the single treatments described above, with this treatment it usually takes 1 to 2 weeks for symptoms to resolve. The maneuver works either by habituation or by dislodging debris from the cupula of the posterior SCC. Vestibular suppressant drugs have no role in the treatment of BPPV unless the patient refuses to do the maneuvers because of excessive vertigo and nausea.

Transient Ischemic Attacks

Spells of vertigo may occur from vertebrobasilar ischemia (VBI). These spells are abrupt and usually last only a few minutes. They frequently are associated with other vertebrobasilar symptoms, most commonly visual disturbance, drop attacks, unsteadiness, and weakness. A small percentage of patients with VBI may present with isolated spells of vertigo, presumably due to ischemia in the distribution of the anterior vestibular artery. This small artery perfuses the anterior and lateral SCC and the utricular macule and spares the cochlea. In order to treat the patient appropriately it is important to recognize that isolated spells of vertigo can occur from VBI. These patients usually have known cerebrovascular disease or risk factors for it. Treatment includes reduction of risk factors for cerebrovascular disease and antiplatelet therapy.

Migraine

Migraine is a common but seldom recognized cause for spells of dizziness. Spells usually last 4 to 60 minutes and may or may not be associated with headache. We use the International Headache Society (IHS) criteria for the diagnosis of migraine. Since this is a diagnosis of exclusion, the diagnosis is confirmed by a positive response to treatment.

Spells of vertigo due to migraine respond to the same types of treatment as those used for headaches. After establishing the diagnosis and reassuring the patient, we give the patient a handout that lists the risk factors and foods that may precipitate an aura. We encourage patients to avoid hypoglycemia by eating every 6 to 8 hours, avoid nicotine, avoid or reduce exogenous estrogen, and try to maintain a regular sleep schedule. If strict avoidance of these risk factors does not

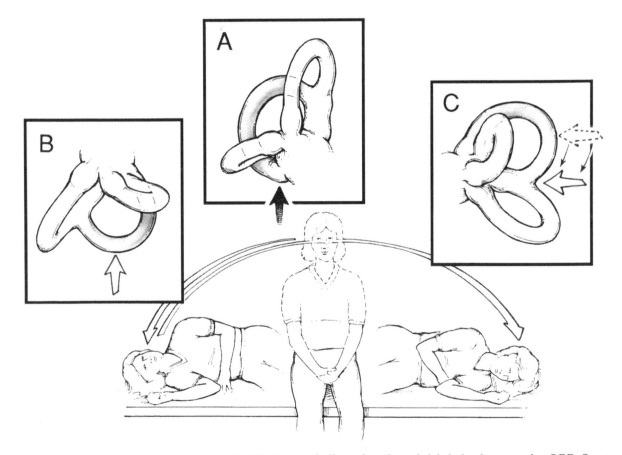

Figure 2 Semont's maneuver for treatment of BPPV. Arrows indicate location of debris in the posterior SCC. See text for description.

significantly reduce their spells, as determined by a diary they keep, then a daily antiserotoninergic medication is used.

Panic Attacks and Hyperventilation

Panic attack is an anxiety disorder that causes intense fear or discomfort that reaches a crescendo within 10 minutes and is frequently associated with dizziness, nausea, shortness of breath, and sweating. It may occur unexpectedly or be situation bound. It may be initiated by an organic cause of vertigo such as BPPV, especially in patients with a family history of panic attacks. Helpful diagnostic criteria can be found in American Psychiatric Association *Diagnostic and Statistical Manual* (DSM-III) *Options Book.* Treatment includes patient education, antidepressants (imipramine), and supportive psychotherapy to help reduce anxiety.

Hyperventilation associated with chronic anxiety can also present with vague complaints of dizziness. Usually this is associated with shortness of breath or chest tightness and paresthesia. A helpful screen for anxiety and depression is the PANAS scale. Treatment includes patient education and stress management through supportive psychotherapy.

Meniere's Disease

A Meniere's attack usually consists of a roaring sound (tinnitus), ear fullness, and hearing loss (often associated with vertigo); it lasts hours to days. With repeat attacks, sustained low-frequency sensorineural hearing loss (SNHL) and constant tinnitus usually develop. The diagnosis depends on documenting fluctuating hearing loss on audiograms. The mechanism is still unclear, but it is believed to be decreased reabsorption of endolymph, or possibly excess secretion, which results in perforation of the membranous labyrinth. This is more likely to occur in an ear previously damaged by trauma or viral infection.

The treatment is primarily prophylactic and includes elimination of alcohol and caffeinated products (including chocolate), and if possible restricting dietary sodium to 2 g or less. To help with this diet we usually give the patient a paperback book entitled the *Complete Guide to Sodium* by Barbara Kraus (Signet, 1987). In addition, a diuretic may help. Diuretics can be given daily, or around the time of the menstrual period to women who suffer attacks during this part of their cycle. Acetazolamide

Table 2 Management of Acute Vertigo

Acute (day 1-3)	Subacute
Vestibular suppressants (see Table 3)	Stop vestibular suppressants
Bed rest	Begin vestibular exercises
Hospitalize if dehydrated or if central defect is suspected	Laboratory tests:
Laboratory tests:	Audiogram (obtain immediately if Meniere's disease is suspected)
Blood tests:	Caloric
FTA-ABS, ESR	Rotary chair test
RF, ANA	
Computed tomography or magnetic resonance imaging of head if central defect is suspected	

FTA-ABS = fluorescent treponemal antibody absorption; ESR = erythrocyte sedimentation rate; RF = rheumatoid factor; ANA = antinuclear antibody.

Table 3 Vestibular Suppressants

Drug	Dosage (mg)
Antivertiginous (sedation)	
Diazepam	5–10 PO, IM, or IV q4–6h
Droperidol	2.5–5 IM q12h
Antiemetics	
Promethazine	25–50 PO, IM, sup q4–6h
Prochlorperazine	5–10 PO or IM q4–6h
	25 sup q12
Meclizine (Bonine)	25 PO q4–6h
Scopolamine	0.5 transderm q3d

Table 4 Physical Findings That Distinguish Peripheral from Central Causes of Acute Vertigo

Finding	Peripheral (Labyrinth or eighth nerve)	Central (Brain Stem, Cerebellum)
Nystagmus		
Direction	Usually mixed (horizontal and rotatory); occasionally horizontal alone	Usually single direction (horizontal, vertical, or rotatory)
Fixation	Usually suppresses	Usually does not suppress
Gaze	Increases with gaze toward direction of quick phase	No change or reverses directions
Other findings		
Caloric (ice water in affected ear)	Nystagmus shows little change	Nystagmus usually increases
Balance	Mild defect, poor tandem, + past point, − Romberg	Severe defect, no tandem, + + past point, + Romberg
Others	Sometimes, hearing loss or tinnitus	Usually, no hearing loss or tinnitus; sometimes, cerebellar and brain stem defects

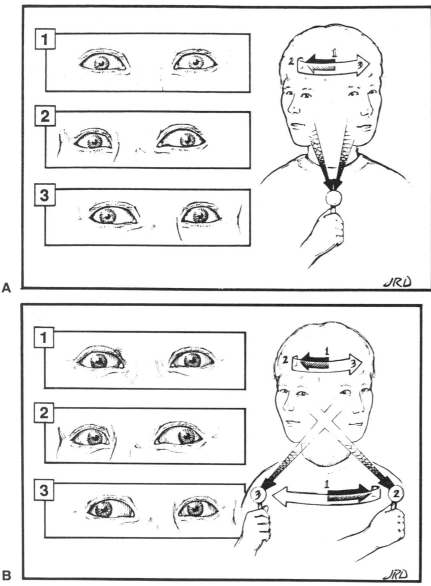

Figure 3 Exercises to enhance the vestibulo-ocular reflex. *A,* Tape or hold a business card in front of you so that you can read it. Move your head back and forth sideways, keeping the words in focus. Move your head faster but keep the words in focus. Continue to do this for 1 to 2 minutes without stopping. Repeat the exercise, moving your head up and down. Do this exercise several times a day. *B,* After this exercise can be easily accomplished move the card and your head back and forth horizontally in *opposite* directions keeping the words in focus. Continue as described above.

may be the optimal diuretic, as it may decrease osmotic pressure in the endolymph. Acute attacks are treated in the same way as any other attack of acute vertigo (see Acute Vertigo), except blood work and vestibular exercises are usually not necessary because the patient recovers quite quickly.

Medical therapy may not control Meniere's disease. Endolymphatic shunts may be used, though they are not always effective or may stop working after a few years. Labyrinthectomy is appropriate for patients who have severe pre-existing hearing loss on the side of the defective labyrinth and no evidence of disease on the other side. Vestibular neurectomy is used in patients whose hearing is preserved.

ACUTE VERTIGO

An acute imbalance of spontaneous neural activity in the vestibular nucleus—due to disease in the laby-rinth, eighth nerve, vestibular nucleus, vestibule-cerebellum (nodulus and flocculus), or central otolith pathways—results in vertigo, nausea, nystagmus, and postural abnormalities. Table 2 lists guidelines for management of acute vertigo. During the first few days, vestibular suppressants should be used (Table 3). If nausea is the primary problem, antiemetics should be used; if vertigo is the primary problem, sedation is more helpful. Patients need hospitalization only if they are dehydrated or if a central lesion is suspected. For central lesions vestibular suppressants often need to be used longer. Guidelines for determining whether the lesion is likely peripheral or central are listed in Table 4.

A common mistake is to keep patients on vestibular suppressants too long. After an acute insult, the imbalance of spontaneous neural activity in the vestibular nucleus usually corrects itself within several days, possibly via commissural pathways. What remains is a dynamic deficit in vestibular function, in which patients perceive vertigo or unsteadiness during head move-

Table 5 Exercises to Improve Postural Stability

Many different balance exercises can be used. These are devised to incorporate head movement and therefore enhance vestibular adaptation or to foster the use of different sensory cues for balance.

Standing with feet as close together as possible the patient turns the head to the right and to the left horizontally while looking straight ahead at a visual target on the wall. This movement is performed for 1 minute without stopping. It is important that the patient keep the visual target in focus during the head movement, in order to foster vestibular adaptation. The patient then tries moving the feet even closer together.

The patient begins to practice turning the head while walking. Because this renders the patient less stable the patient should walk near a wall. Emphasis should be placed on seeing clearly during head movements.

The patient practices turning around while walking, at first making a large circle but gradually making smaller and smaller turns. The patient must be sure to turn in both directions.

The patient can practice attempting to maintain visual fixation of a stationary target while sitting and bouncing on a bed or standing and bouncing on a trampoline. This may facilitate adaptation of the otolith-ocular reflexes.

Out in the community, the patient can practice walking in a mall before it is open (and thus while it is quiet); walking in the mall while walking in the same direction as the flow of traffic; and walking against the flow of traffic. This stresses balance by providing a complex visual environment and increasingly more difficult maneuvering tasks.

The patient stands with the feet shoulder width apart with eyes *open*, looking straight ahead at a target on the wall. The base of support is progressively narrowed from feet apart to feet together to a semi–heel-toe position. Each position is held for 15 seconds before the patient does the next more difficult exercise.

The patient repeats the previous exercise but with eyes *closed*, at first intermittently and then for longer and longer periods. This exercise enhances the use of nonvisual cues for balance.

The patient practices standing on different support surfaces; progressively more difficult tasks might be hard floor (linoleum, wood), thin carpet, shag carpet, thin pillow, sofa cushion. Graded-density foam can also be purchased. This gradually alters somatosensory feedback. The exercises can also be performed with eyes closed to enhance the use of vestibular cues for balance.

The patient practices walking with a narrower base of support. The patient can first touch the wall for support or for tactile cues and then, gradually, can touch only intermittently and then not at all.

Table 6 Exercises to Enhance Substitution of Alternative Strategies to Improve Gaze Stability in Patients with Bilateral Vestibular Deficits

Active eye-head movements between two targets
This exercise is designed to foster the use of saccadic eye movements to regain a visual target after a head movement. This can be performed using two horizontal targets or two vertical targets: Look directly at one target, being sure that your head is also lined up with the target; look at the other target with your eyes and then turn your head to the target [saccades should precede head movement]. Be sure to keep the target in focus during the head movement. Repeat in the opposite direction. Vary the speed of the head movement, but always keep the targets in focus.

Imaginary targets
This exercise is designed to facilitate the central preprogramming of eye-head movements: Look at a target directly in front of you. Close your eyes and turn your head slightly, imagining that you are still looking directly at the target. Open your eyes and check to see if you have been able to keep your eyes on the target. Repeat in the opposite direction. Be as accurate as possible. Vary the speed of the head movement.

---

ments. This dynamic deficit can be repaired only by vestibular adaptation. Because vestibular suppressants delay vestibular adaptation, the patient should stop taking these medications as soon as possible and start vestibular exercises.

Vestibular adaptation occurs when there is a mismatch between head motion as it is sensed by the vestibular system and by the visual system. Adaptation is mediated via cerebellar projections to the vestibular nucleus. To facilitate vestibular adaptation, the patient is taught a series of vestibular exercises that encourage movement of the head while they view a stimulus (Fig. 3). In addition, they are given exercises to improve postural control, at first while standing still and then while the head and body move through space (Table 5).

CHRONIC DYSEQUILIBRIUM

Normal balance depends on integration of sensory input (vision, vestibular, and somatosensory) and appropriate automatic postural responses involving frontal lobe, basal ganglia, cerebellum, spinal cord, and peripheral nerve. Patients with vestibular, somatosensory, or anterior cerebellar lobe defects frequently complain that their balance is worse in the dark. Patients with basal ganglia defects tend to have retropulsion.

Dysequilibrium due to unilateral and or bilateral damage to the vestibular system (peripheral or central) can be significantly decreased with vestibular exercises, but often the diagnosis is missed and appropriate treatment is not given. Thus, it is crucial to recognize a chronic vestibular defect. The clinical examination can be very helpful in the diagnosis. Patients frequently have refixation saccadic eye movements following head thrust due to a decrease in the vestibulo-ocular (VOR) gain. In addition, unilateral defects frequently cause nystagmus following horizontal head shaking, and bilateral lesions usually result in more than a 4 line elevation in visual acuity during 2 Hz head oscillation and oscillopsia. The diagnosis should be secured by demonstrating a decreased VOR response on the Rotary Chair Test and the peripheral nature of the defect identified by a decreased caloric response.

Treatment should include avoidance of all ototoxins that may cause permanent peripheral vestibular damage (gentamicin, streptomycin, tobramycin, ethacrynic acid, furosemide, quinine, cisplatinum) and avoidance of drugs that may transiently impair balance (sedative, antianxiety, antiepileptic, antidepressant). Vestibular exercises should be tailored to the problem. For unilateral defects, exercises described in the section on Acute Vertigo should be used (see Fig. 3, Table 5). For bilateral defects, these same vestibular adaptation exercises can be used to improve the gain of any remaining vestibular function and the cervico-ocular reflex to help reduce oscillopsia. In addition, exercises are given to facilitate the substitution of other ocular motor systems to improve gaze stability (Table 6).

SUGGESTED READING

Baloh RW, Honrubia V. Clinical neurophysiology of the vestibular system. Philadelphia: FA Davis, 1990:301.
Brandt T, Daroff RB. Physical therapy for benign paroxysmal positional vertigo. Arch Otolaryngol 1980; 106:484–485.
Epley JM. The canalith repositioning procedure: For treatment of benign paroxysmal positional vertigo. Otolaryngol Head Neck Surg 1992; 107:399–404.
Herdman SJ, Borello-France D, Whitney S. Treatment of vestibular hypofunction. In: Herdman SJ, ed. Vestibular rehabilitation. Philadelphia: FA Davis, 1993.
Herdman SJ, Tusa RJ, Zee DS, et al. Single treatment approaches to benign paroxysmal positional vertigo. Arch Otolaryn (in press).
(IHS) Headache Classification Committee of the International Headache Society. Classification and diagnostic criteria for headache disorders, cranial neuralgias and facial pain. Cephalalgia 1988; 8(suppl 7):1–96.
Kroenke K, Mangelsdorff D. Common symptoms in ambulatory care: Incidence, evaluation, therapy and outcome. Am J Med 1989; 86:262–266.
Peroutka SJ. The pharmacology of current anti-migraine drugs. Headache 1990; 30(suppl):5–28.
Semont A, Freyss G, Vitte E. Benign paroxysmal positional vertigo and provocative maneuvers. Ann Otolaryngol 1989; 106:473–476.
Shinkawa H, Kimura RS. Effect of diuretics on endolymphatic hydrops. Acta Otolaryngol 1986; 101:43.
Tusa RJ. Diagnosis and management of neuro-otological disorders due to migraine. In: Herdman SJ, ed. Vestibular rehabilitation. Philadelphia: FA Davis, 1993.
Watson D, Clark LA, Tellegen A. Development and validation of brief measures of positive and negative affect: The PANAS scales. J Personal Social Psychol 1988; 6:1063–1070.

PATIENT RESOURCE

Vestibular Disorder Association (VDA)
1015 NW 22nd Avenue, D230
Portland, Oregon 97210-3079
Telephone: (503) 229-7705

SLEEP DISORDERS

CHRISTOPHER J. EARLEY, M.D., Ph.D.

Although the diagnosis of the various sleep disorders is based primarily on clinical manifestations, special investigations are often necessary to verify or further characterize the suspected problem. The two diagnostic procedures central to the evaluation are the polysomnogram (PSG) and the multisleep latency test (MSLT). Although the sleep disorders laboratory or clinic often makes the final decision about which tests to use, the following information is presented to give the referring physician a basic idea of how and why the studies are done and of some of their limitations.

The PSG should be performed as an all-night study. The patient is wired to a multichannel recording unit. The standard PSG usually has two channels designated for electroencephalogram (EEG) and eye movements, one or two channels for limb movements, one channel for the oximeter, and one channel each for chin, thoracic, and diaphragmatic movements. Pressure recordings from an esophageal balloon or temperature recordings from a rectal or nasoesophageal probe are also commonly used in some laboratories. The PSG is limited in the type of answer it can provide about disorders of the sleeping and waking states. These include the frequency of limb movements, disordered breathing, and arousals or awakenings. The degree of oxygen desaturation, latency to sleep onset, and the pattern of sleep stages are also derived from the PSG. The PSG is of limited value for assessing nocturnal seizures, as most laboratories use only two channels for EEG activity. An 18-channel overnight EEG would be the choice for such evaluations. Some laboratories have only a single limb recording as their standard PSG. If periodic limb movements are suspected, the referring physician should make sure testing has been done with recordings from both legs. The PSG is the investigation of choice for verifying or establishing the diagnosis of sleep apnea, periodic limb movements, restless leg syndrome (RLS), and rapid eye movement (REM)–related behavioral disorders.

The MSLT is performed during the day and may run 8 to 10 hours. The patient is monitored only for purposes of sleep staging and is assessed for time to stage 1 sleep (sleep latency), time to stage 2 sleep, and time to REM onset. The patient is required to take several 20 minute naps, which are spaced about 2 hours apart. In order for the MSLT to be sufficiently reliable, the patient should be tested over four or more nap periods. The underlying assumption of the MSLT is that it represents a relatively reliable indicator of sleepiness. The MSLT is performed after an abnormal PSG — for example, secondary to sleep apnea — in order to ascertain how sleepy the person might be in relation to the nocturnal problems. In a person who complains of excessive daytime sleepiness but has a normal PSG, the MSLT may demonstrate reduced sleep latency. A reduced sleep latency of less than 5 minutes in the absence of an abnormal PSG and in the presence of two or more REM onsets on an MSLT is highly suggestive of narcolepsy. Thus, the MSLT may be of value in delineating hypersomnolent states from such conditions as chronic fatigue or depression. The latter conditions are unlikely to be associated with severe reductions in mean sleep latency and do not produce naps with REM activity.

INSOMNIA

Clinical Features

The symptoms associated with insomnia include difficulty in falling asleep or staying asleep and difficulty in getting adequate sleep and feeling tired and fatigued all day. These symptoms may be transient (< 3 weeks) or persistent (> 3 weeks). Psychophysiologic insomnia and insomnia secondary to psychiatric disorders are the most common types of persistent insomnia. Depression and anxiety disorders often present with insomnia. The sleep disturbance commonly seen in depression is frequent awakening, predominantly in the early morning, with subsequent inability to get back to sleep. Difficulty initiating sleep is usually not a prominent component unless there is associated anxiety. Psychophysiologic insomnia may start as minor personal problems, which then lead to major disturbances in the normal sleep pattern. Initially, the patient has a few bad nights of sleep, feels tired during the day, then starts taking naps to compensate. Now he/she is not as tired at night, complains of persistent inability to fall asleep, and continues to feel tired during the day. What was transient insomnia is now persistent. The patient has a psychological fear or frustration about not sleeping plus a disturbed sleep-awake cycle.

Diagnosis

The diagnosis is made primarily on clinical grounds. If the physician feels this is psychologically based insomnia, PSG and MSLT are not required; however, the physician needs to make sure that other potential problems, whose symptoms may appear as an insomnia, are not overlooked. These would include sleep apnea, periodic leg movements of sleep, RLS, narcolepsy, sleep-wake cycle disorders, chronic insufficient sleep, and chronic pain syndromes.

PSG and MSLT may be required to identify secondary causes, though that decision should be left to a sleep disorders clinic to avoid an expensive and unnecessary procedure.

Treatment and Management

Assuming that the potential secondary causes have been excluded, the physician needs to decide about treatment. Patients with clearly defined depression or depression/anxiety disorders require treatment for that disorder. First and foremost, this group of patients have substantial potential for abuse of sedatives or hypnotics. Use of a sedating antidepressant (tricyclic or trazodone) would be recommended. Most of the remaining patients' problems fall into the category of psychophysiologic insomnia. The modification of a patient's behavior is probably the most rewarding and effective therapy for this disorder, but it takes time and effort on the part of both physician and patient to see it through. One should start by re-establishing basic sleep hygiene (Table 1). The next approach is more structured behavioral readjustment; two such approaches are outlined below.

Patients who are unable to initiate sleep or awaken from sleep should leave the bed and go to another room. They can watch TV or read, but they are not to sleep in the other room. When they feel sufficiently tired they can return to bed. Initially, patients lose sleep, but eventually they develop a more positive attitude toward sleep that overrides their previous negative perspective. Another approach for patients who cannot initiate sleep is to have them hold off going to bed until later (e.g., 1:00 AM rather than 11:00 PM). They are not to sleep at all during the day. Again, there is an initial increase in daytime sleepiness, but when it comes time to sleep they are ready. The physician then slowly advances the bedtime towards normal. The wake-up time is held constant so as not to affect the circadian rhythm.

Pharmacologic treatment of insomnia is varied and often less than successful. Some patients with mild or transient insomnia may benefit from over-the-counter medications. However, some of these medications (e.g., diphenhydramine) may produce nocturnal restlessness and subsequent worsening of the insomnia if used long term. If long-term treatment seems likely, an antidepres-

Table 1 Guidelines for Sleep Hygiene

No daytime naps.

More daily exercise; a late evening walk is often very relaxing.

Avoid heavy meals several hours before bedtime, but a light snack before bed may be helpful.

How much sleep is needed should be defined by the patient but then routinely adhered to.

There should be a fixed time for lights out and for awakening.

The bedroom is used only for sleeping; all stimulating or arousing activities should be done elsewhere.

The bedroom should be quiet, comfortable, cool, and dark.

Learn to relax before bed. Meditation, breathing exercise, light reading, or writing down any nagging thoughts are all ways of relaxing before bed.

Take no stimulants shortly before bedtime and if necessary for 6 to 8 hours before bedtime.

Alcohol or sedative medication should not be routinely used to force sleep.

If sleep will not come after 20 to 30 minutes, leave the bedroom; try reading or watching TV or working on relaxing. If you have nagging thoughts, spend time writing them out.

sant or a neuroleptic in small doses should be tried. If a patient presents with a week or two of insomnia and the precipitating condition seems likely to be short lived, a benzodiazepine may be helpful. By treating the insomnia until the transient precipitating condition resolves, one may prevent the cascade of events that lead to persistent insomnia. We rarely advocate benzodiazepines for persistent insomnia, because long-term use is likely to create more problems than it cures.

Long-term use of benzodiazepines can lead to paradoxical worsening of sleep. Usually, there is an initial increase in dose, which gives temporary benefit, but again the patient returns with the complaint. Many patients suffer poor sleep because of chronic use of benzodiazepines but have never had an increment in their dose. Successful treatment of these cases requires very slow withdrawal of the medication. Frequent reassurance from the physician is required during the initial phase. Initially, the insomnia may get worse, but after several weeks the patient should begin to feel improvements. Patients need to know what plans have been made if the insomnia persists after drug withdrawal. Such plans would include psychological or psychiatric therapy or re-evaluation of the insomnia for secondary causes.

PERIODIC LEG MOVEMENTS AND RESTLESS LEG SYNDROME

Clinical Features

Periodic leg movements (PLM) of sleep are frequent, rhythmic or semirhythmic movements of one or both legs. Patients complain of frequent awakenings but are often unaware of the movements. A history from the bed partner may identify the problem as frequent movements. In the absence of such a witness, the disheveled state of the bed in the morning may be the only clue.

The RLS is a clinical subset of PLM. The distinguishing feature is that RLS represents a sensory phenomenon during the waking state as well as nocturnal movements. This sensory phenomena is often described as a deep, uneasy, and constant aching feeling. There is no one "feeling" that can clearly be identified with RLS. Immobility and rest always heighten the sensation. Movements, particularly walking, always bring some, if not total, relief. Patients also find benefit from heat (hot bath or shower or heating pad) and from rubbing the affected limb.

PLM and RLS can be divided into idiopathic and secondary forms. The idiopathic form probably constitutes the largest group. Its prevalence increases with age; it is very uncommon before 40 years of age and rarely demonstrates spontaneous remission. Secondary causes of these two syndromes include anemia, peritoneal/hemodialysis, dopamine agonist and antagonist medications, and tricyclic antidepressants. Secondary RLS often does not have the typical nocturnal or diurnal variation. Remission often is seen when the underlying problem is adequately treated.

Diagnosis

The diagnosis of RLS is based on the clinical history. The leg movements of sleep seen in PLM and RLS, though inferred from the history, need to be identified by PSG. A MSLT is performed the day after the night-time PSG and serves as a guide to how disturbed the sleep has been. Because of the night-to-night variability that may be seen in some patients, a single PSG may appear "normal." This variability also underscores the difficulty in drawing a correlation between the number of kicks at night and clinical symptoms. When in doubt, we use ambulatory monitors for 1 or 2 weeks.

The differential diagnosis for RLS includes fibromyalgia, myopathic processes, arthralgia, and radiculopathies. The differential diagnosis for PLM includes seizures, myoclonus, paroxysmal kinisigenic choreoathetosis, and joint and muscle pain. Back and joint pain commonly cause movements throughout the night that, if frequent enough, can disturb sleep.

Treatment and Management

The first line of treatment is dopaminergic medication. We start with a half tablet of Sinemet 25/100. Every 3 or 4 days we add a half-tablet increment. The increments are based on benefits versus side effects. If benefits are not achieved by four tablets or if side effects occur, we change to another dopamine agonist. The single most common side effect is a "rebound effect." After several days on Sinemet, patients complain of having RLS symptoms during the earlier part of the day. Also, the late night symptoms now become early evening symptoms. Attempts to broaden the treatment schedule rarely succeed. The outcome of such treatment plans is worsening symptoms between doses and shortening of Sinemet's effectiveness. If rebound effects are the primary problem, changing to Sinemet CR at an initial dose of one tablet an hour before bedtime may be of benefit. The maximum dose would be two tablets at night, and this is achieved by making half-tablet increments, as with the Sinemet 25/100. Dopamine medication management is sufficiently complicated that it may well be best done at a sleep disorder center.

Failing to benefit patients with dopamine agonist, one moves to sedative medication. We have used 100 to 300 mg of propoxyphene (and related opiates) or benzodiazepines (starting with short- or intermediate-acting ones). The benefits of sedative medication lie in their ability to suppress arousal induced by leg movements. As far as the daytime symptoms of RLS are concerned, sedative medication may blunt the distress and anxiety but has variable and inconsistent effects on the sensory experience.

There is a long list of drugs that have been used in the past 20 or 30 years for this disorder, all with variable and inconsistent results. This list includes the anticonvulsants and antidepressants, which can be tried if the above regimens fail. However, it is important first to make sure that the diagnosis is correct and that there are no identifiable secondary causes. We have seen concurrent PLM and narcolepsy, and in some of these cases the PLM has not responded well to dopaminergic drugs.

SLEEP APNEA AND SNORING

Clinical Features

Sleep apnea syndromes (SAS) represent disordered breathing events which lead to partial (hypopnea) or complete (apnea) cessation of breathing. Subsequently this may lead to hypoxia and arousal from sleep. It is the frequent occurrence of the two events that is associated with the clinical syndrome. Two distinct forms of SAS can be differentiated, obstructive (OSAS) and central (CSAS). OSAS follows from upper airway limitation of air flow. CSAS follows from a loss of central nervous system control of respiration.

OSAS may present with daytime hypersomnolence, sexual dysfunction, dementia, minor memory difficulties, depression, or early morning headaches. There may be complaints from the bed partner of frequent movements, snoring, or apneic spells. The patient often is totally unaware of these nocturnal events. Patients with CSAS tend to have more complaints of insomnia and frequent awakening, but otherwise CSAS can lead to similar problems to those seen with OSAS.

Alcohol, sedative medications, sleep deprivation, weight gain, and positioning may all exacerbate OSAS. Although it is commonly associated with obesity, cerebrovascular disease, neuromuscular disease, or hypothyroidism may precipitate OSAS. CSAS may be associated with cerebrovascular disease, hydrocephalus, brain tumors, autonomic dysfunction, or cardiovascular dysfunction. Complete lack of respiratory drive during sleep is referred to as *Ondine's curse*.

Diagnosis

The diagnosis of SAS is often suspected on clinical grounds, but the definitive diagnosis is made by PSG and MSLT. The first test identifies the type (central and/or obstructive) and amount of disordered breathing. It also demonstrates how much oxygen desaturation occurs and how frequently the spells cause arousal. The MLST is a good indicator of how tired the patient is and, therefore, usually correlates well with the degree of nocturnal disturbances.

Treatment and Management

Conservative management of OSAS should include weight reduction and the avoidance of alcohol and sedative medication. Often, weight reduction can lead to marked improvement in the apnea, and at times even to resolution of the episodes. Medication has been used with varying success. Protriptyline, 5 or 10 mg at bedtime, has been shown to reduce the number of disturbed breathing events. The anticholinergic side effects may lead to drug withdrawal. Surgical management includes uvulopalatopharyngoplasty (UPPP), tonsillectomy, septoplasty, and tracheostomy. UPPP has been the most widely used of these surgical approaches. There are no clear ways to identify who will and who will not benefit from the procedure, though clearly some patients do. The procedures carry surgical and anesthetic risks. Sometimes problems with swallowing and speech are encountered postoperatively.

Continuous positive airway pressure (CPAP) is the most widely used medical therapy for OSAS. The patient wears a tight fitting mask over the nose and mouth. Air under pressure is delivered continuously while the mask is worn. The major complaints are discomfort from the mask and the pressurized air. Nasal or sinus congestion may occur but is usually remedied by humidifying the air. When CSAS appears in conjunction with OSAS, treating the latter may benefit the former. When CSAS appears as the only disorder or the prominent one, CPAP or surgical management may give little benefit. Treatment, if needed, is with home O_2 in order to maintain blood PaO_2 during the apneic spells or with bi-level positive airway pressure (BiPAP) to assist breathing.

Snoring, independent of sleep apnea, often creates problems for the spouse, who awakens frequently because of the noise. Weight loss, elimination of alcohol and sedative medication, or the use of protriptyline may all bring some benefit. When snoring occurs because of underlying apnea, CPAP therapy for the apnea resolves the snoring. Surgical management by UPPP has been reported to have a high success rate in eliminating snoring. But its risks and complications may be less acceptable for the treatment of snoring. There are also mechanical devices, such as the tongue-retaining device, which can be fitted by a dentist, that when worn during sleep reduces snoring in some patients.

NARCOLEPSY AND IDIOPATHIC HYPERSOMNOLENT STATES

Clinical Features

Narcolepsy is a syndrome in which a tetrad of clinical symptoms may appear. Excessive daytime somnolence (EDS) is the commonest of the four symptoms and it may be the only one. Furthermore, the patient may not always perceive the problem as sleepiness but may complain of being unable to focus the vision or unable to sustain attention while driving or reading.

Cataplexy and sleep paralysis are periods of usually seconds to minutes, during which the patient is unable to move a body part or the entire body because of the atonic state of the muscles involved. The patient is awake and fully aware during this period. Cataplexy is precipitated by emotional states (e.g., laughter, anger), and it becomes worse or less controllable during periods of tiredness. Sleep paralysis usually occurs just before sleep onset but may occur upon awakening. The patient is fully alert but completely paralyzed and unable to talk.

Hypnagogic hallucinations, the fourth set of symptoms, occur just before falling asleep. They are visual in nature, but not uncommonly they involve the auditory system. Tingling or prickly sensation, distorted or complex sensory experiences, or an out-of-body experience may all be described by patients who have experienced hypnagogic sensory hallucinations.

A less well-recognized symptom of narcolepsy is disturbed nocturnal sleep. Patients have little problem falling asleep but often awaken after 2½ to 3 hours. They feel fully awake and unable to sleep for the next 45 to 60 minutes but then fall back to sleep for another 2½ to 3 hours. Often the disturbed nocturnal sleep is perceived as the source of the daytime somnolence, but treatment directed at the nocturnal disturbances has no effect on the daytime problems.

Diagnosis

In the majority of cases the diagnosis of narcolepsy is made from the history. The PSG and MSLT are used to objectify the probable diagnosis. In making the diagnosis on the basis of EDS one must clearly attempt to weed out possible secondary causes of somnolence: sleep apnea, chronic insufficient sleep, insomnia, periodic movements of sleep, sedative medications, depression, chronic fatigue, fibromyalgia, or chronic pain syndrome. In the history, fatigue must be differentiated from sleepiness. In the end, this is difficult; the PSG and MSLT, therefore, become essential for the diagnosis.

After excluding secondary causes, the key differential for primary EDS is idiopathic hypersomnolence syndrome (IHS) versus narcolepsy. With the IHS there is only EDS and none of the other three symptoms of narcolepsy. Often, patients respond poorly to stimulant medications. Short naps, which invigorate narcoleptics, have marginal benefit for patients with IHS. In both conditions, MSLT shows shortened median sleep latency, but only with narcolepsy do two or more REM-onset naps occur in less than 15 minutes.

Treatment and Management

Physician and patient must come to a clear understanding of the goals and expectations of therapy. Not everyone derives full benefit from treatment. Often there is fluctuation in benefits. Some patients' expectations are probably unattainable and therefore bound to create future problems.

Nondrug therapy should be the initial, though not necessarily the only, way to manage EDS. Drug therapy needs to be used in conjunction with nondrug therapy, not as a separate or independent management option. Nondrug therapy has four options: short naps, caffeinated beverages, exercise, and food avoidance. Short naps (10 to 20 minutes) are often superior to drugs in restoring high levels of alertness and attention. Naps

should be taken on a scheduled basis, two or three a day or when the patient is likely to encounter sleep-provoking situations (conferences or driving). Naps can be followed by consumption of caffeinated beverages, or both can be used independently throughout the day. Exercise has a potent arousing and alerting effect. Even a brief walk outside helps break the overwhelming sense of sleepiness. Food, on the other hand, induces somnolence. Light lunches, small portions spread throughout the day, or avoidance of all except high-glucose beverages are the options. Neither naps nor drugs can fully override the somnolent effects of a heavy meal. It is the mixing of these four options throughout the day that often allows patients to function quite well without resorting to drugs. As an example, a patient who has an afternoon meeting can avoid eating lunch, take a 15 minute nap at his desk, have several cups of coffee, and take a short walk at lunch time.

Drug treatment involves the uses of stimulants (Table 2). These include pemoline (Cylert), methylphenidate (Ritalin), dextroamphetamine (Dexedrine) tablets, and methamphetamine (Desoxyn Gradumet) tablets.

Methylphenidate and amphetamine come in short- and long-acting preparations. We usually start with pemoline, 18.75 mg in the morning. Adjustments are made about every week by a further 18.75 mg. The maximum dose is 75 mg in the morning and 37.5 mg at 1:00 PM. Next, we move to Ritalin, then to amphetamine. Once the desired benefits have been achieved with the short-acting preparation, one can change over to a longer-acting formulation if necessary.

Cataplexy is not appreciably affected by the stimulant medications and thus requires separate treatment. We start with protriptyline 10 mg once a day and if necessary move up to two or three times a day. Desipramine 25 mg may be considered next if the side effects of Protriptyline are a concern. We have also found some patients to be very responsive to Prozac, which produces markedly less pronounced side effects. For those unresponsive to the antidepressants, gamma-hydroxybutyrate and yohimbine are being used in clinical trials.

IHS is treated with stimulant medications in a manner similar to narcolepsy; however, IHS frequently does not respond even to very large doses of amphetamine. Nondrug therapy options similarly do not carry a lot of benefit for these patients. Unfortunately, an occasional patient walks out of the clinic as tired as he or she walked in.

Table 2 Stimulant Medication

Medication	Starting Dose	Maximum Dose	Serum Half-life (hr)
Pemoline	18.75 mg qd	112.5 mg qd	12
Methylphenidate	5 mg t.i.d.	30 mg q.i.d.	4–5
Dextroamphetamine	5 mg b.i.d.	40 mg t.i.d.	8–10
Methamphetamine	5 mg t.i.d.	30 mg q.i.d.	4–5

It should be remembered that not all narcoleptics achieve 100 percent benefit from even very large doses of amphetamines. The physician must always be alert to the fact that when a patient who has been stable for a year or more on medication presents with worsening symptoms a thorough re-evaluation of personal, social, and medical status is necessary before changing medication. The reappraisal may identify stressors or lifestyle changes that can be managed directly without resorting to medication changes.

With regard to the nocturnal disturbances sometimes seen in narcolepsy, there are no data to suggest that preventing the awakenings with benzodiazepines improves the EDS. Sometimes sedative medication worsens the EDS, especially during the earlier part of the morning. Therefore, if benzodiazepines must be used, short- or intermediate-acting formulations should be used, with an awareness of the risk of early morning problems, such as accidents on the way to work.

PARASOMNIAS

Clinical Features

The parasomnias are simple or complex movements or behaviors that occur just prior to sleep onset or upon arousal from sleep. Sleepwalking, night terrors, and nocturnal enuresis are parasomnias that are predominately non-REM (NREM) events. These NREM parasomnias present at various times in childhood and only rarely persist or present after adolescence. They are not commonly associated with underlying psychosocial problems. They tend to occur during the earlier part of sleep, when NREM activity is prevalent.

The fourth type of parasomnia of clinical concern is referred to as *REM behavior disorders,* because they occur during the REM phase of sleep. It is almost exclusively an adult phenomena. The patient may be verbally abusive, physically threatening to himself or others, appear severely frightened, or cry uncontrollably. These episodes last as long as several minutes and may recur several times a night and on several consecutive nights. The repeated episodes often have similar characteristics. The patient is unaware of the ongoing event unless awakened during them, in which case the events may be recalled as part of a dream experience.

Diagnosis

The diagnosis for the parasomnias is based almost entirely on history. Difficulties arise when symptoms are present in adulthood. A phenomenon similar to night terrors may affect young adults. The awakenings are experienced as profound fear, dread, or doom. There is accompanying autonomic hyperactivity. The differential diagnosis includes REM behavior disorder, seizure disorder, and anxiety attacks.

Sleepwalking can also present in adult life, and REM behavior disorder would be the alternative condition to rule out. A childhood history of parasomnias and the clustering of events toward the earlier part of sleep make sleepwalking the more likely diagnosis. With REM behavior disorder, the events cluster towards early morning, when REM activity is most concentrated. A PSG is usually helpful in differentiating the two disorders. The PSG may show in which sleep phase the event occurs. Also it may show the presence of brief periods of muscle tonicity and/or twitching during the REM phase. This would be diagnostic of REM-related disorders. As this disorder may be associated with central nervous system disease, a full neurologic examination is required to evaluate secondary causes.

Finally, nocturnal enuresis is often a benign condition of otherwise healthy children. A thorough history, physical, and a few basic blood tests should eliminate possible secondary causes like urinary tract infection, diabetes mellitus, seizures, spina bifida, and psychosocial or behavioral problems.

Treatment and Management

A sleepwalker's family must take certain precautions to prevent injury. These include securing windows and doors and clearing walkways and stairways. It cannot be overemphasized that this is a benign event and that the use of sedative hypnotics should be restricted to situations where personal injury is a real concern. Even then, efforts should be made to change the environment to reduce these risks. Sleepwalking in adults usually reflects underlying stress or use of sedative medication or alcohol. Treatment should therefore address these issues first. The infant or child with sleep terrors awakens screaming uncontrollably. All efforts by parents are futile. The child eventually calms down and goes back to sleep. The child has no memory of the event, though the parents live in dread of the next one. The primary treatment is education of the parents. They need to know that these are benign and common in childhood; that all efforts to stop the child will only make matters worse for them and the child; and that the child will outgrow them. The night terrors that occur in adulthood may reflect psychosocial problems, so efforts should be directed toward identifying such problems. If the problem is likely to be of short duration (e.g., night terrors secondary to bereavement), then benzodiazepines are usually helpful; however, tricyclic antidepressants and neuroleptics should be avoided, since they may intensify the condition.

Nocturnal enuresis represents one of the more challenging parasomnias to treat. There is little in the literature to suggest that emotional problems constitute a major factor in this disorder. Treatments include bladder training, sphincter training, conditioning procedures, motivational techniques, and medication. The initial treatment should be the simplest. Medication is rarely, if ever, needed. The occurrence of nocturnal enuresis in adults suggests an underlying medical or psychosocial problem. Treatment depends on the primary problem.

REM behavior disorders respond very well to benzodiazepines. We usually start with alprazolam and then if necessary move on to a longer-acting preparation (clonazepam). Of all the parasomnia, patients with this disorder are best seen by a sleep disorder specialist in order to confirm the diagnosis and lay out the plans to manage it.

DISORDERS OF THE SLEEP-WAKE CYCLE

Clinical Features

Sleep-wake cycle disorders represent "dis-synchronicity" between the biologically defined sleep period and the social or actual sleep time. The shift worker is the classic example of social demands creating a sleep-wake cycle that is dis-synchronous with normal circadian rhythm. In another situation, persons may appear to keep a normal sleep-wake cycle yet suffer from this disorder because their natural rhythm interval is greater than 24 hours (progressive sleep cycle delay) or because their sleep phase is fixed and out of synchrony with what we consider normal. In the fixed sleep cycle disorder the biologic sleep time may be shifted several hours earlier in the evening (advanced sleep phase) or several hours later in the morning (delayed sleep phase). The latter is the most common.

Patients with a delayed sleep phase retire at a normal time but are unable to fall asleep for several hours. When they awaken at a "normal" hour, they feel tired for the earlier part of the morning. On weekends or during vacations they often go to bed late and get up late. Also during this time, they have no problem falling asleep or staying asleep and they feel refreshed when they awaken. They usually sleep only 7 to 8 hours. Those with an advanced sleep phase demonstrate just the opposite behavior: early to bed and early to rise. Because this lifestyle is more acceptable it is less likely to be considered a problem.

Diagnosis

In order to have a clear idea of the individual biologic and actual sleep-wake cycle, the patient keeps a diary for several weeks to a month. Documentation of bedtime, actual sleep time, awakening time, daily activity, and periods of tiredness or naps are kept in the diary. If the historical data suggest a circadian rhythm disorder,

then a 24 hour ambulatory temperature monitor or a prolonged PSG with temperature monitoring is performed. A shift in the peak and trough temperatures indicate a shift in the circadian rhythm.

The main element in the differential diagnosis is persistent insomnia. With insomnia, sleep remains disturbed despite going to bed later or getting up later. There may be underlying psychiatric problems, which would be more suggestive of insomnia.

Treatment and Management

The primary goal of treatment is to realign the social and biologic sleep phases. For a small minority this can be accomplished by changing their social life. In the majority, however, shifting the circadian rhythm back into a normal pattern is required. Forcing the person to retire early and use of sedative-hypnotics have no benefit.

Attempts to shift the circadian rhythm are, at present, best achieved with light therapy. The concept is that by overemphasizing the light-dark cycle one can influence the biological clock. The patient is exposed to either sunlight or special high-lux (> 2000 lux) lamps for 1 to 2 hours after awakening. Starting at midafternoon, dark glasses (with side and top enclosures) are worn until evening. Using this method for several weeks usually leads to a significant shift in the sleep-wake cycle; however, the procedure needs to be repeated every few weeks.

SUGGESTED READING

Coats, TJ, Thoresen CE. How to sleep better: A drug-free program for overcoming insomnia. Englewood Cliffs, NJ: Prentice-Hall, 1977.
Kryger M, Roth T, Dement WC. Principles and practice of sleep medicine. Philadelphia: WB Saunders, 1989.
Lamberg L. American Medical Association guide to better sleep. New York: Random House, 1984.

PATIENT RESOURCES

Association of Professional Sleep Disorders
604 Second Street S.W.
Rochester, New York 55902

American Narcolepsy Association
Box 5846
Stanford, California 94305

NEUROGENIC ORTHOSTATIC HYPOTENSION

PHILLIP A. LOW, M.D.

Orthostatic hypotension (OH) is a relatively common, if under-recognized, problem in neurologic practice. Symptoms range from a feeling of tiredness, mental slowness, unsteadiness, "dizziness" (ranging from light-headedness to a sense of disequilibrium), nausea, tremulousness, or blurred vision, to a feeling of impending syncope, to syncope. For the purposes of this discussion, OH is defined as an orthostatic reduction of systolic blood pressure (BP) by 30 mm Hg or mean BP (diastolic plus one-third of pulse pressure) of 20 mm Hg, associated with symptoms.

In many of the situations, no further evaluation or treatment is needed, because the mechanism is obvious. For instance, following administration of tricyclic antidepressants, diuretics, or antihypertensive medication or a couple of weeks of bed rest elders often develop OH. In this chapter I focus on the management of neurogenic OH. There are numerous causes of neurogenic OH; the most common causes of severe OH seen in neurologic practice are listed in Table 1.

There is no completely satisfactory generic drug treatment for OH. The optimal dose in one situation is underdosing in another. The best approach is to recognize that, for the majority of patients OH constitutes a chronic problem for which drug treatment is only one component of the management regimen. The patient needs to be educated in the management of OH in the same way that patients with other chronic disorders such as the insulin-dependent diabetic are. They need to understand the mechanisms of the maintenance of postural normotension, the everyday orthostatic stresses, and the full range of countermeasures, including pharmacologic agents.

AIMS OF TREATMENT

The aims of treatment are summarized in Table 2 and described below. It is important to remove the cause of the neurogenic OH if possible or to administer specific treatment when available. The patient with a menigioma compressing neural pathways in the upper cervical cord may be cured of the OH following surgical resection. A patient with arsenical or thallium autonomic neuropathy improves when the cause is removed. Some cases of acute, presumably immune-mediated, acute autonomic neuropathy have improved with treatment with prednisone or intravenous gamma globulin. Patients with the myasthenic syndrome may have OH, and the symptom may improve with the administration of 3,4-diaminopyridine. Tumor resection has infrequently been followed by improvement of the paraneoplastic autonomic neuropathy.

The next aim is to reduce the severity, frequency, and duration of symptoms of orthostatic hypotension. This aim is achievable over short periods. To sustain the benefits requires much fine tuning of the patient's activities and medications and also patient education.

Currently, all effective treatment is associated with supine hypertension and nocturnal hypertension. Indeed, the main side effect of vasoactive drugs is supine hypertension.

All patients with OH can be helped. It is important to set realistic goals. The patient with multiple system atrophy (MSA) with severe bradykinesia has more modest goals than one with pure autonomic failure (PAF, idiopathic OH, Eggleston-Bradbury syndrome), which has a much better prognosis. For all patients, the aim is to increase and improve performance of activities of daily living. For young patients with PAF the goal might be to continue with work and activities of home and leisure. Such patients require aggressive therapy with close attention to detail. Older patients with severe extrapyramidal signs might have a more limited goal (e.g., to extend standing time from 10 seconds to 2 minutes).

Table 1 Common Causes of Generalized Autonomic Failure

Pure autonomic failure
Multiple system atrophy
Diabetic autonomic neuropathy
Amyloid neuropathy
Guillain-Barré syndrome
Sjögren's syndrome
Acute panautonomic neuropathy (idiopathic, paraneoplastic)

Table 2 Aims of Treatment of Orthostatic Hypotension

Remove cause, if possible.
Administer specific treatment if available.
Reduce severity, frequency, and duration of symptoms of orthostatic hypotension.
Improve orthostatic BP without undue supine hypertension.
Set realistic goals.

APPROACH TO THE MANAGEMENT OF ESTABLISHED NEUROGENIC ORTHOSTATIC HYPOTENSION

I approach management in a series of sequential steps.

Step 1: Is Treatment Warranted?

The first step is to decide if the patient needs treatment. An asymptomatic patient with OH may not need treatment, since cerebral autoregulation is enhanced in such patients. However, it is important to recognize the repertoire of orthostatic symptoms and their severity and temporal pattern. Symptoms may be a lot more subtle than syncope or presyncope. Sometimes it is only after correction of OH that the patient becomes aware of symptoms of OH. In general, patients whose BP is no higher than 80/50 are usually symptomatic. The type and severity of symptoms depend on a number of factors, including acuteness of OH, time of day, orthostatic stress, and age of the patient. Younger subjects with recent-onset OH have lightheadedness, blurred vision, weakness, nausea, ataxia, and occasional vertigo followed seconds later by syncope. In contrast, older subjects typically do not complain of lightheadedness or other florid symptoms. Instead, they are slower mentally and faint without apparent warning. The symptoms need not be just orthostatic dizziness. Some patients feel tired, others unsteady, and still others mentally slow.

An important consideration is the effect of OH on the patient's activities of daily living (i.e., work, home life, recreational activities). Such an evaluation needs to be done over a significant period of the day, and the symptoms need to be considered relative to the orthostatic stress. Such an evaluation involves a consideration of orthostatic stresses, symptoms, and BP.

Different types of OH may produce different symptoms. Patients with generalized autonomic failure, such as PAF, have different symptoms than patients with postural orthostatic tachycardia syndrome (POTS) (Table 3). The rest of the chapter focuses on non-POTS OH.

Step 2: Treat Reversible Factors

The second step is to seek treatable causes such as diuretic therapy, dehydration, deconditioning, or antidepressant or hypotensive therapy. If OH is due to any of these mechanisms removing the cause or reconditioning the subject should reverse the OH.

Step 3: Try Simple Measures First

For patients who have symptomatic OH, the next step is expansion of the plasma volume by hydration and increasing salt intake and retention (with fludrocortisone). The patient should drink a minimum of five glasses or cups of fluid per day and consume a generous amount of added salt in the diet. The patient should be taking in 150 to 250 mEq of salt (10 to 20 g).

Patients should try sleeping with the head of the bed elevated 6 to 10 inches. Some patients with autonomic failure lose much salt and water during the night; this can be prevented by head-up tilt, which appears to work by stimulating the renin-angiotensin-aldosterone mechanism. Patients who cannot tolerate this degree of tilt should use less; even a tilt of 20 degrees has been shown to work. In my experience, most patients do not benefit substantially from nocturnal head-up tilt, at least as evaluated by reduction of urine output in the morning or weight change. Nevertheless, I continue to recommend it for a different reason. Patients with generalized autonomic failure lose their BP-buffering mechanisms and their diurnal variation in BP. They become hypertensive by day and especially at night. It is often necessary to accept supine BP that does not exceed 180/105 or 180/110 much of the time. Raising the head of the bed reduces arterial pressure to the brain.

Step 4: Pharmacologic Treatment

Drug treatment is an important part of the overall therapeutic regimen, and if used well greatly enhances BP control. The first-line therapeutic agents are listed in Table 4.

The first drug should be fludrocortisone (Florinef), 0.1 mg once or twice daily, to provide volume expansion and sensitize vascular smooth muscle. The dose may be increased to 0.4 or 0.6 mg per day. This is the essential first step. Because the regulatory reflexes are much impaired, it is necessary to slightly overexpand the plasma volume of these patients. Mild dependent edema is usually present and expected, but care must be taken to avoid congestive cardiac failure in elderly patients. The goal is a weight gain of 3 to 5 pounds.

The next drug to be considered is ibuprofen (Motrin), 400 mg four times a day. Although most

Table 3 Comparison of Generalized Autonomic Neuropathy and Postural Orthostatic Tachycardia Syndrome (POTS)

Parameter	Generalized Autonomic Neuropathy	POTS
Orthostatic dizziness	Immediate	Delayed
Orthostatic tremulousness	Absent	Present
Orthostatic palpitations	Absent	Present
Orthostatic hypotension	Consistent	Variable; delayed
Orthostatic tachycardia	Reduced	Exaggerated
Supine norepinephrine	Usually reduced	Normal
Standing norepinephrine	Reduced	Increased or normal
HR to deep breathing	Reduced	Normal
Valsalva ratio	Reduced	Normal or increased
BP_{BB} to VM:		
Early phase II	Markedly increased	Increased
Late phase II	Absent	Normal of reduced
Phase IV	Absent	Increased

experience has been accumulated with indomethacin (Indocin), 25 to 50 mg three times a day, I prefer the former, which appears to have fewer gastric irritant problems. It probably works by inhibiting prostaglandin synthesis. These nonsteroidal anti-inflammatory drugs have also been shown to increase the sensitivity of infused norepinephrine and angiotensin II. The drug should be taken with meals or with a glass of milk to reduce the gastric irritant effect.

The next drug I would use is phenylpropanolamine (Propagest), a direct-acting alpha-agonist. The drug is available in 25 mg tablets. The beginning dose is 12.5 to 25 mg. The usual dose is 25 mg three times a day. Maximal dose is about 50 mg three times a day. Sustained-release phenylpropanolamine is available over the counter (e.g., Dexatrim). My choice of the preparation depends on the indication. For patients who are about to face a relatively brief orthostatic stress, say for an hour or two, the short-acting drug is preferred. For patients who need longer action, the sustained-release preparation is indicated.

The most reliable alpha-agonist is Midodrine, an alpha-agonist on both arterioles and the venous capacitance bed. It causes less supine hypertension than other alpha-agonists. It is better absorbed and has a longer duration of action than phenylpropanolamine. Currently, it is an investigational drug.

Alternative or Second-Line Pharmacologic Agents

Second-line drugs that I would consider are ephedrine, methylphenidate, desmopressin, dihydroergotamine, and intranasal ergotamine.

Ephedrine. Ephedrine is an indirect-acting alpha-agonist with beta-agonist effects. The drug is less effective than phenylpropanolamine or Midodrine and is less reliably absorbed. It has central stimulant effects (beta-agonist), and tachyphylaxis is a problem. The usual dose is 25 to 50 mg three times a day.

Methylphenidate. Methylphenidate (Ritalin) or dexamphetamine, both in doses of 5 to 10 mg three times a day, can be beneficial in reducing OH. These drugs have central effects, including stimulation and addiction.

Desmopressin. Desmopressin is a vasopressin analogue that is given by the intranasal or intramuscular route. The drug may be useful in reducing nocturnal fluid loss. Especially in patients with high sodium and fluid intake who also take fludrocortisone, caution is necessary to avoid water intoxication.

Dihydroergotamine. Dihydroergotamine (DHE-45) may be given in a dose of 2.5 to 10 mg up to four times a day. The drug is poorly absorbed, causes supine

Table 4 First-Line Treatment of Orthostatic Hypotension

High-salt diet (10–20 g/day)
Large-volume fluid intake ($\geq$ 20 oz/day)
Fludrocortisone 0.1–0.6 mg/day
Ibuprofen, 400 mg t.i.d.
Phenylpropanolamine 25 mg t.i.d.

hypertension, and has the theoretical problem of ergotism. It is not currently approved for this indication. One benefit is its significant effects on the venous capacitance bed.

Intranasal Ergotamine. Related to DHE is the use of intranasal ergotamine, 1 or 2 puffs per dose. The agent is best used for severe postprandial OH. The drug should be used with caution and has the same contraindications as when used for migraine.

Usually Less Useful Drug Combinations

Beta-Blockers. A nonspecific beta-blocker such as propranolol (Inderal) is started at a dose of 20 mg twice a day and increased. An alternative approach is to use a beta-blocker with partial agonist effects, such as pindolol. The initial dose of pindolol (Viskin) is 10 mg twice a day and it is adjusted upward. The drugs are thought to act by blocking beta-mediated vasodilatation and by their agonist effects. Newer analogues include prenalterol and zamoterol. I have not found beta-blockers to be effective in patients with OH-associated with PAF. In patients with POTS with beta-receptor supersensitivity beta-blockers are very useful.

Clonidine. Clonidine (Catapres), 0.1 to 0.6 mg per day is a centrally acting alpha$_2$-agonist and a partial peripheral alpha$_1$-agonist. The central effect results in hypotension, and the drug is used as a central-acting antihypertensive agent. In patients with decentralized central sympathetic traffic, however, as in patients with tetraplegia or MSA, clonidine may work by its peripheral alpha-agonist effect on supersensitive postsynaptic alpha-receptors without a central inhibitory action. Side effects are dry mouth, dizziness, and constipation. The drug should be withdrawn slowly. It can be effective in patients with paroxysmal sympathetic sudomotor overactivity but is usually ineffective for OH.

Metoclopramide. Metoclopramide (Reglan), 10 mg three or four times daily taken an hour ante cibum, has been used to treat OH, presumably because it blocks the vasodilator effects of dopamine. Extrapyramidal side effects may be a problem. The drug is sometimes beneficial for gastroparesis.

Levodopa. Levodopa (without dopa decarboxylase inhibitor) combined with fludrocortisone is occasionally beneficial, but the effect is modest and is superseded by more effective vasoactive agents.

Chlorpheniramine with Cimetidine. The combination of these H$_1$ and H$_2$ antagonists has been suggested to be effective. This combination is used for mastocytosis. For OH these have been superseded by more effective ones.

Dihydroxylphenylserine. Also known as L-DOPS, this is an investigational drug of modest benefit in PAF. It is very useful in the rare deficiency of dopamine-beta-hydroxylase syndrome.

Yohimbine. Yohimbine (Yohimex) is an alpha$_2$-antagonist used in a dose of 8 mg PO two or three times daily for partial adrenergic failure. Side effects are anxiety, nervousness, and diarrhea.

Treatment of Postprandial Orthostatic Hypotension

Patients with OH often experience postprandial exacerbations. The approach to management is summarized in Table 5. Most of these patients do not need specific additional medication. Some find that the exacerbations can be reduced by eating frequent small meals. Some find that certain foods are more troublesome and avoid these. Some need to avoid hot drinks or food.

If symptoms are troublesome and need additional treatment, my approach is to next suggest having two cups of strong coffee or tea (containing about 250 mg of caffeine) with the meal. This dose causes a significant increase in standing BP.

The next step is to use ibuprofen, 400 mg, or indomethacin, 25 to 50 mg, with the meal. The next step is to take phenylpropanolamine, 25 mg, with the meal. If these measures are inadequate, I would proceed to using intranasal ergotamine, 1 or 2 puffs with the meal, or the meal that is followed by the most severe orthostatic symptoms.

If all these approaches are inadequate, the somatostatin analogue, octreotide, in a dose of 25 μg by SC injection, can be used, and the dose may be increased if necessary to 100 to 200 μg.

Treatment for Periods of Increased Orthostatic Stress

It is not possible to maintain postural normotension in patients with OH. A reasonable goal is a regimen that maintains reasonable BP control without undue supine hypertension; the patient is then provided the means to handle periods of increased orthostatic stress. The following approaches are recommended for patients who need several hours of enhanced orthostatic BP:

1. An elastic body stocking may be beneficial. These must be well-fitted and put on prior to arising. They work by reducing the venous capacitance bed. Disadvantages are the cumbersome application and discomfort in hot weather. I find these stockings to be of very limited benefit and reserve them for situations of increased orthostatic stress. Available sources are Jobst, Barton-Carey, Sigvaris, and Camp.
2. Phenylpropanolamine, 25 mg an hour before and as needed. The dose and formulation depend on how long the patient must remain upright. Some patients need to take the drug every 2 to 3 hours for as many as three or four doses. Some patients

Table 5 Treatment of Postprandial Orthostatic Hypotension

Frequent small meals
Dietary modifications
Caffeine, 250 mg
Ibuprofen, 400 mg
Phenylpropanolamine, 25 mg
Intranasal ergotamine, 1 or 2 puffs
Octreotide, 25–200 μg SC

do better with the 75 mg sustained-release preparation.
3. Ibuprofen, 400 mg four times a day, can be used if effective.
4. Other drugs to be considered include intranasal ergotamine, DHE-45, and octreotide.

Treatment of Nocturnal Hypertension

Normal subjects have a diurnal variation in BP, which is lower at night. Patients with neurogenic OH have nocturnal hypertension. To minimize this problem, pressor medications should not be given after 6:00 PM. The head of the bed should be elevated, resulting in lower intracranial BP. A nighttime snack with a glass of fluid (not coffee or tea) produces some postprandial hypotension and can be used to increase fluid intake and reduce nocturnal hypertension. Patients who enjoy a glass of wine should have it at this time for its vasodilator effect.

Occasionally, it is not possible to control OH without producing significant nocturnal hypertension. To these patients, hydralazine (Apresoline) 25 mg, can be given at night. This drug, with its sodium-retaining properties, is especially suitable. Procardia, 10 mg, is an alternative.

PATIENT EDUCATION

Guidelines for Patient Management of Orthostatic Hypotension

Patient education is critically important and lack of it is probably the single most important factor in the relatively poor control of OH. The physician treating OH needs to be cognizant of the fact that the level of OH fluctuates. A key charge on the management team is to educate the patient in the day-by-day management of the fluctuating OH. Key elements in the education program are described in the following paragraphs.

Education About the Mechanisms of the Maintenance of Postural Normotension

The patient has to recognize that the normal mechanisms of maintenance of postural normotension have failed. The patients need to know the three sets of factors essential in the regulation of postural normotension (Table 6). Generalized autonomic failure resulting

Table 6 Factors That Maintain Postural Normotension

Normal blood volume
Normal neurovascular reflexes
Arterial baroreflexes
Low-pressure baroreflexes
Venoarteriolar reflexes
Cerebellar reflexes
Humoral mechanisms
Norepinephrine
Vasopressin
Renin-angiotensin-aldosterone

in OH results from a failure of all three components. They have normal plasma volume, but this is *relatively reduced* because denervation results in an increased vascular capacity. Their neurovascular reflexes are defective, so that the dynamic regulation of total peripheral resistance is impaired, as is sustained regulation. Their humoral mechanisms are the least impaired.

Against this background they need to know that perfect moment-to-moment orthostatic BP regulation is impossible. Instead, they need to achieve the best compromise by slightly overexpanding their plasma volume, optimizing their residual reflexes, simulating these with vasoactive agents, and maintaining sufficient stress to stimulate the humoral defense mechanisms. To ensure plasma volume, the patient is taught to drink a minimum of one glass of fluid with every meal and two additional glasses apart from meals. Patients should add salt to each meal and have a good working knowledge of what foods have high salt content (see below). The patient with a slightly expanded plasma volume may have mild ankle edema but should not have pitting edema extending above the ankles. They should have an accurate scale. One of the best simple guides to the volume status is the weight of the subject, taken on arising. The aim of the salt and fludrocortisone regimen is a weight gain of 3 to 5 pounds. Patients should avoid the supine posture and instead use recliners or chairs.

Education About Orthostatic Stresses and Countermeasures

The patient should recognize that OH varies throughout the day, depending on the time of day, activities (exercise, coughing, straining), posture, eating, fluid intake, and medications. They have to titrate orthostatic stress with countermeasures from moment to moment. To adequately do this, they need to recognize their major orthostatic stresses and their most effective countermeasures. During a training session patients gain insights into some of these mechanisms. Fine tuning requires a longer period of observation and trial and error.

Modification of Activities of Daily Living

Patients follow up on some of the insights gained in step 2 by regulating their level of activity, food intake, and other orthostatic stresses. Many patients feel worse when they first arise, and they benefit from drinking two strong cups of coffee or tea before arising. If they need vasoconstrictors, these can be also taken on first awakening, and the patient defers getting up for 30 minutes to an hour. During times of maximal symptoms patients should approach arising in two phases. They sit up for 5 minutes, then stand, and only after they feel stable on their feet do they walk. This is also the time when they may need to employ orthostatic first aid measures (see below). They may need to identify their periods of maximal orthostatic tolerance and undertake their more

strenuous activities then. For each patient, the most troublesome orthostatic stresses and the most effective countermeasures need to be defined.

Keeping a Blood Pressure and Symptom Log

During the evaluation period, the patient should keep a log to study the relationships among orthostatic symptoms, BP, activities, relationship to meals, time of day, and medication. They should also keep a daily record of their weight taken with an accurate scale. The most convenient BP system is an automated digital one. These are reasonably accurate. For a period of about 2 weeks, the patient, or preferably a spouse or other support person, should take the BP while the patient sits and after the patient has been standing for 1 minute. Recordings should be taken (1) on awakening, (2) after a meal, (3) during a time of maximal orthostatic tolerance, (4) during a time of poor orthostatic tolerance, and (5) before and 1 hour after medication.

Some physicians are concerned that patients thus instructed might develop a "BP neurosis." With appropriate education, this is not a problem. Instead, the patients develop a better understanding of their symptoms and their significance and learn to better regulate their activities and utilize orthostatic countermeasures. After optimal control is attained, it is not necessary to routinely measure BP or continue keeping a log.

Medications to Avoid

The patient needs to be educated to avoid over-the-counter cough/cold medications that contain vasopressor agents. Phenylpropanolamine is an ingredient in many cough/cold medications and may cause severe hypertension in patients with denervation supersensitivity. Patients also learn the importance of avoiding drugs such as diuretics that reduce blood volume.

Recognizing Orthostatic Symptoms

With the aid of BP recordings and a symptom log, patients soon recognize that they have good days and bad days. For often inexplicable reasons they have days when they are more orthostatically intolerant. With training and experience, they learn to distinguish orthostatic symptoms from nonorthostatic ones. The former are recognized as those that are related to posture and duration of standing and that are worse shortly before the next dose of medication and better an hour after they take the drug.

Learning to Prevent Presyncope and Syncope

Some techniques are very helpful in extending the patient's tolerance for being upright. Patients need to identify the mechanical first aid maneuvers that prevent syncope and to incorporate them into their repertoire. Some patients carry a derby chair, a cane that, when unfolded, opens out into a seat. When presyncopal symptoms arise, the patient can open the device and sit until the symptoms subside.

Dietary Education

Patients need to be familiar with the sodium content of common food items and be conscientious about a high sodium intake. There is a close relation between salt intake and BP. Some patients are intensely sensitive to salt intake and can fine-tune their plasma volume and BP by controlling salt intake alone. Foods rich in salt include fast foods like hamburgers, hotdogs, chicken pieces, French fries and fish fries. Canned soups, chili, ham, bacon, sausage, additives like soya sauce, and commercially processed canned products also contain a lot of sodium. The patient should have at least one glass or cup of fluids with each meal and at least two at other times each day; total daily fluid intake should be 2 to 2.5 L.

Patients need to be on a high-potassium diet because of their heavy sodium intake and fludrocortisone. Fruits such as bananas and vegetables contain a lot of potassium. Patients should have a snack with more fluids at night. The postprandial OH will reduce some of the nocturnal hypertension.

Laboratory Training of Patients with Orthostatic Hypotension

The nurse educator undertakes some important tasks.

Guidelines in Patient Management of Orthostatic Hypotension

The patient is taught the guidelines for patient management of orthostatic hypotension described above.

Instructions on the Keeping of a Blood Pressure and Orthostatic Symptom Log

Patients are taught how to take BP and how to log their symptoms for the period of home evaluation. It is helpful to have the patient grade the symptoms as well as describe them. We use a 10 point scale (Table 7).

Table 7 Symptom Scale for Orthostatic Hypotension

0	Absence of orthostatic symptoms
2	Tiredness; momentary lightheadedness
4	Mental sluggishness, difficulty concentrating
6	Dizziness, unsteadiness
8	Blurred vision, feeling of faintness
10	Syncope or presyncope

Instructions on First Aid Measures to Prevent Syncope

Patients are taught a number of first aid measures to prevent syncope or increase orthostatic tolerance. Where facilities are available, it is very helpful to teach patients these maneuvers while they watch a beat-to-beat BP display, so they can recognize the relationship of posture to symptoms and BP. They are taught a number of orthostatic countermeasures, some of which are more effective for some persons than for others. Patients learn which ones best serve them personally:

- Contraction of lower limb muscles: Some patients find that shifting balance from leg to leg reduces symptoms. Others prefer to simultaneously contract muscles of both lower limbs in a forced extension maneuver.
- Leg crossing is a favorite of many patients.
- Raising one or both legs on a stool
- Forward flexion of the neck
- Squatting
- Abdominal contraction: Some patients find it effective to combine this maneuver with neck flexion.

Instruction on Medications to Avoid

Medications are usually prescribed without evaluating their efficacy firsthand. It is very helpful to compare orthostatic BP and symptom evaluation before and 1 hour after the patient takes the drug. I prefer to incorporate this evaluation into the patient education program with continuous recordings of BP. For most other physicians, it would be adequate to check the BP before and after the patient takes the medication.

SUGGESTED READING

Fealey RD, Robertson D. Treatment of orthostatic hypotension. In: Low PA, ed. Clinical autonomic disorders: Evaluation and management. Boston: Little, Brown, 1993.

Hoeldtke RD, Davis KM. Orthostatic tachycardia syndrome: Evaluation of autonomic function and treatment with octreotide and ergot alkaloids. Clin Endocrinol Metab 1991; 73:132–139.

Khurana RK. Paraneoplastic neuropathies. In: Low PA, ed. Clinical autonomic disorders: Evaluation and management. Boston: Little, Brown, 1993.

Low PA. Autonomic neuropathy. Semin Neurol 1987; 7:49–84.

Low PA, McLeod JG. The autonomic neuropathies, In: Low PA, ed. Clinical autonomic disorders: Evaluation and management. Boston: Little, Brown, 1993.

Schondorf R, Low PA. Idiopathic postural tachycardia syndrome. In: Low PA, ed. Clinical autonomic disorders: Evaluation and management. Boston: Little, Brown, 1993.

SEIZURE DISORDERS

NEONATAL SEIZURES AND INFANTILE SPASMS

WILLIAM D. BROWN, M.D.
O. CARTER SNEAD III, M.D.

NEONATAL SEIZURES

One of the most vexing problems in neurology is the diagnosis and treatment of seizures in newborns. The difficulty lies in the fact that the neonate typically does not have the kind of seizure that is familiar to us. Observed seizures include an often bewildering array of incomplete behaviors, such as multifocal myoclonic jerks, bicycling, sucking, and mouthing movements, and abrupt cessations in movement often associated with apnea. Typical generalized tonic-clonic seizures are usually not seen because the developing brain has a number of features that conspire to make it remarkably resistant to initiating, propagating, and sustaining generalized seizure activity.

The neonatal brain is immature at birth. Organization and development of the brain continue well into childhood, and some pathways that co-ordinate cortical and brain stem activity are not myelinated until some time after birth. The most mature portions of the neonatal brain are the deep cortical and limbic structures; this may explain the protean seizure types and difficulties in the interpretation of the electroencephalogram (EEG) in this age group. In addition, there is a relative excess of inhibitory synapses in the neonatal brain, which helps to confer on the neonate's brain an inherent resistance to seizure activity.

The leading causes of recurrent seizures that have their origin in the neonatal period are congenital brain abnormalities and prenatal/perinatal insults, which account for nearly 85 percent of all recurrent seizures. Many common adverse perinatal events may affect the newborn brain: prolonged labor, fetal distress or bradycardia, precipitous or arrested delivery, umbilical cord compression, aspiration of meconium, poor initiation or effectiveness of respiration, inadequate or delayed conversion from fetal to adult type circulation, and acidosis or hypoxemia (not to mention the more severe complications of sepsis, maternal substance abuse, gestational diabetes, hypothyroidism, or ecclampsia).

Classification

Various classification schemes for neonatal seizures have been proposed, but the most common easily distinguishable seizures are shown in Table 1.

Three behaviors that are often confused with seizures in the newborn period are apnea, jitteriness, and spontaneous clonus. It is important to remember that apnea associated with bradycardia is a very common finding in normal premature infants of less than 32 weeks gestational age. Usually, *convulsive apnea is not associated with bradycardia* unless the seizure is prolonged and brain hypoxia ensues. "Apnea of prematurity" tends to disappear after 32 to 34 weeks gestational age, when brain stem autoregulatory centers mature.

Jitteriness is sometimes confused with seizure activity in the newborn. It is a common abnormal movement disorder characterized by rhythmic, symmetric tremors of equal amplitude that can be stopped by passive flexion. While suggestive of central nervous system hyperirritability due to encephalopathy, hypocalcemia,

Table 1 Classification of Neonatal Seizures

Seizure Type	Identifying Features
Motor automatisms	• Abnormal eye movements predominate • Oral-buccal-lingual movements • Swimming, bicycling movements, apnea • EEG may be normal
Generalized tonic	• Tonic extension of extremities • Often seen in premature infants • May herald intracerebral hemorrhage • EEG may be normal
Multifocal clonic	• Migratory clonic movements of extremities • Usually seen in term infants • EEG abnormal
Focal clonic	• Localized clonus • No alteration of consciousness • Often associated with focal brain injury • EEG normal
Myoclonic	• Single or multiple myoclonic jerks • May involve arms or legs • EEG is usually normal

hypoglycemia, or drug withdrawal, jitteriness is not epileptic and should not be treated with anticonvulsants. It may persist beyond infancy; in this setting, and in the absence of other demonstrable neurologic abnormalities, persistent jitteriness is associated with an excellent prognosis.

Spontaneous clonus also may be misinterpreted as seizures, but it is stopped by passive flexion. While not representative of seizure activity, spontaneous clonus is always abnormal and indicates aberrant brain function.

Treatment

While certain metabolic and infectious causes for neonatal seizures have specific treatments that do not necessarily include anticonvulsant therapy, the final common pathway for the clinical expression of seizure remains the same in all cases. Since the pharmacologic armamentarium for the treatment of seizures in neonates is limited, treatment for seizures in this group of patients is likely to be similar whatever their cause, and in practice it matters little whether the practitioner attempts to differentiate among specific seizure types.

Rationale

A safe way to approach this diagnostic and management problem is to assume that *any behavioral activity that looks like a seizure probably is and should be treated as such, once a treatable (e.g., metabolic) cause has been excluded.* Rationale for this policy is based on four tenets:

1. Seizures Are Related to a Specific Illness, Which May Have Its Own Specific Therapy. Such illnesses include metabolic disorders such as hypoglycemia, hypocalcemia, hypomagnesemia, hyponatremia, or hypokalemia, pyridoxine or vitamin cofactor deficiency, drug withdrawal, and some aminoacidurias as well as the more common infectious problems of bacterial or viral sepsis that are easily treated without anticonvulsant drugs. Other specific illnesses that require only symptomatic and supportive seizure management include developmental abnormalities, intracerebral hemorrhage or thrombosis, "anoxic encephalopathy," structural cerebral damage as a result of "birth trauma," and meningoencephalitis due to bacteria, toxoplasmosis, cytomegalovirus, or herpes simplex virus.

2. Neonatal Seizures May Go Unrecognized. Failure to recognize seizures is a particular hazard when a sick neonate is being mechanically ventilated and has been sedated or is receiving neuromuscular blockade drugs. Isolated seizures or status epilepticus may go unrecognized for minutes, hours, or days and may interfere with supportive therapy such as intravenous fluid administration or mechanical ventilation. A high index of suspicion should be maintained in this setting and careful attention paid to alterations in blood pressure, responsiveness, or heart rate, since these may be the only clue to the presence of seizures. An extremely useful tool in this setting is EEG; a better tool

is video-EEG monitoring. Clinical correlation of unusual behavior with EEG abnormalities makes the diagnosis of seizure nearly certain. Several caveats must be emphasized, however: (1) The EEG must be interpreted by an experienced clinical neurophysiologist who is familiar with neonatal tracings. (2) The limitations of the technique of EEG make its use as a diagnostic tool difficult. An EEG is generally considered to be "normal" if it lacks abnormal patterns, but a normal EEG does not exclude the possibility of electrographically "silent" clinical seizures. (3) Conversely, an abnormal EEG does not always mean that the unusual behavior is a seizure. The EEG is best used to validate a clinical impression and as a prognostic tool.

It should be noted that there is controversy over the value of a silent EEG in the diagnosis and treatment of seizures in the newborn period. Some authorities do not consider certain abnormal movements currently classified as seizures in the neonatal period to be "epileptic" unless the EEG correlates with the clinical activity in question. In this context, tonic posturing and motor automatisms are regarded as primitive brain stem and spinal motor patterns that are "released" from the tonic inhibitory influence of forebrain structures. These two types of seizures, it is argued, should not be treated with anticonvulsant drugs because they do not originate from cortical structures.

Nevertheless, paroxysmal EEG tracings associated with a variety of clinical behaviors such as multifocal migratory clonus, generalized tonic posturing, myoclonus, and apnea have been reported even in hydranencephalic babies who lack cortical tissues. The origin for both the clinical seizure activity and the paroxysmal EEG in one of these infants had to be the brain stem: no brain substance above the mesencephalon was found at autopsy. A variety of behaviors are known to originate from the brain stem, and some of these may represent seizures. The mechanisms that underlie such behaviors and paroxysmal EEG activity are unknown; until they are better understood, stereotyped behaviors and unusual movements are best considered to be seizures and treated accordingly.

3. Seizures Themselves Have the Potential to Cause Brain Injury. Recurrent seizures in the newborn may be associated with hypoventilation, apnea, hypertension, and depletion of adenosine triphosphate (ATP) and phosphocreatine as well as excessive release of excitatory and neurotoxic neurotransmitters such as glutamate and aspartate. Each of these has potential to cause direct and lasting injury to neurons.

4. Uncontrolled Neonatal Seizures Have a Poor Outcome. As many as 90 percent of infants whose seizures last 4 days or longer have a poor developmental and neurologic outcome.

Pretreatment Evaluation

Appropriate management of seizures in neonates should be directed by historical, clinical, and laboratory findings. The evaluation of all such patients includes a detailed history (complications of pregnancy and delivery, maternal substance abuse, heritable diseases), physical examination (including neurologic, ophthalmologic, and dermatologic examinations), and laboratory investigation. This should include serum glucose, calcium, and magnesium as well as sodium and potassium, bicarbonate, urea nitrogen, creatinine, ammonia, and arterial blood gas determinations. Also, a complete blood count with differential and blood cultures as well as urine and cerebrospinal fluid (CSF) cultures are indicated as are CSF protein, glucose, cell count, and Gram stain. Further directed investigation may include urine organic and serum amino acid determinations, cranial ultrasound, and computed tomography (CT) to evaluate the possibilities of infarction, hemorrhage, or calcification. STORCH (Syphilis Toxoplasmosis Rubella Cytomegalovirus Herpes Simplex) titers should be obtained to investigate the possibility of congenital infection.

Treatable metabolic disorders that typically do not respond to standard anticonvulsants are listed in Table 2.

Anticonvulsant Drugs

Once the diagnosis of seizures in a neonate is established and treatable metabolic causes are eliminated, anticonvulsant drug therapy is indicated to stop the seizures. Phenobarbital, the preferred drug for the management of virtually all neonatal seizures, is extremely effective as an anticonvulsant and has few serious side effects. It has a long half-life in neonates, 100 hours or longer; though the desired therapeutic range is 15 to 40 µg per deciliter, individual patients may require markedly higher levels to establish seizure control. The intravenous loading dose is 20 mg per kilogram (maximum rate of administration 100 mg per minute). This is followed by intravenous boluses of 5 to 10 mg per kilogram until seizures stop. A second anticonvulsant should be considered when phenobarbital levels reach 50 to 60 µg per deciliter but seizures continue. At that point, serious consideration must be given to the possibility of a metabolic disorder that may be unresponsive to anticonvulsant therapy but would quickly respond to administration, of, say, glucose or calcium. The phenobarbital maintenance dose is usually 3 to 5 mg per kilogram per day, given in two doses.

If in the face of very high serum levels of phenobarbital seizures persist, benzodiazepines or phenytoin may be considered. Lorazepam may be given in a 0.1 mg per kilogram IV bolus over 2 minutes; it may be repeated once for status epilepticus; lorazepam should be used rather than diazepam, because it has fewer effects on respiratory drive and longer duration of action. Diazepam is given as a 0.05 to 0.5 mg per kilogram IV bolus at a rate below 1 to 2 mg per minute IV; diazepam is extremely effective acutely but is impractical as a long-term anticonvulsant because of its short duration of action and undesirable effects on level of arousal.

Phenytoin is a very effective anticonvulsant but must be given intravenously to maintain therapeutic levels in infants. Its absorption after oral administration is highly variable and unpredictable. The loading dose is 15 to 20 mg per kilogram IV given at a maximum rate of 10 to 20 mg per minute. The maintenance dose is 3 to 8 mg per kilogram per day IV. Serum levels between 10 and 20 µg/dl should be maintained. Phenytoin is formulated in a propylene glycol vehicle with a pH of 12 and must only be given intravenously, never IM. It should be administered in a saline venous line without glucose, which would cause the drug to precipitate.

Paraldehyde is a very effective anticonvulsant that has been used extensively in the past. It may be given rectally or orally at a dose of 0.3 to 0.6 cc per kilogram per dose. If it is to be given rectally, it should be mixed in a vegetable oil (e.g., peanut, cottonseed, olive) in a 4:1 ratio, to minimize mucosal irritation. More than 25 percent of the drug is excreted through the lungs, and paraldehyde is contraindicated in any neonate with pulmonary compromise.

The duration of treatment for neonatal seizures is controversial. It seems reasonable to believe that long-term exposure of the developing brain to anticonvulsant drugs should be avoided if possible, and the decision to withdraw therapy should be balanced against the risk of recurrent seizures. Neonates who have an acute onset of seizures that are easily controlled, a normal neurologic examination, and a normal EEG may be tapered off anticonvulsants within a month of the onset of their illness. Phenytoin should be discontinued before phenobarbital.

The more problematic patient is the one who suffers recurrent clinical seizures despite anticonvulsant ther-

Table 2 Treatment of Metabolic Disorders That Cause Seizures

Disorder: Treatment	Initial Treatment	Maintenance Therapy
Hypoglycemia: glucose	2 cc/kg 10% solution IV	5–8 µg/kg/min IV
Hypocalcemia: calcium	4 cc/kg 5% solution IV	200–250 mg/kg/day ÷ q6°
Hypomagnesemia: magnesium	0.2 cc/kg 50% Mg sulfate IV	0.2 cc/kg/day IM, IV
Vitamin deficiency:		
Pyridoxine	100 mg IV	100 mg/day
Carnitine	50–500 mg/kg/day ÷ b.i.d.	50–500 mg/kg/day ÷ b.i.d.
Cyanocobalamin	100 µg IM, SC ÷ qd	100 µg IM, SC ÷ qd
Thiamine	10–25 mg/dose qd, IM, IV	
Inborn errors of metabolism	Protein restriction, elemental or special formulas	

apy. The physician should try to be as aggressive as possible without resorting to polypharmacy, the goal being no clinical seizures. Electrographic seizure activity may indicate a higher risk for clinical seizures, but the goal need not be to "treat the EEG" unless the patient actually has a clinical seizure. For recurrent seizures that begin in the neonatal period, anticonvulsant therapy should be continued for a period of 2 to 3 months after the last clinical seizure before consideration may be given to termination of therapy.

INFANTILE SPASMS

The entity termed *infantile spasms* is a relatively rare form of epilepsy that occurs nearly exclusively in infancy and early childhood (onset before the first 4 to 8 months of life, sometimes in a previously normal baby). The disorder takes several different forms, but distinguishing one from another makes little diagnostic or therapeutic difference. Their distinction from other types of seizures that occur in infancy and early childhood is quite important, however, because infantile spasms are notoriously refractory to standard anticonvulsant therapy and are commonly treated with a completely different class of drugs: corticosteroids.

Clinical Description

The first and best clinical description of infantile spasms was made in 1841 by West, who in a letter to *The Lancet* described an unusual affliction of his own son that consisted of "bobbings of the head . . . bowings and relaxings" in clusters of "ten to twenty or more times at each attack," and a progressive deterioration of intellect such that he "never smiles or takes any notice but looks placid and pitiful." The spasms may occur at any time of the day or night but occur least frequently when the infant is asleep and most frequently upon awakening.

Clinically, spasms may be classified as flexor (uncommon), extensor (least common), or mixed (most common). Flexor spasms primarily involve flexion of the neck, trunk, and extremities. Truncal flexion may be quite dramatic, giving rise to a sudden "jack-knifing" or "salaam" movement that is nearly pathognomonic for infantile spasms. Extensor spasms involve sudden, brief extensor posturing in the same distribution, whereas the mixed type of spasms involve flexion of the arms, trunk, and neck with extension of the legs.

Prognosis

It is important to establish the diagnosis with a relatively high degree of certainty, because a diagnosis of infantile spasms carries with it profound implications for both prognosis and treatment. Infantile spasms are associated with a morbidity rate of 75 to 90 percent and a mortality rate as high as 20 percent. The primary morbidity consists of moderate to severe mental retar-

dation. The spasms are quite age specific: peak incidence is at 6 months of age and incidence rapidly declines after 12 months of age. There are isolated reports of spasms occurring in children up to 4 years of age but these are exceedingly rare.

Infants with the best outcome are those who are between 3 and 12 months of age and are developmentally and neurologically normal at the time of diagnosis and treatment, who have no other type of seizures, who have no identifiable cause for their spasms, and who do not lose the ability to follow visually during their illness. These are classified as "cryptogenic" infantile spasms; about 35 percent of these patients have a normal outcome. Those with the worst outcome are older babies who had a pre-existing seizure disorder, poor developmental achievement, and abnormal findings on neurologic examination. The prognosis for this group of patients is grim. They are referred to as "symptomatic," and they account for up to 90 percent of all patients with infantile spasms, 90 percent of whom suffer severe to profound neurologic compromise. As many as 25 percent of all infants with infantile spasms, however, exhibit spontaneous remission after the first 12 months of seizures.

Patient Evaluation

Prognosis depends somewhat on identifying a cause for the spasms. An identifiable pre- or perinatal cause may be documented in as many as half of all patients. This is usually related to cerebral malformations, a genetic or heritable metabolic disorder, intrauterine infection, perinatal insult, postnatal infection, intracerebral hemorrhage or infarction, and head trauma. A complete history, family history, and physical and neurologic examinations are important parts of the initial evaluation.

Electrolytes, complete blood count, urinalysis, calcium, phosphorus, serum glucose, metabolic screening, endocrine and chromosome studies, and examination of CSF are indicated when the initial evaluation so directs. Serum and CSF lactate and pyruvate determinations are easy to perform and helpful, but often overlooked. Magnetic resonance imaging of the brain is not absolutely indicated, but it is the best method currently available to assess the integrity of cerebral gray and white matter and congenital malformations.

Use of Electroencephalography

The diagnosis of infantile spasms is much facilitated by EEG. When a hypsarrhythmic pattern (high-voltage, chaotic slowing with multifocal spiking and marked asynchrony) is seen, the diagnosis is confirmed. Unfortunately, classic hypsarrhythmia is not always observed and the criteria for hypsarrhythmia have been broadened to allow for areas of focal abnormality, synchrony, asymmetry, and burst suppression. As infantile spasms may occur only a few times in a day, a single EEG is not enough to exclude the diagnosis. It is our practice to make use of continuous video EEG monitoring over 8 to 24 hours to help establish the diagnosis in difficult or atypical cases.

Therapy

A variety of drugs has been used to treat infantile spasms, none of which has been particularly effective. These include valproate, benzodiazepines, pyridoxine, immunglobulin, thyrotropin-releasing hormone (TRH), and a number of experimental drugs including vigabatrin (an irreversible inhibitor of the catabolic enzyme for gamma-aminobutyric acid), typhoid vaccine, serotonergic compounds, and naloxone.

Adrenocorticotropic Hormone and Prednisone

In 1958 Sorel and Dusaucy-Bauloye were the first to report a "spectacular" response of infantile spasms to adrenocorticotropic hormone (ACTH) as manifested by normalization of behavior, control of seizures, and improved EEG. Prednisone was shown to be effective the same year. These have been the mainstays of therapy for infantile spasms for the last 35 years; however, the medical treatment of this condition is nearly anecdotal, as neither the mechanism of disease nor the mode of action of any of the many drugs that have been used to treat this disorder is understood. In addition, numerous, often contradictory studies using markedly different doses for both ACTH and prednisone have not helped to clear up the confusion. Nevertheless, the goals for treatment are clear: seizure control and improved cognitive outcome.

Large doses of ACTH are the best treatment for infantile spasms and have been shown to control seizures in as many as 90 percent of children if an initial dose of 150 U per square meter ACTH gel is used IM in two divided doses for the first week, 75 U per square meter in one daily dose for the second week, then 75 U per square meter every other day for the third week. The ACTH is gradually tapered over the next 9 weeks. Usually a rather abrupt response to treatment is seen within 7 days, but a high (50 percent) relapse rate is common during the tapering period, especially in the "symptomatic" group of patients. When relapse occurs, the dose is increased to the previously effective dose for two weeks (150 U per square meter per day if seizures recur despite that increase) then tapered again.

Prednisone may be used when oral administration is desired. It has fewer side effects than ACTH, but the same pretreatment evaluation is indicated. The initial dose is 3 mg per kilogram per day in four divided doses for 2 weeks, followed by a 10 week taper. The reason for such frequent dosing is to try to duplicate the sustained elevation of plasma cortisol that is seen in children who receive the ACTH regimen already described; prednisone has a short half-life and if given infrequently gives inconstant cortisol levels.

The patient should always be hospitalized for the institution of ACTH therapy. Monitoring of blood pressure, urine glucose, and serum electrolytes and teaching parents how to give the injections, to measure urine glucose three times a day, and to recognize spasms so that they can help monitor effectiveness with a seizure record all warrant admission. ACTH and steroids are dangerous drugs, especially in large doses. Most children develop cushingoid features. Many become hyperirritable and some develop hypertension. Blood pressure, electrolytes, serum glucose, calcium, and phosphorus should be monitored regularly. Rare effects are congestive heart failure, cerebral ventriculomegaly, and hypothalamic-pituitary or adrenocortical dysfunction. Immunosuppression and the increased risk of sepsis require vigilance.

The patient may be discharged from the hospital on day 3 of therapy. Monitoring of blood pressure must occur during the ensuing week, either by having the patient return to the hospital or, preferably, through the use of visiting nurse services. Hypertension is treated first with salt restriction and diuretic therapy rather than cessation of ACTH. Follow-up is mandatory. Serial EEGs help determine treatment response.

Benzodiazepines

When ACTH and prednisone fail, there are alternatives, although none is as effective as ACTH. These include benzodiazepines and valproic acid. The most useful benzodiazepine in this regard is clonazepam, started at 0.01 to 0.03 mg per kilogram per day divided into two or three doses and increased by 0.25 to 0.5 mg every 3 days until a maintenance dose of 0.1 to 0.3 mg per kilogram is reached. Nitrazepam (0.5 to 1.0 mg per kilogram per day) and several other drugs, such as clobazam and chlorazepate, have been reported to have some beneficial effect, but clonazepam and nitrazepam have demonstrated better efficacy.

Valproic Acid

Valproic acid has been reported to be effective for infantile spasms, but its use is limited mainly by very toxic side effects in this age group, including hepatotoxicity and pancreatitis. It should not be used unless it is used alone and liver function studies are monitored before and regularly during its use. The initial dose is 20 mg per kilogram. Maintenance doses are increased gradually to 30 to 60 mg per kilogram divided into two or three doses per day.

Experimental Therapy

Pyridoxine (30 to 400 mg per kilogram per day), immunoglobulin, and the TRH analogue TRH-t (0.5 to 1.0 mg IV or IM) have been reported in isolated trials to have a beneficial effect on infantile spasms. These are not accepted medical therapy, but they may prove to help us understand the disorder.

SUGGESTED READING

Ferguson JH, et al. Brainstem seizures in hydranencephaly. Neurology 1974; 24:1152–1157.
Haenggeli CA, et al. Pyridoxine-dependent seizures, clinical and therapeutic aspects. Eur J Pediatr 1991; 150:452–455.
Hrachovy RA, et al. Hypsarrhythmia: Variations on the theme. Epilepsia 1984; 25:317–325.
Mizrahi EM. Characterization and classification of neonatal seizures. Neurology 1987; 37:1837–1844.
Shuper A, et al. Jitteriness beyond the newborn period: A benign pattern of movement in infancy. J Child Neurol 1991; 6:243–245.
Snead OC. Other antiepileptic drugs: Adrenocorticotropic hormone (ACTH). In: Levy R, Mattson R, Meldrum B, et al. Antiepileptic drugs. 3rd ed. New York: Raven Press, 1989.
Sorel L, Dusaucy-Bauloye A. A propos de cas d'hypsarhythmie de Gibbs: Son traitement spectulaire par l'ACTH. Acta Neurol Belg 1958; 58:130–141.
Volpe JJ. Neonatal seizures. In: Neurology of the newborn. 2nd ed. Philadelphia: WB Saunders, 1987:129.
West WJ. On a peculiar form of infantile convulsions. Lancet 1841; 1:724–725.

PATIENT RESOURCE

Ms. Patricia Gibson
Director, Epilepsy Information Service
Department of Neurology
Bowman Gray School of Medicine
Medical Center Boulevard
Winston-Salem, NC 27157-1078
(800) 642-0500
(919) 748-2319

FEBRILE SEIZURES

S. ROBERT SNODGRASS, M.D.

Febrile seizures have been recognized since classical times. Hippocrates noted that they were most common near the time of eruption of the canine teeth (about age 18 months). Febrile seizures occur in 3 to 6 percent of children and often run in families. The diagnosis of a febrile seizure requires evidence of infection before the seizure, fever lasting more than 8 hours after the seizure, or clear evidence of infection, such as an exanthem or pharyngeal exudate. Because seizures themselves cause transient fever and because screaming may cause red eardrums (erroneously suggesting otitis media), the diagnosis of febrile seizures may be ambiguous in some cases. An accurate history is the single most important part of febrile seizure evaluation. Unfortunately, this history is often lacking because the physician may have limited access to eyewitnesses. Taking the time to speak directly with eyewitnesses may change the diagnosis. For example, a history suggesting autonomic syncope (characterized by observers as *seizure* or *collapse* preceded by screaming or minor injury) is important. In the absence of such a history, imaging studies, electroencephalography (EEG), and extensive blood chemistry studies only mislead the physician.

Most childhood fevers are not associated with a seizure, and most seizures associated with febrile illness are restricted to the first 24 to 36 hours of fever. Infection causes fever indirectly, by release of cytokines, which act on the brain to produce fever. The main "endogenous pyrogen" appears to be interleukin 1, which induces fever and sleep when injected into the lateral ventricles of animals. Tumor necrosis factor and interleukin 6 may also contribute to fever. The risk of febrile seizures increases with body temperature, but there is reason to doubt that fever is the direct cause. Similarly, benign seizures sometimes occur *without fever* in the context of obvious viral illnesses or after immunization. *Reactive seizures* may be a better name than febrile seizures. Although it is commonly assumed that genetic differences in febrile seizure susceptibility must be due to brain differences, differences in the immune system, cytokine secretion, and receptors may be equally important.

FEATURES OF FEBRILE SEIZURES AND IMPLICATIONS FOR THERAPY

The potential for death and disability concerns parents of children with febrile seizures. The medical literature of past centuries spoke of death from febrile seizures (or *teething convulsions*). Those deaths were probably due to bacteremia, meningitis, and dehydration. Given our present understanding of febrile seizures, affected children have no increased risk of death and little risk of retardation or major handicap assuming previous development was normal. Older literature also frequently refers to children with febrile seizures as having a disproportionate incidence of developmental and school problems. Recent prospective studies have shown that children with febrile seizures do not differ from siblings in intelligence or neurologic status when studied years later. Further, modern controlled studies show no increased incidence of abnormal pregnancies, birth injuries, or other risk factors when febrile seizure patients were compared to matched controls. Prospective studies show that even febrile status epilepticus usually has an excellent prognosis when it occurs in children without meningitis or evidence of a pre-existing handicap. Verity, for example, found that even 50 minutes of febrile seizure had no permanent harmful effect in a cohort of British children. Nevertheless, we try to stop seizures before 50—or even 30—minutes has passed.

Parents may find it hard to believe that febrile seizures are benign. They may have been told that high fever is brain damaging even in the absence of seizures, and the color changes and erratic respiration associated with many febrile seizures suggest the possibility of a catastrophic outcome. Some experienced physicians feel that the modern view of febrile seizures is too casual and that bad outcomes are relatively frequent. Sheila Wallace's book presents the view that febrile seizures often indicate significant neurologic problems. I believe that this reflects selection bias, because specialists and referral centers see patients selected by peculiar manifestations or severity of disease. Since some patients with severe myoclonic epilepsy of infancy begin with more or less typical febrile seizures, intuition may suggest that in an individual case the febrile seizure caused the myoclonic disorder. Even experienced physicians may be influenced by such unusual cases and find it hard to think in probabilistic terms. Actuarial prediction thus has a much better track record than clinical prediction, which is tailored to individual patients.

Most children who suffer a febrile seizure never develop epilepsy or recurrent afebrile seizures. The subgroup with long seizures, highly focal seizures, and abnormal development are more likely to develop epilepsy. However, only a few prospective studies of the incidence of epilepsy after febrile seizures are available, and retrospective series from epilepsy clinics are likely to be inherently misleading. The study by Verity of English children born in 1970 (Table 1) demonstrates that the child who suffers a simple febrile seizure has a very low risk for epilepsy, little more than that of the general population.

Controlled studies show that maintenance therapy with *certain* anticonvulsants (see below) reduces the incidence of recurrent febrile seizures, *if and only if strong measures are taken to ensure compliance.* Anticonvulsants do not appear to reduce the already low incidence of late epilepsy and mental retardation. While death and disability rarely follow febrile seizures, some children experience repeated hospitalizations. These are undesirable because of expense, psychological trauma,

and the possibility of iatrogenic complications. Only children with prolonged or multiple seizures whose control requires so much medication that the child cannot eat or drink require hospitalization. Exceptions are patients with serious infections, possible meningitis, or other diagnostic problems. A child usually develops a pattern of seizure characteristics. For example, children with brief simple seizures with fever usually have similar seizures if they have any recurrence. The unusual child who is prone to long seizures or clusters of multiple seizures typically exhibits these characteristics early. Such patients can usually be kept out of hospital if parents are taught to administer benzodiazepine (BDZ) suppositories after the first seizure of the day.

Most febrile seizures occur during ordinary febrile illnesses. Any febrile illness, however, may provoke seizures in susceptible children—meningitis, bacteremia, tuberculosis, and other serious illnesses. Relatively typical febrile seizures may also be the first sign of myoclonic epilepsy of infancy. The possibility that a child's fourth febrile seizure is due to meningitis limits home use of suppositories. Therefore, a child who does not improve rapidly must be seen.

A child with febrile seizures who is taken to a new hospital or seen by a physician lacking the history is likely to undergo multiple expensive tests, including imaging studies. The risks of meningitis and serious infection do not usually require imaging and extensive blood chemistry studies. In general, emergency room (ER) studies of electrolytes, glucose, and calcium are uninformative in patients with febrile seizures unless there has been a history of vomiting, diarrhea, or several days during which the child did not eat. Parents should be urged to be sure that babysitters and day care providers know the physician's name and that the child be taken to the same hospital, if at all possible. This is a counsel of perfection when most families have no primary physician and often mistrust physicians, but it saves time and money. Returning to a physician who knows the child and family facilitates follow-up arrangements and is less costly.

Details are important in the evaluation and care of febrile seizure patients. Casual arrangements concerning febrile seizure management may result in patients' running the risks of drug treatment (monetary and psychological costs, hepatic enzyme induction) without the benefits (reduced number of seizures and risk of hospitalization). I doubt that anticonvulsants can prevent subsequent development of epilepsy. Written protocols and algorithms, such as that presented here, are particularly useful if the consultant is not likely to follow the patient. Longitudinal follow-up by one physician or group is essential to identify the occasional child whose febrile seizures antedate development of myoclonic epilepsy or other serious problems.

Finally, I am always uneasy about apparent febrile seizures in children younger than 6 months. They are more likely than older children to merit specialist referral and more extensive studies. The same is true for children who have been febrile for more than 24 hours before the seizure.

Table 1 Risk of Epilepsy After Febrile Seizure

Population	Febrile Seizure Subtype*	Later Epilepsy No. (%)
398	All	9 (2.2)
287	Simple febrile seizures	2 (1)
95	One or more complex febrile seizures	6 (6.3)

*Complex seizure is defined as longer than 15 minutes, clearly focal, or multiple seizures in 1 day.

THERAPY

Protocol for Acute Management of Children with Possible Febrile Seizures

Initial Telephone Contact

1. Has the child had more than one seizure?
   Has the child not recovered consciousness quickly?
   Is the child younger than 6 months old?
   Has the child been ill for more than 36 hours?
   Has the child been vomiting?

   If the answer to any of these questions is yes, the child should be seen promptly.

2. Is the seizure prolonged beyond 10 to 15 minutes or ongoing?
   If yes, transport by ambulance to nearest ER. If the child is at hospital, give parenteral or rectal BDZ.

3. Does the child have a history of febrile seizures?
   If so, and if the seizure was brief and the child promptly recovered and is taking fluids, the child can wait to be seen. If not better the following day, the child should be evaluated, even if there are no further seizures.
   If not, the child should be evaluated even if the seizure is over and consciousness is recovered quickly.

Emergency Room Evaluation

1. Do you have a good eyewitness account of the seizure?

   If not, consider the possibility of other diagnoses as well as seizures.

2. Is the child febrile? Is infection evident?

   Either condition increases the probability that the event was a febrile seizure.

3. Is meningitis likely?

   If it is, or if the child has been ill more than 36 hours, and especially if the child is receiving an antibiotic, proceed to lumbar puncture. If the history suggests increasing intracranial pressure (vomiting or obtundity for days before the seizure), or if the head is unduly large, perform an imaging study or obtain consultation before lumbar puncture. Obtain blood cultures while waiting for the test or consultant. If meningitis is probable, begin high-dose antibiotic therapy after obtaining blood for culture.

4. Is the child improving?

   Do not send a child home until alertness is clearly improved.

5. Is there a history of vomiting or diarrhea? Is the child dehydrated?

If so, measure electrolytes and glucose, and treat the dehydration.

6. Has the child had more than two seizures or is seizure ongoing?

   If so, give parenteral or rectal BDZ. I prefer lorazepam, 0.1 mg per kilogram. Children who have two or more seizures in one day are likely to have more.

7. What was the response to the BDZ?

   If the seizure recurred or continued despite treatment, repeat the dose one time. If seizures continue, give phenobarbital IV, 10 mg per kilogram slowly. Obtain electrolyte, glucose, creatinine, and calcium values, if this has not already been done. Admit or transfer the patient to a pediatric intensive care unit, and treat for status epilepticus. Be certain that either lumbar puncture (LP) findings are normal or that high-dose antibiotic treatment for meningitis has been instituted. If the seizures are controlled, be certain there is no evidence for meningitis or other serious infection. A dose of BDZ does not commit to hospitalization, as long as the child clearly recovers after a seizure. Lumbar puncture is indicated if the fever is increasing or if the child fails to recover quickly. The child may be discharged home if LP findings are normal, vital signs stable, and the child is alert. Oral antibiotics should be prescribed if bacterial infection is likely. Any child receiving BDZ for seizures should be followed-up by telephone or evaluated by the physician the next day.

Protocol for Long-Term Management of Children with Febrile Seizures

A point system approximates the prognosis for subsequent hospitalization and the development of epilepsy. Patients who have more than three febrile seizures, any one seizure that lasts longer than 15 minutes, or a first-degree relative with epilepsy should have an EEG. The score can then be tallied as shown in Table 2.

A score of 4 points or more suggests chronic anticonvulsant therapy may be warranted. Treatment is thus largely reserved for those with neurologic deficit, multiple hospitalizations, or many very focal seizures. A score of 2 or 3 points in a child who suffers multiple daily seizures or prolonged seizures suggests rectal BDZ after seizures may be worthwhile.

The purpose of these treatments (long-term oral anticonvulsant or rectal BDZ after a seizure) is to avoid hospitalization. Neither is appropriate when hospitalization is unlikely. In some cases (very many febrile seizures or a very worried parent of a child with some continuing febrile seizures), a more vigorous treatment may be selected if it will be properly carried out. Failure to properly carry out treatment is especially likely when someone other than the parent must administer post-seizure rectal BDZ suppositories.

General Measures Appropriate for All Patients

We must prepare parents for seizure recurrences. I have found it useful for the parents of all children with seizures to meet with a nurse and review what to do when a seizure occurs or if medication problems arise, as well as other issues. Having a knowledgeable second person review these issues with parents is useful, because parents may find it easier to admit their confusion or worries to a nurse than to the doctor. Parents should learn how to respond to a seizure. We instruct them to roll the child to one side and not to put anything in the mouth. Most seizures last less than 3 minutes. The distinction between seizure and postictal lethargy should be clear. Criteria for when and how to seek help should be reviewed. The local facility best suited for 24 hour emergency care should be identified ahead of time. If only one adult is present, that person should call paramedics rather than drive the child alone.

Treating fever more vigorously decreases the number of recurrences of febrile seizures. The family must own a thermometer and know how to use it. A rectal temperature of less than 100°F requires no acetamino-

Table 2 Scoring System for Determining Prognosis of Children With Febrile Seizures

Variable	Points
Status epilepticus or serial seizures requiring hospitalization:	
Within the last 12 months	3
Within 12–24 months	2
More than 24 months ago	1
Definitely focal seizures associated with:	
Age >12 months	2
Age 6–12 months, not followed by Todd's paralysis	1
Three or more seizures in one day or a total of five previous seizures	1
Definite spasticity, hemiparesis, or microcephaly	2
Developmental delay without positive findings	1
Definitely epileptogenic EEG findings	1

phen, but the child should be observed closely, as the temperature may rise further. Any degree of fever warrants loosening of clothing. If the child seems uninterested in food and play, increased fluid intake is desirable. Children with a febrile illness who are sleeping peacefully should not be awakened to have their temperature taken.

If the temperature is in excess of 100°F, acetaminophen can be given, but not more than four times daily. If in spite of acetaminophen and removal of clothing the temperature exceeds 102°F, the child should be rubbed vigorously with a dry towel to increase skin blood flow. Sponging with a warm cloth is acceptable, but cold water causes shivering, which tends to increase the temperature. Alcohol rubs should be avoided because of percutaneous absorption of alcohol. Solids in the diet are reduced, and liquids offered frequently. Any febrile child should be examined for a rash. If the child is vomiting, solids are withheld at least 3 hours. Parents should contact a physician if fever persists longer than 24 hours, regardless of whether a seizure occurs.

Parents are reminded that fever control measures do not apply to other children without febrile seizures and that fever is usually beneficial (see Schmitt for discussion of fever phobia, which we seek to avoid). Children with febrile seizures should receive all immunizations, including pertussis, but those who have had more than four seizures or seizures protracted enough to cause hospitalization may be given prophylactic acetaminophen for 36 hours after the immunization.

Special instructions should be left for the babysitter (Table 3).

Treatment with Rectal Benzodiazepines During or After a Febrile Seizure

BDZ are rapidly absorbed from the rectum and can easily be administered in suppository form. Unfortunately, BDZ suppositories are not currently a commercial formulation. Some pharmacies specially prepare a suppository that remains solid in the refrigerator and melts at body temperature. BDZ solutions, which are more rapidly absorbed, may be given per rectum using a plastic syringe, but this method is more complex for the care giver. We prefer lorazepam to diazepam suppositories but have used both. I prefer lorazepam to diazepam for intravenous use because of less apnea and longer duration of action, but apnea has not occurred in

Table 3 Instructions for Babysitter or Child Care Center

1. Telephone parents if child appears significantly ill (runny nose and cough do not count if child is interested in food or play).
2. Know which hospital and physician care for child and all medications that child is currently receiving. These can be written on an index card.
3. Place child on one side during a seizure. Most seizures last 3 minutes or less. Do not place anything in the mouth, nor permit others to insert anything into the mouth (injuries of the teeth and palate are common when people do this). Be aware of distinction between seizure and postictal lethargy.
4. If seizure lasts >5 minutes or child has multiple seizures, call paramedics or emergency squad. Advise such helpers that child is known to have febrile seizures and provide name of physician, hospital, and medications (if any). Even if paramedics take child to a different hospital, child's physician or hospital record room can be contacted by telephone and provide important information.
5. If child is taken to hospital, call parents and ask them to go to hospital.

any of my patients treated with diazepam suppositories or rectal solution. By either route, the lorazepam dose is 0.1 mg per kilogram, and the diazepam dose is 0.3 to 0.4 mg per kilogram not to exceed 2 mg lorazepam and 15 mg diazepam, no matter how large the child. Big children need proportionately less medication than tiny babies, and repeat doses should never be given at home: they may be ineffective because of acute drug tolerance, but more important, the child may have a complicating problem.

Before rectal BDZ is prescribed for prolonged or repeated febrile seizures, parents or care givers should be carefully prepared. This may often be arranged with a nurse specialist during the most recent hospitalization for seizures. A kit containing disposable glove, suppository, or solution with plastic syringe is kept in a box in a refrigerator where it is immediately available. The parents should mark the syringe at the level of the proper dose. After each use, the box is replenished. The parents are instructed to first attend to the same general issues of care during a seizure: rolling to one side and ensuring a clear airway. Then the suppository or solution can be given, holding the buttocks together to prevent escape of the medicine. If the first dose of medicine fails to promptly control seizures, or obtundity persists after the seizures are controlled, the parents should bring the child promptly to an ER. Either response may signal a serious underlying condition.

Maintenance Anticonvulsant Therapy

Some children with serious brain abnormalities, prolonged seizures, or both febrile and afebrile seizures do better on an *effective maintenance anticonvulsant* program. This requires daily medication and special measures to ensure compliance. Only phenobarbital, BDZ, and valproic acid are effective in reducing febrile seizure recurrence. Phenobarbital is usually preferred because it is cheaper (Table 4) and need be given only once daily. If the child is intolerant of phenobarbital, I change to clonazepam or valproic acid. Phenytoin and carbamazepine are *ineffective* as treatment for febrile seizures.

Anticonvulsant Medications

Phenobarbital. When indicated, phenobarbital is prescribed at a dose of 2.5 to 3.0 mg per kilogram given once daily. It is my experience that tablets are preferable

Table 4 Wholesale Cost of Anticonvulsants*

	Formulation (No.)	Cost ($)
Phenobarbital	30 mg tablets (30)	0.20
Klonopin	0.5 mg tablets (30)	17.50
Depakote sprinkles	125 mg capsules (60)	16.00

*One month supply, Southern California 1992

to liquids over time. Tablets contain no alcohol and dosing is more accurate. Children tend to spit out some of a liquid dose, or parents may try to "sneak" the medicine in by adding the elixir to a juice bottle, which is then only partially consumed. I give phenobarbital elixir to parents who insist that they are unable to give the tablets, but I make them try the tablets first. Parents may need instruction in giving tablets to a willful child and may find it easier to give crushed tablets with a bit of soft food. I obtain a single blood level study 4 to 6 weeks after starting the medication and aim for a level between 15 and 25 μg per milliliter. My experience is that children whom I do not see in follow-up rarely get the medication reliably.

Interested pediatricians can take over the follow-up care. I recommend that the child is seen after 4 to 6 weeks, then every 3 months until there has passed a 6 to 9 month seizure-free interval. If seizures continue, I make a small increase in dosage (usually 20 to 25 percent). I do not obtain blood levels later unless the child has many seizures or I doubt that the parents are giving the medication. Although I want an initial blood level to ensure compliance and may repeat it, I treat to a clinical end point rather than to a particular blood level.

If a child who is behaviorally intolerant or allergic to phenobarbital is younger than 12 months or has parents who appear less than fully reliable, I change to clonazepam; otherwise I change to valproic acid. Unless there is a strong indication for long-term anticonvulsants, however, I offer the parents the option of withdrawing all long-term anticonvulsant therapy. *A strong indication is typically a combination of substantial neurologic deficit with a tendency for status epilepticus.*

Clonazepam. The usual starting dose of clonazepam is 0.25 mg (half of a 0.5 mg tablet) every 12 hours for children who weigh less than 12 kg, and 0.5 mg every 12 hours for heavier ones. The child is followed at similar intervals as in phenobarbital treatment. Blood levels are less useful, as they are expensive to measure and difficult to interpret. If the child is unduly sleepy, I reduce the dose. After 6 to 9 seizure-free months, the dose is tapered. If the child is intolerant to clonazepam, I consider changing to valproic acid.

Valproic Acid. I try to avoid using the syrup, as it is often poorly tolerated. I give Depakote tablets or sprinkles every 12 hours at a dose of 20 to 30 mg per kilogram per day. I obtain blood and serum glutamic-oxaloacetic transaminase levels SGOT at the 4 to 6 week follow-up and caution the parents to contact me any time the child is inexplicably obtunded or unable to eat for more than 6 hours. Hepatotoxicity from valproic acid is much more likely when a child is fasting, possibly because even modest levels of valproic acid impair the beta-oxidation of free fatty acids that are mobilized in response to diminished carbohydrate reserve. I do not usually give carnitine or check carnitine levels, but if a child on valproic acid is not growing satisfactorily I check a carnitine level, and may prescribe it.

Dose Adjustments and Side Effects

I use ERs to check patients, to be sure intravenous fluids are not needed, and to exclude serious infections. I do not want the basic treatment plan to be altered by ER physicians but do not object to blood tests or any tests they deem necessary to be assured of compliance with the drug regimen. If seizures persist, I always increase the dose of a drug that is well-tolerated in preference to starting a new drug. A single brief febrile seizure usually does not require a change in dose.

At least half of patients taking anticonvulsants have real or perceived side effects. Before prescribing any anticonvulsant, I explain that side effects are common, mostly transient, and not serious and that physicians and family together, rather than family alone, should make any decision about altering the plan. *I point out that side effects are common in children with febrile seizures treated with placebos and that the body often takes some time to adjust to any psychoactive medication.* If parents report a rash, I ask a physician to look at the child before deciding that the rash is due to medication allergy. *If parents report the child is irritable and has difficulty sleeping, I ask them to continue 10 days more, explaining that most patients are back to baseline by that time.* If significant side effects occur, I change to a second anticonvulsant or discontinue the medication. I tell parents how difficult it is for a physician who does not know the child to determine the origin of undesirable behavioral effects, and that continuity of care is more valuable to a child's well-being than fancy or expensive tests.

THE WORRIED PARENT

I hope to persuade parents of children with a good prognosis (the majority) that simple antipyretic management is adequate and that the risk of maintenance anticonvulsants exceeds their benefits. I also hope to decrease doctor shopping and unrealistic fears about injury from seizures. Some perspective on the evolution of our thinking about febrile seizures is helpful. In the old days, we thought of febrile seizures as indicators of "brain-damaged children" and predicted trouble for them. In some cases, these predictions fostered undesirable changes in the parent-child relationship. I may give them copies of this chapter, and for the subset of parents who want to know all about medical details, photocopies of Farwell's paper. I am always willing to order an EEG if pressed. *If that EEG shows major epileptic features, such as spike-wave bursts, I will agree to*

maintenance phenobarbital therapy once the child has had four febrile seizures, even in the absence of other risk factors. I offer the parents a follow-up appointment in 2 to 3 months, to see if anything has changed.

RECOMMENDATIONS

Febrile seizures are frightening but rarely cause serious injury. As with asthma, it is important to plan for future crises. The role of anticonvulsant medication in children with febrile seizures is principally to prevent hospitalization. Most parents can be convinced that barbiturates and other anticonvulsants are more hazardous than febrile seizures. When maintenance anticonvulsant therapy is justified, I always start with phenobarbital as the cheapest and easiest drug to use. Enormous individual differences occur between patients, and many children do not tolerate barbiturates. Most symptoms of medication intolerance resolve over a few weeks. If they continue, medication should be changed. Some additional precautions are needed for safe use of valproic acid in children younger than 2 years, but I have had no life-threatening problems giving small dose valproic acid for febrile seizures. Support for the primary care physician is very important and helps patient and family. Talking with parents and having the neurology nurse meet with them is cheaper and more reassuring than scans and EEGs.

SUGGESTED READING

Annegers JF, Jauser WA, Elveback LR, Kurland LY. The risk of epilepsy following febrile convulsions. Neurology 1979; 29:297–305.

Dawes RM, Faust D, Meehl PE. Clinical versus actuarial judgement. Science 1989; 243:1668–1674.

Farwell JR, Lee YJ, Jirtz DG, et al. Phenobarbital for febrile seizures: Effects on intelligence and seizure recurrence. N Engl J Med 1990; 322:364–368.

Maytal J, Sinnar S. Febrile status epilepticus. Pediatrics 1990; 86:611.

Nelson K, Ellenberg J. Prognosis in children with febrile seizures. Pediatrics 1978; 61:720–727.

Schmitt BD. Fever phobia. Am J Dis Child 1980; 134:176–181.

Verity CM, Butler NR, Golding J. Febrile convulsions in a national cohort followed up from birth. II—Medical history and intellectual ability at 5 years of age. Br Med J 1985; 290:1311–1314.

Verity CM, Golding J. Risk of epilepsy after febrile convulsions: A national cohort study. Br Med J 1991; 303:1373–1376.

Wallace SJ. The child with febrile seizures. London: John Wright, 1988.

Wolf SM, Forsythe A. Epilepsy and mental retardation following febrile seizures in childhood. Acta Pediatr Scand 1989; 78:291–295.

EPILEPSY WITH ABSENCE SEIZURES

W. EDWIN DODSON, M.D.

Absence seizures are manifested by brief episodes of staring that begin and end abruptly. During absence seizures there may be fluttering of the eyelids, minimal clonic movements, automatisms, and slight alterations of tone, but posture is largely unaffected. Typical absence seizures usually are associated with patterns of generalized spike and wave on the electroencephalogram (EEG). Atypical absence seizures differ from typical ones primarily in that they occur in patients who have other types of seizures and who have encephalopathy with mental impairment and that they are more likely to produce postural alterations such as head nodding. Atypical absence seizures usually are associated with more complex, asymmetric and irregular EEG patterns such as poly–spike and wave.

DIFFERENTIAL DIAGNOSIS

The differential diagnosis of staring spells includes daydreaming, absence seizures, and complex partial seizures (Table 1). Confirming that consciousness is interrupted is the principal means of distinguishing seizures from daydreaming. During complex partial seizures and absence seizures the mental status is altered to a variable extent, depending on the duration of the seizure. Complex partial seizures usually last more than 30 seconds, which is time enough to confirm that consciousness is impaired. In contrast, many absence seizures are so brief that they go undetected. Even if absence seizures are suspected, they can be difficult to substantiate because they are so brief. Most lay persons and many health professionals without specific training do not know how to ascertain brief alterations of consciousness.

Clinical detection of absence-associated alterations of consciousness is easy after the patient and the observer are taught how. The approach is to teach the patient to repeat a series of spoken words on command. When the observer suspects that the patient is having an absence seizure, the observer should speak aloud a series of four or five words such as fox, ball, bike, cat, radio, which the primed patient is then asked to repeat promptly. Omitting one or more of the just presented words signifies an interruption of consciousness. Asking the patient, "Are you all right?" almost never resolves the question, because this approach does not temporally resolve brief episodes. The observer usually cannot be sure that the patient understood the question before the spell is over.

When the diagnosis is in doubt, an ictal video-EEG is the best way to answer the question. Video recording is indispensable here, because absence seizures are so brief that precise correlation of behavior with the EEG pattern is essential. Repeatedly viewing the spells also helps with proper analysis.

EPILEPSY WITH ABSENCE SEIZURES

Absence seizures are a central feature of several forms of generalized epilepsy, especially childhood absence epilepsy and juvenile myoclonic epilepsy (JME), two of the most common generalized epilepsies (Table 2).

Childhood absence epilepsy is characterized by absence seizures that tend to occur in clusters. The seizures are associated with an ictal EEG pattern of regular, monotonous 3 Hz spike and wave patterns. The disorder is relatively rare, accounting for 2 to 4 percent of childhood epilepsy. Affected children usually are intellectually normal, but frequent absence seizures can lead to erratic school performance. The disorder remits in at least 40 percent of patients as they enter adolescence, so lifelong therapy may not be needed. Because this condition is benign, ethosuximide is recommended first; valproic acid is recommended when ethosuximide is insufficient or when the patient also has generalized tonic-clonic seizures. Other effective drugs include acetazolamide, the ketogenic diet, clonazepam, and trimethadione.

JME should be suspected when absence seizures begin in late childhood or early adolescence. Myoclonic

Table 1 Features of Absence Seizures, Complex Partial Seizures, and Daydreaming

Feature	Absence Seizures	Complex Partial Seizures	Daydreaming
Altered consciousness	Yes	Yes	No
Aura	No	Maybe	No
Automatisms	Yes	Yes	No
Duration	< 30 sec	> 30 sec	Variable
Amnesia	Variable	Usually	No
Postictal state	No	Maybe	No
Precipitated by HV	Yes	Usually no	No
Ictal electroencephalogram	3 Hz spike and wave	Focal spikes	Normal

seizures are a diagnostic *sine qua non,* but they often are inconspicuous and are ascertained only by pointed questioning about early morning clumsiness. Both absence and generalized tonic-clonic seizures occur in this disorder. This results in considerable overlap with both childhood absence epilepsy and the syndrome of generalized tonic-clonic seizures (grand mal) on awakening. The ictal EEG pattern in juvenile myoclonic epilepsy sometimes demonstrates polyspikes and poly–spike and wave complexes with frequencies faster than 4 Hz. Valproic acid is the drug of choice.

Differentiating childhood absence and JME can be difficult. Childhood absence epilepsy tends to begin in the middle years of childhood, whereas JME more often begins in later childhood or in preadolescence. However, there is much variation in the age of onset of both disorders, and both may be manifested solely by absence seizures in young children. The natural history of the two disorders differs considerably and has implications for how long drug treatment should be continued. Whereas many patients with childhood absence epilepsy experience remission and can discontinue antiepileptic drugs, patients with juvenile myoclonic epilepsy do not outgrow their propensity to have seizures and, therefore, need antiepileptic therapy perpetually.

The atypical absence seizures that occur in severe childhood epilepsies are more difficult to prevent. *Myoclonic astatic epilepsy with slow spike-wave* (Lennox-Gastaut syndrome) is the most common form of severe myoclonic epilepsy that affects young children. Criteria for the diagnosis of Lennox-Gastaut syndrome include

these: multiple types of seizures, usually including nocturnal tonic seizures, atypical absence seizures, and atonic seizures (astatic seizures or drop attacks); mental subnormality; EEG pattern of slow spike and wave (< 2.5 Hz). The syndrome can be symptomatic or idiopathic. Compared with the symptomatic variant, the idiopathic or primary form responds to medication better and has a better prognosis. In this disorder absence and atypical absence seizures can occur with extremely great frequency (several hundred seizures daily).

Lennox-Gastaut syndrome is difficult to treat. Traditionally, antiepileptic drugs have been selected on the basis of the patient's most common seizure type. It is important to recognize that anticonvulsants such as carbamazepine, phenytoin, and phenobarbital sometimes worsen the astatic and atypical absence seizures. When this happens, one should consider starting valproic acid and discontinuing the anticonvulsant. Benzodiazepines, especially clonazepam, are useful in Lennox-Gastaut syndrome, but usually any benefit from clonazepam comes at the price of neurotoxicity.

TREATMENT OF ABSENCE SEIZURES IN PRIMARY GENERALIZED EPILEPSIES

Differentiating absence seizures, complex partial seizures, and daydreaming is very important because different antiepileptic medications are indicated for the different types of seizures. Of course, antiepileptic therapy is not warranted for daydreaming. Ethosuximide is ineffective in complex partial seizures. Anticonvulsants that are appropriate for complex partial seizures such as carbamazepine often exacerbate absence seizures.

Childhood absence epilepsy (petit mal epilepsy) often responds to ethosuximide, whereas juvenile myoclonic epilepsy should be treated with valproic acid because of the sizeable risk of generalized tonic-clonic seizures (Table 3). In a child younger than 8 years who begins to have only absence seizures, I start treatment with ethosuximide if the EEG shows a classical pattern of 3 Hz monotonous spike and wave. I start with valproate if the child has a history of generalized tonic-clonic seizures or has any of the following EEG

Table 2 Epilepsies with Absence Seizures

Primary epilepsies
 Childhood absence epilepsy (pyknolepsy; petit mal)
 JME
 Epilepsy with myoclonic absences
 Epilepsy with continuous spikes and waves during sleep
 Eyelid myoclonia with absences
 Juvenile absence epilepsy

Symptomatic epilepsies
 Early myoclonic encephalopathy
 Early infantile epileptic encephalopathy with suppression-burst
 West's syndrome (infantile spasms)
 Severe myoclonic epilepsy in infants
 Lennox-Gastaut syndrome

Table 3 Features of Juvenile Myoclonic Epilepsy and Childhood Absence Epilepsy

Feature	Childhood Absence	JME
Age at onset	Early–mid-childhood	Puberty
Myoclonus	Rare	Required for diagnosis
Tonic-clonic seizures	Rare in 50% of patients	Common, early AM
EEG	3 Hz, spike and wave	Poly–spike and wave, 4–6 or 8–12 Hz
Genetics	Autosomal-dominant	Autosomal-dominant
Treatment	Ethosuximide or valproic acid	Valproic acid
Prognosis	40% remission	Life long

features: a spike and wave frequency faster than 3.5 Hz or slower than 2.5 Hz; a poly–spike and wave pattern or a slow background. For children who begin to have absence seizures after age 8 years, I usually begin with valproate. If there is a family history of other types of seizures such as generalized tonic-clonic or myoclonic seizures, or if there are any features that suggest JME, I begin with valproate.

Ethosuximide is the drug of first choice for childhood absence epilepsy. Starting with ethosuximide here avoids any risk of valproate-associated hepatotoxicity, although the risk of this lethal adverse effect in these patients appears to be vanishingly low. Most of the children who have developed this side effect have had a progressive neurologic disease (Alper's disease) or inborn errors of organic acid metabolism, not a primary generalized epilepsy with absence seizures.

Whether generalized spike and wave discharges on EEG in and of itself defines an absence seizure is controversial. Studies done in the mid-1970s suggested that all generalized spike and wave bursts are associated with some degree of altered mental processing; however, more recent investigations revealed that these cause significant alterations of consciousness only 40 percent of the time. I do not prescribe medication for patients whose EEG contains generalized spike and wave patterns but no clinical seizures.

Patients with JME should be advised that a healthy lifestyle can reduce the chance of seizures. Before the advent of effective drug therapy, behavioral manipulations were the principal means of modifying the frequency of seizures in JME. Sleep deprivation and alcohol use increase the frequency of myoclonic seizures, which can culminate in clonic-tonic-clonic seizures.

Most patients' progress can be monitored clinically. The goal of therapy is no seizures and no side effects. If hyperventilation elicits absence seizures while the patient is taking drug therapy, most authorities recommend increasing the dose of medication. Drug levels should not be treated per se, because some of these patients respond to relatively small doses and low concentrations of medication. Thus, if the patient's seizures are controlled with drug concentrations that are below the "therapeutic range," the dosage should not be increased.

Even though children with childhood absence epilepsy can have above average intelligence, some of them still run aground academically. If absence seizures are suspected, it is important to make certain that the child clearly understands assignments. When absence seizures affect school performance, they usually result in misunderstanding of assignments or instructions rather than global intellectual deficits. The affected child may do the wrong assignment or fail to complete the test, rather than failing to grasp the conceptual basis of the work.

Principal Medications for Absence Seizures

The principal antiepileptic medications used to treat epilepsies with absence seizures include ethosuximide, valproic acid, trimethadione, acetazolamide, and benzo-

diazepines such as clonazepam. The anticonvulsants carbamazepine, methsuximide, phenobarbital, mephobarbital, primidone, and phenytoin are not effective for absence seizures and, in fact, may exacerbate them.

Monotherapy is feasible for a large percentage of patients with primary generalized epilepsy with absence seizures. Here, as in other forms of epilepsy, it is best to give as few drugs as possible because polytherapy usually increases the risk of side effects to a greater extent than it increases the chance of seizure control. In symptomatic and encephalopathic epilepsies where atypical absence seizures are common, monotherapy is less likely to succeed.

The general approach is to increase the first medication incrementally until seizures are controlled or intolerable side effects occur. I add a second drug if the initial drug is ineffective or only partially effective. If the first drug was altogether ineffective, it should be discontinued as the second is started. If the first drug was partially effective, it should be retained while the second is started. If seizures are controlled at this point with two drug therapy, one should next attempt to withdraw the first drug. Multiple drug therapy should be continued only after establishing that both drugs are required to prevent seizures.

Ethosuximide is effective against absence seizures but not against partial or generalized tonic-clonic seizures. Thus, it is sufficient for most children with childhood absence epilepsy but insufficient for those with JME. Once or twice daily dosing is sufficient, because the half-life of ethosuximide is 24 to 42 hours. I prefer twice daily administration because the family has two chances to remember. The dosage ranges from 10 to 70 mg per kilogram daily. The therapeutic range is 45 to 100 µg per milliliter. Hiccups and hallucinations are the major neurologic side effects of ethosuximide. Idiosyncratic rashes prohibit long-term administration of this agent in as many as 10 percent of patients. Less often there may be transient depression of the white blood cell count.

Valproic acid is effective in absence, generalized tonic-clonic, and myoclonic seizures; it is also useful as an adjunct in complex partial seizures. For unknown reasons the full effect of valproate may be delayed several weeks, or even months. Thus, the drug should be administered for several months and at the maximally tolerated dose before it is judged ineffective.

Valproic acid is the drug of choice for JME. The dosage ranges from 10 to 70 mg per kilogram per day. The half-life of valproic acid is 4 to 15 hours; shortest in children and in patients on polytherapy. Whenever possible, a formulation with delayed or slowed absorption such as Depakote should be prescribed. The most frequently published therapeutic range is 50 to 100 µg per milliliter but many patients tolerate a considerably higher concentration.

Valproate has a low incidence of neurotoxicity. Common systemic side effects include transient alopecia, gastrointestinal upset, skin rash, and alterations of appetite. Drug interactions are common. It consistently causes phenobarbital levels to increase, and phenobarbital doses should be reduced if valproate is added. Valproate decreases the total, but not unbound (free), phenytoin level, owing to a drug–protein-binding interaction; these changes usually do not necessitate adjustment of phenytoin dosage. Because valproic acid has a short half-life, it usually must be given in three or more daily doses.

The most serious though rare side effect of valproic acid is hepatic failure. This idiosyncratic problem usually occurs in the first 6 months of therapy, most often among children who are taking other anticonvulsant drugs and who have progressive neurologic disease with refractory partial seizures. This drug probably should be avoided in patients with recurrent status epilepticus due to partial seizures or epilepsia partialis continua, unless the patient's liver biopsy specimen is normal. Liver function tests should be obtained before starting valproic acid and periodically during the first months of treatment. Unfortunately, it is not clear which test of liver function is best for early detection of this adverse effect. Transaminase values are mildly elevated in 15 to 30 percent of children who take other anticonvulsants, and they may be only modestly increased with valproate-associated hepatotoxicity.

Acetazolamide is a carbonic anhydrase inhibitor that is effective in some patients with minor motor seizures. Because it is a sulfonamide, it should be avoided in patients who are allergic to sulfa. The usual dosage is 10 to 20 mg per kilogram per day. Long-term therapy with this drug causes renal tubular acidosis, osteopenia, and rarely rickets.

Trimethadione has a spectrum of activity like that of ethosuximide but is used less frequently. The demethylated metabolite dimethadione has a very long half-life, (estimated to be 10 days), making this a convenient therapeutic agent. However, because trimethadione is highly teratogenic and is contraindicated in pregnancy, it should be a drug of last resort in women who have child-bearing potential. Other adverse effects include nephrotoxicity, hematopoetic suppression, and rash.

Among the *benzodiazepines, clonazepam* is the one most frequently used for long-term treatment of epilepsy in the United States. Although the half-life of clonazepam is 16 to 60 hours, three or four daily doses is recommended to minimize side effects. The range of doses is 0.03 to 0.1 mg per kilogram per day. Drug concentrations correlate poorly with drug action, but concentrations of 0.02 to 0.07 µg per milliliter have been reported to be effective and tolerated reasonably well.

Although clonazepam is effective for absence seizures, it is used infrequently in childhood absence epilepsy because it very frequently causes sedation and behavioral side effects. Other drugs are less neurotoxic. Drooling, irritability, disobedience, reduced attention span, and depression are common complaints with clonazepam; in very high concentrations it can precipitate absence status (minor motor status). Clonazepam is used most often in severe childhood epilepsy with multiple types of seizures such as infantile spasms and the Lennox-Gastaut syndrome. When it is given long-term for these disorders, the dose should be increased slowly, allowing the patient to become tolerant to the adverse drug actions. Unfortunately, patients also develop tolerance to its antiepileptic actions. When ineffective, clonazepam must be withdrawn very slowly, usually over weeks or months, because of the hazard of withdrawal seizures. For these reasons, I use clonazepam as a last resort and I prescribe it in the smallest dose possible.

Patient Follow-Up

Patients taking anticonvulsants must be re-evaluated periodically to determine if their medication is effective and if there are side effects. When problems occur — either continued seizures or toxicity — drug level measurement is an adjunct to individualizing the dose.

Drug levels should be measured whenever the patient develops side effects or fails to respond to average-sized doses. If an initial low average dose is effective, drug levels are necessary only as a baseline for the future assessment of compliance. However, many patients will not be adequately treated with the first, small dose. Thus, as the dose is increased, follow-up examinations are essential. When seizures persist or when patients develop symptoms that may be due to side effects, drug levels can help the physician individualize each patient's dose with greater insight than can be achieved by clinical examination alone. Repeated drug measurements also encourage and document compliance.

SUGGESTED READING

Bancaud J, Talairach J. Clinical semiology of frontal lobe seizures. In Chauvel P, Delgado-Escueta AV, et al. eds.: Advances in neurology. Vol 57. New York: Raven, 1992: 3.

Dodson WE. Special pharmacokinetic considerations in children. Epilepsia 1987; 28(suppl 1):S56–S70.

Dodson WE, Pellock JM, eds. Pediatric epilepsy: diagnosis and therapy. New York: Demos, 1993.

Levy RH, Dreifuss FE, Mattson RH, et al, eds. Antiepileptic drugs. 3rd ed. New York: Raven, 1989.

Roger J, Dravet C, Bureau M, et al. Epileptic syndromes in infancy, childhood, and adolescence. London: John Libbey and Company, 1985.

TREATMENT AND PROPHYLAXIS OF A FIRST TONIC-CLONIC SEIZURE

JOHN M. FREEMAN, M.D.

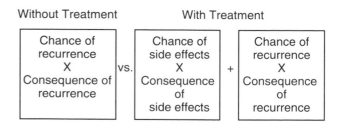

Figure 1 Febrile Seizures: Analysis of risks and consequences.

A person, child or adult, who has had a single seizure, whether febrile or afebrile, does not *necessarily* need to be started on anticonvulsant medication. Decisions about treatment should be based on an analysis of the chances and consequences of another seizure *for that individual* and an analysis of how, for that person, the risks and benefits of treatment compare to the risks and benefits of remaining free of medication. Though the risk-benefit analysis discussed below is based on our knowledge of the natural history of febrile seizures in children, a growing body of information suggests that the process applies equally well to decisions about treatment of afebrile seizures in children. Though the natural history and the consequences of first tonic-clonic seizures in adults are less well-defined, the decision-making process involved, and the dialogue between the physician and the patient are similar for adults and children. Because the risks and consequences of another seizure are the patient's and the side effects of treatment are also the patient's, the ultimate decision should be the patient's as well. The physician should be the provider of up-to-date information and a counselor and interpreter for the patient.

DIAGNOSIS OF SEIZURES AND EPILEPSY

A seizure is defined as a paroxysmal electrical discharge of neurons in the brain that results in alteration of function or behavior. It is important to remember that an electrical event on the electroencephalogram (EEG) is not a seizure unless it is simultaneously accompanied by clinical manifestations. Unless the EEG is recorded during an event that the physician personally sees and interprets as a seizure, the only way to diagnose a seizure is by interpretation of the clinical history. A meticulously detailed history of the event taken from an observer is thus critical for both the diagnosis and the classification of the seizure.

If, at the end of that history the physician cannot be certain of the diagnosis the proper action is to reserve diagnosis and forbear treating. If more events occur, the physician should be able to improve the observations and be more certain of the diagnosis. If no more events occur, the initial one was of no importance.

Epilepsy is defined as two or more seizures not immediately provoked by specific events such as fever, trauma, infection, or chemical changes. Two or more seizures occurring on the same day, or during the same episode, still are not considered epilepsy. As you will see

from our decision-making process, we rarely treat after a single seizure (or episode). We usually treat recurrent seizures — epilepsy.

RISK-BENEFIT ANALYSIS

Formal decision making requires calculating the chance that an event will occur and the consequences of that event. A decision then is made by comparing the value derived from these two numbers to the value of the chance and consequences of the alternatives. For the person who has had one or more seizures this means understanding the chance of having another one and the consequences of another such episode. The value derived is compared to the chance of side effects of treatment with an anticonvulsant and the consequences of those side effects. A diagram of such a risk-benefit ratio is shown in Figure 1.

MANAGEMENT OF SEIZURES

In making decisions about management after an initial seizure it is necessary to identify the seizure type and the seizure pattern (or type of epilepsy). Some types of seizures, such as most neonatal seizures, are benign and usually self-limited. Others, such as infantile spasms, are age dependent, and "malignant" in that they cause or are associated with other types of neurologic dysfunction. Absence seizures are pattern-dependent, are easily recognized from their description, and are relatively benign. Benign rolandic seizures, with their signature of focal facial twitching, may not need therapy at all. Still others, such as juvenile myoclonic epilepsy of Janz, which is marked by early morning myoclonic jerks, is a genetic epilepsy that responds best to valproate and requires treatment for many years. These various types, their recognition, and their management were recently reviewed (see Suggested Reading). Each type, owing to its peculiar severity and natural history, affects the physician's recommendations and the patient's decision about treatment differently.

In this chapter I concentrate on the factors in the decision-making process that is set in motion by the occurrence of a single generalized tonic-clonic seizure. I focus on the process rather than the decision itself, because various decisions are acceptable. The same process can—and should—be applied to other seizure types, but for each type and each individual, the weight given to the various factors is different. I start with febrile seizures as the model for the decision-making process, because febrile seizures are relatively homogeneous and their natural history is the best-defined.

Febrile Seizures in Children

Chance of Recurrence

Should a child who has had a single convulsion with fever be started on anticonvulsant medication? To assist in making that decision, the physician should know the chance of a recurrence of a febrile seizure and the consequences of such a recurrence. The chance of further febrile seizures, and of subsequent afebrile seizures, is shown in Table 1.

Consequence of Recurrence

Contrary to popular belief, there are few if any consequences of one, or even of many, febrile seizures. There is *no* increased risk of death, *no* increased risk of injury, *no* increased risk of brain damage, and *no* evidence of an increased risk of learning disorders. Since most children (70 percent) do not have a recurrence of the febrile seizure, and since there are virtually *no* consequences of a recurrence for a child who has had a febrile seizure, all the side effects of therapy, even those with a low incidence, are worse than the virtually nonexistent consequences of another febrile seizure (see Table 1).

There is therefore general consensus among most pediatric neurologists that initial febrile seizures rarely require treatment. Although the chance of a recurrence may increase after the initial febrile seizure, the consequences of these recurrences remain unchanged. For this reason, we rarely treat children who suffer recurrent febrile seizures.

Risk of Afebrile Seizures and Epilepsy. A child who has had a single febrile seizure has a slightly greater chance of having future afebrile seizures (2.0 percent) than a child who has never had a febrile seizure (0.1 percent). Even within this "higher-risk group" there are predictive factors (see Table 1). Even a child who has all of the risk factors has a 90 percent chance of *not* having afebrile seizures. There is no evidence that anticonvulsant treatment of afebrile seizures in this higher-risk group prevents later epilepsy.

Afebrile Seizures in Children

The chance of a recurrence after a child has a first afebrile seizure is shown in Table 2. As with a first febrile seizure, the overall risk of recurrence is in the range of 30 percent. Most recurrences occur in the year after the first seizure, and 90 percent within 2 years. The risk of recurrence is greater if the child has a static encephalopathy or shows evidence of prior neurologic damage. A

Table 1 Chance and Consequences of Recurrent Febrile Seizures

Chance of recurrence	(%)
After first seizure	30
After second seizure	40
After third seizure	40
Consequence of recurrence	
Mental retardation	No greater than
Cerebral palsy	for children
Learning disorder	without febrile
Death	seizures.
Epilepsy risk (%)	
If no febrile seizures	0.1
If one febrile seizure	2.0
Risk factors for later epilepsy:	
Seizures prolonged > 15 min, one-sided, or two or more during the same day	
Parent, brother or sister with epilepsy	
Neurologic disorder or developmental delay	
Risk of epilepsy after one febrile seizure	(%)
With 0 risk factors	0.1
With 1 risk factor	2.5
With 3 risk factors	5–10

Table 2 Chance of Recurrence After One Afebrile Seizure as a Function of Seizure-Free Interval

	Risk (%)		
	By 12 mo	By 24 mo	By 36 mo
Overall recurrence rate	26	36	40
Remote symptomatic seizure (with static encephalopathy)	37	53	60
Ideopathic seizure	24	33	36
Abnormal EEG	41	54	56
Normal EEG	15	23	26

Treatment did not affect chance of recurrence.

From Shinnar S, et al. Risk of a seizure recurrence following a first unprovoked seizure in childhood. Pediatrics 1990; 85:1076–1085; with permission.

child who has an idiopathic, unprovoked seizure has a smaller chance of recurrence if the initial EEG is normal than if it is abnormal.

What are the consequences if an afebrile seizure should recur? We are often told that seizures need to be treated because they may result in death, injury, more seizures, or neurologic damage. But, as with febrile seizures, there appears to be virtually *no* risk of the child's dying, *no* risk of injury, *no* risk of brain damage, and *no* evidence that the higher incidence of learning disorders seen in association with seizures is caused by the seizures rather than by their treatment. And yet, these are the reasons why initial tonic-clonic seizures are often treated. Let us examine them one at a time.

Death

Though a slightly increased risk of dying is associated with epilepsy, there is no evidence that treatment decreases that risk. Indeed, the studies of deaths in persons with epilepsy are studies of persons with known epilepsy, all of whom were being treated at the time. Stopping medication may have played a role in some of the deaths. In any event, for a child (or adult) who has had a single seizure, the chance of dying during the next seizure must be vanishingly small.

Injury, Risks, and Overprotection

Children are often given medication after a single seizure in order to prevent injury during another seizure. For the same reason they are often overprotected by physicians, parents, and schools. The concern is raised, "What if one of those things happens while the child is riding a bike, swimming, or crossing the street?" But this is the wrong question. Children are injured far too often in just these activities, whether or not they have seizures. Take swimming for example. Children drown far too frequently, but we do not prohibit them from swimming. Rather, we try to insist that they swim under supervision and in safe circumstances. If those restrictions extend to all children, the question we should be asking is, "Is the child who has had a seizure at greater risk for injury than the child who has not had seizures? How much additional risk attends a child who has had seizures?" The degree of *increased risk* depends on the child's age, the seizure type and frequency, and whether there is an aura to the seizures. The risk also increases in proportion to the amount of time the child spends at a "risky" activity (e.g., in the water).

A child who has had a single seizure has only about a 30 percent chance of ever having another. If he swims 1 hour each day for 3 months each summer, you can calculate the minuscule increased chance of that child's having a seizure in the water. Because the consequences of that seizure, if it did occur in the water, could be enormous, the child should be supervised when in the water, just as every other child should be supervised, to minimize those consequences. This makes far more sense than prohibiting a child who has seizures from swimming.

When this line of reasoning and analysis of risks and benefits is pursued the following recommendations can be made:

- We do *not* recommend starting medication after a single seizure to prevent injury.
- We place virtually *no* restrictions on a child who has had a single seizure.

If a child has many absence or partial complex seizures, some restrictions may be reasonable until the seizures are brought under better control with medication. Like medication, restrictions should be imposed in the smallest possible "dose" and for the shortest reasonable period. Most children can live with time-limited restrictions.

There are some risks that an individual might take for him- or herself, such as sky diving, flying, or scuba diving. Another person might find these risks unacceptable. As long as the risk is only to the individual and not to others, the individual and/or the family should be the ones to decide the magnitude of risk that is acceptable to them and the magnitude of the benefits that they derive. Since the risk and the benefit belong to the individual, the decision should be the individual's as well. Driving, which places others at risk, is a different matter. The privilege of driving and the increased risk that society is willing to assume are matters for society to decide. The decision cannot be left to the driver alone; however, society must be reasonable and proportional in its self-protection.

Overprotection and restrictions on activities, whether self-imposed or imposed by parents or by physicians, may ultimately become the patient's major handicap, particularly if the seizures are later controlled.

Brain Damage

There is no evidence that a single seizure, or even recurrent seizures, damage the brain. Recent studies have shown that even status epilepticus, which was once widely and mistakenly believed to cause brain damage, does not cause such damage in children *when it is properly treated.* Rather, it is the events that caused the status epilepticus—the meningitis, encephalitis, head trauma, or anoxia—that both precipitated the status *and* left the resultant damage. When status epilepticus is associated with febrile seizures or when the child who has epilepsy has an episode of status because medication is stopped, there is no evidence that that child will suffer brain damage. Although the studies have not been performed, presumably the same is true of adult seizures.

Kindling

Kindling is an animal model of epilepsy that does not appear to occur in primates or humans. Whether kindling plays a role in the causation of seizures and epilepsy after a local brain injury may be a different question.

Thus, because a single seizure causes no permanent damage, and because serial seizures and even status epilepticus do not damage the brain, and because the electrical activity of kindling has no effect in humans, there is no evidence to support the old thinking that seizures beget seizures.

Learning Problems

Learning problems and behavioral problems are more likely due to the side effects of anticonvulsant medications than to the seizures themselves. All anticonvulsant medications probably have some neuropsychologic effects. Clearly, some have more side effects than others.

Seizures in Adults

The decision-making process about treating an adult who has had a single seizure should be similar to that applied for children.

- The *chance of recurrence* after a single, idiopathic, simple tonic-clonic seizure is similar for adults and children.
- The *consequences of a recurrence* are, in most respects, similar:
  (1) The risk of death from a seizure recurrence remains minimal.
  (2) The risk of injury is similarly low.
  (3) The risk of brain damage from seizures is no different than for children.
  (4) Although the effects of treatment on learning are different than in children, few adults function at "optimal" capacity while taking medication. Some medications such as phenobarbital have more and better-documented effects on cognitive function than others.

No anticonvulsant is good for the brain! The effects of medication are only better or worse than the effects and consequences of the seizures themselves.

The major consequences of seizure recurrence are psychosocial. The psychosocial consequences of a recurrent seizure or seizures may be age dependent, job dependent, and family dependent. Driving, for example, is of no importance to children, whereas it is a mark of maturity and independence for adolescents, and it is of critical importance to most adults, who may have to drive to, or for, their employment.

Despite the lack of physical consequences of another seizure, the loss of driving privileges, should another seizure occur, may be sufficient reason for treating an adult after a single seizure. It may also explain the reluctance of adults who have had a seizure (or seizures), and of their physician, to discontinue medication. This is one reason why we endeavor to get adolescents off medication *before* they begin to drive. It is also why efforts are being made to reduce the amount of time that patients must be seizure-free before they may drive.

But even with the issue of driving, one individual may attach far more consequence to a recurrent seizure than another. A city dweller may have less trouble finding other transportation than someone who lives in a suburban or rural area. Patients who have access to good public transportation may be less likely to request medication than others. The type of work a person performs may also play a major role in the decision to start or continue medication.

DECISION MAKING AFTER A FIRST SEIZURE

In our decision-making process and in our dialogue with our patients and their families we believe that the crucial question becomes, What is the worst that could happen if . . . .

- What is the worst that could happen *if* we decide not to start medication? The worst is another seizure, and we can estimate the chance of recurrence. What would be the *consequences* of another seizure? That may depend on the person's age, seizure type and frequency, and on the parents, the spouse, or the employer.
- What is the worst that could happen *if* we started medication? We know the chance of allergic, idiosyncratic, or dose-related side effects and their consequences. Even with medication, the patient could still have another seizure.
- What is the worst that could happen *if* medication were discontinued? That again depends on the age, the job, the area where the patient lives, lifestyle, and other factors.

These worst case scenarios are meant to keep risk-taking in proper perspective. If the person who has had a seizure can accept the worst, then every other alternative is also acceptable. This perspective improves physicians' ability to help the child, the individual, and the family in a joint decision-making process. As we assess the chances of this worst case scenario occurring, we also independently assess, together with affected individuals, the importance of the consequences, *if* they occur. Together we compare the risks of treatment with the risks of waiting to see if there will be more seizures.

In many situations there is not a single correct decision but rather a variety of options. It is the physician's role to provide good information and to express opinions about which of these options are thought to be "the best." The best decision is usually the one that has the patient, the parent, and the physician on the same team.

Sometimes it is best to start medication. Sometimes it is best to wait. When medication is to be started, the decision about which medication to use depends both on the seizure type and on the patient's (or family's) willingness to accept the risks and the side effects of the medication.

Treatment of Seizures

The anticonvulsant medication that is selected should be the one most effective for that seizure type, should have the fewest side effects, and should be the least expensive. The physician should use the medication that meets those criteria, and prescribe the smallest effective dose for the shortest period of time. *Smallest*, *shortest*, and *effective* should be determined through considerable discussion between the patient, the family, and the physician. A summary of commonly used medications, their side effects, and their dosages is shown in Table 3.

Table 3 Use of Specific Anticonvulsant Drugs in Different Seizure Types

	Indications					
Drug	Partial (focal)	Absence	Tonic-Clonic	Usual Dose (mg/kg per day)	Half-Life (hr)	Side Effects
Carbamazepine	+		+	10–40	10–30	Headache, drowsiness, dizziness, diplopia, blood dyscrasia, hepatotoxicity, arrhythmia
Clonazepam		+	+	0.05–0.10	24–36	Drowsiness, ataxia, secretions, hypotonia, behavioral problems
Ethosuximide		+		20–40	24–42	Gastrointestinal distress, rash, drowsiness, dizziness, systemic lupus erythematosus, blood dyscrasia
Phenobarbital	+		+	2–8	48–100	Drowsiness, rash, ataxia, behavioral and cognitive problems
Phenytoin	+		+	4–8	6–30	Drowsiness, gum hyperplasia, rash, anemia, ataxia, hirsutism, folate deficiency
Primidone	+		+	12–25	6–12	Drowsiness, dizziness, rash, anemia, ataxia, diplopia
Valproic acid	+	+	+	10–60	6–18	Gastrointestinal distress, hepatitis, alopecia, drowsiness, atasia, tremors, pancreatitis, thrombocytopenia

From Freeman JM, Vining EPG. Decision making and seizures. Pediatrics in Review 1992; 13:298; with permission.

Discontinuing Medication

If medication is started, how long does a patient have to continue taking it? Using the same line of reasoning, the decision to discontinue medication depends on the risks that the person is willing to undertake and the consequences for that individual of another seizure, should one occur. With adults, as with children, *if* the patient has been seizure free for 2 years *and* the EEG is better than at the start of treatment, that person may have a better than 75 percent chance of remaining seizure free if the medication is tapered over several months. Are those odds good enough? Almost certainly they are for a child or young adolescent, for whom the consequences of another seizure are less grave. They are probably acceptable for a teenager who can defer driving for 6 months to a year. Are they good enough for a working person who has a family to support, who needs to drive and needs the job?

The decision to continue or discontinue medication depends on the individual's assessment of the risks of another seizure and the consequences, should one occur. The decision also depends on the individual's assessment of the benefits of being free of medication. There is no correct answer about discontinuing medication. Patients should be given the opportunity to make that decision for themselves, based on the physician's best information about the risks and benefits and the individual's personal priorities. The answer may be different for a woman who, desiring a child, must consider the additional potential consequences of the anticonvulsant to the fetus than for a father who has a family to support.

Epilepsy Prophylaxis

There is virtually *no* evidence that anticonvulsants afford prophylaxis against epilepsy. There is no evidence that anticonvulsant treatment prevents afebrile seizures in children who have had febrile seizures. There is no evidence that the use of medication (usually phenytoin) during and in the days after neurosurgery or in the days after head trauma prevents later epilepsy. Phenytoin given in appropriate therapeutic doses during the 7 days after head trauma does suppress seizures. This suppression could be important during the time when the brain is already swollen, the theory being that a prolonged seizure at that time could produce further swelling and compromise cerebral blood flow. A similar rationale could be used to support treatment in the perioperative period. However, since most survivors of head trauma or brain surgery do not develop epilepsy, and since there is no evidence that anticonvulsants prevent later epilepsy, we see no reason for long-term prophylaxis for these patients.

SUGGESTED READING

Callaghan N, Garrett A, Goggin T. Withdrawal of anticonvulsant drugs in patients free of seizures for two years: A prospective study. N Engl J Med 1988;318:942–946.

Delgado-Escueda AV, Janz D, Beck-Mannagetta G. Pregnancy and teratogenesis in epilepsy. Neurology 1992;42(Suppl 5):7–160.

Freeman JM, Vining EPG. Decision making and seizures. Pediatr Rev 1992; 13:298–311.

Freeman JM, Vining EPG, Pillas DJ. Seizures and epilepsy in childhood: A guide for parents. Baltimore: Johns Hopkins University Press, 1990.

Lippman I, et al. Epilepsy Foundation of America consensus statement on drivers licensing and epilepsy. Neurology 1992, in press.

Shinnar S, Berg AT, Moshe SL, et al. Risk of a seizure recurrence following a first unprovoked seizure in childhood. Pediatrics 1990;85:1076–1085.

PATIENT RESOURCES

The Epilepsy Foundation of America
4351 Garden City Drive
Landover, Maryland 20785
(800)EFA-4050

The Epilepsy Foundation of America maintains an extensive information service for both patients and physicians. This information service responds to individual queries from patients and maintains an extensive file of free brochures on specific topics. Physicians may receive, free of charge, access to computerized searches on various topics related to epilepsy and copies of individual articles.

NEUROLEPTIC DRUGS

BARNEY J. STERN, M.D.
JANET R. FARHIE, M.D.

Neuroleptic medications are the mainstay of treatment for psychotic disorders. Target symptoms that respond to these drugs are disorders of thinking such as delusions, paranoid ideation, and fragmented or disorganized thought and perceptual disturbances such as hallucinations and illusions, with hyperresponsiveness to unrealistic interpretations of environmental or internal stimuli. Resultant behavioral changes, including agitation, aggression, or catatonic withdrawal, and undue emotional disturbances of fear, depression, or elation are also responsive to these medications. As beneficial as antipsychotics are, potential side effects can be irreversibly disabling or even life threatening.

PHARMACOLOGY

It is postulated that the antipsychotic effects of neuroleptics are mediated by depolarization blockade, which reduces neuronal firing in the mesolimbic dopamine system. Antagonism of dopamine transmission in the nigrostriatal system results in extrapyramidal side effects. Tuberoinfundibular dopamine blockade accounts for excessive prolactin release and alterations in appetite and body temperature regulation.

Table 1 lists the chemical classes of commonly used agents, their relative potency, and the doses ordinarily prescribed. Drug potency refers to the milligram equivalence that produces the same antipsychotic effect as a standard 100 mg dose of chlorpromazine. All drugs have equal efficacy, although some patients may show clinical responsiveness to some drugs but not others, even at equivalent doses.

Before a neuroleptic is prescribed, evidence for pre-existing movement disorders should be sought.

Relative contraindications to using these drugs are psychotic symptoms caused by anticholinergic toxicity, intoxication with central nervous system (CNS) depressants, impaired hepatic function, severe cardiac disease or very recent myocardial infarction, and bone marrow depression or blood dyscrasia. Baseline complete blood count, liver and renal function studies, and, for patients older than 40 years, an electrocardiogram, are suggested.

It is useful to think of antipsychotics as a spectrum of drugs with low-potency agents (large doses, e.g., chlorpromazine) at one end and high-potency drugs (small doses, e.g., haloperidol) at the other. Which antipsychotic to use depends largely on the side effect profile, considered together with the patient's history of response. What was helpful for alleviating symptoms in the past? What did not work? What side effects did the patient experience and were they severe enough to result in noncompliance or force discontinuation of the medication? Therapy is best confined to the briefest course of the smallest possible dose.

Intramuscular depot forms of haloperidol and fluphenazine are available, and there is increasing evidence that these preparations reduce psychotic relapse rates and are better for refractory symptoms. It may be advantageous to measure the plasma level of any antipsychotic when response is inadequate, to document noncompliance or rapid drug metabolism.

More potent agents have more extrapyramidal side effects but fewer sedative, anticholinergic, and cardiovascular problems. This makes high-potency drugs a better choice for geriatric patients, for whom sedation and cognitive impairment are undesirable. Low-potency agents may be more helpful in sedating agitated patients, and for treating males and young patients, who are generally more susceptible to extrapyramidal reactions.

Peripheral anticholinergic side effects include decreased bronchial secretions, dry mouth with increased dental caries, impaired visual accommodation, increased pupillary size, decreased gastrointestinal motility with constipation, increased heart rate, decreased sweating, and urinary retention. The latter may respond to a trial of bethanechol, 25 to 50 mg three times a day.

Patients can develop an anticholinergic delirium

Table 1 Selected Antipsychotic Drugs and Dosages

Class, Generic, and Proprietary Name	Dose Equivalence (mg)	Commonly Prescribed Daily Dose (mg)
Phenothiazines		
Aliphatics		
Chlorpromazine (Thorazine)	100	200–1000
Triflupromazine (Vesprin)	26–35	50–200
Piperidines		
Thioridazine (Mellaril)	100	200–800
Mesoridazine (Serentil)	50–60	100–500
Piperazines		
Perphenazine (Trilafon)	8–10	8–64
Trifluoperazine (Stelazine)	3–5	5–60
Fluphenazine (Prolixin)	1–2	2–40
Fluphenazine decanoate	–	12.5–100 IM q 2–4 wk
Thioxanthenes		
Thiothixene (Navane)	2–5	10–60
Butyrophenones		
Haloperidol (Haldol)	1–3	2–60
Haloperidol decanoate	–	25–200 IM q 3–4 wk
Droperidol (Inapsine)	1–2	5–10
Dibenzoxazepines		
Loxapine (Loxitane)	10–20	50–250
Dihydroindolones		
Molindone (Moban)	6–10	20–200
Pimozide (Orap)	–	1–10
Dibenzodiazepine		
Clozapine (Clozaril)	–	50–800

characterized by disorientation, intense confusion, agitation, and visual hallucinations. Physostigmine, 1 to 2 mg IV or IM, given over several minutes, reverses the toxicity for diagnostic purposes but the improvement is not sustained. The clinician needs to consider the additive effects of prescribing neuroleptics and anticholinergic agents for extrapyramidal side effects (see below). It often helps to warn patients that they can expect anticholinergic side effects and that they indicate that the medicine is getting into their system.

Neuroleptic induced alpha-adrenergic blockade can produce orthostatic hypotension, which is frequently alleviated by dose reduction or by switching to a higher-potency drug.

Drug-related hyperprolactinemia causes amenorrhea, breast tenderness, gynecomastia and galactorrhea, all of which may respond to amantadine treatment. Sexual dysfunction—decreased libido, retrograde ejaculation, or inability to attain or maintain an erection or reach orgasm—can sometimes be eliminated by converting to a different class of medication. If weight gain is troublesome, molindone is recommended.

Neuroleptics lower the threshold for seizures and could antagonize the effects of anticonvulsants, but clinically this happens infrequently. An important exception is clozapine, which carries a much greater seizure risk, 4 to 5 percent. Fluphenazine and molindone may be less likely to aggravate seizures.

Transient leukopenia is very common and should be distinguished from rare, idiosyncratic agranulocytosis. Neuroleptic-induced hepatic dysfunction, with increases in alkaline phosphatase and bilirubin, warrants discontinuation of medication. Finally, patients should be advised to avoid intense sun exposure and to use UV skin block that contains para-aminobenzoic acid.

Clozapine

Clozapine is an atypical antipsychotic that does not decrease dopaminergic neuronal activity in the nigrostriatal system. Increasingly, clozapine is used for patients who cannot tolerate or do not respond to typical agents. Its efficacy for psychosis is thought to be superior to that of other neuroleptics. Clozapine has not been found to cause extrapyramidal or tardive syndromes. Because of a 1 to 2 percent incidence of rapidly progressive agranulocytosis, patients must have a weekly blood count and be registered with a national clozapine data bank. Further information is available from the Clozaril National Registry (800/448-5938).

INDICATIONS

The Psychotic Patient

The therapeutic goals for patients with psychiatric illness are treatment of acute psychotic decompensations and maintenance therapy to prevent psychotic relapse. Diagnoses that frequently require antipsychotic therapy include schizophrenia, schizoaffective disorder, mania or depression with psychotic features, primary delusional disorders, head injury syndromes, mental retardation with psychosis, and other brain disorders associated with delusions and hallucinations. Psychotic ideation and perceptual disturbances in patients with personality disorders also may be responsive to neuroleptics.

One approach to treatment is to start with a moderate-potency medicine like perphenazine, or the particularly inexpensive trifluoperazine. Benztropine, 0.5 to 2.0 mg twice a day, or amantadine, 100 mg twice a day, is often prescribed to minimize extrapyramidal side effects that to some patients (who may already be paranoid and delusional) can be so disturbing that they decide they are "allergic" or are being poisoned by their doctor.

For acute psychosis, small doses are used initially, and the dose is increased to moderate size over 2 to 4 weeks. For example, one might start with perphenazine, 4 to 8 mg twice a day, and increase to 8 to 15 mg twice a day or with trifluoperazine, 4 to 5 mg twice a day, increasing to 5 to 15 mg twice a day. For inadequate response, larger doses, 32 to 64 mg perphenazine or 30 to 60 mg trifluoperazine, may be necessary. If symptoms are not better by 6 to 8 weeks, the medication should be tapered off and a different class of antipsychotic used for the next trial. It is important to note that 3 to 4 weeks often must pass before improvement occurs. Large or rapid increases in dose are best avoided, because larger doses do not necessarily produce a better response. Only a small proportion of patients require very large doses (e.g., haloperidol, 100 mg per day) for a good response. Unfortunately, the ultimate dose for any individual cannot be readily predicted. Patients with a similar clinical picture may do well on a 5 mg daily dose of haloperidol or may need upwards of 100 mg.

Doses used for treatment of acute episodes are larger than those used to manage chronic symptoms. The antipsychotic can be tapered gradually over a period of several months, while the patient is carefully observed for subtle relapse signs: suspiciousness, irritability, sleep or appetite changes, agitation, or withdrawal. For maintenance the minimum necessary amount of neuroleptic is advised. In many cases adjuvant agents such as lithium, carbamazepine, or benzodiazepines may enable the patient to take smaller doses of neuroleptics.

The Acutely Agitated Patient

Patients with a metabolic encephalopathy or a focal cerebral disturbance from trauma, stroke, tumor, or infection, to name only a few conditions, can suffer from hyperkinetic delirium. Treatment is directed toward correcting the underlying problem; however, patients can benefit from the calming effect of neuroleptics, which reduce misperceptions and hallucinations. Haloperidol can be administered in doses ranging from 0.5 to 5 mg IM or IV. Young, otherwise healthy persons are usually given larger doses, whereas elderly, infirm patients are provided smaller doses, at least initially. The key aspect in management is to adjust the dose and timing of medication to the patient's condition; a fixed dosing regimen should be avoided. Once the patient's condition is stabilized, a relatively small dose of medication given once or twice daily is often sufficient to maintain the desired effect. The intensity of treatment should not lead to obtundation or coma; the need to individualize management cannot be overemphasized. As the underlying problem remits or stabilizes, the neuroleptic can often be tapered slowly and discontinued.

Patients are often encountered who have been given multiple sedating agents, often by multiple routes of administration. We recommend switching medications so that one agent is provided by a single route. Again, fixed dosing schedules should be avoided. A neuroleptic can then be used to obtain the desired calming effect without producing undue sedation.

The Chronically Agitated Patient

Patients with conditions that affect cognition, such as Alzheimer's disease, Parkinson's disease, and stroke, can be chronically confused and agitated. Hallucinations, delusions, and disordered sleep can develop. These symptoms can often be treated with small doses of neuroleptic drugs. Haloperidol, 0.5 to 1.0 mg at bedtime, can be very effective. When extrapyramidal side effects are unwanted, thioridazine, 10 to 25 mg at bedtime, can be used. Minimal doses are given at first and the dose is increased every 3 to 5 days, as needed. Not infrequently, a bedtime dose alone is not sufficient and a morning dose roughly half the size of the nighttime one can be used. Often, once the patient has been stabilized for a week or so, a smaller maintenance dose suffices. Depending on the patient's clinical course, the neuroleptic should be tapered and discontinued every few months, to determine whether drug therapy is still necessary.

Parkinson's disease is a particular challenge. Confusion, agitation, and hallucinations can be related to the underlying disease as well as to anti-Parkinson's medications. If possible, medication regimens should be adjusted to minimize drug effects. If a neuroleptic is necessary, the extrapyramidal effects of thioridazine, the most commonly used agent, may be unacceptable, in which case a trial of clozapine should be considered. Initially a dose of 6.25 mg can be given at bedtime, and the dose is then adjusted slowly and incrementally to levels as high as 400 mg daily, given in divided doses to avoid seizures. Alternate-day therapy can be tried to minimize sedation. The medication should be continued for 1 month before it is judged ineffectual. Anti-Parkinson's medications can be increased to optimize motor activity while the patient is taking clozapine. Delirious patients with other extrapyramidal disorders can also be managed with clozapine when more traditional neuroleptics have undesirable side effects.

ADVERSE EFFECTS

Acute Dystonia

Acute dystonic reactions most frequently occur within hours, days, or weeks of starting treatment, but they can also develop in the context of long-term therapy. The patient experiences sudden, uncontrollable spasms and contractions of the face, jaw, tongue, neck, head, or extraocular muscles, sometimes with oculogyric crisis. Laryngeal spasm, though rare, can impair respiration. Other manifestations include sustained dystonia of the limbs or trunk.

Treatment consists of IV, IM, or PO anticholinergics. Benztropine, 1 mg, or diphenhydramine, 50 mg, IV or IM, usually produces relief within minutes, but the effects also wear off quickly. Several injections are sometimes needed, and oral anticholinergics should then be prescribed for several days to weeks.

Parkinsonism

Neuroleptics produce a parkinsonian state in 15 to 40 percent of treated patients. Parkinsonian signs alone do no warrant treatment. When the neuroleptic-induced extrapyramidal symptoms interfere with the patient's desired activities, the neuroleptic dose should be decreased or the drug discontinued. At times, another neuroleptic that is less likely to cause extrapyramidal side effects can be used. If the patient is taking other agents that can cause a parkinsonian state, such as metoclopramide, those drug regimens should also be modified. Often, these options are not available because of underlying psychiatric or medical disorders. If symptoms persist in spite of adjustments in medications, an anticholinergic such as benztropine can be administered in progressively larger doses. Unfortunately, anticholinergic therapy can cause a host of undesirable side effects, including impaired memory, and so may not be tolerated, especially by elderly patients. If anticholinergic therapy is unsuccessful, a trial of amantadine, 100 to 300 mg daily, can be started. Another option is to give a carbidopa/levodopa preparation in progressively larger doses. There are concerns that a carbidopa/levodopa preparation might exacerbate psychosis, but usually this is not a major problem. If the neuroleptic-induced parkinsonian state is refractory to treatment, clozapine therapy should be considered.

Akathisia

Antipsychotic-induced akathisia is a state of observable motor restlessness accompanied by a sensation of unpleasant, dysphoric inner tension or anxiety. Patients often appear unable to sit still, shifting in their seats, rocking, shaking their legs, or pacing. A common error is to mistake akathisia for worsening psychosis and to increase the patient's medication. It is important to diagnose and treat akathisia aggressively, as severe cases can result in self-mutilation or suicide.

Some 20 to 40 percent of patients who take antipsychotic drugs develop akathisia, which is thought to be an extrapyramidal reaction due to dopamine blockade. Most often, it appears early in the course of treatment, but it has been known to develop after a period of years.

Though other extrapyramidal syndromes respond well to anticholinergics, akathisia frequently does not. Our first approach is to lower the antipsychotic dose. If the patient's mental status precludes this, switching to a lower-potency medicine may be beneficial. Though all commonly used neuroleptics carry an akathisia risk, its prevalence is usually greatest with high-potency agents. If changing the patient's neuroleptic protocol is ineffective, significant improvement can be obtained with benzodiazepine treatment, notably clonazepam, 0.25 to 2.0 mg twice daily. Beta-adrenergic antagonists have also been used with some degree of success. Propranolol, 20 to 160 mg per day, is the most consistently effective; certain other beta-blockers such as nadolol show little or no benefit.

The improvement seen with benzodiazepines or beta-blockers may be enhanced when these drugs are combined with anticholinergics. Certain patients derive relief from anticholinergics alone. If no relief is forthcoming, a trial of clonidine, 0.15 to 0.40 mg per day, or amantadine, 200 to 300 mg per day, is worthwhile.

Tardive Syndromes

Tardive dyskinesia is a syndrome of involuntary hyperkinetic movements involving orofacial, truncal, and limb musculature. Some 15 to 50 percent of patients treated with antipsychotics longer than 3 months develop tardive syndromes. Dyskinesias may be permanent in more than 50 to 60 percent of patients who develop them. Proposed risk factors for tardive syndromes are advanced age, large doses or prolonged treatment with neuroleptics, coexisting parkinsonism, presence of affective disorders, and pre-existing brain damage. Nonetheless, all exposed patients are at risk, and a documented discussion of this risk is indicated as soon as the patient's mental state permits. Preventive measures consist of using the smallest possible neuroleptic dose and monitoring the patient with the Abnormal Involuntary Movement Scale (AIMS).

Management of tardive dyskinesia is a challenge. Tapering off and discontinuing the antipsychotic can result in slow, gradual improvement, but can also cause temporary exacerbation (withdrawal dyskinesia). Patients who require antipsychotic drugs have several therapeutic options aimed at the postulated mechanism for tardive dyskinesia: a neuroleptic-induced reduction in gamma-aminobutyric acid (GABA) neurotransmission. Consequently, benzodiazepines, which are indirect $GABA_A$ agonists, are being utilized with excellent results. Clonazepam, 1 to 4 mg per day (up to 10 mg for some few patients), has been especially effective. Diazepam, 5 to 40 mg per day, and alprazolam, are also useful, though not as thoroughly studied. Should the antidyskinetic effects of benzodiazepines wear off, tapering and stopping these agents and subsequently restarting them often produces a robust response. The GABA-ergic drug valproic acid has not been found to be helpful.

Among the older but less efficacious treatments for tardive dyskinesia are propranolol, 60 to 180 mg per day; clonidine, 0.15 to 0.9 mg per day; and reserpine, 0.1 to 1.0 mg per day. Anticholinergics may help some patients; paradoxically, other patients may observe improvement in tardive dyskinesia when their anticholinergic is withdrawn.

Tardive dystonia is a disorder of abnormal sustained posture that follows months to years of antipsychotic drug therapy. Tardive dystonias are probably more prevalent in younger patients and may arise after relatively brief exposure to the medication. The rate of spontaneous remission is less than 5 percent. Tardive myoclonus presents as brief, involuntary, jerky contractions of the limbs, usually the arms.

Anticholinergic agents, clonazepam, and bromocriptine have been used successfully in many cases. Patients who have serious dystonic symptoms but who continue to require neuroleptics can be treated with clozapine. With clozapine, dystonias often improve and the patient is spared further risk of developing other tardive disorders.

Rabbit Syndrome

Fine, rhythmic lip movements that resemble a rabbit's chewing occur with a prevalence of 2 to 5 percent in populations treated over the long term with neuroleptics. This extrapyramidal side effect generally resolves with anticholinergic medication.

Neuroleptic Malignant Syndrome

Neuroleptic malignant syndrome (NMS) may occur at any time during the course of therapy in as many as 1 percent of persons who take neuroleptics, particularly haloperidol. Characteristic signs include marked rigidity, fever (as high as 41°C), and tachycardia. Extremes of blood pressure, tachypnea, diaphoresis, tremulousness, and impaired consciousness can occur. Elevation of the creatine phosphokinase value and leukocytosis are common. The differential diagnosis includes sepsis, meningitis or encephalitis, heat stroke, malignant hyperthermia, hyperthyroidism, tetany, tetanus, strychnine poisoning, anticholinergic drug toxicity, and lethal catatonia. With supportive treatment alone, mortality is approximately 20 percent.

Interference with dopamine neurotransmission by a neuroleptic probably leads to the rigidity, fever, and obtundation of NMS. Profound muscle contraction may also contribute to hyperthermia.

General supportive measures include withdrawal of neuroleptic and anticholinergic medications, aggressive hydration, antipyretics, use of a cooling blanket, and cardiopulmonary stabilization. Rhabdomyolysis can occur because of rigidity and tremulousness; renal dysfunction may contribute to mortality. Specific therapy often utilizes bromocriptine, a direct dopamine agonist, and dantrolene, a muscle relaxant. Patients treated with these agents, alone or in combination, may enjoy more rapid clinical improvement and a smaller risk of death (5 to 10 percent) than patients managed with supportive measures alone. Enteral bromocriptine, 2.5 to 7.5 mg every 8 hours, can improve rigidity, fever, and obtundation within a day; occasionally larger doses are required. Intravenous dantrolene, 0.8 to 3 mg/kg, every 6 hours, can help control hyperthermia and rhabdomyolysis. Amantadine and carbidopa/levodopa combinations have also been used successfully to treat NMS.

SUGGESTED READING

Factor SA, Brown D. Clozapine prevents recurrence of psychosis in Parkinson's disease. Movement Disorders 1992;7:125–131.

Fleischhacker WW, Roth S, Kure J. The pharmacologic treatment of neuroleptic-induced akathisia. J Clin Psychopharmacol 1990;10:12–21.

Hardie RJ, Lees AJ. Neuroleptic-induced Parkinson's syndrome: Clinical features and results of treatment with levodopa. J Neurol Neurosurg Psychiatry 1988;51:850–854.

National Institute of Mental Health. Abnormal involuntary movement scale. In: Guy W, ed: ECDEV Assessment Manual. Rockville, MD: U.S. Department of Health, Education, and Welfare, 1976.

Rosenberg MR, Green M. Neuroleptic malignant syndrome. Review of response to therapy. Arch Intern Med 1989;149:1927–1931.

Thaker G, Nhuyen J. Clonazepam treatment of tardive dyskinesia. Am J Psychiatry 1990;147:445–451.

STATUS EPILEPTICUS

DAVID M. TREIMAN, M.D.

Treatment of status epilepticus (SE) begins with its diagnosis. The International League Against Epilepsy in the *International Classification of Epileptic Seizures,* (1981) states, "The term 'status epilepticus' is used whenever a seizure persists for a sufficient length of time or is repeated frequently enough that recovery between attacks does not occur." Operationally, most neurologists now define SE as two or more epileptic seizures without full recovery of neurologic function between seizures or more or less continuous seizure activity lasting longer than 30 minutes. I consider a patient to be in SE if there is even slight residual impairment of neurologic function before the next seizure occurs. Furthermore, for treatment purposes I think therapy should be instituted whenever generalized convulsive seizure activity lasts more than 10 minutes. Roger Porter and his colleagues at the National Institutes of Health recently studied 123 generalized convulsions on telemetry and observed that all of the generalized tonic-clonic seizure activity lasted less than 2 minutes. Thus, when generalized convulsive activity persists longer than 2 minutes it is likely to be something other than a single, discrete seizure. A benzodiazepine (diazepam or lorazepam) can be drawn up for intravenous injection, and if the patient is still in seizure when the syringe is prepared (usually at least 10 minutes) SE can be presumed and treatment initiated.

GENERALIZED CONVULSIVE STATUS EPILEPTICUS

Generalized convulsive status epilepticus (GCSE) is the most common and most threatening form of SE. In the past, this term has been considered to apply to repeated generalized tonic-clonic or major motor convulsions without full recovery of consciousness between seizures. However, over the last decade my colleagues and I have come to recognize that GCSE is a dynamic entity that if allowed to continue without treatment or with inadequate treatment has a predictable progression of both behavioral and electrographic features. GCSE usually begins with discrete generalized tonic-clonic seizures that recur one after another without full recovery of consciousness between seizures. If status persists without adequate treatment, an electromechanical dissociation develops, so that as the patient becomes increasingly encephalopathic from the ongoing status, the convulsive activity becomes increasingly subtle, even though seizure activity in the brain continues. When the underlying cause of the episode of SE is a severe encephalopathy, only one or two generalized convulsions may occur before subtle GCSE develops. Occasionally,

the underlying encephalopathy may be so severe, as in anoxic brain damage after cardiac arrest, that the patient never does experience a generalized convulsion before subtle GCSE. Nonetheless, in my opinion such a patient should be considered to be in GCSE and should be treated as vigorously as the patient who presents with overt GCSE.

Just as there is a progression from overt to increasingly subtle motor manifestations of GCSE, we now know that there is a predictable series of progressive electroencephalogram (EEG) changes if GCSE is allowed to persist without treatment adequate to stop all electrical as well as motor activity. Initially, seizures are electrographically discrete and have characteristics similar to isolated generalized convulsions recorded on EEG. However, if GCSE is allowed to progress without treatment or with inadequate treatment, the discrete EEG seizures begin to merge together to form a waxing and waning pattern of rhythmic discharges that eventually become continuous and monomorphic. If status is not stopped, this continuous activity begins to be punctuated by flat periods, which lengthen as the ictal discharges shorten, until finally, in late SE, the EEG exhibits periodic epileptiform discharges on a relatively flat background. These EEG patterns are important, because the demonstration of any one of them in a profoundly comatose patient should lead to the diagnosis of GCSE and institution of a vigorous treatment protocol.

Approach to Treatment

I have found the protocol outlined in Table 1 to be useful in the management of GCSE. Treatment should be instituted whenever the diagnosis of GCSE can be made with confidence. For overt GCSE this usually required the observation of one additional generalized convulsion in a patient who presents with a history suggestive of GCSE. The reason for observing an additional seizure is to preclude treatment of hysterical or psychogenic seizures with potentially dangerous drugs. Of course, if a repeated seizure has been confirmed by a reliable observer, treatment should be initiated immediately. For subtle GCSE, the diagnosis is based on the demonstration of ictal EEG activity in a patient with convulsive movements so subtle that the diagnosis of GCSE cannot be made with certainty without EEG confirmation.

We manage all cases of SE with simultaneous EEG recording. However, when the diagnosis of SE can be made by clinical observation, treatment should never be delayed while awaiting the arrival of the EEG technician. In many hospitals, emergency EEG is difficult to arrange. EEG monitoring is not absolutely essential in the management of SE unless the patient fails to recover consciousness rapidly after convulsive activity has stopped. In this situation emergency EEG recording is required to verify complete cessation of ongoing electrical seizure activity. There is now abundant evidence that electrical seizure activity, even in the absence of motor convulsions, if allowed to continue during SE may cause profound neuronal damage and thus result in prolonged or permanent neurologic deficits.

Once the diagnosis of GCSE is made and the physician has ensured an adequate airway, respiratory effort, and cardiac function, blood should be drawn for hematology, serum chemistry, and antiepileptic drug concentration studies. An intravenous line should be established using normal saline, because a dextrose solution may cause phenytoin to precipitate. If hypoglycemia is a possible cause of SE, the blood glucose concentrations can be determined accurately enough by a glucose test strip after a fingerstick to decide if a bolus injection of glucose is necessary. Glucose should not be given unless there is clear evidence the patient is hypoglycemic, because hyperglycemia may exacerbate neuronal damage caused by seizure activity in the brain. If supplemental glucose is required, 100 mg of thiamine must be given first, at least to adults, to prevent the rare but devastating development of Wernicke's encephalopathy in a thiamine-deficient patient. Many adult patients who develop SE because of hypoglycemia are hypoglycemic because of chronic alcoholism and are likely also to be thiamine deficient. Ordinarily, administration of bicarbonate, even in the presence of significant acidosis, is not necessary. Once the seizure activity is controlled the serum pH normalizes rapidly.

Pharmacologic Management

Pharmacologic management of SE can be initiated with an intravenous injection of a benzodiazepine, phenytoin, or phenobarbital. I prefer lorazepam, because it can be administered quickly, it enters the brain relatively rapidly, and yet it has a prolonged duration of action against SE. Diazepam enters the brain exceedingly rapidly, but because it is extremely lipid soluble it is rapidly redistributed to body fat stores, and the serum concentration (and thus the brain concentration) falls, allowing SE to resume in 20 to 30 minutes in many cases. Lorazepam is less lipid soluble and also appears to be actively retained in the brain; thus it offers prolonged protection against SE.

SE should always be treated via intravenous injection, at least in a medical setting. Intramuscular injection should never be used to treat SE, because the rate of absorption from intramuscular sites is too slow and thus drug concentrations adequate to stop SE are rarely achieved by intramuscular injections. Rectal administration of benzodiazepines for the treatment of SE is used in Europe and is undergoing testing in this country, but is not yet accepted as a standard of care. It may be useful for preventing development of SE in children who have frequent episodes of serial seizures, which sometimes evolve into SE. Because of its prolonged duration of action against SE (at least 24 hours in our studies), if lorazepam stops SE the patient's routine antiepilepsy drug can be resumed or a new antiepilepsy drug, such as phenytoin, can be instituted in an orderly manner, perhaps even after the patient has awakened.

If SE does not stop after lorazepam, intravenous administration of phenytoin should be initiated. Ten to twenty minutes from the start of lorazepam infusion is a reasonable time to start intravenous phenytoin. All of the lorazepam will have been administered and peak brain concentration should have been achieved by 10 to 20 minutes. Phenytoin should not be given faster than 50 mg per minute. ECG and blood pressure should be monitored carefully during phenytoin infusion and the rate of infusion slowed if hypotension develops. Although some authors have advocated diluting phenytoin in 100 mg of saline solution and administering it by intravenous drip from a burette chamber, I prefer that the physician push phenytoin by syringe into the intravenous port nearest the patient and that the ECG and blood pressure be continuously monitored throughout the infusion.

If 20 mg per kilogram of phenytoin fails to stop SE, an additional 5 mg per kilogram — or if necessary, 10 mg per kilogram — should be given, because for many patients a very high concentration (30 to 40 μg per milliliter) is necessary to stop ongoing SE, particularly when it fails to respond initially to intravenous lorazepam. In my experience, 50 percent of patients who fail initial lorazepam treatment subsequently respond to phenytoin.

If phenytoin is not successful, phenobarbital should be given. Because the patient already has been given a benzodiazepine, respiratory status must be observed closely and the physician should be prepared to provide respiratory assistance, including endotracheal intubation if necessary. The addition of phenobarbital is likely to be effective at stopping SE in 40 percent of the patients who require a third drug. Intravenous paraldehyde, in a 4 percent saline solution, was, until recently, a good alternative to phenobarbital at this stage of the treatment of refractory status. Unfortunately, at the present time paraldehyde is not available in the United States for parenteral administration. Intramuscular injection causes sterile abscesses, and rectal administration results in variable absorption.

REFRACTORY STATUS EPILEPTICUS

A small number of patients with truly refractory SE who fail to respond to triple therapy, require general anesthesia sufficient to eliminate all epileptiform activity on the EEG. This is best accomplished by barbiturate coma induced by intravenous administration of additional phenobarbital sufficient to suppress all epileptiform activity or by thiopental or pentobarbital. We have used pentobarbital successfully to manage refractory GCSE, using initial doses outlined in Table 1. Although most authors have called for the achievement of a burst suppression pattern on the EEG, in my opinion it is necessary only to suppress all epileptiform activity on the EEG. Failure to do so inevitably leads to recurrence of the ictal pattern when the rate of pentobarbital infusion is slowed. Barbiturate coma may cause significant

Table 1 Treatment Protocol for Generalized Convulsive Status Epilepticus

Time (min)	Treatment Protocol
0	Make the diagnosis by observing one additional seizure in a patient with a history of recent seizures or impaired consciousness or by observing continuous seizure activity for more than 10 minutes.
	Call EEG technician and start EEG as soon as possible, but do not delay treatment while waiting for the EEG unless necessary to verify diagnosis.
5	Establish intravenous catheter with normal saline (dextrose solutions may precipitate phenytoin).
	Draw blood for serum chemistry and hematology studies and antiepilepsy drug concentrations. If hypoglycemia is suspected confirm by fingerstick, then administer 100 mg thiamine followed by 50 ml of 50 percent dextrose by direct push into the intravenous line.
10	Administer lorazepam, 0.1 mg/kg by intravenous push (< 2 mg/min).
25	If status does not stop, start phenytoin, 20 mg/kg by slow intravenous push (< 50 mg/min), directly into intravenous port closest to patient. Monitor blood pressure and electrocardiogram closely during infusion.
	If status does not stop after 20 mg/kg phenytoin, give an additional 5 mg/kg and, if necessary, another 5 mg/kg, to a maximum dose of 30 mg/kg.
60	If status persists, consider intubation before giving phenobarbital, 20 mg/kg, by intravenous push (< 100 mg/min).
90	If status persists, start barbiturate coma. Either administer more phenobarbital or give pentobarbital, 5 mg/kg, slowly as initial intravenous dose to suppress all epileptiform activity. Continue 0.5–2 mg/kg/hr to maintain EEG suppression. Slow rate of infusion periodically to see if seizures have stopped. Monitor blood pressure, electrocardiogram, and respiratory function closely.

hypotension and the use of pressor agents may be necessary.

It has become increasing clear that the longer SE persists and the later the EEG stage the more difficult it is to stop. Most patients with discrete electrographic seizures on their EEG are responsive to one or more drugs for the treatment of SE, whereas, in our experience, fewer than one-third of patients with a periodic epileptiform pattern on the EEG can have epileptiform activity completely eliminated. Furthermore, the prognosis for patients in SE is largely dependent on the underlying cause. More than two-thirds of patients who present initially with subtle generalized SE die before discharge after an episode of subtle GCSE (SGCSE). This high mortality rate is discouraging, but because one-third of patients who present in late SE with periodic epileptiform discharges on the EEG respond to treatment and one-third of patients who present with SGCSE recover sufficiently to leave the hospital, I continue to be very aggressive in my treatment of all patients with either overt or subtle GCSE.

FOLLOW-UP

When patients do recover from an episode of GCSE I consider it appropriate to continue antiepilepsy therapy. If the patient had known epilepsy and developed SE because of low antiepilepsy drug concentrations I prescribe the antiepilepsy drug again. If SE developed in the presence of the maximum tolerated concentration of the drug, I consider *adding* another antiepilepsy drug or *switching to* a different one.

Sometimes it is necessary to administer a "miniload" of a drug after SE has been successfully treated. This is most common when phenytoin is being used to provide protection against recurrence of SE. The size of the miniload can be easily calculated, because for most antiepilepsy drugs the volume of distribution is close to 1 L per kilogram. For a drug with a volume of distribution of approximately 1 L per kilogram a rule of thumb close enough for clinical purposes is that the loading dose in milligrams per kilogram is equal to the desired increase in serum concentration in micrograms per milliliter. Thus, if a patient is found the day after an episode of SE to have a phenytoin level of 12 μg per milliliter and the physician wishes to maintain the phenytoin at 20 μg per milliliter, the miniload dose required is 8 mg per kilogram.

After successful treatment it is also important to evaluate the patient for the cause of the episode of SE. The nature and extent of the evaluation depend on the circumstances of the individual case. If the episode of SE is the first occurrence of seizure activity in an otherwise healthy patient, a thorough evaluation for a precipitating cause such as brain tumor or arteriovenous malformation is essential. If the episode of SE is a complication of an ongoing medical disease, then further evaluation depends on known complications of that condition that can cause SE (e.g., infection, cerebrovascular compromise, metabolic encephalopathy). If the episode occurs in a patient with known epilepsy then the reason for the episode of SE must be considered.

TREATMENT OF OTHER TYPES OF STATUS EPILEPTICUS

This discussion of the treatment of SE has focused on the treatment of GCSE. However, the protocol that has been presented is equally appropriate for the treatment of complex partial SE, particularly if such an episode has been allowed to persist for some time before vigorous therapy is started and the impairment of the patient's contact with the environment is significant. A number of cases of prolonged complex partial SE have been reported that have resulted in long-term neurologic deficits. In these cases, it is likely the neurologic impairment would not have occurred had the episode of SE been treated rapidly and successfully.

The proper treatment of spike wave stupor (absence SE) and simple partial SE is far less clear. Certainly, spike wave stupor should be treated early and aggressively with benzodiazepines. However, because drugs such as phenytoin and phenobarbital may exacerbate primary generalized seizures it is not clear that such drugs should be used in the rare refractory case of spike wave stupor. Valproate may be a better choice in this situation, especially when the parenteral form becomes available. Simple partial SE, because it is cortical in its localization, should respond to benzodiazepines, phenytoin, or barbiturates, though by definition such patients have no impairment of consciousness. Phenytoin, if necessary, in very large doses, is the treatment of choice for simple partial SE. Benzodiazepines or barbiturates ordinarily should not be used for simple partial SE because it is undesirable, and usually contraindicated, to make a conscious patient comatose.

The protocol described in this chapter is based on my clinical experience and what is written about the treatment of SE in the medical literature. However, at present there are insufficient data on which to base a truly rational selection of one treatment regimen over another for the initial management of GCSE. This is why I have initiated a nationwide DVA Cooperative Study to compare four treatments (phenytoin, diazepam followed by phenytoin, lorazepam, phenobarbital) in the initial management of GCSE. When that study is completed, it may be that my approach to the treatment of SE will be substantially modified.

SUGGESTED READING

Delgado-Escueta AV, Wasterlain C, Treiman DM, Porter RJ, eds. Advances in neurology. Vol 34. Status epilepticus. New York: Raven, 1983.

Treiman DM. General principles of treatment: Responsive and intractable status epilepticus in adults. In: Delgado-Escueta AV, Wasterlain C, Treiman DM, Porter RJ, eds. Advances in neurology. Vol 34. Status Epilepticus. New York: Raven, 1983:377.

Treiman DM. Pharmacokinetics and clinical use of benzodiazepines in the management of status epilepticus. Epilepsia 1989; 30(suppl 2):S4–S10.

Treiman DM. Status epilepticus. In: Resor SR Jr, Kutt H, eds. The medical treatment of epilepsy. New York: Marcel Dekker, 1992.

Treiman DM, Walton NY, Kendrick C. A progressive sequence of electroencephalographic changes during generalized convulsive status epilepticus. Epilepsy Res 1990; 5:49–60.

RECURRENT GENERALIZED AND PARTIAL SEIZURES

GREGORY KENT BERGEY, M.D.

After a full evaluation, the decision to treat epileptic seizures is based on several factors. If seizures are recurrent or if the evaluation suggests a propensity to recur (e.g., a prominent focal abnormality on electroencephalography [EEG]), treatment is usually indicated, at least for some time. If, however, the cause of the seizure or seizures is self-limited (e.g., hypoglycemia, posttraumatic impact seizures, alcohol withdrawal) antiepileptic treatment may not be indicated. Indeed, perhaps 10 percent of the population experience a single seizure during their lifetime, whereas only 1 to 2 percent of the population have the diagnosis of epilepsy, with recurrent seizures.

SEIZURE CLASSIFICATION AND EVALUATION

There are classifications of seizure types and classifications of epilepsies. The seizure type is defined by the patient's behavior during the event and by the associated EEG pattern. Epileptic syndromes include other factors, such as the natural history, genetics (if known), ictal and interictal EEG patterns, and response

Table 1 Classification of Epileptic Seizures

Partial seizures (seizures that begin locally)
  Simple partial (preserved consciousness)
  Complex partial (altered consciousness)
  Secondarily generalized (simple or complex seizures that spread to bilateral involvement)

Generalized seizures (generalized from onset)
  Tonic-clonic
  Tonic
  Clonic
  Myoclonic
  Absence
  Atonic
  Myoclonic

Modified from the 1981 International League Against Epilepsy Classification Epilepsia 1981; 22:489–501; with permission.

to medications, and provide for a much more specific classification of some episodes. Appreciation of the shorter classification of seizure types (Table 1) allows physicians to treat the great majority of their patients appropriately. With a few exceptions (juvenile myoclonic epilepsy, benign rolandic seizures of childhood) that should be recognized, most of the epileptic syndromes fall more appropriately into the purview of the epileptologist, who sees patients whose seizures are difficult to diagnose or to manage. Accurate classification of the type of seizures a patient is experiencing is the keystone to determining appropriate therapy.

Simple partial seizures do not produce alteration of consciousness. The clinical manifestations reflect which region of the brain is affected. Focal motor seizures are the most commonly recognized simple partial seizures, but focal seizures originating from sensory, visual, or other cortical regions also occur. The aura preceding a complex partial seizure is one type of simple partial seizure.

Complex partial seizures, previously referred to as psychomotor or temporal lobe seizures, can originate from frontal, parietal, or (in the majority of instances) temporal lobe regions. Complex partial seizures are nonconvulsive seizures that produce alteration of consciousness. These seizures can be some of the more difficult seizures to diagnose, because of their complex symptoms and broad range of manifestations. Complex partial seizures may be confused with absence (petit mal) seizures because of the presence of a prominent stare and their nonconvulsive nature. The presence of an aura and a postictal state in the complex partial seizure may be important differentiating points.

Any partial seizure may generalize secondarily. Primary generalized seizures, however, are seizures that appear (clinically and on EEG) to begin bilaterally, affecting both sides of the brain simultaneously. Despite this similar bilateral involvement, the various primary generalized seizure types have widely different clinical manifestations, from the brief nonconvulsive staring of absence seizures to the dramatic drop attacks of atonic seizures or the generalized motor manifestations of tonic-clonic seizures.

Because the cause of a seizure disorder can have important treatment implications, full evaluation of all patients with seizure disorders is warranted. This evaluation includes a careful history (including use of medications, alcohol, and drugs) and a general and a neurologic examination and general blood chemistry studies. If a central nervous system infection (viral or bacterial) or inflammation (vasculitis) is suspected, lumbar puncture should be performed, (after a neuroimaging study, if there are focal findings or significant alteration of consciousness). While computed tomography (CT) is often the emergency imaging study performed, magnetic resonance imaging (MRI) is the neuroimaging procedure of choice for evaluation of new-onset partial or generalized seizures. MRI may detect as many as three times as many lesions (many of them static) in patients whose complex partial seizures originate from the temporal lobe regions. Patients with absence seizures may not require neuroimaging studies.

The EEG remains an important component of the evaluation of a seizure disorder, assisting in the diagnosis and classification. Only 70 to 80 percent of patients with known epilepsy have abnormal interictal EEG results. Therefore, if the EEG is normal, it is quite appropriate to begin therapy based on a good history of recurrent seizures.

There are other seizures that may not require antiepileptic drug (AED) treatment. Uncomplicated febrile seizures, benign familial neonatal seizures, occipital seizures, and some benign rolandic seizures of childhood may not require treatment. Absence seizures and myoclonic seizures characteristically recur, and

partial seizures (simple and complex) are usually also recurrent. Most seizures recur within the first year. If a person has a single generalized tonic-clonic seizure and the evaluation findings (neurologic examination, EEG, MRI) are all unremarkable, the chance for a recurrence in the next 2 to 5 years may be as small as 15 to 30 percent. For this reason, many neurologists do not treat a single idiopathic tonic-clonic seizure in children, or in many adults, although in the adult population treatment decisions may need to be individualized because of social and vocational considerations. If the decision is made to treat a single seizure in a person with a negative evaluation, these patients should be candidates for trials off medication if they remain seizure free.

PRINCIPLES OF ANTIEPILEPTIC DRUG THERAPY

The principles of AED therapy for recurrent seizures are several. First and foremost is accurate determination of the seizure type. A single antiepileptic medication should be selected for initial therapy; polypharmacy should be reserved for seizures that are refractory to a single medication. The use of sedative AEDs (phenobarbital, primidone, benzodiazepines) should be restricted, if possible. Seizure frequency should be monitored carefully; a patient diary is often very helpful. Acute and chronic drug toxicity should be minimized. AEDs should be withdrawn gradually, to avoid rebound seizures unless the situation (e.g., a severe allergic reaction) dictates otherwise. The goal of treatment is the fewest seizures on the smallest amount of medication.

The most important factors in selection of an AED for a specific seizure type are efficacy and safety (Table 2). Other factors of less importance are dosing requirements, need for monitoring, side effect profile, and cost. The two Veterans Administration (VA) co-operative studies published in 1985 and 1992 provide some of the most relevant data for the treatment of partial and secondarily generalized tonic-clonic seizures. In the first of these studies, carbamazepine and phenytoin were found to be the preferred agents for treatment of partial seizures (simple and complex). Carbamazepine, phenytoin, and phenobarbital were equally efficacious in the treatment of secondarily generalized seizures; primidone was less successful principally because of increased side effects. In the most recent VA co-operative study, valproate was compared with carbamazepine. Both agents were equally effective in the treatment of secondarily generalized seizures, but carbamazepine (and phenytoin by inference from the first VA study) was more efficacious than valproate (which was effective) in the treatment of complex partial seizures.

Primary generalized tonic-clonic seizures are readily controlled in perhaps 80 percent of patients. The selection of medication is based on dosing requirements and side effect profiles. Primary generalized absence seizures are best treated with either ethosuximide or valproate. If the patient has associated tonic-clonic seizures or myoclonic seizures, valproate is clearly

Table 2 Antiepileptic Drugs of Choice for Specific Seizure Types*

Partial Seizures (Simple and Complex)	Secondary Generalized Tonic-Clonic Seizures	Primary Generalized Tonic-Clonic Seizures	Primary Generalized Absence Seizures	Myoclonic Seizures
Carbamazepine	Carbamazepine	Carbamazepine	Ethosuximide	Valproate
Phenytoin	Phenytoin	Phenytoin	Valproate†	
	Valproate	Valproate		Clonazepam
Valproate			Clonazepam	
	Phenobarbital	Phenobarbital		
Phenobarbital				
Primidone	Primidone	Primidone		

*AEDs are listed in order of general preference based on efficacy and side effects. AEDs listed together are roughly equivalent; the specific medication for a given patient should be chosen based on the patient profile. Sedative AEDs of equal efficacy are listed below those AEDs that are generally less sedating. Not all AEDs listed are FDA approved for the specific seizure types.

†Valproate is first choice when primary generalized absence seizures coexist with primary generalized tonic-clonic seizures.

preferred, because ethosuximide has no significant effect on tonic-clonic seizures and is not as effective for myoclonic seizures. Indeed, in any epileptic syndrome that includes myoclonic seizures, valproate is usually the agent of first choice.

PHARMACOKINETICS OF ANTIEPILEPTIC DRUGS

An understanding of the pharmacokinetics of the various AEDs is helpful in administering them (Table 3). Their half-lives are dramatically different. These AED half-lives determine both dosing requirements and the time to steady-state kinetics after a medication adjustment. It takes five half-lives to reach a new steady state in the blood. While in the case of valproate or phenytoin this may be only days, with phenobarbital it takes 3 weeks. AED blood levels drawn before the new steady state is achieved are of little value and can be misleading.

The AED half-lives determine the dosing regimen. Because of its very long half-life, phenobarbital can be given once a day. In readily controlled patients the proprietary sustained-release preparation of phenytoin (Dilantin) can also often be given once daily; if seizures are not totally controlled, twice daily dosing is preferred. Generic phenytoin is not a sustained-release preparation and three times daily dosing is recommended. Primidone, carbamazepine, and valproate generally require three times daily dosing to provide relatively steady serum levels. When higher doses are used, four times dosing is sometimes advantageous, to avoid transient dose-related toxicity, realizing that as dosing becomes more frequent, compliance may suffer. The proprietary form of carbamazepine (Tegretol) and the enteric coated divalproex sodium (Depakote) tend to be absorbed more gradually than generic carbamazepine or valproic acid (generic or Depakene). This may allow twice daily dosing in readily controlled patients where variability of blood levels may not be critical, a particular advantage for school children to avoid mid-day dosing. The enteric coated valproate preparation (Depakote), although originally touted as a sustained-release preparation, may only have delayed rather than prolonged

absorption in many patients, so three or four times daily dosing may be required. The proprietary "sprinkle preparation" acts more as a sustained-release form, allowing twice daily dosing more frequently. Ethosuximide can be given twice daily.

INSTITUTING ANTIEPILEPTIC THERAPY

It is important to avoid initial drug toxicity. A loading dose of phenytoin can be given orally or intravenously and be well tolerated. Generally, phenobarbital and valproate are first given in low maintenance doses, although in some cases valproate can be given in larger doses. Higher initial doses of phenobarbital cause significant sedation. Both primidone and carbamazepine must usually be started in very low doses, typically a single tablet, and gradually increased every 3 to 4 days to avoid side effects. This is required for carbamazepine, because the half-life is much longer initially; autoinduction takes several weeks. Patients often say they have been given a trial of carbamazepine or primidone and could not tolerate them when they were started on a full maintenance dose.

ANTIEPILEPTIC DRUG LEVELS

Therapeutic drug levels (see Table 3) are designed to be guides to ranges that, in theory, provide a good chance for reducing or controlling seizures while avoiding dose-related AED side effects. In actuality these levels are somewhat arbitrary and should be individualized for the given patient. There are patients whose seizures are well-controlled at levels below the therapeutic range; there is usually little need to increase their medication unless they have additional seizures. There are also patients who clearly benefit from levels above the therapeutic range. Indeed, in attempting to control patients with monotherapy whenever possible, it is reasonable to increase the dose of nonsedating AEDs (carbamazepine, phenytoin, valproate) to such levels (e.g., 100 to 150 μg per milliliter for valproate; 20 to 25 μg per milliliter for phenytoin; 12 to 14 μg per milliliter

Table 3 Pharmacokinetics of Common Antiepileptic Drugs

Drug	Half-Life (hr)	Therapeutic Range (μg/ml)	Usual Frequency of Dosing (per day)	Usual Daily Doses (mg/kg)
Carbamazepine	10–35*	4–12	3–4	10–20
Ethosuximide	30–60	40–100	1–2	15–30
Phenobarbital	80–120	10–35	1–3	1.5–3
Phenytoin	10–35†	10–20	1–3	4–7
Primidone	6–12	5–12	3–4	10–20
Valproate	8–12	50–100	2–4	15–30

*Longer half-life at initiation of therapy before autoinduction.
†Half-life is concentration dependent; higher levels may inhibit metabolism.

for carbamazepine) if they are tolerated without significant toxicity.

All of the AEDs except phenytoin obey first-order kinetics. Therefore with each dose increment there is a relatively proportional increase in the blood level. Phenytoin's kinetics are nonlinear: with further dose increments there are progressively greater, nonproportional increases in blood levels. This has important implications for clinical practice. If a patient has a low blood level (e.g., 5 μg per milliliter) increments of 100 mg per day can be added with little risk of toxicity. When titrations of dose are made in the therapeutic window (10 to 20 μg per milliliter), they should be made with the 30 mg capsules; adding a 100 mg capsule can risk toxicity if the patient has a steep, nonlinear dose-response curve. Titrations of phenytoin should be made with preparations that have similar kinetics; only the proprietary 100 mg and 30 mg capsules (Dilantin) are sustained-release preparations. The proprietary 50 mg tablets (Infatabs) and generic phenytoin are both prompt-release preparations.

AED levels are helpful in guiding adjustments in the refractory patient, when toxicity is suspected, to monitor compliance, and when interacting medications are prescribed concurrently. Often, however, AED levels (typical cost $35 to $40 per assay) are obtained more frequently than is necessary. There is little to be gained from obtaining quarterly AED levels on a well-controlled patient who continues to require medication and is experiencing no signs of toxicity. Similarly, much of the frequent random laboratory screening for hepatic or hematologic abnormalities (e.g., monthly CBCs and LFTs) produced by AEDs does little to increase the detection rate of these rare complications above that provided by the patients' histories combined with indicated or occasional blood screening.

BENEFITS OF MONOTHERAPY

In the past it was popular to begin patients with seizure disorders (especially generalized tonic-clonic seizures) on two AEDs (typically phenytoin and phenobarbital). The theory behind this treatment was to maximize the chance of preventing subsequent seizures by employing multiple agents with different mechanisms

Table 4 Antiepileptic Drug Interactions

Interacting AED	Affected AED	Change in AED Level
Carbamazepine	Phenytoin	Higher
	Valproate	Lower
Phenobarbital	Phenytoin	Lower
	Valproate	Lower
	Carbamazepine	Lower
Phenytoin	Carbamazepine	Lower
	Valproate	Lower
	Phenobarbital	Variable
Valproate	Carbamazepine	Higher epoxide
	Phenobarbital	Higher
	Phenytoin	Higher free

of action. Though some patients with seizures that are refractory to a single agent can benefit from the addition of a second or even a third AED, probably no more than 50 percent of patients actually have fewer seizures following the addition of a second AED. Polypharmacy typically results in increased side effects, more pills, increased cost, and poorer compliance. Therefore, the improvement with polypharmacy should be documented. Too often, patients are given multiple medications that increase toxicity and provide questionable benefit. Such patients may benefit from switching to monotherapy, reporting fewer side effects and no increase in seizure frequency.

All of the AEDs interact with each other (Table 4), complicating multiple drug regimens. Most of these interactions result in lower drug levels. The exception is polypharmacy with valproate. Valproate increases the phenobarbital level, sometimes dramatically. If the steady state level of phenobarbital is at or near toxicity, reducing the dose by one-third with the institution of valproate cotherapy is appropriate. Valproate also increases the amount of the carbamazepine epoxide metabolite; this may result in increased toxicity that is not apparent in routine AED levels. One of the most common interactions is that between valproate and phenytoin. Both valproate and phenytoin are highly protein bound (in the range of 90 percent), and cotherapy results in displacement with increased free fractions of each but often little change in total serum

Table 5 Common Side Effects of Antiepileptic Drugs

Drug	Side Effect
Carbamazepine	Double or blurred vision, vertigo, gastrointestinal upset, diarrhea
Phenobarbital	Sedation/lethargy, cognitive impairment, behavioral changes, hyperactivity, nystagmus, ataxia
Phenytoin	Nystagmus, cosmetic changes, gingival hyperplasia, ataxia
Valproate	Gastrointestinal upset, weight gain, hair loss, tremor

Table 6 Rare Side Effects of Antiepileptic Drugs

Drug	Side Effect
Carbamazepine	Aplastic anemia, agranulocytosis, thrombocytopenia, hepatitis, syndrome of inappropriate secretion of antidiuretic hormone, Stevens-Johnson syndrome, pancreatitis
Phenobarbital	Agranulocytosis, hepatitis, aplastic anemia, Stevens-Johnson syndrome
Phenytoin	Agranulocytosis, aplastic anemia, hepatitis, hypocalcemia, peripheral neuropathy, pseudolymphoma, Stevens-Johnson syndrome
Valproate	Hepatitis, pancreatitis, platelet dysfunction, thrombocytopenia, agranulocytosis, aplastic anemia, Stevens-Johnson syndrome

concentrations. Therefore, patients may show signs of phenytoin toxicity after the addition of valproate cotherapy, yet the total phenytoin levels may be relatively unchanged and still be in the therapeutic range. Because of the displacement by valproate, the free fraction of phenytoin increases and signs of toxicity become manifest. Although free drug fractions are now readily available, recognition of this interaction may be sufficient to guide alterations in therapy. Increased free phenytoin is also seen in renal failure, other hypoproteinemic states, and pregnancy.

SIDE EFFECTS OF ANTIEPILEPTIC DRUGS

All medications have potential side effects, and AEDs are no exception (Tables 5 and 6). Side effects can be classified as acute or transient (see above), dose-related, cognitive, idiosyncratic, or teratogenic. Dose-related side effects can be reduced by reducing the dose; these may occur in some patients even when levels are "therapeutic," particularly if polypharmacy is being used. Cognitive side effects are some of the most important long-term considerations. Various recent analyses controlling for drug levels suggest that carbamazepine, phenytoin, and valproate all have similar effects on cognitive function and these effects are generally less profound than those produced by the sedative antiepi-

leptics, phenobarbital, primidone, and the benzodiazepines.

Idiosyncratic drug side effects, although generally rare, can be important. Aplastic anemia and agranulocytosis can be produced by any of the antiepileptic drugs, although carbamazepine may be associated with a slightly higher incidence of these very rare blood dyscrasias. Even with carbamazepine, the risk of aplastic anemia is only about 1 in 200,000 per year or 1 in 50,000 to 1 in 100,000 for long-term therapy (the incidence of agranulocytosis is even lower). The role of routine blood counts in predicting these dyscrasias in asymptomatic persons is not established; the commonly seen mild to moderate reductions in total white cell counts seen with carbamazepine therapy do not predict the more severe reactions.

Although valproate has been associated with fatal hepatotoxicity, recent analyses now indicate that age and polytherapy are important determining factors. Indeed, for a teenager or adult taking valproate monotherapy the risk of hepatotoxicity is extremely small (<1 in 200,000), and even polypharmacy increases the risk only to 1 in 40,000. Conversely, for infants younger than 2 years taking polypharmacy the risk approaches 1 in 600. This susceptibility may reflect either enzyme or cofactor deficiencies that have yet to be fully elucidated. The hepatotoxicity with valproate generally occurs in the first 6 months of therapy. Slight, transient elevations (less than threefold) in liver function tests following initiation of valproate therapy are not uncommon and do not require discontinuation of the medication.

Although a full discussion of the use of AEDs during pregnancy is beyond the scope of this chapter, prescription of antiepileptic medication for a female of childbearing age needs to anticipate future pregnancies. The antiabsence drug trimethadione is the one known highly teratogenic agent. Other AEDs generally increase the risk of fetal malformations only slightly (i.e., several percent over control value), and many malformations are relatively minor (e.g., nail hypoplasia). Polypharmacy increases the risk of malformations. Neural tube defects, one of the more serious malformations, may occur in 1 to 2 percent of infants of mothers taking valproate and perhaps as many as 0.9 percent of mothers on carbamazepine. Although amniocentesis (checking for elevated level of alpha-fetoprotein) detects virtually all these malformations, simple screening with a combination of measurements of maternal serum alpha-fetoprotein and sophisticated level-two ultrasonography at about 20 weeks' gestation can reduce the risk of an undetected neural tube defect to about 1 in 1000 to 1 in 1500 (the risk in control populations) if these two test results are unremarkable. Folate has been shown to reduce the incidence of non–drug related neural tube defects and should be given before conception to women taking AEDs. Whenever possible, it is wise to anticipate pregnancy and minimize AED polypharmacy. It is desirable to have the lowest drug level necessary to control seizures, particularly in the important, formative first trimester. Some nonconvulsive seizures, particularly simple partial seizures, can often be tolerated during pregnancy, as the risk to the fetus is much less than with convulsive seizures.

GENERIC PREPARATIONS

Generic preparations are available for most of the major AEDs. Theoretically, generic preparations provide bioequivalency between ±20 percent of the proprietary formulations. Unfortunately, some epileptic patients may be sensitive to these fluctuations and experience breakthrough seizures. The generic AED situation has been further confounded by drug recalls, multiple sourcing, anecdotal reports of drug failures, and incomplete or overtly fraudulent bioequivalency testing. Phenobarbital is the one universally acceptable generic preparation. No generic preparations exist for the proprietary enteric coated divalproex sodium preparation (Depakote) or for the proprietary sustained-release phenytoin (Dilantin); generic phenytoin preparations are all prompt acting. Generic preparations may cost one-third to one-half what proprietary forms do (although sometimes the differences are much less), but these savings are eliminated if the patient requires more frequent blood monitoring or emergency visits. Equivalent generic preparations can be used appropriately in selected patients with well-controlled seizures; preparations from a single manufacturer are preferred.

REFRACTORY SEIZURES

Approximately 80 percent of patients with primary generalized seizures achieve control of their seizures with AED therapy. This success rate drops to about 50 percent for patients with partial seizures and below 30 percent for some of the complicated epileptic syndromes such as Lennox-Gastaut. Whenever seizures are not controlled, it is important to review the history. Is the classification of the seizure type appropriate? Sometimes prolonged or video EEG monitoring of actual seizures can provide clarification of a difficult diagnosis. Indeed, 10 to 40 percent of all patients referred to major epilepsy centers with the diagnosis of refractory epilepsy are found to have nonepileptic events (see the chapter on *Pseudoepileptic and Psychogenic Seizures*). AED levels, dosing, and combinations should be carefully reviewed. Interacting medications or substances (e.g., alcohol) should be identified. Sequential trials of the various antiepileptic agents should be tried alone and in combination, with each agent increased to the point of maximum benefit or early toxicity. Sometimes it is a benefit to try some less frequently used AED (clorazepate, methsuximide, ethotoin, acetazolamide, methylphenobarbital), but usually these agents are more toxic and offer little additional benefit for refractory seizures. Fortunately, in the next decade a number of new agents currently in the latter stages of testing should become available. The physician should keep in mind that although an occasional seizure (particularly nonconvulsive) may not compromise the life of an institutionalized patient, even one or two complex partial seizures per year may keep an active young adult from having a driver's license. For many patients whose seizures remain refractory to medical therapy, surgical treatment (particularly of partial epilepsy) is now a more common and earlier alternative consideration (see the chapter *Complex Partial Seizures* in this volume).

DISCONTINUATION OF MEDICATION

Just as the first goal of treatment of epilepsy should be seizure control, the physician should be regularly reassessing the need for continued AED therapy. Some childhood epilepsies may remit in adolescence. About 75 percent of patients with absence seizures have no more seizures after becoming adults. Benign rolandic seizures of childhood, as the name implies, universally remit by the early to mid-teenage years, and these former patients have no increased risk of subsequent epilepsy. Similarly, idiopathic generalized tonic-clonic seizures in children and adults may remit. Seizures occurring in the setting of some acute cerebral insults (e.g., trauma, infection, subarachnoid hemorrhage) may not recur, particularly if there is no residual brain damage. For instance, only 25 percent of people who experience early post-traumatic seizures in the first week after head trauma develop late post-traumatic epilepsy.

Patients who have persistently abnormal EEG studies (particularly if epileptogenic) have a much greater risk of seizure recurrence when medications are discontinued. The symptomatic epilepsies (i.e., those in patients with structural lesions) are less likely to remit. Patients who have been seizure free for 2 years or more and who have normal interictal EEGs are the best candidates for withdrawal of medication. For children who have had few seizures, are neurologically normal, and fulfill these criteria, the risk of relapse may be as low as about 10 percent. One important exception to these criteria is patients with juvenile myoclonic epilepsy. Their seizures are often readily controlled, and their EEGs frequently normalize with therapy. Nevertheless, 80 percent of them suffer a relapse, and long-term therapy typically is required.

AEDs should be withdrawn slowly, typically over weeks to months. During the withdrawal period, the patient should reduce or minimize activities that might be dangerous (e.g., driving) should the seizures recur. For some patients, particularly those with symptomatic epilepsy, the risk of recurrence may be great enough (approaching or exceeding 50 percent) to warrant continuation of medication. Some other patients in more favorable categories may also be unwilling to accept even the small risk of seizure recurrence if they stop taking medication.

SUGGESTED READING

Engel JE Jr. Seizures and epilepsy. Philadelphia: FA Davis, 1989.

Levy RH, Dreifuss FE, Mattson RH, et al, eds. Antiepileptic drugs. New York: Raven, 1989.

Mattson RH, Cramer JA, Collins JF, et al. Comparison of carbamazepine, phenobarbital, phenytoin, and primidone in partial and secondarily generalized tonic-clonic seizures. N Engl J Med 1985; 313:145–151.

Mattson RH, Cramer JA, Collins JF, et al. A comparison of valproate with carbamazepine for the treatment of complex partial seizures and secondarily generalized tonic-clonic seizures in adults. N Engl J Med 1992; 327:765–771.

PATIENT RESOURCE

Epilepsy Foundation of America
National Epilepsy Library
4351 Garden City Drive
Landover, Maryland 20785
Telephone: (800) EFA-4050

COMPLEX PARTIAL SEIZURES

GREGORY L. KRAUSS, M.D.

In most cases, complex partial seizures (CPS) are relatively easy to control. In about 30 percent of patients, however, seizures are difficult to control, and careful manipulation of anticonvulsants is necessary to avoid side effects. The treatment of CPS is similar to that of simple partial and secondarily generalized seizures, but it may differ from treatment for primary generalized epilepsy and other epilepsy syndromes. CPS are partial seizures (due to focal ictal discharges) that produce alterations in awareness. CPS usually involve the temporal or frontal lobes, although they may originate in other brain regions.

TREATMENT

A sequence of steps can be followed in treating CPS.

Carefully establish the diagnosis of CPS. Observers' reports are very useful in establishing a history of recurring, brief confusional spells, often accompanied by motor automatisms (fumbling, blinking, lip movements) and mild clonic limb movements. Common alternate diagnoses are psychogenic seizures and anxiety or hyperventilation attacks, migraines, vertigo, intoxication states, and syncope. Focal epileptiform activity on a routine electroencephalography (EEG) study helps confirm the diagnosis of CPS, although a normal interictal EEG does not rule out the diagnosis. Repeated or prolonged outpatient EEGs may increase the yield in detecting epileptiform activity when the diagnosis is in doubt.

Begin treatment with first-line anticonvulsants for CPS, carbamazepine and phenytoin. Valproic acid is effective for CPS, though, compared to first-line agents, it more frequently produces side effects such as nausea, weight gain, and tremor. Phenobarbital and primidone are useful second-line agents, but they are slightly less effective than other partial seizure medications and may produce sedation. I prefer carbamazepine over phenytoin for treating children and young women because of the risks of gingival hypertrophy and cosmetic side effects with phenytoin therapy.

For patients whose seizures are infrequent, begin anticonvulsants at small doses, in order to minimize "adjustment" side effects. These include sedation, imbalance, dizziness and diplopia, toxicity symptoms that may occur with large doses but that also occur when anticonvulsant therapy is instituted or the dose is increased.

I ask patients to call promptly if they develop severe side effects or if after several days milder intoxication symptoms do not subside. If they are not warned of adjustment side-effects, many patients discontinue anticonvulsants after only several days.

Adjustment side effects can usually be dealt with by decreasing doses for 1 or 2 days and then attempting very gradual dose increases. If severe symptoms do not improve after several days despite small doses of medication, or if mild intoxication symptoms persist several weeks, I usually switch to another anticonvulsant. It is sometimes worthwhile to have a patient endure up to 2 weeks' *mild* intoxication symptoms before discontinuing an anticonvulsant, because the symptoms often subside. Frequently, patients who do not tolerate a drug turn out to have tried it for only a few days, and it can be tried again using small initial doses.

Increase anticonvulsants gradually to target dose ranges. For patients who have very frequent seizures the initial dose can be adjusted according to seizure control rather than the blood level of the drug. Carbamazepine is usually started at a dose of 200 mg twice daily, and then increased every 3 to 4 days to 600 to 800 mg total, in three doses (larger doses for larger patients). Phenytoin doses may be increased more abruptly (e.g., 300 mg per day or 100 mg twice daily for 3 days, then 200 mg twice daily or 300 mg at bedtime). Phenytoin may also be loaded orally, if needed (e.g., for acute treatment 300 mg every 4 hours for three doses, then 300 or 400 mg per day). Initial doses are influenced by the patient's size, a history of sedation in response to other anticonvulsants, and the need for rapid seizure prophylaxis. Valproic acid produces nausea if increased rapidly and is usually begun at twice daily doses of 125 mg or 250 mg, and then increased to 750 or 1,000 mg daily in three doses.

About a week after the patient reaches a stable starting dose (longer for barbiturates), obtain target drug blood levels and adjust doses if necessary. Once an approximate target blood level dose is reached, anticonvulsant doses should be individualized in order to control seizures and minimize side effects. For example, phenytoin can be started 300 mg at bedtime, and if the blood level is slightly low (e.g., 7 to 9 mg per liter) a week later, it can be increased to 400 mg per day or 200 mg twice daily. Valproic acid blood levels (recommended 50 to 100 mg per liter) are less predictive of treatment response than they are for other anticonvulsants.

It is important to explain to patients that there is much individual variability in the dose of anticonvulsant that is needed to control seizures. I also explain that because there is increased risk of side-effects with large doses, they start taking small to moderate-sized doses, which will be increased if they experience "breakthrough" seizures. For patients for whom it is socially important to avoid any seizures, I initially aim for medium to high blood levels. Someone whose employment would be threatened by recurring seizures, for example, might have the phenytoin dose adjusted to produce a blood level of 15 to 20 mg per liter or carbamazepine to produce levels of 8 to 11 mg per liter.

The incidence of side effects in individual patients varies markedly. Patients may do well on carbamazepine but may not tolerate phenytoin, and vice versa. If carbamazepine or phenytoin is not tolerated, then valproic acid, primidone, or phenobarbital may be tried. I usually overlap medications. The new anticonvulsant is slowly started, and when I reach a target level or obtain seizure reduction, I taper the first anticonvulsant. If side-effects occur during this switch, then I taper the first anticonvulsant early, before reaching a full dose on the new drug.

If seizures recur despite adequate treatment with single drugs, anticonvulsant combinations may be used. Typical combinations are carbamazepine or phenytoin plus valproic acid or primidone.

The incidence of side effects is high with combinations of anticonvulsants, and anticonvulsant blood levels are helpful for sorting out which drug may be producing side effects. The side effects produced by adding a new drug can often be mitigated by decreasing the dose of the first drug. For example, if a patient is sedated when valproate is added to carbamazepine and clorazepate, sedation may be reduced by decreasing clorazepate.

If combinations of anticonvulsants do not control seizures, I often add clorazepate or lorazepam to the patient's most effective anticonvulsant. If seizures have been difficult to control and come under control on an atypical regimen, I do not taper or change anticonvulsants unless it is necessary. If a patient has a prolonged flurry of seizures, I sometimes add small doses of lorazepam or clorazepate twice or thrice daily for several days, as the regular anticonvulsant is adjusted. For example, if a patient has five seizures over 2 days, I may add lorazepam, 1 mg twice a day for 4 days, as carbamazepine or valproic acid is being adjusted.

TREATMENT ERRORS

Failing to Educate Patients

Failing to educate patients adequately about epilepsy and about the strategy for treatment is a major cause of poor medication compliance. Before initiating long-term epilepsy treatment, it is important to discuss what is known about the causes of the epilepsy, how epilepsy is defined, what lifestyle restrictions should be observed (e.g., driving, swimming and bathing alone, working at heights), and how important it is to minimize the effects of epilepsy on employment and personal goals. Parents and family frequently require as much counseling as patients do: patients may be unaware of their seizures, and families sometimes place unreasonable restrictions on persons with epilepsy.

Women need to be told about issues of pregnancy and epilepsy. Women taking carbamazepine should be warned that it may interfere with the effectivness of oral contraceptives and at least 50 μg of estradiol should be given.

Adjusting Anticonvulsant Doses Based on Target Drug Levels Alone

When target levels are slightly "high" or "low" and the patient is doing well, dosages do not necessarily require adjustment.

Failing to Tailor Anticonvulsants to Individual Factors

Some patients who do not reliably take medications three times a day do best on phenytoin in a single daily dose. Those taking carbamazepine or valproate may need to take it twice a day rather than risk missing a dose if it is prescribed three times per day. Pillboxes are helpful for patients who have cognitive impairments.

Failure to Reassess a Patient When Treatment Fails

Some patients have alternative diagnoses, such as hyperventilation attacks or migraines. Some patients have progressive disease (e.g., tumor). The possibility of a conversion disorder should be explored if a patient has had multiple normal EEGs and has emotional difficulties.

Overreacting to Slight Hepatic Enzyme Elevations or Slight White Blood Cell Reductions.

Carbamazepine and phenytoin frequently produce minor elevations of alanine aminotransferase (ALT) and aspartate amino-transferase (AST) and often greater increases in gamma-glutamyltransferase. Carbamazepine often produces mild leukopenia. These effects are rarely progressive or associated with clinical symptoms. Clinical monitoring and repeated laboratory screening are usually reassuring. If AST or ALT increases to four times normal or the leukocyte count drops below 2000 per cubic millimeter, I usually adjust medications. Amylase should be checked if the alkaline phosphatase value is markedly elevated.

SPECIFIC THERAPEUTIC APPROACHES FOR SPECIFIC SITUATIONS

Catamenial (Triggered by Menses) Epilepsy

Some patients have menstruation-related seizures, but a seizure diary should be examined for several months, since this association is often not as strong as patients suspect. Predictable catamenial seizures can be treated with lorazepam, 1 mg twice or thrice daily for the several-day risk period, or the patient's regular anticonvulsant dose can be boosted slightly during this period.

Seizure Flurries

Many patients' seizures occur as predictable flurries of three or more. *Pulse* treatment with lorazepam or an extra dose of the standard medication may help block recurrence of seizures. For example, after two seizures in a single day, such patients can take lorazepam, 1 mg two or three times a day, or one or two extra phenytoin or carbamazepine tablets.

Nocturnal Seizures

Patients who have nocturnal seizures can be given imbalanced dosing schedules, as large doses are often tolerated when given at bedtime. For example, a patient who suffers early morning seizures might be given carbamazepine 200 mg in the morning, 200 mg in the afternoon, and 600 mg at bedtime.

Phenytoin Allergy or Toxicity

Ethotoin is useful for patients who develop side effects or allergic reactions with phenytoin, particularly if their seizures were controlled by phenytoin. For example, a patient whose seizures were controlled on phenytoin but who developed gingivitis and did not respond to carbamazepine, may benefit from ethotoin. The manufacturer's recommended treatment is 2,000 to 3,000 mg in four doses.

Several other anticonvulsants less frequently used do not have significant advantages over standard medications. Phenacemide is effective for treating CPS, but because of psychiatric, renal, and hepatic effects should be prescribed carefully, probably by an epilepsy specialist. Although phenacemide usually increases serum Cr, renal scan measurement of glomerular filtration rate usually demonstrates normal renal function.

Investigational Agents and Epilepsy Surgery

Clinical trials of new anticonvulsants are available to patients with CPS who live near a study center. Most study designs include only a 5 to 7 month period of randomization into placebo or treatment period and then allow open-label investigational drug treatment. Compassionate-use protocols may also be available for individual patients. Some patients obtain treatment in Europe with newer anticonvulsants before they are introduced in the United States.

Patients who have medically intractable, frequent seizures (usually at least 1 per month) are candidates for epilepsy surgery. Video EEG epilepsy screening is needed to determine whether focal resection surgery is feasible.

Counseling

Patients with epilepsy face a variety of personal and social difficulties and often benefit from counseling. For example, many employers and insurers discriminate against patients with epilepsy. Specific driving restrictions must be followed in each state. A chronic condition may trigger emotional issues centered around self-image and dependence. Women need to be counseled about how to manage the risks of epilepsy and pregnancy. Some patients may have psychiatric disorders due to linked conditions (e.g., post-traumatic, organic mental disorders and epilepsy). It is important to respond to these issues and to refer patients to a psychiatrist when appropriate. Neurologic nurses trained in epilepsy often act as excellent counselors and can help patients deal with many of these emotional and social issues. Local epilepsy centers often provide vocational and personal counseling. Information for patients can be obtained from state epilepsy associations and from the Epilepsy Foundation of America.

SUGGESTED READING

Epilepsy octet. Lancet 1990; 336:93, 161, 231, 291, 350, 423, 486, 551.
Resor SR Jr, Kutt H, eds. The medical treatment of epilepsy. New York: Marcel Dekker, 1992.
Scheuer ML, Pedley TA. The evaluation and treatment of seizures. N Engl J Med 1990; 323:1468–1474.

PATIENT RESOURCE

Epilepsy Foundation of America
4351 Garden City Drive
Landover, Maryland 20785
(800) 492-2523.

PSEUDOEPILEPTIC AND PSYCHOGENIC SEIZURES

ALLAN KRUMHOLZ, M.D.
LYNN M. GRATTAN, Ph.D.

Pseudoepileptic or psychogenic seizures pose major problems for physicians, particularly neurologists, who care for patients with intractable seizures. Indeed, pseudoepileptic seizures account for approximately 20 percent of all intractable seizure referrals to comprehensive epilepsy centers in the United States. Although recent advances in video electroencephalography (EEG) monitoring have much improved our ability to diagnose this condition correctly, management remains a problem. Therefore, our approach to the management of patients with pseudoepileptic seizures emphasizes both proper diagnosis and effective therapy.

DEFINITIONS

Although the term *epilepsy* should be reserved for well-defined disorders of the brain caused by electrical disturbances of normal brain function, *seizure* can be used in a more general sense. Consequently, we refer to disorders that are mistaken for epilepsy but are not due to abnormal electrical discharges in the brain as *pseudoepileptic seizures*. Historically, many other terms have been used to describe such events: hysterical seizures, hysteroepilepsy, pseudoseizures, nonepileptic seizures, and psychogenic seizures, among others. These are similar disorders, but they are not equivalent.

Pseudoepileptic Seizures

The term *pseudoepileptic seizure* describes all conditions, both physiologic and psychological, that are mistaken for epilepsy (Table 1). Indeed, the clinical manifestations of epilepsy are so varied that many disorders can be mistaken for epileptic seizures. In children, some of these physiologic disorders are breath-holding spells, pallid infantile syncope, gastroesophageal reflux, night terrors, and other parasomnias. In adults, physiologic pseudoepileptic disorders that may imitate epilepsy include syncope, migraine, and transient ischemic attacks (TIAs). Such physiologic disorders, however, are responsible for only a small proportion of the patients we see with pseudoepileptic seizures.

Psychogenic Seizures

The majority of pseudoepileptic seizures are psychogenic pseudoepileptic seizures or, more simply, psychogenic seizures. In general any psychological disorder that mimics epilepsy can be considered a psy-

Table 1 Classification of Pseudoepileptic Seizures

Physiologic pseudoepileptic seizures (e.g., syncope, TIA, complicated migraine, narcolepsy, night terrors, breath-holding spells)
Psychogenic seizures
  Somatoform disorder (e.g., somatization disorder, conversion disorder)
  Misinterpretation disorder (e.g., hyperventilation syndrome, panic attack, dissociative disorder)
  Stress and coping disorder (associated with post-traumatic stress disorder, mental retardation, and true epilepsy)
  Factitious disorder (e.g., chronic factitious disorder or Munchausen's syndrome)
  Malingering

chogenic seizure. In contemporary thought, the notion that all psychogenic seizures are a result of "hysteria" has been abandoned in favor of a growing appreciation for the heterogeneity and diversity of the patients.

Rather than treating psychogenic seizure patients uniformly as one group, we have found it more useful to classify the causes of psychogenic seizures into five major categories (see Table 1): (1) somatoform disorders, (2) misrepresentation disorders, (3) stress and coping disorders, (4) factitious disorders, and (5) malingering. This classification is based on a heuristic model; the subgroups are not mutually exclusive, as we recognize that the causes of psychogenic seizures are multifactorial.

Somatoform Disorders

The principal somatoform disorders that are associated with psychogenic seizures are somatization disorders, conversion disorders, and undifferentiated somatoform disorders, as classified by the *Diagnostic and Statistical Manual of Mental Disorders–Revised* (DSM-III-R). The essential feature for a diagnosis of somatization disorder is a history of recurrent and multiple somatic complaints of early onset and long duration. In contrast, conversion disorder involves a more restricted range of somatic complaints, the expression of which is based on unconscious psychodynamic processes and is typically symbolic of a psychological conflict or need. Undifferentiated somatoform disorders include those whose clinical profile is similar to that of other somatization disorders but does not meet all necessary criteria.

Misinterpretation Disorders

Misinterpretation disorders describe genuine physical, neurologic, or psychological symptoms that for some reason are misinterpreted. Either through misunderstanding, exaggeration, or amplification, symptoms such as paresthesias secondary to hyperventilation, panic attacks, experiences of derealization or depersonalization, or attentional disturbances are incorrectly interpreted as epilepsy by the patient or physician.

Stress and Coping Disorders

Psychogenic seizure patients who have stress and coping disorders lack the capacity to cope with the stresses in their lives. This may be because they have a predisposing vulnerability that lowers the threshold for coping with stress and anxiety (e.g., mental retardation, learning disability, or cognitive changes associated with head injury) or because their lives have been burdened by extraordinary stress (e.g., post-traumatic stress disorder, multiple losses, or true epilepsy). Their psychogenic events are not volitional but are usually temporally related to certain stressful life events.

Factitious Disorders and Malingering

The shared feature of these two psychogenic seizure precipitants is the conscious fabrication of seizure-like symptoms. An important difference between factitious disorders and malingering is the *goal* of the intentionally induced or simulated seizure symptoms. The goal of the psychogenic seizure patient with *factitious disorder* (e.g., Munchausen's syndrome) is to maintain him- or herself in the role of patient. To that end, they fake symptoms, exaggerate existing physical symptoms, or self-induce symptoms. The goal of the *malingerer* is to obtain a recognizable external benefit (e.g., financial gain or release from prison).

DIAGNOSIS

Clinical observation has long been the basis for distinguishing psychogenic seizures from epileptic seizures, but, in recent years, clinical observation has been much aided by the use of video EEG monitoring, serum prolactin levels, and neuropsychological assessments.

A complicating factor in diagnosis is that both psychogenic and epileptic seizures may occur in a single patient. Indeed, approximately 10 to 40 percent of patients identified to have psychogenic seizures have been reported also to have true epileptic seizures. There are several possible explanations for this. Some patients with epilepsy may learn that seizures get attention and fill certain psychological needs. Alternatively, they may have concomitant neurologic problems, personality disorders, cognitive deficits, or impaired coping mechanisms that predispose them to psychogenic symptoms. In our experience with these combined seizure types, the epileptic seizures are usually well-controlled or of only historical relevance at the time the patient develops psychogenic seizures.

Clinical Observations

There are no pathognomonic clinical signs that allow an observer to distinguish pseudoepileptic or psychogenic seizures from epileptic seizures. Pseudoepileptic or psychogenic seizures are varied and may present with generalized convulsive manifestations, signs of altered consciousness or loss of consciousness, and focal motor or sensory symptoms.

Some clinical observations are useful for distinguishing psychogenic from epileptic seizures. In particular, psychogenic seizures often last considerably longer than epileptic seizures, which typically persist less than 3 minutes, excluding the postictal state. Also, the nature of the convulsive activity in psychogenic seizures differs from that of generalized convulsive epilepsy. With psychogenic seizures, the movements are more often purposeful or semipurposeful, asymmetric, or asynchronous, such as thrashing or writhing motions, rather than the tonic-clonic activity of epileptic seizures. (It is more difficult to distinguish the movements of psychogenic seizures from the automatisms of complex partial epileptic seizures.)

There are other clinical differences between psychogenic and epileptic seizures. For example, consciousness and responsiveness may be surprisingly retained during psychogenic seizures. Also, incontinence can occur but is relatively unusual, as is serious self-injury. In addition, unlike epileptic seizures, psychogenic seizures characteristically do not respond well to antiepileptic drug treatment. Psychogenic seizures are also more likely to be provoked by emotional stimuli or suggestion. In fact, provocative procedures may be useful for reproducing events during EEG recording.

Video EEG Monitoring

A diagnosis of pseudoepileptic or psychogenic seizures is most secure when a characteristic seizure is recorded during simultaneous EEG and video monitoring and demonstrates no evidence of epileptic activity. Patients with generalized convulsive epileptic seizures invariably demonstrate significant EEG changes on ictal EEG recordings. Even persons with partial seizures, who may have small or deep seizure foci, should still show significant ictal EEG abnormalities in perhaps 85 to 95 percent of true epileptic seizures. The ictal EEG recording is particularly important, because occasionally interictal or routine EEGs are actually misleading. For example, interictally, some patients with epilepsy may have normal EEGs, and some patients with psychogenic seizures may have minor EEG abnormalities.

There are several ways to capture a clinical seizure during EEG monitoring. Outpatient monitoring is particularly useful for patients who have daily events or seizures that can be provoked by suggestion. Patients with less frequent events may require extended inpatient video EEG monitoring. Simultaneous video EEG recording offers the advantage of permitting careful observation and review of the clinical manifestations of seizures. This can be especially useful when assessing patients with psychogenic seizures, because video EEG recordings are particularly helpful for distinguishing epileptic seizure discharges from movement and muscle artifacts. For these reasons, we favor video EEG recordings over ambulatory recording systems without video capability in the evaluation of patients with intractable seizures.

Prolactin Levels

The serum prolactin level is a useful test for suspected psychogenic seizures. Prolactin levels rise approximately 5- to 10-fold after generalized convulsive epileptic seizures—and somewhat less but still significantly (typically at least two- to threefold) after complex partial seizures. This prolactin increase is maximal in the initial 20 minutes to 1 hour after a seizure. We caution that, although prolactin measures may be useful in distinguishing pseudoepileptic and true epileptic seizures, some false positive and false negative results occur. In particular, simple partial seizures or mild complex partial seizures, particularly those with little motor activity, may not raise the prolactin level significantly.

Neuropsychological Testing

Another important consideration in evaluating patients with suspected psychogenic seizures is their psychological status. Such an assessment requires referral to mental health professionals experienced in psychological and psychiatric assessment, psychometric assessment, and psychotherapeutic intervention with patients with neurologic disorders. We have found neuropsychologists most helpful in this regard. However, if such a specialist is not available, referral to a clinical psychologist or a psychiatrist may be beneficial.

Neuropsychological evaluations are useful by (1) determining the potential or likelihood of significant contributing psychopathology or cognitive difficulties, (2) by defining the nature of those associated psychological or psychosocial issues, and (3) by determining whether the patient would benefit from a psychologically based intervention.

With respect to specific neuropsychological tests, the clinical interview is most valuable, but it is also very subjective. Therefore, we recommend in addition standardized and more objective psychometric assessments of personality (Minnesota Multiphasic Personality Inventory-2 [MMPI-2]), intellect (Wechsler Adult Intelligence Scale-Revised [WAIS-R]), and basic neuropsychological functions (e.g., psychomotor speed, attention, memory, language, visual-spatial perception, constructional praxis, and cognitive flexibility). The utility of additional psychological diagnostic procedures is best individualized and may include more detailed studies of depression (e.g., Beck Depression Inventory), stressful life events (e.g., Life Events Questionnaire), anxiety (e.g., State-Trait Anxiety Scale), personality (Millon Clinical Multiaxial Inventory-II [MCMI-II]), or higher level cognition (e.g., executive functions or problem-solving ability).

Mental health professionals should not be expected to determine whether seizures are psychogenic rather than epileptic, because they generally lack the necessary training or experience in clinical diagnosis of epilepsy. The distinction between psychogenic and epileptic seizures is best made by neurologists, particularly those with special expertise in epilepsy, and it is based on consideration of both clinical data and neuropsychological assessments.

TREATMENT

Even after a diagnosis of psychogenic seizures is established, neurologists can and should continue to take an active role in the care of these patients (Table 2). Actually, psychological interventions need not be very prolonged, elaborate, or mystical processes. In fact, many psychogenic seizure patients benefit from education and support, which can be readily provided by the neurologist. If the neuropsychological assessment suggests a clinical profile that requires a mental health professional's intervention, then an appropriate referral should be made. Some ways in which neurologists or primary care physicians may facilitate treatment are described below.

Physiologic Pseudoepileptic Seizures

For persons with physiologic pseudoepileptic seizures such as syncope, complicated migraine, or TIAs, therapy, clinical course, and prognosis vary depending on the disorder that has been mistaken for epilepsy. For example, patients with cardiac syncope may need placement of a pacemaker, and their prognosis will depend on the nature of their cardiac disease.

Psychogenic Seizures

In contrast, optimal management of patients with psychogenic seizures requires attention to their psychological and social problems, though obtaining good psychological care and support for these patients can be

Table 2 Psychotherapeutic Interventions for the Neurologist Treating Patients with Psychogenic Seizures

Present the diagnosis of psychogenic seizures positively, emphasizing the potential for seizure control.

Follow patients after referral to mental health professionals, and try to co-ordinate your efforts with theirs.

Schedule regular follow-up visits, and do not make visits contingent only on new or worsening problems.

Give patients attention when they are doing well, and encourage them to talk about their life situation instead of their seizures or somatic complaints.

Avoid prescribing unnecessary medications.

Avoid unnecessary testing and excessive referral to specialists.

Permit the patient to have some symptoms. The patent's well-being and function, rather than complete eradication of seizures, should be the ultimate goal.

difficult. Most neurologists or primary care physicians are not experienced or comfortable diagnosing and treating psychiatric or psychological disorders. Consequently, once psychogenic seizures are diagnosed, neurologists often attempt to shift responsibility for management to a psychiatrist or mental health professional. In our experience, however, few mental health professionals are confident caring for such patients, and the patients often suffer. This problem can be addressed by trying to identify mental health professionals who are capable and comfortable caring for patients with such disorders and supporting these professionals during the patient's psychotherapy.

General Treatment Considerations

We advise that patients with psychogenic seizures be managed similarly to patients with other types of so-called abnormal illness behavior (see Table 2). The first consideration should be the manner in which the diagnosis of psychogenic seizures is presented to the patient and family. We stress honesty with the patient and a positive attitude toward the diagnosis. We emphasize as favorable or good news the fact that the patient does not have epilepsy. We also underscore that this disorder, although serious and "real," does not require treatment with antiepileptic medications and that, as stress or emotional issues are resolved, the patient has the potential to obtain control of these events and discontinue medications.

Not all patients readily accept this diagnosis or this approach. Some seek other opinions, and this move can be supported. An adversarial relationship with the patient should be avoided. In fact, the patient should be encouraged to return, if desired, and records should be made available to avoid duplication of services.

After the diagnosis of psychogenic seizure is presented, supportive measures should be instituted. We prefer to schedule regular neurologic follow-up visits for the patient, even if a mental health professional is involved. This allows the patient to get medical attention without demonstrating illness behavior. Moreover, it offers support to the involved mental health professional. Patient education and support are stressed at these visits. Because family issues are often important contributing factors, physicians should consider involving family members.

A special effort should be made to give these patients attention, not only for complaints but also—perhaps even moreso—when they are doing well. In particular, we encourage patients with psychogenic seizures to talk about their life situation instead of their somatic complaints.

If symptoms worsen or new ones develop, they should receive appropriate attention. Still, it is important to avoid unnecessary testing, uncalled for prescribing of medications, and excessive referral to specialists. Also, it is advised the patients be allowed to have some symptoms, even psychogenic seizures. The goal of treatment should be to maximize the patient's well-being and functioning, not just to eliminate seizures. More specific individualized treatment strategies are discussed below.

Specific Therapeutic Strategies

In planning treatment, we feel it is important to focus not only on a narrow psychological diagnosis but to consider other factors, such as the individual's personality structure, coping mechanisms, related psychosocial stressors, and associated cognitive problems. This type of approach is supported by current psychiatric theory, as reflected in DSM-III-R, which attempts to consider these various factors as stratified axes. We consider this a useful approach, because it emphasizes the multifactorial nature of psychogenic seizures and the fact that these various factors may prove to be additive. We believe that from the intervention perspective patients with psychogenic seizures lend themselves to a somewhat different and more specific approach that is based on our classification of psychogenic seizures (see Table 1) and is outlined in Table 3.

Somatoform Disorders

Somatoform psychiatric disorders are best treated with psychotherapy. Since the seizures are unconsciously driven, direct patient confrontation typically is fruitless. In fact, it may only serve to alienate the patient from seeking treatment or weaken their psychiatric status. For instance, if the patient has associated depression, their feelings of helplessness and hopelessness may increase with confrontation and they may become suicidal. Major psychosis is unusual in patients with psychogenic seizures.

Misinterpretation Disorders

Patients who are misinterpreting or exaggerating genuine symptoms typically benefit from being provided accurate information about neurologic or psychological symptoms and appropriate treatment alternatives.

Stress and Coping Disorders

For psychogenic seizures that stem from stress and coping disorders, the goal of therapy is to enhance patients' capacity to cope with life stresses. This may be done by encouraging patients to make lifestyle or environmental changes and by referring them to a mental health professional to improve the strength and repertoire of their coping resources. A psychologist or psychiatrist may effectively employ a variety of cognitive behavioral methods to treat these patients. These could include, but are not limited to, education, coping skills training, and stress management techniques. Some patients may need more intensive insight-oriented psychotherapy to help them manage the psychological effects of significant past traumas.

Table 3 Suggested Diagnostic Assessment and Treatment Interventions for Psychogenic Seizure Disorders

Psychogenic Seizure Category	Diagnostic Procedures	Interventions
Somatoform disorders	Clinical interview, MMPI-2, Millon Clinical Multiaxial Inventory, physical symptom checklist	Motivate patient to seek and maintain active involvement in psychotherapy
Misinterpretation disorders	Clinical interview, MMPI-2, cognitive assessments, WAIS-R	Information and education to help patients properly reinterpret symptoms
Stress and coping disorders	Clinical interview, MMPI-2, cognitive assessments, WAIS-R, Life Events Scale, coping inventory	Cognitive-behavioral and educational interventions to reduce stress and improve coping skills
Factitious disorders and malingering	Clinical interview; MMPI-2; documented medical, accident and legal history; family history	Psychotherapy with supportive confrontation to help patients obtain desired goals in a more adaptive fashion. Remove objects of primary and secondary gain.

Factitious Disorders and Malingering

Treating a patient with a factitious disorder is very difficult. Typically, patients with factitious disorders present with a vague and inconsistent medical history, and when confronted with evidence that their symptoms are faked, deny the allegation and seek medical services elsewhere. Chances for successful treatment are best if they can be motivated to see a mental health professional who can provide psychotherapy to address their need to seek and maintain the patient role and who can help them obtain desired goals in a more adaptive fashion. Patients who are malingering typically desist if their opportunity for gain is removed. Thus, facilitating speedy resolution of court cases or other proceedings is recommended. Fortunately, neither factitious disorders nor malingering are common causes of psychogenic seizures.

Sexual Abuse

A history of sexual abuse in patients with psychogenic seizures is an emerging issue whose relevance has yet to be fully established. From a diagnosis and treatment perspective, it is noteworthy that psychogenic seizures are more common in women, and several recent studies emphasize that a history of sexual abuse may be very common in patients with psychogenic seizures. In light of this observation, we advise that the issue be explored by the neurologist or consulting mental health professional and integrated into the treatment plan as necessary.

Patients with psychogenic seizures are a diverse group, and some fail to respond even to optimal therapy. In some such situations, psychiatric hospitalization may be necessary. Inpatient treatment offers the advantage of removing the patient from an unhealthy environment, family, or social situation, and it may provide a better therapeutic milieu.

PROGNOSIS

The outcome for patients with psychogenic seizures varies from one to another. Long-term follow-up studies show that about half of all patients with psychogenic seizures function reasonably well following appropriate diagnosis. However, only about one-third stop having psychogenic seizures or related problems entirely, and approximately half the patients have poor functional outcomes. When the diagnosis of psychogenic seizures is based on reliable criteria such as video EEG monitoring, misdiagnosis is unlikely. Instead, the usual cause for a poor outcome is related to a patient's chronic psychological and social problems.

It is noteworthy that children with psychogenic seizures appear to have a much better prognosis than adults. This may relate to the fact that children's psychogenic seizures are more likely to be related to transient stress and coping disorders, whereas adults psychogenic seizures are more likely to occur in the context of a more chronic psychological maladjustment, such as personality disorders.

Indeed, we have observed that patients with stress and coping disorders or misinterpretation disorders (see Tables 1 and 3) respond relatively well to supportive educative or behavioral therapeutic approaches. In contrast, patients with somatoform disorders and factitious disorders more often have associated chronic personality problems and a poorer prognosis. We are hopeful that as such information about the nature of psychogenic seizures and their associated psychopathology is clarified, better treatment strategies can be developed that will improve the care and prognosis of these difficult and challenging disorders.

SUGGESTED READING

Cohen RJ, Suter C. Hysterical seizures: Suggestion as a provocative EEG test. Ann Neurol 1982; 391–395.

Gates JR, Ramani V, Whalen S, Loewenson R. Ictal characteristics of pseudoseizures. Arch Neurol 1985; 42:1183–1187.

Krumholz A, Niedermeyer E. Psychogenic seizures: A clinical study with follow-up data. Neurology 1983; 33:498–502.

Laxer KD, Mullooly JP, Howell B. Prolactin changes after seizures classified by EEG monitoring. Neurology 1985; 35:31–35.

Shen W, Bowman ES, Markand ON. Presenting the diagnosis of pseudoseizure. Neurology 1990; 40:756–759.

Wilkus RJ, Dodrill CB. Factors affecting the outcome of MMPI and neuropsychological assessments of psychogenic and epileptic seizure patients. Epilepsia 1989; 30:339–347.

Wyllie E, Friedman D, Luders H, et al. Outcome of psychogenic seizures in children and adolescents compared with adults. Neurology 1991; 41:742–744.

PAIN

PAIN: GENERAL RECOMMENDATIONS

ROBERT R. ALLEN, M.D.
KENNETH L. CASEY, M.D.

Pain is the most frequent chief complaint. Every clinician is obliged to treat pain in the course of normal clinical experience. Fortunately, although we are often unable to cure the underlying disease, we can usually treat the pain. Correct treatment requires a correct diagnosis. Pain may be caused by neurologic injury or by injury to extraneural tissue, and therapeutic options vary accordingly. We focus here on the general principles of pain treatment and make specific reference to some of the more common painful conditions seen in neurologic practice. Headache and back pain are not discussed because they are addressed in individual chapters.

Rational therapeutic choices can be made only after identifying the site of the pain-producing lesion and recognizing the basic pathophysiologic mechanisms involved (Figure 1). Therapeutic strategies then vary according to the type, location, and duration of painful symptoms. Multiple pathophysiologic mechanisms may contribute to certain painful conditions—a rational basis for combined or adjuvant therapy. Although pharmacologic therapy remains the primary mode of treatment, nonpharmacologic measures such as cooling, local or regional anesthesia, transcutaneous electric nerve stimulation (TENS), and gentle physical therapy may be useful in specific cases. In all cases, but especially with chronic pain, strong psychological support from the treating physician is essential.

IDENTIFY THE SITE OF PAIN-PRODUCING INJURY

Pain caused by *extraneural tissue injury* is usually described as a nearly continuous or frequently recurring sensation involving localized or multifocal regions. Symptoms are commonly aggravated by activity and relieved by rest. Physical examination usually reveals focal tenderness, often associated with signs of inflammation. Pain onset typically is abrupt.

In contrast, pain caused by *neural tissue injury* may occur immediately, develop gradually, or be delayed several months. Pain following injury to the peripheral nervous system is often described as (1) continuous, "burning," dysesthesia, commonly present in toxic or metabolic neuropathy caused by diabetes or alcohol abuse, or (2) paroxysmal, "sharp," or lancinating pain, like that experienced with compressive mononeuropathy, plexopathy, or radiculopathy. The two symptoms may occur together. A distinguishing feature of peripheral nerve lesions is pain that is worse at rest or during the night. Examination may reveal allodynia (pain elicited by normally innocuous stimuli), hyperalgesia (reduced pain threshold), or hyperpathia (abnormally prolonged, intense response to a mildly noxious stimulus) and sensory loss, usually without obvious signs of inflammation. These findings also may be associated with pain due to lesions in the central nervous system. Central pain typically is described as deep, burning or aching, and usually constant but often associated with superimposed paroxysms exacerbated by movement or cold. Neurologic examination typically reveals elevated thresholds for pain and temperature in the region of the pain complaint. Central pain syndromes are commonly seen following traumatic spinal cord injuries but are also associated with stroke, multiple sclerosis, or other neurologic disease. Delayed onset of pain is the rule rather than the exception in these cases, although most begin within the first year after injury.

DIRECT TREATMENT TO THE SITE OF PAINFUL INJURY

Extraneural Injury

Acute treatment of extraneural tissue injury should be directed at relieving the underlying cause of inflammation. When pain is due to tissue inflammation, nonsteroidal anti-inflammatory drugs (NSAIDs), and occasionally corticosteroids, are most useful. Nonpharmacologic therapies such as ice, rest, and elevation should also be applied when swelling and inflammation

Receptor Sensitization	Abnormal Impulse Generation	Hyperexcitable Central Nociceptive Neurons

1. Tissue inflammation
2. Sympathetic efferents
	1. Nerve, root inflammation
	2. Nerve, root compression
	3. Axonal De/Regeneration
	4. Demyelination
	5. Sympathetic efferents
		1. Peripheral degeneration
		2. CNS Lesions:
		   Vascular
		   Demyelinating
		   Traumatic
		   Neoplastic
		3. Psychological mechanisms

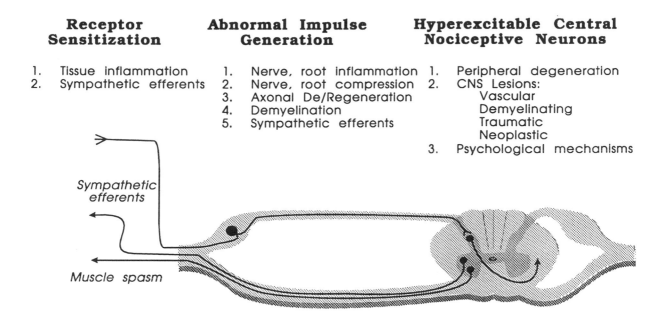

Figure 1 *Pathophysiologic processes in pain.* Three major pain-causing pathologic conditions are shown at the principal neurologic levels of their occurrence. Some of the pathologic processes that contribute to these conditions are listed below each example.

are associated. For mild to moderate pain, NSAIDs or non-narcotic analgesics alone may be effective; for more severe pain, opioids are the drugs of choice (Table 1).

NSAIDs act peripherally by inhibiting prostaglandin synthesis and are most effective for inflammatory conditions without neurologic involvement. For anti-inflammatory affects, aspirin, 650 mg every 4 to 6 hours (maximum 6000 mg per day), is our drug of choice because it has anti-inflammatory, analgesic, and antipyretic effects. Acetaminophen is a poor choice for inflammatory conditions but is an equally good analgesic and does not cause the gastric irritation commonly seen with aspirin. Further choice of an NSAID is based on the relative toxicities of individual drugs, the major limiting side effects being gastric irritation, platelet dysfunction and, rarely, interstitial nephritis. For patients with a history of gastritis or peptic ulcer disease, concurrent treatment with misoprostol (Cytotec), a prostaglandin derivative, may be protective. Similar protection is not seen with sucralfate, cimetidine, or ranitidine. Once an ulcer has formed, however, no agent is protective, and NSAIDs should not be used. For cancer patients expected to have hematologic problems we initially use a non-narcotic with minimal platelet toxicity (choline magnesium trisalicylate or acetaminophen).

Indomethacin may have more gastric side effects but greater analgesic strength and should be considered when other NSAIDs have failed. Greater analgesia may be obtained with the newest of the NSAIDs (Keterolac), but long-term use is not advised because of the increased risk of gastrointestinal side effects.

Corticosteroids are helpful when pain is caused by bone involvement, as with cancer and in certain rheumatic conditions. Treatment should consist of a short (2 week) tapered course of dexamethasone or prednisone.

Short-term side effects include hyperglycemia, increased risk of infection, impaired wound healing, and hypokalemia. Long-term use for pain alone is seldom, if ever, indicated in neurologic practice.

Opioids are the drugs of choice for more immediate relief of moderate to severe pain. Aggressive use of opioids is indicated when an organic cause for pain is evident and other medications are ineffective. Fear of addiction or tolerance in the acute setting are often unwarranted, and the hazard may be exaggerated even in the treatment of more chronic nonmalignant pain syndromes. We have seen chronic pain controlled with "nonescalating"—stable, small—doses of these drugs. Dose-limiting side effects include sedation, constipation, nausea, and respiratory depression. When opioids are combined with peripherally acting agents such as NSAIDs there may be an additive, or even synergistic, analgesic effect. This combination may also help to minimize side effects common to both drugs when they are given in larger doses.

Sympathetically Maintained Pain

Sympathetically maintained pain (SMP) most commonly follows trauma, and it can occur *with or without associated neural injury.* In the early stages of this condition, pain may be present even though findings suggestive of sympathetic involvement (sweating, vasoconstriction) are not. Hyperpathia or allodynia to light touch or cold may be present on examination. The definitive diagnosis of SMP, however, relies on the documentation of pain relief following sympathetic interruption to the affected area. This can be achieved by (1) sympathetic ganglion blocks with local anesthetic, (2) regional alpha-adrenergic block with guanethidine,

Table 1 NSAIDs and Opioids Used to Treat Pain

Drug	Oral Dosage for 70 kg patient (mg)	Estimated Duration of Action (hr)	Comments
Acetaminophen	650 q4h	3–5	Not anti-inflammatory
Aspirin	650 q4h	3–5	
Choline magnesium trisalicylate	750 t.i.d.	8–12	No platelet toxicity
Ibuprofen	400 q.i.d.	4–6	
Naproxyn	250–500 b.i.d.	8–12	
Indomethacin	25 q.i.d.	4–6	
Ketoprofen	75 t.i.d.	6–8	
Codeine	30–60 q4–6h	4–6	
Oxycodone	5–10 q4–6h	3–5	
Morphine sulfate	25 q4h	4–6	Watch for cumulative effects
(MS Contin)	30 b.i.d.	8–12	with repeated dosing
Methadone	2.5–10 q6–8h	12–18	
Levorphanol	2 q6h	6–8	

or (3) the recently described systemic alpha-adrenergic blockade with IV phentolamine.

Once SMP has been documented, pharmacologic or surgical therapy may be necessary to relieve pain. Initial treatment might consist of a trial with phenoxybenzamine, a systemic alpha-adrenergic receptor antagonist. The initial dose is 10 mg twice a day; each week it is increased by 10 mg per day until therapeutic effects or unacceptable side effects appear. The maximal effective dose range is usually 20 to 120 mg per day. The side effects of impotence and postural hypotension often limit use of this drug. Alternate therapy with clonidine, 0.1 mg two or three times daily, or prazosin, 2 mg twice a day, may also be effective, although these drugs can cause hypotension. If pharmacologic therapy fails, repeated regional blocks with guanethidine, or more permanent surgical sympathectomy, may be necessary. Before surgery is considered, signs of improvement should be sought. SMP can resolve spontaneously. Following surgical sympathectomy, as many as 20 to 40 percent of patients may have pain (sympathalgia). Fortunately, this pain is usually self-remitting or easily controlled with phenytoin or carbamazepine.

Neural Injury

Peripheral Nervous System

The first step in treating pain associated with injury to the peripheral nervous system is to consider all possible reversible causes, such as nerve root compression or correctable metabolic or immune system abnormalities (plasmapheresis for the denervation pain of Guillain-Barré syndrome, insulin for acute diabetic neuropathy). When such treatments fail to alleviate painful symptoms, several therapeutic options are available.

Tricyclic antidepressants (TCAs) are thought to act by potentiating central inhibitory mechanisms mediated by norepinephrine and serotonin and are most effective in relieving the *continuous, dysesthetic neuropathic pains* that are common in toxic or metabolic neuropathy (uremic, diabetic, alcoholic). The treatment with TCAs should be based on analgesic effectiveness and on individual medication side effect profiles (Table 2). We recommend amitriptyline, in an initial dose of 10 to 25 mg daily (lower for elders) and increased slowly over a 2 to 3 week period to a daily dose of 75 to 100 mg. The drug is often best tolerated when given at bedtime. If amitriptyline is poorly tolerated or contraindicated owing to anticholinergic side effects, we begin with nortriptyline (Pamelor) or desipramine (Norpramin).

We recommend the following guidelines for use of TCAs:

1. Start with small doses, particularly for elderly patients, and increase slowly.
2. Advise the patient to expect certain side effects such as sedation, dry mouth, blurred vision (which are often self-limited), and warn of the more serious side effects such as urinary retention or irregular heartbeats.
3. If unacceptable side effects develop, consider maintaining the present dose or decreasing the dose. If adverse symptoms persist, consider changing to an alternate TCA such as nortriptyline or desipramine.
4. Be alert to evidence of serious depression and suicidal tendencies and dispense only a 1 to 2 months' supply.

If TCAs are only partially effective, we consider combined treatment with capsaicin (0.075 percent) applied topically three or four times daily. Relief is commonly seen only when higher concentrations are used. The need for frequent daily applications can be burdensome to many patients. In our experience, capsaicin appears most effective for pain associated with diabetic sensory neuropathy and is much less effective with postherpetic neuralgia (PHN). Aspirin (750 to 1500 mg), crushed and dissolved in 20 to 30 ml diethyl ether or chloroform, was recently enthusiastically recommended as a topical treatment for acute herpetic neuralgia or PHN. We have had no experience with this method but would recommend trying it based on the published reports.

Anticonvulsants suppress spontaneous high-

Table 2 Effects of Tricyclic Antidepressants Used to Treat Pain

Drug	Sedative	Anticholinergic Effects	Orthostatic Hypotension	Cardiac Toxicity
Amitriptyline	+ + +	+ + +	+ +	+ + +
Nortriptyline	+ +	+	+/−	+ +
Desipramine	+	+	+	+ +

Modified from Drug Evaluation Annual. Chicago: ©American Medical Association, 1991; with permission.

frequency bursts of neuronal firing and are therefore effective in relieving the *paroxysmal sharp or lancinating pains* common in trigeminal neuralgia. We begin treatment with carbamazepine, starting at a dose of 100 to 200 mg per day and gradually increasing as needed to a maintenance dose of 800 to 1200 mg per day. Pain relief appears to be dose dependent, but there is considerable interpatient variability and there are no clear dosing guidelines or target serum levels. Common side effects include ataxia, sedation, and blurred vision. Nausea may be experienced at the initiation of treatment, but it is usually self-limited and can be avoided by gradually increasing the dose.

NSAIDs and corticosteroids can be effective against the pain of acute neurologic injury when inflammation is involved. Corticosteroids appear most effective for pain associated with tumor involvement of nerves or nerve roots and offer the advantage over NSAIDs of causing fewer symptomatic gastrointestinal side effects. A short (10 to 14 day) course of tapering steroid such as dexamethasone, starting with a dose of 6 mg four times daily, is usually tolerated well and can provide temporary analgesia pending the effect of planned chemotherapy or radiation therapy.

Despite the treatment options described above, many provide little or no significant relief for neuropathic pain. In some cases (phantom limb or postamputation pain), special attention should be given to the proper fitting of prosthetic devices, which can cause local irritation or pain. Significant incremental pain relief may also be achieved by using noninvasive nonpharmacological adjuncts such as physical therapy and TENS. Strong psychological support from the treating physician is most important. Every effort should be made to avoid using multiple medications because of the risks of complex interactions and side effects.

Surgery specifically for pain is beneficial in selected cases. Surgical analgesic procedures should be undertaken only after adequate pharmacological trials have failed. Of the various procedures that are being attempted, dorsal root entry zone (DREZ) lesions appear to be the most effective in selected cases of postherpetic neuralgia and brachial plexus avulsions.

Central Nervous System

The treatment of central nervous system pain is difficult, but satisfactory results may be obtained with agents that enhance central transmission of norepineph-

rine and serotonin. Clinically significant improvement is most frequently obtained with tricyclic antidepressants, and less often with anticonvulsant agents.

For treating central pain, we recommend starting with amitriptyline, using the guidelines given for the treatment of peripheral neuropathy or other chronic pain syndromes. Nevertheless, therapeutic benefit may be obtained only with large doses (150 mg per day). If satisfactory relief is not obtained and the diagnosis of central pain syndrome is secure, we consider using a small dose of a long-acting narcotic such as methadone, 5 mg per day, or levorphanol, 2 mg per day, with analgesia augmented by dextroamphetamine, 2.5 to 5 mg twice a day. In combination therapy, these medications may achieve adequate analgesia with smaller doses of opioids, thus reducing or avoiding constipation and sedation. Baclofen, by enhancing gamma-aminobutyric acid–inhibitory neurotransmission, may relieve certain aspects of central pain such as allodynia, but treatment is commonly limited by sedative side effects.

Neuroablative procedures for central pain have yielded inconsistent results and may produce additional permanent neurologic deficits. Epidural electrical stimulation of the spinal cord or focally within the ventral posterior thalamus has relieved central pain in some cases, but these approaches should be considered only for severe, intractable pain.

TREAT PAIN AGGRESSIVELY AND EARLY

Early, aggressive treatment may help prevent peripherally induced central nervous system changes that may intensify or prolong the pain. For severe, acute pain, opioids are the drug of choice, and they provide analgesia superior to that afforded by other medications. Once a choice is made to use opioids, the doses should be adjusted according to the analgesic effect achieved; limited only by undesirable side effects. Once an organic cause of pain has been identified, opioids should be used if other medications are ineffective. Only when the analgesic of first choice is *totally* ineffective at the maximal acceptable dose should it be discontinued. When an analgesic is *partially* effective, it may be continued along with the addition of an adjunctive analgesic agent. For example, for refractory acute pain an NSAID could be combined with an opioid. Severe neuropathic pain may require treatment with an opioid whose analgesic effect is augmented by combination with TCAs, amphetamine, or hydroxyzine.

DISTINGUISH BETWEEN PAIN AND PSYCHOPATHOLOGY

With few exceptions, such as some headache and musculoskeletal syndromes, *pain in the absence of corroborative evidence of organic disease should receive only mild symptomatic treatment, if any.* If depression or another psychiatric disorder is thought to be the only cause of the pain complaint, the patient should be referred for psychological evaluation and counseling. Many patients with chronic nonorganic pain complaints resist the idea of psychotherapy, but short-term treatment with antidepressants alone is of little value. Tricyclic antidepressants are effective in many pathologic pain conditions, but alone they will not cure serious depression and they introduce the risk of complications from side effects.

AVOID "AS-NEEDED" DOSING

Constant or frequently recurring pain requires continuous analgesia. Pain should be treated with scheduled doses and intervals determined by the expected duration of action of the specific medications used (see Table 1). Avoid "as needed" dosing for chronic or frequently recurring pain. Patient feedback about analgesic adequacy is important and should be encouraged, but this does not mean that the patient should have to plead repeatedly for pain relief. Regularly scheduled analgesic dosing leads to better pain control, helps to alleviate the anxiety associated with painful conditions, and preserves the patient's dignity.

RELY ON THE FAMILIAR

Analgesic therapies may be expected to increase in number and complexity, paced by scientific advances that reveal a host of new pathophysiologic mechanisms and novel neuromodulators of pain transmission and inhibition. New treatments should be tried if they are based on a sound and scientific rationale. However, there is much to recommend an adequate trial of more conventional therapy, keeping in mind that the full range of side effects or complications of new treatments may not yet be realized. A mentor of one of us (RRA) once expressed this more eloquently:

Experience teaches us that today's truths are often tomorrow's misconceptions.

SET REALISTIC GOALS AND BE SUPPORTIVE

Despite recent advances in research, there is no single effective pharmacotherapy for many pain syndromes. Consequently, realistic goals should be substituted for complete analgesia. These should focus on functional recovery, including attention to sleep, appetite, and sexual activity. If complete analgesia is the only goal, supportive therapies may be overlooked or deemed ineffective. Substituting pharmacology for the complete care of patients with pain will ultimately fail and result in patient dissatisfaction and additional suffering. The valuable anxiolytic and analgesic effects of explanation, reassurance, and support by the treating physician cannot be overemphasized.

SUGGESTED READING

Benedettis, et al. A new topical treatment for acute herpetic neuralgia and post-herpetic neuralgia. Pain 1992;48:383–390.
Casey K. Pain and central nervous system disease. New York: Raven Press, 1991.
Fields H. Pain syndromes in neurology. Stoneham, Mass.: Butterworth, 1990.
Foley K, Payne R. Current therapy of pain. Toronto: BC Decker, 1989.
King RB. Concerning the management of pain associated with herpes zoster and post-herpetic neuralgia. Pain 1988;33:73–78.
Raj PP. Practical management of pain. 2nd ed. St. Louis: Mosby–Year Book, 1992.
Raskin NH, et al. Postsympathectomy neuralgia: Amelioration with diphenylhydantoin and carbamazepine. Am J Surg 1974;128:75–78.
Stanton-Hicks M. Pain and the sympathetic nervous system. Norwell: Kluwer Academic Publishers, 1990.

PATIENT RESOURCES

American Pain Society
5700 Old Orchard Road
Skokie, IL 60077
(708) 966-5595

American Chronic Pain Association (ACPA)
Box 850
Rocklin, CA 95677
(916) 632-0922

National Chronic Pain Outreach Association (NCPOA)
7979 Old Georgetown Road, Suite 100
Bethesda, MD 20814
(301) 652-4948
Fax: (301) 907-0745

LOW BACK PAIN AND LUMBAR DISC HERNIATION

JOHN DEAN RYBOCK, M.D.

Low back pain is a common problem. Sixty to eighty percent of the population experience a significant episode at some time, and surveys find a 10 to 20 percent prevalence at any point in time. In many cases, the low back pain represents a simple strain, self-limited and requiring no medical attention. In other cases, the pain may be severe and immobilizing, needing urgent attention. In still others, the pain may be long standing and permanently disabling; one-third of workmen's compensation costs result from back problems.

It is important to remember that low back pain is a symptom not a disease. There are syndromes that include low back pain for which a disease model and therapeutic course have been defined, but for the majority of cases of low back pain, there is no such model and treatment is largely empirical, utilizing sequential therapeutic trials. Because of the difficulty (and intellectual frustration) inherent in treating a symptom without a specific diagnosis, the common approach to the patient with low back pain is to try to make a diagnosis. This often leads to prolonged and excessive testing and delay in initiating any treatment; it also may have the effect of fitting a patient into an inappropriate diagnostic category and giving inappropriate treatment. There are good data to suggest that a substantial number of the more than 200,000 patients who undergo discectomy each year are not appropriate surgical candidates.

EVALUATION

The patient with acute back pain has most likely suffered a strain or soft tissue injury. The patient can usually identify a specific event that precipitated the pain (e.g., lifting a heavy weight or twisting) or an unusual activity within the day or so before the onset of the pain (e.g., painting a ceiling, putting in a garden). If there is any relationship to work or an accident, it is wise to document the history in detail, for legal purposes. If the patient cannot identify a precipitating event, the possibility of other causes increases. In a patient younger than 55 or 60, the pain may be the first sign of lumbar disc herniation. In older patients, the possibility of either osteoporotic compression fracture, pathologic vertebral body fracture, or abdominal aortic aneurysm must be considered and plain x-ray films should usually be taken.

The pattern of back pain itself is of little diagnostic use; virtually all acute back pain of any cause is characterized by spasm and pain in the low back muscles, usually bilateral, that radiates into the gluteal region. The pain may radiate up the spine into the thoracic region. When severe, it may even radiate into the posterior thighs. In exploring the patient's pain pattern, the physician is looking for radiation and symptoms outside these regions, most specifically for evidence of nerve root irritation.

With lumbar disc herniation, the pain at onset may be simple nonspecific back pain, but nerve root irritation usually manifests itself within 8 to 12 hours. Because more than 95 percent of lumbar disc herniations irritate either the L5 or S1 nerve roots, pain radiating to the ankle, called sciatica, is particularly significant. When present, it is often associated with paresthesias in the foot itself. When upper lumbar nerve roots are irritated, the pain is largely confined to the anterior thigh, seldom reaching below the knee. The rare upper lumbar disc herniation, compression fracture, and tumors are all possible causes of such pain. It should be noted that groin pain is rarely a sign of lumbar spine disease.

Certain aspects of the pain are helpful in seeking a cause. In disc herniation, the pain is frequently increased by raising the intra-abdominal pressure (coughing, sneezing, Valsalva's maneuver) and relieved by lying with a pillow under the knees. Pain due to an intraspinal tumor is usually much worse at night.

As the pattern of back pain itself is of little diagnostic value, so are the findings referable to the back. Muscle spasm, as determined by palpation, tenderness, and limitation of motion, is the common component of back pain from any cause. The degree of loss of motion in each plane should be documented, however, to provide a gauge for monitoring response to treatment.

Most important in the evaluation of low back pain is the status of nerve root function, as determined by the standard sensory, motor, and reflex examination. An additional component of the neural examination is the search for "nerve root tension signs." Because traction on a compressed nerve root produces increased pain along its distribution, sciatic nerve stretch (straight leg raising) and femoral nerve stretch are utilized. It is important to note that such tests are significant only if they reproduce the patient's radicular pain.

When a patient first presents with acute back pain, radiography is indicated in only a few specific situations. An elderly patient with spontaneous-onset pain should undergo plain radiography, as noted above. A patient with a major neurologic deficit, such as complete foot drop or loss of bladder control, requires urgent evaluation, usually with magnetic resonance imaging (MRI); minor deficits, such as an absent reflex, should be followed clinically.

TREATMENT

Following the initial evaluation, a tentative diagnosis of either probable disc herniation or probable back strain should be made. In the absence of major leg pain and nerve root tension signs, the latter diagnosis is preferred. Initial treatment is the same, but assignment to the appropriate category facilitates the beginning of patient education, which is important to long-term outcome for both groups.

Back Strain

The patient with back strain is reassured that the problem is unlikely to be serious or long lasting and that the goal is to let the acute injury settle down for a few days, then to begin rehabilitating the back. It is explained that the back muscles have been overstressed and that, as a result, they have tightened up. If the patient stays inactive for a long time, the muscles may relax on their own, but by then they will be too weak to work well and the patient has a new cause of pain. The best course is to rest for a few days, so the acute inflammation can subside, and then begin gentle back stretching and strengthening exercises; the sooner the patient resumes normal activity, the quicker the back will recover. It sometimes takes quite an effort to get this message across, as many people think they should rest until complete recovery has occurred; this is even more difficult if the pain is the result of a work injury and the patient feels entitled to time off until the back completely returns to normal. In this group of patients, any narcotic use should be limited to a few days and an early switch to a nonsteroidal anti-inflammatory drug is in order.

If the episode is relatively mild and short lived, the patient can often be given a printed set of instructions in lumbar flexion exercises and in back care, to help prevent recurrence. More severe cases may benefit from referral to a physical therapist for specific exercise training and education in proper body mechanics.

Disc Herniation

Patients with probable disc herniation are also reassured that the chances for a complete recovery are good with conservative therapy, but they must also understand that such therapy may take weeks or longer. They should be discouraged from viewing surgery as a quick fix and understand that they are likely to do better in the long run if they recover without surgery. The initial recommendation is to rest at home; complete bed rest is not necessary, but the patient should specifically avoid any activity that aggravates the leg pain. The patient has to understand that no prediction can be made about the length of time required for resolution, as each case is different. Progress is then monitored regularly. The straight leg–raising test is probably the best indicator of the amount of nerve root impingement and is used to assess progress. It is best to monitor the patient by telephone in the early stages, to minimize the stress involved in car travel.

The pain associated with lumbar disc herniation can be quite severe and often requires narcotic analgesics; oxycodone compounds usually suffice. If muscle spasm is severe or the patient has much difficulty resting, diazepam may be helpful.

As the pain decreases and the straight leg–raising test becomes less positive, the patient can gradually increase activity. Once the patient is free from positive nerve root tension signs and normal mobility is restored, the same exercise instruction or physical therapy referral made for back strain patients is advisable.

Disc Surgery

Surgery for a herniated lumbar disc is indicated in three situations. If the patient has bowel or bladder impairment, immediate consideration should be given to surgery. If the neurologic deficit is severe, as with complete foot drop, early surgery may be indicated to reverse the deficit. Finally, if the patient fails to show improvement with conservative therapy over a period of at least 3 weeks, surgery is an option. Before surgery, the diagnosis is confirmed by MRI.

Several techniques are used to treat disc herniations, both open and percutaneous, and the surgeon must select the best technique for the specific case. The standard operation, simple discectomy, is done by removing a small area of non-structural bone (laminotomy), retracting the nerve root, and excising the herniated disc fragment. Any other loose fragments in the disc itself are then removed. A variation is microlumbar discectomy, in which an operating microscope is utilized, bone is not removed, and only the herniated fragment is excised. In properly selected patients, the outcome appears to be about the same by either technique; I personally find that simple discectomy, with loupe magnification, allows the best root decompression with a small incision.

A new technique utilizes a closed approach. The automated percutaneous lumbar discectomy is done by inserting, under local anesthesia, a suction-cutting cannula into the center of the disc and removing a portion of it. The reduction in internal tension may allow a bulging disc to resolve. A similar technique, which utilizes a laser to internally decompress a disc, has been developed. However, such closed techniques are not effective if a fragment of disc has become separated (free-fragment herniation), and my experience suggests that the majority of patients who need surgery have free-fragment herniations.

There is no need for a fusion as part of an operation for simple disc herniation, nor is there reason for prolonged postoperative immobility. Patients should begin ambulation on the first postoperation day and progress to adequate activity for self-care within a few days. Simple stretching exercises for the back muscles may be started in the second week after operation, progressing to return to work in 4 to 6 weeks.

CERVICAL SPONDYLOSIS

HOWARD MOSES, M.D., M.S.

Cervical spondylosis refers to that collection of conditions of the cervical spine consisting of degenerative disc disease and the attendant adjacent spondylotic ridges and osteophytes, facet joint arthritis, uncovertebral joint arthritis, ossified posterior longitudinal ligaments (OPLL), redundant ligamentum flavum, and vertebral body listheses. Although often felt to be the concern of orthopaedists and neurosurgeons, in fact some neurologists play key roles in the diagnosis and management of these patients, especially when they also have other neurologic diseases, and the differential diagnosis of their condition includes cervical spondylosis.

The incidence of cervical spondylosis is not known. It probably begins in the second or third decade, and is often accentuated by genetic factors and trauma and becomes common after the fourth or fifth decade.

The main considerations concern the neurologic syndromes that result from spinal cord and root compression. Rarely, the vertebral artery or esophagus is compressed. Cervical spondylotic myelopathy (CSM) and cervical spondylotic radiculopathy (CSR) result from cord or root compression by the factors noted above. Effects of pressure may be sudden and abrupt, as with disc rupture, or slowly progressive and insidious, as in spondylotic ridges or OPLL.

DIAGNOSTIC EVALUATION

If CSM is slowly progressive, pain may or may not be present, but when it is, it may be localized or diffuse and may radiate to one or both upper extremities, the scapula, or the anterior chest. The area to which it radiates may help to localize the myelopathy. Pain does not necessarily correlate with the degree of cord or root compression. The differential diagnosis is that of segmental cervical cord and root disease. In CSR, patients usually present with symptoms and signs of root compression without long tract involvement. The findings include the segmental signs of specific muscle weakness, softness and wasting, specific decreases in deep tendon reflexes and dermatomal sensory loss. Long tract signs such as increased reflexes, flexor spasms, and extensor plantar response suggest associated myelopathy and help define the level of the lesion.

Workup of patients with suspected spondylosis begins with a careful history, and physical and neurologic examination. Plain films of the cervical spine remain the first imaging study. Magnetic resonance imaging (MRI) of the cervical spine with gadolinium enhancement is now an essential study, because of its capacity to visualize the spinal cord roots, and their relationship to surrounding stenoses. On occasion, imaging studies done for other conditions reveal some degree of cervical spondylosis. If the patient has no neurologic symptoms or signs due to the cervical spondylosis, further workup and treatment need not be pursued.

If there is a correlation between the history and examination findings and the cervical spine MRI study, indications for further imaging studies depend on other considerations. If the patient has a free fragment of disc without significant spondylotic changes and needs surgery because of root or cord compression, further imaging studies may not be necessary.

If, however, the workup indicates significant cord or root compression at one or more levels and eventual surgery is a consideration, a cervical myelogram with computed tomography (CT) is the next diagnostic step. Myelography should cover the entire cervical spine from C1 through T1 and not merely look at selected levels, because the cervical myelogram and CT study may reveal lesions that were either poorly visualized or not seen at all on MRI.

In the absence of a good correlation between the clinical presentation and the imaging studies, the diagnosis may in fact be something other than (or in addition to) spondylitic myelopathy or radiculopathy; possibilities include cerebral lesions (parasagittal), thoracic lesions, or even a degenerative disease such as amyotrophic lateral sclerosis or multiple sclerosis. Further diagnostic tests may be necessary to explore those possibilities.

Electromyography and nerve conduction studies are of little value in the diagnosis of CSM or CSR but can help to recognize motor neuron disease and to identify confounding neuropathy. They can confirm the presence of radiculopathy or other denervating disease. I do not feel that discography is of any benefit in the diagnostic workup of spondylotic patients.

CONSERVATIVE MANAGEMENT

For patients whose cord or root compression is not particularly severe or who do not desire or cannot tolerate surgery, conservative approaches are instituted. These consist of the use of a soft cervical collar, nonsteroidal antiinflammatory agents, muscle relaxants, and physical therapy. There are physical therapists who are particularly gifted in the management of the subjective and objective features of CSM and CSR and one such should be sought. They may help to defer aggressive management of these patients, temporarily or permanently. These therapists use many modalities, including neck muscle strengthening, traction, and various hot and cold packs. Some patients prefer to work with chiropractors, who may afford them some measure of relief. I will not refer patients to these practitioners unless I am convinced that their manipulations pose no significant risk of cord or root compression. Facet joint injection is of questionable value. I personally feel that transcutaneous electronic nerve stimulation units and acupuncture have primarily a placebo effect.

If initial conservative management with physical therapy proves unsatisfactory the patient may be referred for surgical management if there are signs and symptoms that correlate with findings of the imaging studies. In the absence of imaging or physical evidence of myelopathy or radiculopathy, failure to relieve neck pain by conservative management is not, by itself, justification for an aggressive surgical approach.

SURGICAL MANAGEMENT

When evaluating patients with CSM or CSR for surgery it is important that there not only be a correlation between structural changes in the cervical spine and symptoms and signs on examination, but that those structural changes be sufficiently prominent to explain the clinical presentation. Such patients may then be referred for surgical management. Accurate localization of all levels of cord and root compression before surgery is essential. Cervical spine surgery should be done by neurosurgeons and orthopaedists who specialize in spine work, are specially trained, and have extensive experience in such.

The procedure of choice is anterior cervical discectomy (ACD), possibly including corpectomy (partial or total) and anterior cervical fusion (ACF) using an iliac crest or tibial strut graft. Osteophytectomy and resection of OPLL are critical to the success of this approach, and when not accompanying the ACF, may result in persistent signs of root and cord compression. ACD and ACF is the primary surgical approach because all of the disease that compresses the roots or cord is anterior to them. Posterior cervical laminectomies with discectomy or osteophytectomy may be successful in cases of radiculopathy, but if done for myelopathy they relieve cord compression only temporarily, and signs and symptoms of myelopathy may reappear within 1 or 2 years.

If there are multiple levels of cord compression, there are particular surgeons who are skillful in handling up to three or four levels of ACF. If at least the upper one or two levels of cord compression are addressed surgically, the chances of successfully relieving the signs and symptoms are greater. When possible, I always examine my patients postoperatively to determine whether in fact the signs of cord or root compression have been relieved. If not, the reason may be that the wrong levels were operated on, that the decompression was not adequate, or that some other disease process is present.

I do not refer my patients for percutaneous lysis of discs at any level of the spine.

OTHER CONSIDERATIONS

Certain aspects of cervical spondylosis merit special comment. Litigation is an important element in the presentation of many patients with this disease entity. If personal injury is involved and there is insufficient correlation between the symptoms and the findings on examination and imaging this may in fact be "a pain syndrome." The physician should be particularly careful about referring such patients to surgeons, as the success rate is very poor.

Thoracic outlet syndrome is diagnosed more often than it is present. It cannot be diagnosed simply by electrodiagnostic studies. It is a very rare entity in my practice, although often part of the differential diagnosis of other conditions, such as CSR.

Patients with cerebral palsy who present with onset of progressive weakness at almost any age should be suspect of having CSM; there is a high incidence of cervical spondylosis among these patients. If surgery is appropriate, they can respond very well to it. Because of the movement disorders involving neck muscles they may need both ACF and posterior fixation.

Patients with CSM often fall into the same age group as those with motor neuron disease (amyotrophic lateral sclerosis). Because of the poor prognosis of these patients with ALS, I do not refer them for surgery, no matter how severe their CSM. I have, however, referred patients with CSM and multiple sclerosis for ACF.

There is a high coincidence of patients with CSM and lumbosacral spondylotic radiculopathy. The latter may be associated with significant lumbosacral canal and neural foramen stenoses. The management of the cervical cord disease usually takes precedence over the lumbar disease. A large number of patients may enjoy spontaneous relief of the symptoms of lumbosacral radiculopathy after ACF, though at some future date the lumbar disease may need to be addressed surgically.

Although vascular compression syndromes involving the cervical spine are often suspected, they are very rare. Patients with CSM or CSR may present with head and neck pain, but in these patients the pain almost invariably begins in the neck and radiates to the head, and there are signs and symptoms of root and cord disease. Correction of the cervical spine problem may relieve headache, but many of these patients have associated migraine as well.

RHEUMATOID ARTHRITIS

Although rheumatoid arthritis is, strictly speaking, not cervical spondylosis, patients with rheumatoid arthritis involving the cervical spine often have spondylotic changes as well and warrant attention here. Conditions of the cervical spine caused by rheumatoid arthritis consist of rheumatoid pannus with upper cervical cord compression, subluxation of the odontoid, and impaction of the upper cervical spine and dens up into the cranial cavity with resultant cord and lower brain stem compression. The surgical management of these patients is often difficult. In a large number of cases pannus responds simply to fusion of the upper cervical spine, often to the occiput. Disimpaction of the upper cervical spine may require a combination of traction, stabilization with fusion (often involving instrumentation), and in more severe cases, odontoidectomy. This should be attempted only by surgeons who have extensive experience in it.

SUGGESTED READING

The Cervical Spine Research Society. The cervical spine. Philadelphia: JB Lippincott, 1989.
Murray KJ, Dudley AH III, Moses H. Cervical spondylosis: A therapeutic update. Md Med J 1990; 39:947–949.

HEADACHE AND FACIAL PAIN

MIGRAINE AND CLUSTER HEADACHES

NABIH M. RAMADAN, M.D.
K.M.A. WELCH, M.D.

Descriptions of migraine headache, and possibly cluster headache, date back several hundred years, yet appropriate management of these debilitating conditions was not devised until late in this century, when a better understanding of the mechanisms of these headaches emerged. Accurate diagnosis of the migraine syndrome and differentiation of migraine from cluster contributed to the development of new and effective treatment strategies. We describe the approaches and protocols we use at the Headache Center, Henry Ford Hospital, in treating patients suffering from migraine and cluster headache.

DEFINITIONS AND CLASSIFICATION OF HEADACHE

Recognizing the type of headache is an important first step toward effective and appropriate treatment. Since 1988, we have adopted the International Headache Society (IHS) definitions and criteria for the diagnosis of head pain disorders. These phenomenologic definitions describe migraine as an episodic, recurrent, and throbbing headache that is usually, but not always, unilateral and lasts 4 to 72 hours. Commonly, photophobia, phonophobia (sonophobia), and gastrointestinal distress accompany the pain, and the headache is frequently aggravated by physical activity. When the headache is preceded or, less frequently, accompanied by a transient focal neurologic deficit (visual, sensory, linguistic, or vestibular) and the deficit lasts 5 to 60 minutes, migraine with aura is diagnosed.

Cluster headache is almost always unilateral, does not shift sides during an attack, and lasts 15 to 180 minutes. Frequently, eyelid edema, ptosis, miosis, conjunctival injection, and rhinorrhea develop ipsilateral to the head pain. Cluster headaches typically occur in cluster periods for several weeks and rarely becomes chronic when no remission is experienced in 1 year.

TREATMENT OF ACUTE MIGRAINE HEADACHE

General Considerations

Migraineurs frequently complain of severe head pain, which is aggravated by light, noise, and physical activity. Providing a quiet, dark environment and allowing the patient to relax and sleep are important initial therapeutic steps. While Dr. Wilkinson at the Headache Clinic in London uses short-acting benzodiazepines to induce sleep, we and others do not advocate the outpatient use of such medications in migraineurs.

Anorexia, nausea, and/or vomiting are frequently associated with migraine. Also, some studies have shown that the absorption of oral medications is delayed during a migraine ictus, partly owing to gastroparesis. Thus, initiating therapy with agents like metoclopramide, 10 mg, not only ameliorates the gastrointestinal manifestations of migraine but also improves gastric peristalsis for quicker and more complete absorption of more specific analgesic drugs.

It is crucial to treat an attack of migraine headache at the earliest sign (e.g., onset of the aura), because delaying therapy makes aborting the attack more difficult, even with powerful analgesics. Patients with migraine aura are at an advantage, as the headache is heralded by the neurologic aura. Many patients who do not develop the aura experience prodromal or premonitory symptoms like mood swings, craving for sweets, or heightened sensitivity to light, noise, or odors. Patients should be made aware of these paroxysms, which in some instances occur as long as 24 hours before the headache, so that therapy can be instituted as early as possible.

Another consideration in the treatment of acute migraine attacks is to use the most effective medication that has the fewest reported side effects. In other words, nonsteroidal anti-inflammatory drugs (NSAIDs) or Midrin (isomethoptene, dichloralphenazone, and acetaminophen) should be tried first when patients suffer mild to moderate headache. Stronger agents, like the ergot alkaloids or sumatriptan, should be reserved for moderately severe to severe headache or when NSAIDs fail after one or two attacks.

Finally, it is recommended that the maximal safe and effective dose of a certain drug be used at the onset of the symptoms rather than giving repeated small doses.

Pharmacologic Treatment

Several classes of medications are used to treat acute attacks of migraine. NSAIDs (Table 1) are usually the drugs of choice for mild to moderate attacks, but they are often ineffective in treating severe attacks. Figures 1 and 2 summarize our practice of acute migraine therapy. Figure 3 describes the therapeutic approach to refractory migraine or status migrainosus, defined according to the IHS as an attack of severe migraine headache lasting longer than 72 hours despite treatment.

Table 1 Nonsteroidal Anti-inflammatory Drugs for Acute Migraine

Drug	Initial Dose and Route	Effectiveness
Aspirin	650 mg PO	+
Ibuprofen	800 mg PO	+
Naproxen-Na	825 mg PO	+ +
Ketoproten	150 mg PO	+
Ketorolac	30 mg IM	+ + +

+ = slightly effective; + + = moderately effective; + + + = very effective.

In addition to the drugs listed in the algorithms, alternative agents can be tried. Phenothiazines have been used to treat severe attacks of migraine, both orally and parenterally. Recently, it has been shown that 0.1 mg per kilogram doses of chlorpromazine given intravenously (maximum of three doses per day) or prochlorperazine, 5 to 10 mg, also given intravenously every 8 to 12 hours, can abort a severe migraine attack. Sumatriptan, the newest acute migraine drug, has been released for use in the United Kingdom, Canada, and some European countries, but not in the United States. Sumatriptan is a highly effective pain agent when given orally (100 mg) or subcutaneously (6 mg). Other major advantages of sumatriptan, a serotonin receptor type 1 agonist (5 HT_1-like, 5 HT_{1D}), include rapid onset of action (even when given during a fully developed attack), amelioration of the gastrointestinal symptoms and the photophobia/phonophobia associated with the migraine ictus, and lack of sedating side effects. Sumatriptan therapy, however, has been associated with a relatively high rate of rebound headache. Multiple dose strategies, patches, slow-release formulas, intranasal, and rectal preparations are under investigation.

Side Effects of Agents for Acute Migraine

NSAIDs commonly cause gastrointestinal distress; occasionally it is severe enough to necessitate stopping the drug. Hypersensitivity skin reactions and impaired

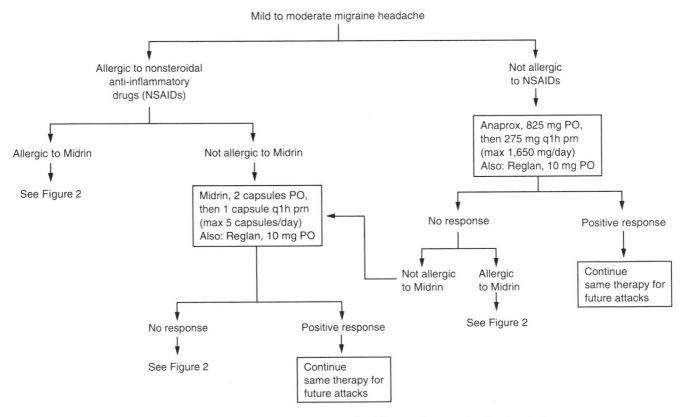

Figure 1 Algorithm for the treatment of mild to moderate migraine headache.

platelet function with potential for excessive bleeding are other potential NSAID side effects. Midrin occasionally causes transient dizziness and skin rashes, which resolve on discontinuation of the drug. Ergot preparations often cause anorexia, nausea, and occasionally vomiting, thus worsening the gastrointestinal symptoms of the migraine ictus. Transient cardiac palpitations, ac-

roparesthesias, and restlessness (probably related to the caffeine in most ergot preparations) are less frequent side effects. Dihydroergotamine has the mildest side effects of any of the ergot drugs. Patients with cardiac disease should not be considered for ergot treatment. Phenothiazines and narcotics cause sedation, which limits out-of-hospital use, especially in the workplace. Phe-

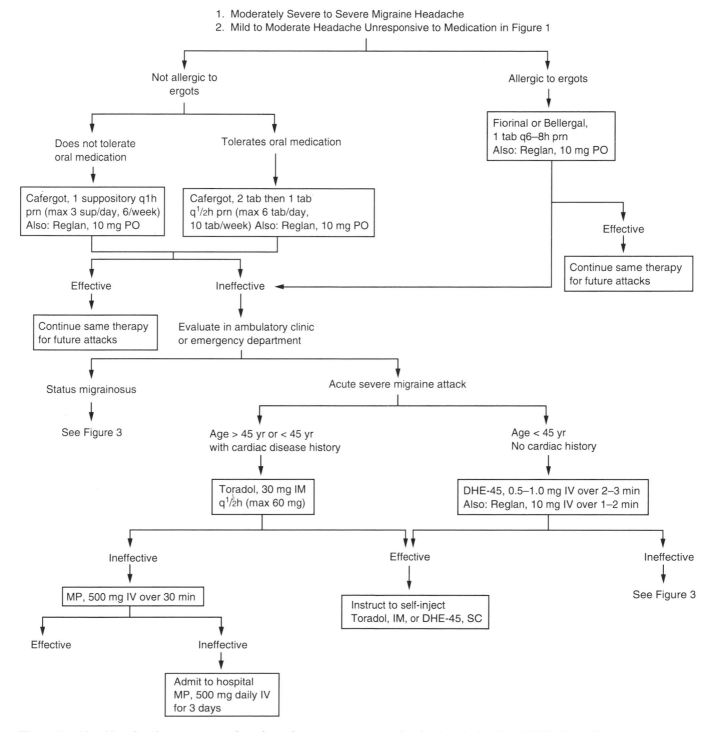

Figure 2 Algorithm for the treatment of moderately severe to severe migraine headache. Key: DHE-45 = dihydroergotamine; IM = intramuscular; IV = intravenous; MP = methylprednisolone; SQ = subcutaneous.

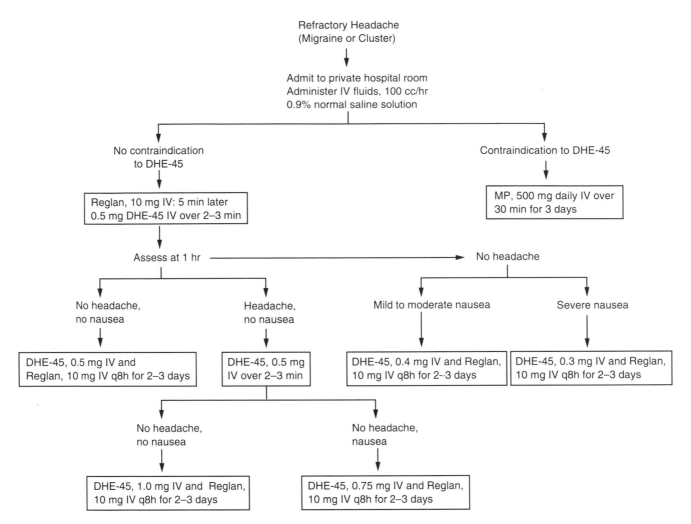

Figure 3 Algorithm for the treatment of refractory headache. Key: DHE-45 = dihydroergotamine; IV = intravenous; MP = methylprednisolone. (Adapted in part from Raskin NH. Treatment of status migrainosus: The American experience. Headache 1990; 30:550–553; with permission.)

nothiazines can cause idiosyncratic extrapyramidal side effects, including oculogyric crises, which respond to antihistamines. Short-term steroid use does not produce the cushingoid features associated with long-term administration. Transient hypotension could develop after intravenous methylprednisolone. Sumatriptan causes transient facial flushing, acroparesthesias, and pain at the subcutaneous injection site. Sumatriptan does not cause the gastrointestinal symptoms commonly associated with other antimigraine drugs.

MIGRAINE PROPHYLAXIS

General Considerations

For some migraineurs who suffer frequent attacks of headache a preventive approach is indicated, in addition to the conventional acute treatment. Generally, patients who suffer two or more migraine attacks per month should be considered for prophylactic therapy. Some patients have one severe attack per month, which can last several days and cost significant loss of time from the job. Such patients might also choose to receive prophylactic therapy. Patients who do not respond to acute treatment or who experience severe side effects may require prophylaxis. Occasional patients are psychologically unable to cope with one or two severe attacks a month, and they may be candidates for prophylaxis. Patients who suffer from menstrual migraine — attacks of headache more than 90 percent of the time clustered around the menses — should be given a trial of an NSAID such as naproxen sodium, 550 mg twice daily, or ibuprofen, 600 mg three times daily, for the week before and for 7 to 10 days after the first day of the menses. Such regimens have been quite effective in preventing attacks of menstrual migraine.

Another important rule in migraine prophylaxis is to avoid polytherapy and institute treatment with a single agent in the smallest possible dose. Gradual increase of the dose should be attempted if the patient does not respond to the small dose, provided no side effects develop. Switching to another agent is in order when over 2 to 3 months the maximal tolerable dose has produced no benefit.

Patients and their treating primary physician should be alerted to potential drug interactions when prophylactic and abortive medications are used in combination. For example, NSAIDs used for acute attacks can increase the risk of gastrointestinal distress and hemorrhage when drugs of the same class are administered for prophylaxis. Rarely, methysergide combined with ergot preparations used for acute therapy could result in psychiatric, behavioral, or vasoconstrictive complications, probably owing to ergot overdose. Fatigue could become pronounced when beta-blockers and tricyclic antidepressants are used in combination.

Patients with migraine frequently identify triggers to the headache attacks. Lack of sleep, skipping meals, overexposure to bright light, foods like cheese, onions, citrus compounds, chocolate, and alcohol (especially red wine), are common migraine triggers. Keeping a diary of the headaches and the circumstances surrounding them helps to track the migraine triggers to be avoided. Recently, several reports were published on the relative deficiency of magnesium in the brain, saliva, and red blood cells of migraineurs. We recommend supplementing the diet of migraineurs with magnesium gluconate, commonly available in health food stores.

Finally, pregnant women should not be offered migraine prophylactic pharmacotherapy because of the known or experimentally demonstrated teratogenic effects of all antimigraine drugs.

Pharmacotherapy of Migraine Prophylaxis

Antiprostaglandins

Several NSAIDs have been tried in migraine prophylaxis, including naproxen sodium, ibuprofen, ketoprofen, mefenamic acid, and aspirin. The mechanism of action of this class of drugs in migraine is unclear, but it could be related to the inhibition of the sterile inflammatory reaction and its painful sequelae. Aspirin is an effective prophylactic drug for childhood migraine, and a recent report has shown its antimigraine efficacy in adults (650 mg daily). Naproxen sodium and ibuprofen are the drugs of first choice for menstrual migraine (see above) and mild to moderate migraine without aura attacks that recur less frequently than once per week. Patients who suffer from arthritic cervical spine conditions and migraine might also benefit from NSAIDs. Gastrointestinal distress, bleeding diatheses, hypersensitivity skin reactions, and, rarely, kidney dysfunction are potential side effects.

Adrenergic Beta-Receptor Blockers (Table 2)

Propranolol, nadolol, timolol, and atenolol have all been used for migraine prophylaxis. The mechanism of

Table 2 Beta-Blockers for Treatment of Migraine

Generic Name	Proprietary Name	Daily Dose (mg)
Atenolol	Tenormin	50–150
Nadolol	Corgard	40–240
Propranolol	Inderal	80–240
Timolol	Blocadren	10–30

action of these drugs in migraine prevention is also unknown but is clearly unrelated to the beta-blocking property. Beta-blocking drugs that have added sympathomimetic agonist activity are ineffective. A recent meta-analysis of all published reports on the use of propranolol in migraine prevention has confirmed the efficacy of this agent for short-term (<6 months) prophylaxis. We have found the medication to be consistently effective over time. Based on the literature, propranolol is the most recommended drug for migraine with aura, basilar migraine, and severe and frequent (>1 per week) migraine of any type. Beta-blockers are contraindicated in patients with congestive heart failure, diabetes, and asthma. Side effects of these agents include slowed mentation, fatigue, hypotension, and bradycardia. Anecdotal reports of migraine-induced stroke in "migraine-with-aura patients" have raised concerns about the use of this drug, as it may impair cerebral autoregulation in ischemic foci, but there are no data to indicate that beta blockade increases the risk for migraine-induced stroke.

Calcium Channel Blockers

Verapamil, nifedipine, and flunarizine (not available in the United States) belong to this class of drugs that have been tried in migraine prophylaxis. One proposed mechanism of action of these agents is prevention of calcium entry into neurons with subsequent neuronal depolarization, release of neuroexcitatory amino acids, spreading depression, and ultimately migraine. Other possible mechanisms include the purely vascular effects of calcium blockade. Nifedipine was popular for migraine prevention in the 1980s, but a recent well-designed and controlled study has shown that nifedipine is ineffective for migraine prevention. In fact, patients treated with the active drug had more headache than the placebo-treated group. Verapamil, 160 to 320 mg daily, has been proposed as the drug of second choice after propranolol for migraine with aura and for severe, frequent migraine headaches of any type. Verapamil is the drug of first choice for patients who cannot tolerate propranolol. Congestive heart failure, atrial flutter or fibrillation, cardiac blocks, and sick sinus syndrome are contraindications to calcium channel blockers. Constipation, nausea, hypotension, headache, rashes, atrioventricular blocks, and dizziness are some side effects of calcium channel blockers.

Table 3 Antidepressants for Migraine

Generic Name	Proprietary Name	Daily Dose (mg)
Amitriptyline	Elavil	50–150
Doxepin	Sinequan	25–150
Fluoxetine	Prozac	20–60
Nortriptyline	Pamelor	25–125
Trazodone	Desyrel	50–150

Antidepressants (Table 3)

Amitriptyline is the antidepressant most commonly used in migraine therapy. Other tricyclics like nortriptyline, trazodone, and doxepin, and nontricyclic antidepressants like fluoxetine are alternative choices. In migraine, antidepressants probably act by inhibiting the 5-HT$_2$ serotonin receptor subtype. Their antimigraine action is independent of the antidepressant effects. Amitriptyline is the drug of choice for the "mixed headache" syndrome (migraine and tension type). It is the drug of third choice after propranolol and verapamil and can be used in conjunction with propranolol (50 to 100 mg amitriptyline and 80 to 160 mg propranolol) in patients who do not respond to beta-blocker monotherapy and cannot tolerate calcium channel blockers. Nortriptyline has fewer anticholinergic and sedative side effects than amitriptyline and can be used by patients who cannot tolerate amitriptyline. Anecdotal experience has suggested that trazodone and doxepin are only occasionally helpful. We have had mixed responses using fluoxetine in migraine prophylaxis, and some have tried this in combination with amitriptyline. No results of large controlled studies are available to support the anecdotal reports of effectiveness. The onset of action of antidepressants is frequently delayed 2 to 3 weeks from the initiation of therapy, and side effects, including headache, are usually more pronounced during this period. Explaining this to the patient is important, so that compliance will continue. Side effects of the tricyclics include sedation, and anticholinergic symptoms like constipation, dry mouth, urine retention, and weight gain. Occasionally, some of these side effects are severe enough to force discontinuation of the drug. Fluoxetine causes restlessness and jitters instead of sedation and has fewer anticholinergic side effects than the tricyclics.

Antiserotonin Agents

Cyproheptadine, methysergide, and pizotifen (not available in the United States) are direct antagonists of the 5-HT$_2$ receptors are effective in migraine prevention. Cyproheptadine is an ideal drug for children with migraine, especially those who also suffer from hyperactivity and are underweight. We only occasionally use cyproheptadine, 4 mg three or four times daily, in adults, when the choices described above have failed. We do not advocate the use of methysergide because of the potential serious side effects of retroperitoneal, cardiac, and pulmonary fibrosis. Other side effects of the 5-HT$_2$ receptor–blocking agents include sedation, weight gain, nausea, and muscle cramps.

Miscellaneous Drugs

Recent interest in the role of *sodium valproate* led to the initiation of a placebo-controlled trial of this medication: moderate benefit was reported in as many as 60 percent of cases. We have tried this medication in a limited number of patients who are refractory to the drugs described above and have had mixed success. *Clonidine,* popular in the 1970s, is an ineffective antimigraine agent. *Phenelzine,* 30 to 45 mg, a monoamine oxidase inhibitor, is rarely used for migraine prophylaxis and only when other options have failed.

ABORTIVE THERAPY FOR ACUTE CLUSTER HEADACHE

General Considerations

Unlike the patients with migraine, cluster headache sufferers do not search for a quiet environment in which to relax. They tend to pace the floor and bang their heads against hard surfaces hoping to relieve the excruciating pain. Rarely, patients with cluster headache are photophobic and/or phonophobic and require a dark room to reduce the pain. Furthermore, alcohol, cold, high altitude, and smoke can trigger an attack of cluster headache, particularly during the cluster period. Such triggers should always be avoided.

Pharmacologic Treatment

Figure 4 summarizes our approach to the treatment of acute cluster attacks. We, like others, have found that *oxygen* is effective for about 70 percent of patients. Unless they stop smoking, smokers should not be prescribed oxygen, because of the danger associated with the use of gas under pressure close to a burning cigarette. Oxygen therapy has no side effects.

Ergotamine inhalers are sometimes difficult to use, and some patients prefer the sublingual preparation, which takes slightly longer to produce the peak blood level. We commonly ask the patient first to attempt to use the inhaler, and we replace it with the sublingual preparation if necessary. The side effects of ergot preparations were outlined earlier in the chapter.

Lidocaine (2 percent) intranasal drops, or occasionally lidocaine gel, is sometimes beneficial in acute cluster attacks. We ask the patients to keep the head back and tilted to the side of the headache when applying the anesthetic.

Finally, the subcutaneous *sumatriptan* trials have produced encouraging data on acute cluster headache treatment. Sumatriptan has rapid onset of action, making it ideal for the treatment of short-lived, severe headaches, of which cluster headache is one.

The mechanism(s) of action of the anti–cluster headache drugs are speculative.

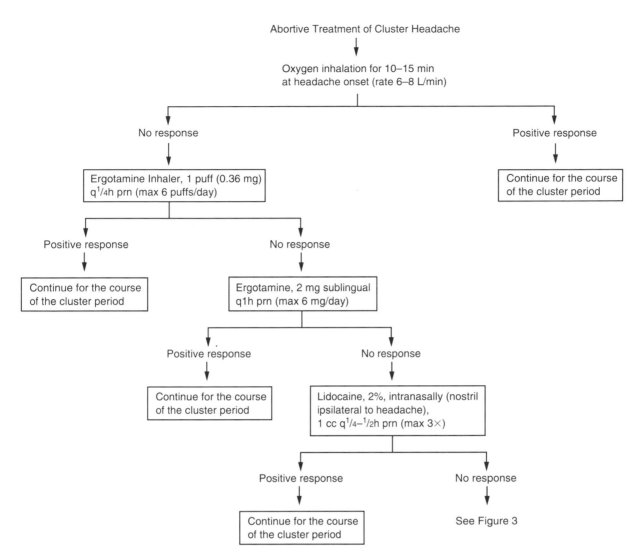

Figure 4 Algorithm for abortive treatment of cluster headache.

PROPHYLAXIS OF CLUSTER HEADACHE

General Considerations

Patients who suffer episodic cluster or chronic cluster headache should receive prophylaxis. It is important that patients keep taking the effective agent for a minimum of 2 weeks after remission has been achieved (2 to 3 months in cases of chronic cluster headache). A dose-tapering schedule should always be provided when remission is achieved. In patients with episodic cluster, once the effective prophylactic regimen has been found it should be used during subsequent cluster periods.

Pharmacotherapy

Figure 5 summarizes the approach to prophylaxis in patients with cluster headache. *Methylprednisolone* is our drug of first choice for episodic cluster headache prophylaxis. As mentioned in the section on migraine,

short-term use of methylprednisolone has not been associated with the untoward side effects observed with long-term treatment. *Verapamil* has been effective in 50 to 75 percent of patients when steroids failed. The response to verapamil has been more favorable in episodic cluster headache than in the chronic type. In our practice, *lithium* has been the more effective prophylactic agent in chronic cluster headache. The blood level of lithium has correlated not with its anticluster activity but with the side effects. Symptoms of cerebellar dysfunction, including tremors, ataxia, and nystagmus, mental confusion, blurred vision, and slurred speech, are some of the known side effects of lithium. Severe extrapyramidal signs and symptoms as well as seizures can occur at toxic drug levels. Long-term lithium therapy has been associated with hypothyroidism, and thyroid function should be monitored every 6 to 12 months while the drug is administered. Limited experience with *nimodipine,* a calcium channel blocker, has suggested a role for the drug in chronic cluster headache

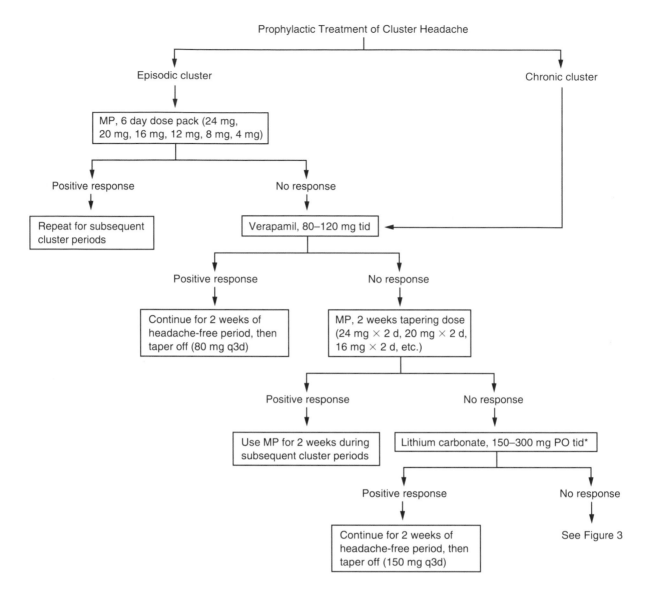

* If patient cannot tolerate lithium, nimodipine, 30 mg PO tid or qid, can be used.

Figure 5   Algorithm for prophylactic treatment of cluster headache. Key: MP = methylprednisolone.

prophylaxis when patients cannot tolerate lithium. The side effects of nimodipine are similar to those of verapamil. Finally, patients with predominantly early morning cluster headache attacks benefit from 2 mg *ergotamine* taken at bed time.

FINAL REMARKS

We have reviewed our management strategies of migraine and cluster headaches, two severe but benign head pain conditions whose pathogeneses remains unclear. These conditions are chronic, and strong rapport between the physician and the patient is the most important therapeutic step. We encourage treating physicians to spend significant time with the patient explaining what these headaches are and discussing at length the treatment options and their rationales. Such a holistic approach results in better compliance and less frustration.

SUGGESTED READING

Headache Classification Committee of the International Headache Society. Classification and diagnostic criteria for headache disorders, cranial neuralgias and facial pain. Cephalalgia 1988; 8(suppl 7):19–28.
Holroyd KA, Penzien DB, Cordingley GE. Propranolol in the management of recurrent migraine: A meta-analytic review. Headache 1991; 31:333–340.
Mathew NT. Cluster headache. Neurology 1992; 42(suppl 2):22–31.
Moskowitz MA. Basic mechanisms of vascular headache. Neurol Clin 1990; 8:801–815.

The Oral Sumatriptan International Multiple-Dose Study Group. Evaluation of a multiple-dose regimen of oral sumatriptan for acute treatment of migraine. Eur Neurol 1991; 31:306–313.

Raskin NH. Treatment of status migrainosus: The American experience. Headache 1990; 30(suppl 2):550–553.

The Subcutaneous Sumatriptan International Study Group. Treatment of migraine attacks with sumatriptan. N Engl J Med 1991; 325:316–321.

The Sumatriptan Cluster Headache Study Group. Treatment of acute cluster headache with sumatriptan. N Engl J Med 1991; 325: 322–326.

Wilkinson M. Treatment of acute migraine: The British experience. Headache 1990; 30(suppl 2):545–549.

IDIOPATHIC INTRACRANIAL HYPERTENSION (PSEUDOTUMOR CEREBRI)

JAMES J. CORBETT, M.D.

DIAGNOSIS

Before the advent of arteriography (AG) and pneumoencephalography (PEG) the diagnosis of pseudotumor cerebri (idiopathic intracranial hypertension, or IIH) depended on lumbar puncture with findings of high cerebrospinal fluid (CSF) pressure and normal chemistry and cytology, skull radiography, and careful re-examination to be sure that a tumor or hydrocephalus was not missed. It was largely an act of faith. Even when AG and PEG were introduced, IIH was still considered to be more often tumor than pseudotumor. Computed tomography (CT), magnetic resonance imaging (MRI), and magnetic resonance angiography (MRA) have changed this. The diagnosis of IIH is on firm footing, because it is unlikely that a tumor or ventriculomegaly will be missed when these studies are used.

IIH is a condition that occurs in 19 of 100,000 obese women of childbearing age; 90 percent of patients are obese and are between ages 15 and 45 years. A much smaller number of men have this condition, and it is even less common in children, who show no sex predilection. Increased CSF pressure occurs as a result of venous sinus occlusions (intravascular thrombosis or extravascular compression) and is anecdotally associated with a number of exogenous agents such as steroid withdrawal, vitamin A toxicity, lithium, nalidixic acid, and the use of tetracyclines.

The need to do complete neuroimaging of these patients cannot be overstated (Table 1). It is still necessary to do a lumbar puncture, because a normal CT or MR picture cannot predict the protein concentration or the number of white cells in the CSF. Neuroimaging and lumbar puncture are clearly complementary studies.

Table 1 Rationale for Imaging When Idiopathic Intracranial Hypertension Is Suspected

To look for brain tumor
To look for hydrocephalus
To look at venous sinuses
To look at the sella turcica
To look for Arnold-Chiari malformation
To look at the perimesencephalic and collicular cisterns

Choice of Study

Magnetic Resonance Imaging

MRI is more expensive but does not miss the occasional astrocytoma or rare case of gliomatosis cerebri, which may masquerade as IIH. Unfortunately, MRI cannot be recommended for all patients, because of weight constraints (most machines cannot support patients who weigh more than 300 pounds) and the ever-present problem of claustrophobia, a particular difficulty with short, obese women, even those who weigh less than 300 pounds. Theoretically, MRI is a better tool for identifying venous sinus occlusion, but, unfortunately, MRI alone misses as many as 25 percent of venous sinus occlusions. In men, postpartum women, and children, venous sinus occlusion is a major diagnostic concern and should be sought with MRA, or with digital subtraction angiography (DSA) if MRA is not available.

MRI is particularly useful in identifying empty sella, a very common concomitant of IIH. The combination parasagittal and coronal cuts also afford assessment of the location of the optic chiasm and optic nerves, since these structures occasionally descend into the sella with deleterious effects on vision.

MRI provides an unparalleled view of the posterior fossa, and particularly of the cerebellar tonsils. The comorbidity of the Arnold-Chiari type I malformation (ACM) and IIH was first brought to my attention in 1988 by Dr. John Harbison. Since then, I have seen a handful of such patients.

I have no firm denominator on which to base the prevalence of the ACM type I in patients with IIH as compared to an unselected population of "normals." The occurrence of ACM is important when lumbar peritoneal (LP) shunt is considered for treatment of CSF hypertension. Lowering the pressure in the spinal canal may cause the cerebellar tonsils to descend and induce (acquired) ACM. Two new problems then arise. Headaches that were bifrontotemporal or holocranial become occipitonuchal: the hindbrain herniation headache. The other problem is the development of a cervical syrinx. I have seen this syrinx and occipital headache problem arise in patients with LP shunt on three occasions, but in each case the lack of both before and after MRI studies made it difficult to be sure whether this was a new problem or a pre-existing condition that worsened. I suspect that the LP shunt was causal.

Computed Tomography

CT using thin cuts and contrast is a useful way to examine the patient with IIH when MRI cannot be used. Special attention should be paid to the superior sagittal, straight, and lateral venous sinuses for the *empty delta sign* of major venous sinus occlusion. This sign is commonly missed by those who have not seen it before or do not understand its significance. It is possible to identify an empty sella using CT even without intrathecal contrast medium, if a combination of thin axial cuts and lateral reconstruction is used.

IIH is probably responsible for most cases of what is known as idiopathic CSF rhinorrhea. Persistent intracranial pressure (ICP) elevation, which occurs in most patients with IIH, causes remolding and erosion of the bones of the skull base, especially the sella turcica and the cribriform plate. CSF drainage through these fenestrated areas is always difficult to demonstrate, but thin cut bone window CT is the ideal way to demonstrate such fenestrae in the bones of the skull.

Angiography

DSA should be used only in patients whose sex, body habitus, or symptoms other than headache and papilledema suggest that this is not a typical IIH patient (Table 2). MRA provides the answer for those who fit in the machine and are not claustrophobic. It is important to establish whether a venous sinus is occluded, in order to provide anticoagulation. Use of diuretics or steroids in this setting would only exacerbate the problem, and this justifies the small risk of angiography.

Special Tests

In the past, patients with IIH have been investigated with scintigraphic studies of CSF flow (isotope cisternography). These studies showed a significant delay in the absorption of the isotope over the vertex of the skull; however, cisternography findings add nothing to the routine management of the IIH patient.

If the patient weighs more than 300 lb or is claustrophobic, CT with contrast medium, using intra-

Table 2 Patients to be Considered for Angiography

Men
Thin women
Children
Patients with prominent cranial bruits, lupus erythematosus, or Behçet's disease

venous, double dose with thin cuts through the sella turcica and bone windows, should be done. The venous sinuses should be scrutinized before and after contrast for evidence of clot. If the hypothetical patient is not obese in habitus, as one would expect of an IIH patient, angiography should be seriously considered.

Special Circumstances

The patient who is being considered for LP shunt should be imaged carefully for evidence of cerebellar tonsillar herniation, both before and after shunting. The final use of neuroimaging in patients with IIH, is lumbar, or even cervical, spinal puncture under fluoroscopic control to measure the spinal fluid pressure and obtain a spinal fluid sample for study.

A patient who for years has had IIH and has signs of CSF rhinorrhea should be evaluated with thin cut axial and coronal bone window CT scans. These studies should focus on the sella and the cribriform plate. Intrathecal radioisotopes and nasal pledgets placed by an otolaryngologist occasionally make it possible to identify the source of CSF rhinorrhea.

The "typical" patient who presents to the neurologist with headache, papilledema, transient visual obscurations, and no focal neurologic signs is an obese woman of childbearing age. If she is not claustrophobic, the ideal neuroimaging study is MRI and MRA. If MRI is available but not MRA, that would be the next best choice. If that study is normal, only a lumbar puncture needs to be done. Evidence of an empty sella and ACM Type I should always be sought (Table 3).

The choice of imaging study in IIH depends on availability of the study and the ability to study the particular patient. Obesity is a central feature of this condition, and the patient's body habitus may dictate whether MRI or MRA can be performed. In the case of the patient who cannot undergo MRI or MRA, an alternative approach that uses CT and DSA provides another route for radiographic assessment. The posterior fossa of patients who are being considered for LP shunt should be imaged very carefully. Above all, a negative or normal imaging study in any patient with the presumed diagnosis of IIH should not be treated as a substitute for lumbar puncture.

Ventricular Size

Dan Jacobsen and colleagues at Marshfield Clinic have shown clearly that it is not possible to distinguish the "slit ventricles" said to be characteristic of patients with IIH from small ventricles of normal persons or

Table 3 Reasons to Order Studies and What to Look for on CT or MRI

Evidence of mass compressing a venous sinus
Major venous sinus occlusion: empty delta sign on CT; bright signal in a venous sinus on MRI
Arteriovenous malformation
Tumor
Hydrocephalus
Tonsillar herniation: Examine parasaggital MRI sections; on CT look at the low cuts using bone windows and observe the tonsils hugging the medulla
Empty sella: evidence of longstanding increased ICP
The presence or absence of ambient cisterns and collicular plate cisterns

non-IIH patients. Whether ventricles in IIH patients actually become larger as a result of treatment is a matter of controversy. On the other hand, large ventricles are never a feature of IIH. Ventriculomegaly in a patient with papilledema, headache, and increased ICP must always be considered a sign of hydrocephalus with some underlying block to flow in the CSF pathways.

TREATMENT

When preliminary radiologic, laboratory, CSF, and visual studies have been completed, treatment of IIH depends on the patient's symptoms, the severity of vision loss, and the presence of other underlying conditions such as glaucoma, systemic hypertension, episodic hypotension, renal disease, pregnancy, or another medical condition. Characteristic treatment settings include the following ones:

The *asymptomatic patient* who has no identifiable cause, no vision loss, and whose condition was discovered accidentally does not need to be treated. Such patients should be followed at 1 to 3 month intervals with neuro-ophthalmologic studies. If vision loss occurs, treatment is acetazolamide, 500 to 1,000 mg twice a day, or furosemide. If vision loss continues to progress, surgery should be considered.

When the patient has only *headache* and vision loss is trivial or nil, the treatment is standard headache medications. Severe, persistent headache may respond to lumbar puncture. Paradoxically, though headaches are relieved frequently with lumbar puncture, long-term ICP monitoring in patients with pseudotumor has produced no evidence of a direct correlation between the CSF pressure and the severity of headaches. Severe, chronic headache as a major symptom of pseudotumor may, on rare occasion, require LP shunt. LP shunt should be used infrequently and the entire range of prophylactic migraine medications should be exhausted in an effort to control headache before recommending shunt. If headaches are postural and remit when the patient is recumbent, the physician should consider using a blood patch, since patients with pseudotumor may also develop post–lumbar puncture headaches.

The patient with *serious loss of visual fields or loss of visual acuity* should not be subjected to multiple medications before surgery is contemplated. Optic nerve sheath fenestration, the procedure of choice, should be done early rather than late if vision loss is a major complaint, especially if visual fields and visual acuities corroborate the symptom. Multiple medications and medication changes have not been effective in preventing progressive vision loss. Surgery may not always prevent blindness, especially when vision loss is severe or precipitous or has been present many days or weeks.

Careful documentation of visual acuity, visual fields, and the photographic appearance of the fundus is crucial, because patients with serious vision loss may actually believe that the treatment caused the problem.

Rapidly progressive vision loss with pseudotumor cerebri is seen rarely, but on occasion a patient may become blind within a few days. Such patients are, paradoxically, disproportionately men, usually black, who have high blood pressure. These patients do not have hypertensive encephalopathy, but the management of their high blood pressure and their increased ICP poses a serious treatment challenge. To date, all patients I have seen with this constellation of severe hypertension, pseudotumor cerebri, and rapid vision failure have developed severe vision loss or blindness despite LP shunt, optic nerve sheath fenestration, and multiple medications. The concurrent attempts to regulate systemic blood pressure may well be responsible by producing decreased blood flow at the optic disc and resultant ischemic infarction on top of papilledema.

A *pregnant patient with severe headache* is best treated with repeat lumbar punctures or with beta-blockers. These are relatively safe methods during pregnancy and should relieve headache. If headache is incapacitating, bed rest and, as a last resort, LP shunt could be considered. If *vision loss* begins or progresses during the pregnancy, optic nerve sheath fenestration is the safest way to preserve vision. Pregnancy is not a contraindication to any treatment. IIH is not an indication for therapeutic abortion.

If the patient has *renal disease* that requires hemodialysis, recurrent drop in blood pressure with volume shifts are common. Hypotension is poorly tolerated by a swollen optic disc and may result in compound vision loss due to papilledema and to ischemic infarction. Vision loss can be safely prevented with optic nerve sheath fenestration.

Specific Treatment Modalities

A *weight reduction diet* is recommended for any obese patient with IIH. For the asymptomatic obese patient, dieting may be the only recommended therapy. Patients should be encouraged to lose weight, not coerced with threats of blindness. A commercial weight reduction program such as Weight Watchers can also be helpful.

Diuretics have been used to treat IIH for years. Those used most commonly are acetazolamide, 1,000 to 2,000 mg daily in the sequel form (500 mg two or three times per day), or furosemide, 40 to 160 mg a day. Both drugs can reduce headache frequency and severity and may diminish transient vision obscurations; however, none of the diuretics has ever been subjected to a randomized prospective trial of therapy. Side effects of acetazolamide include numbness of the hands and feet and circumoral region, and, rarely, renal stones, and all patients develop mild metabolic acidosis, which is never serious. A serum bicarbonate value of 14 to 18 mEq per liter is objective evidence of compliance. In addition to somatosensory symptoms, patients taking acetazolamide complain that carbonated beverages taste metallic. Such patients occasionally become anorectic or depressed. These symptoms may cause a patient to stop taking the medication. Potassium wasting is the rule, and substantial potassium chloride replacement may be required.

Furosemide may be used: 20 to 80 mg daily in two doses. The problem of potassium wasting is even greater here, but it can be controlled. The frequency of urination may present a practical problem; a secretary with IIH lost her job because the furosemide caused her to go to the bathroom too frequently. These drugs may be used for months to years.

Steroids are commonly used and, initially, are effective. When they are given for 2 to 8 weeks and discontinued (a commonly advocated regimen), however, papilledema usually recurs. One is then tempted to prolong steroid administration. The patient is propelled into a long bout of steroid use with all of the attendant complications. I personally avoid giving steroids. Their administration does not reliably relieve CSF pressure, and it adds new problems to patient management. Results are not proven to be better than those with acetazolamide or furosemide.

Frequent lumbar puncture is advocated by some, but I have had the most success with this modality when the objective of the therapy was headache relief and the patient requested it. Repeated lumbar taps are difficult and painful for obese patients and patient compliance is problematic. Occasionally, post–lumbar puncture headaches add a new dimension to patients' headache problem.

SUGGESTED READING

Baker RS, Carter D, Hendrick EB, et al. Visual loss in pseudotumor cerebri of childhood. A follow-up study. Arch Ophthalmol 1985; 103:1681–1686.

Corbett JJ. The 1982 Silversides lecture. Problems in the diagnosis and treatment of pseudotumor cerebri. Can J Neurol Sci 1983; 10: 221–229.

Corbett JJ. Diagnosis and management of idiopathic intracranial hypertension (pseudotumor cerebri). Presented at 1989.

Corbett JJ, Nerad JA, Tse DT, et al. Results of optic nerve sheath fenestration for pseudotumor cerebri. The lateral orbitotomy approach. Arch Ophthalmol 1988; 106:1391–1397.

Corbett JJ, Savino PJ, Thompson HS, et al. Visual loss in pseudotumor cerebri. Follow-up of 57 patients from five to 41 years and a profile of 14 patients with permanent severe visual loss. Arch Neurol 1982; 39:461–474.

Corbett JJ, Thompson HS. The rational management of idiopathic intracranial hypertension. Arch Neurol 1989; 46:1049–1051.

Digre KB, Varner MY, Corbett JJ. Pseudotumor cerebri and pregnancy. Neurology 1984; 34:721–729.

Orcutt JC, Page NG, Sanders MD. Factors affecting visual loss in benign intracranial hypertension. Ophthalmology 1984; 91: 1303–1312.

Sergott RC, Savino PJ, Bosley TM. Modified optic nerve sheath decompression provides long-term visual improvement for pseudotumor cerebri. Arch Ophthalmol 1988; 106:1384–1390.

Wall M, George D. Visual loss in pseudotumor cerebri. Incidence and defects related to visual field strategy. Arch Neurol 1987; 44: 170–175.

HEADACHE IN CHILDREN

GERALD M. FENICHEL, M.D.

Headache is a "normal" life event for people of all ages. Among adolescents, 12 percent report that headache caused them to miss at least 1 day of school during the past month; 13 percent of male and 20 percent of female teenagers have seen a doctor for headache. Medical attention is usually sought because of one or more of the following factors: (1) headache is new and severe, (2) symptoms such as nausea or transitory neurologic disturbances are associated, (3) head injury occurred prior to headache's onset, (4) frequent school absence, and (5) history of brain tumor in a family member.

Parents who seek medical attention for a child with headache look not only for symptomatic relief but to be assured that headache is not a malevolent sign of an intracranial disease such as brain tumor. It is not always necessary, or possible, to identify the cause of headache, only to provide assurance that it is not a sign of serious illness. Such assurance may be therapeutic, and computed tomography (CT) of the brain is often a cost-effective measure.

APPROACH TO HEADACHE

The treatment of headache depends on its cause. I classify non–life-threatening headaches of childhood into five types that are operational for my treatment alternatives: (1) chronic mixed headache, (2) common vascular headache, (3) migraine, (4) situational headache, and (5) unexplained headache. This classification would not be supported by any international organization. Intentionally missing from the classification are such highly regarded causes of childhood headache as sinusitis, allergy, and eyestrain. I believe that sinusitis causes sinus tenderness and nasal congestion but does not cause chronic headache. My experience in evaluating children for dementia is that more than 50 percent of head CT examinations show evidence of sinusitis. It may be that sinusitis is the most common cause of dementia in children, but it seems more likely that radiographic evidence of sinusitis is a relatively common finding that has no clinical correlation. Much the same can be said about "allergy" as defined by a skin reaction to injection of a foreign substance. Whenever a parent reports that a child's headache correlates with eating a specific food substance, usually chocolate, I always agree that the foodstuff should be avoided (chocolate is not an essential nutrient). Almost everybody who engages in prolonged binocular work experiences orbital pain; the cause is obvious, and relief comes rapidly when the eyes are closed.

I usually begin my evaluation by asking, "How many different kinds of headache do you have?" This is especially useful in children who report continuous headache for weeks or months. The usual response is that there are two kinds of headache: the bad headache, of which the child complains spontaneously, and the mild headache, of which the child complains when asked, "Are you having a headache?" When such a history is obtained, the physician should direct further inquiry to the bad headache and give short shrift to the other. An alternative explanation for the complaint of daily headaches of long duration is that the child has had a flurry of headaches over a week or two, and after a prolonged headache-free interval experiences another flurry of daily headaches. Other questions to ask to determine the chronicity and severity of headache are, "When and how long was your longest headache-free interval?" and "How many days of school have you missed because of headache?"

CHRONIC MIXED HEADACHES

Chronic mixed headaches are of uncertain cause and probably represent a somatic response to life stress. *Tension headache* is an alternative term, but it is not always clear that the child is experiencing tension. I distinguish chronic mixed headache from *situational headache,* described later. The former is treated by teaching the child more constructive adaptive mechanisms, the latter by removing the child from a bad situation. Almost 50 percent of adults with chronic tension headache date the onset before 20 years of age, and 15 percent before 10 years of age.

Females are affected three times more frequently than males. Pain is almost always bilateral and diffuse, and the site of most intense pain may shift during a day. Much of the time, headache is dull and aching, but sometimes the pain has a pounding, vascular quality and then is more intense. Headache is generally present upon awakening and may continue all day. Most children describe an undulating course characterized by long periods during which headache occurs almost every day and shorter intervals when they are headache free. Nausea, vomiting, and transitory neurologic disturbances are not associated. When these features are present, they usually occur only a few times a month and suggest that the patient has both intermittent migraine and chronic mixed headache. Neurologic findings should be normal. Chronic mixed headache is, by definition, difficult to treat; otherwise it would not be chronic. Before consulting a physician, most children have tried several over-the-counter analgesics and received no benefit. The use of more powerful analgesics or analgesic–muscle relaxant combinations has limited value. Long-term use of analgesics usually adds an upset stomach to the child's distress.

Amitriptyline is the most useful drug for chronic mixed headache. It has analgesic properties beyond its effect as an antidepressant. I always start with a small bedtime dose, usually 25 mg, and slowly increase the dose as tolerated.

Many children with chronic mixed headache benefit from relaxation exercises or biofeedback. When the response to amitriptyline is unsatisfactory, I routinely refer children for such therapy.

COMMON VASCULAR HEADACHE

Vasodilatation in the carotid circulation causes headache that is usually bitemporal or diffuse and is described as pounding, throbbing, or pulsating. The pain is made worse by sudden jarring or movement of the head. Differentiating migraine from common vascular headache by the description of pain can be difficult. Furthermore, many factors that trigger vascular headache in nonmigraineurs also trigger migraine in migraineurs. Most vascular headaches respond to simple analgesics such as aspirin or acetaminophen. Those that require specific treatment are described below.

Benign Exertional Headache

Exertion, especially during competitive sports, is a known trigger for migraine in predisposed persons. Others who are not migraineus may have vascular headaches only during exertion. Physical exertion is more likely to produce headache when effort is prolonged and sufficiently strenuous to sustain the pulse at twice its resting rate for 10 minutes or longer. Pain begins during or just after exercise and may last as long as 4 hours. It is throbbing and bitemporal. The association between exertion and headache is easily recognized.

Exertional headache can sometimes be prevented by taking indomethacin before engaging in activities known to induce benign exertional headache. The prophylactic use of indomethacin, 25 mg three times a day, or propranolol, 1 to 2 mg/kg/day in divided doses, may reduce the incidence of attacks.

Drugs and Toxins

Many psychotropic drugs, analgesics, and cardiovascular agents have vasodilator properties. Cocaine use produces a migrainelike headache in persons who do not have migraine at other times. Drug-induced headache should be suspected in a child who has vascular headache following the use of any drug.

Many children, especially adolescents, drink large volumes of diet carbonated beverages containing caffeine each day for weight control. Caffeine has vasoconstricting properties and does not by itself cause headache; however, rebound vasodilatation occurs when the blood caffeine concentration drops. Persons who regularly drink large amounts of beverages containing caffeine often notice a dull frontotemporal headache an hour or more after the last beverage. More caffeine is taken to relieve the headache, and caffeine addiction is initiated. Withdrawal symptoms eventually become severe and include throbbing headache, anxiety, and malaise.

Caffeine addiction, like other addictions, is often hard to break. Some patients can be weaned from caffeine, but most require abrupt cessation and experience withdrawal symptoms. Hospitalization and sedation are sometimes necessary to help patients through withdrawal.

MIGRAINE

Migraine is the most common cause of headache in children who are referred for neurologic consultation. It is a hereditary disorder transmitted by autosomal-dominant inheritance. A history of migraine in at least one parent is reported 90 percent of the time when both parents are interviewed personally and 80 percent of the time when only one parent is interviewed. The prevalence of migraine in children under age 7 years is 2.5 percent (both sexes are affected equally), 5 percent from age 7 to puberty (female-to-male ratio of 3:2), and 5 percent in postpubertal males and 10 percent in postpubertal females. The prevalence of migraine in preschool children is probably higher than the recorded figure, because at this age migraine symptoms tend to be atypical. The higher incidence of migraine in pubertal *females* is probably related to the triggering effect of the menstrual cycle on migraine attacks.

The essential caveat for the treatment of migraine in children is that, regardless of treatment, about half of all patients experience more than a 50 percent reduction in headache frequency in the 6 months following the initial visit to a neurologist.

It is important for the child and the family to develop a sense of learning how to live with migraine: (1) avoid, when possible, activities that are known to trigger attacks, (2) when attacks occur, give in and go to bed, (3) use as little medication as possible, because repeated doses only lead to further gastrointestinal upset, and (4) do not use narcotics or other addicting drugs.

Treating the Acute Attack

Although aspirin and other common analgesics may provide relief of pain in children who suffer from only mild headache, treatment with non-narcotic analgesics is not successful for most patients. The response to ergotamine is variable and should never be used for the purpose of diagnosis. In double-blind studies, ergot is not better than placebo.

My approach to treating severe migraine attacks is to put the child to sleep. This can usually be accomplished with oral or rectal promethazine hydrochloride, 0.5 mg per kilogram body weight.

Migraine Prophylaxis

Propranolol is the only agent that is consistently better than placebo for migraine prophylaxis. The dosage in children is 2 mg per kilogram divided into three doses. Because depression is a dose-related adverse reaction, treatment should be initiated at 1 mg per kilogram per day. Depression is the most common reason to discontinue therapy, and parents should be warned of this reaction when the drug is started. The drug should not be used in children who have asthma, because it may provoke an attack. Once a maintenance dose is established, the sustained-release tablet can be used by increasing the daily dose by one-third.

SITUATIONAL HEADACHES

Children who develop headaches because of an intolerable circumstance (e.g., divorce with custody proceedings, sexual abuse) are considered separately, because nothing short of changing the behavior of others will stop the headache. When a mother asks for a letter requesting that a judge curtail the father's visitation rights because they provoke the child's headaches, the physician should neither write a letter nor expect to help the child with analgesics.

Situational headaches are chronic, diffuse, and difficult to characterize. Insomnia and depression are associated features and should be treated with bedtime amitriptyline. Extracting a child from a bad situation and changing adult behavior are always difficult; however, the physician should not do anything that diverts attention from the real problems that must be resolved.

UNEXPLAINED HEADACHES

Some children complain of headaches that cannot be explained by any known pain mechanism. Seizures as a cause of headache should be considered in children with truly paroxysmal head pain; however, sudden headache that lasts only seconds is not a sign of serious disease.

Reassurance is the best treatment option for children with headache syndromes that seem genuine but are inexplicable. Better to say, "I cannot explain your headache, but I feel certain that it is not caused by any serious underlying disease," than to make a psychiatric diagnosis or referral. Brain-imaging studies are comforting in this regard.

SUGGESTED READING

Chu ML, Shinnar S. Headaches in children younger than 7 years of age. Arch Neurol 1992;49:79–82.

Dhuna A, Pascuel-Leone A, Belgrade M. Cocaine-related vascular headaches. J Neurol Neurosurg Psychiatry 1991;54:803–806.

Linet MS, Stewart WF, Celentano DD, et al. An epidemiologic study of headache among adolescents and young children. JAMA 1989; 261:2211–2216.

Prensky AL, Sommer D. Diagnosis and treatment of migraine in children. Neurology 1979;29:506–510.

Silbert PL, et al. Benign vascular sexual headache and exertional headache. Br Med J 1991;54:417–421.

DEVELOPMENTAL ABNORMALITIES

HYDROCEPHALUS

JOHN ARYANPUR, M.D.

Hydrocephalus is a common clinical problem in both pediatric and adult populations. The many different clinical manifestations of hydrocephalus require a variety of different treatment approaches, which are reviewed here.

Hydrocephalus may be divided into two broad categories: obstructive and nonobstructive. Obstructive hydrocephalus is caused by an obstruction to cerebrospinal fluid (CSF) flow between the ventricles and the subarachnoid space or between the ventricles themselves. This is usually caused by obstruction of the foramen of Monroe or the aqueduct of Sylvius. Communicating hydrocephalus occurs when absorption of CSF by arachnoid villi in the subarachnoid space is blocked. Both obstructive and communicating hydrocephalus take congenital and acquired forms.

Congenital hydrocephalus implies an error of neurulation, which leads to impaired CSF circulation and drainage. The vast majority of cases of congenital hydrocephalus are obstructive in nature. Congenital aqueductal stenosis, Chiari malformation, and Dandy-Walker malformation are all examples of obstructive congenital hydrocephalus. Communicating hydrocephalus, which implies normal communication between the ventricles and the subarachnoid space, is a much less common type of congenital hydrocephalus.

Acquired hydrocephalus refers to hydrocephalus resulting from secondary trauma to the nervous system. Although commonly considered a form of congenital hydrocephalus, the neonatal hydrocephalus that results from intraventricular hemorrhage in the premature infant is best considered a variant of communicating acquired hydrocephalus. Other examples of acquired hydrocephalus include post-traumatic hydrocephalus, and hydrocephalus following subarachnoid hemorrhage (both usually communicating hydrocephalus), hydrocephalus caused by tumors of the third or fourth ventricles (usually obstructive hydrocephalus), and normal-pressure hydrocephalus.

DIAGNOSIS

The diagnosis of hydrocephalus is based on both clinical and radiologic features. In a neonate, a head circumference greater than the 95th percentile, or progressive enlargement of the head circumference that crosses percentile lines is an indication for further radiographic evaluation. Although ultrasonography is a good screening tool, it seldom provides the anatomic detail necessary to fully evaluate the ventricles and to determine optimal shunt placement. For this reason, it is our policy to obtain head computed tomography (CT) or magnetic resonance images (MRI) of all infants for whom the diagnosis of hydrocephalus is entertained. The improved anatomic resolution and multiplanar imaging capacity of MRI also has been useful in seeking coexisting congenital nervous system anomalies. For this reason, MRI is favored whenever possible for evaluation of these children. The radiographic picture of ventriculomegaly, when combined with the clinical picture of progressive enlargement of head circumference or an already abnormally large head, establishes the diagnosis of hydrocephalus.

In older children and adults, the diagnosis of hydrocephalus rests more on clinical signs and symptoms. The onset of severe headaches, nausea, lethargy, and decline in cognitive abilities in a patient whose clinical history carries risk of hydrocephalus should be evaluated radiographically with CT or MR imaging. A difficult subgroup of patients are those with arrested hydrocephalus. In this group, neonatal hydrocephalus may have existed but eventually was compensated for by the development of a new set point or equilibrium between normal CSF production and absorption. These persons may present with incidental radiographic evidence of ventriculomegaly, with or without signs suggestive of increased intracranial pressure. Obviously, the child who has isolated ventriculomegaly but no other signs or symptoms of increased intracranial pressure needs no further treatment. All too frequently, however, a history of headache or other nonspecific complaints is elicited; the dilemma then is to determine whether shunting is indicated. In these cases we have occasionally found monitoring of intracranial or lumbar intrathecal pressure in an intensive care unit to be useful for correlating intracranial pressure with the patient's symptoms and for predicting the ultimate response to shunting. This approach is also useful for establishing the diagnosis of normal-pressure hydrocephalus. In this group of patients the classic clinical triad of gait disturbance, urinary incontinence, and memory deterioration, as well as the positive cisternogram, can be supplemented by a trial of therapeutic CSF drainage. Almost every patient who satisfies all these criteria responds positively to shunt placement.

SPECIFIC HYDROCEPHALUS SYNDROMES

In Utero Hydrocephalus

The management of hydrocephalus discovered in utero requires constant weighing of the potential for neurologic damage against the need for pulmonary maturity. The vast majority of fetuses with intrauterine hydrocephalus present with other central nervous system (CNS) abnormalities. In such children, it is these abnormalities, rather than the hydrocephalus itself, that is the limiting factor to intellectual development. For this reason, we have tended to recommend delaying treatment until after delivery in the majority of such cases. Serial ultrasonographic evaluation in utero is useful for delineating the progression of hydrocephalus. Early delivery by caesarean section is warranted if the sonogram shows evidence of progressive hydrocephalus and if pulmonary maturity is confirmed. Only in rare cases, when no other major nervous system abnormalities are noted and hydrocephalus is progressing too rapidly to allow delay until pulmonary maturity, is treatment in utero, in the form of transcutaneous cephalocentesis considered.

Neonatal Hydrocephalus

The vast majority of infants with neonatal hydrocephalus have suffered intraventricular hemorrhage secondary to prematurity. In this case, blood and blood breakdown products in the CSF result in elevated CSF protein levels and obstruction of arachnoid villi and a communicating form of hydrocephalus. In the initial stages, the management of such children is often problematic, owing principally to their extremely small size and their weight. Serial lumbar puncture is useful for promoting CSF drainage and removing blood and blood byproducts, though typically this is only a temporizing measure. Medical treatment of the hydrocephalus with Lasix and Diamox is often advantageous. These measures reduce the volume of CSF production and often slow progression of hydrocephalus. As a temporizing measure, this may allow control of the hydrocephalus until the child is old enough to undergo a more definitive shunting procedure. Unfortunately, in our experience, medical management of hydrocephalus rarely has been definitive treatment. Should such measures fail to control the hydrocephalus in a child who is still too small for shunting, serial ventricular taps may be

performed. Such maneuvers are to be avoided if at all possible, because the risk of iatrogenic meningitis is a real threat. At our institution, the weight cutoff point for consideration for shunting is about 1 kg. Infants smaller than this seldom have enough skin integrity or subcutaneous tissue mass to prevent skin breakdown over the shunt bulb assembly.

In an older child with closed sutures, the diagnosis of hydrocephalus depends more on symptoms of increased intracranial pressure than on enlarging head circumference. The reduced intracranial compliance caused by the rigid boundaries of the skull can bring about symptoms of increased intracranial pressure with hydrocephalus. Headaches, emesis, lethargy, papilledema, and focal neurologic deficits, all may be seen. In such cases, the concordance of symptoms, neurologic findings, and radiographic evidence of hydrocephalus are indications for shunting. Difficulties arise when patients with arrested hydrocephalus present with nonspecific symptoms such as headaches. In such cases, it is worthwhile to carefully consider all nonsurgical options before committing the patient to a lifetime of shunts.

Hydrocephalus in Adults

Hydrocephalus in adults is usually a consequence of some trauma or other injury to the nervous system. Closed head trauma may cause subarachnoid hemorrhage and scarring of the aqueducts, which may lead to obstructive hydrocephalus. Likewise, subarachnoid hemorrhage or meningitis may lead to nonobstructive hydrocephalus. In such cases, the diagnosis of hydrocephalus is usually made when following an insult to the CNS the patient fails to improve to the expected baseline level. Progressive dilatation of the ventricles on radiographic studies without evidence of cerebral atrophy is evidence of hydrocephalus. In cases where the hydrocephalus appears to be communicating (as assessed by uniform dilatation of the third, fourth, and lateral ventricles), serial lumbar punctures may be worthwhile as an attempt to clear the blood and protein breakdown products from the CSF and to temporize until a new equilibrium point is set. Occasionally, by this measure patients may avoid shunting entirely. In general, however, if serial lumbar punctures continue to be necessary after 10 days to 2 weeks, then placement of a permanent shunt is indicated.

SHUNT PLACEMENT

The choice of shunt system and shunt placement are idiosyncratic to each institution and operating surgeon. Shunt types commonly used are ventriculoperitoneal, ventriculoatrial, or lumboperitoneal shunts. While lumboperitoneal shunts have been advocated as an easy and low-risk form of permanent CSF diversion, several factors have led us to prefer ventriculoperitoneal shunting for both children and adults. First, we have had a high incidence of radiculopathy following placement of lumboperitoneal shunts, particularly in the stenotic spinal canal of an elderly patient. Second, it has been our experience that lumboperitoneal shunts have a higher failure rate than ventriculoperitoneal shunts. Third, *properly performed* ventriculoperitoneal shunts have an extremely low rate of morbidity that in our experience parallels that of lumboperitoneal shunts. Finally, lumboperitoneal shunts are contraindicated in cases of obstructive hydrocephalus. For these reasons, we generally prefer ventricular shunting for all cases of hydrocephalus. At our institution, the ventriculoperitoneal shunt is preferred for its ease of placement and of assessment. For patients who have low absorptive capacity in the peritoneum, such as those with peritonitis or a colostomy or other bowel problem, a ventriculoatrial or ventriculopleural shunt is an acceptable option. Perioperative administration of antibiotics is essential to reduce the operative infection rate. It should be emphasized that shunts are technically demanding procedures that require a high degree of expertise if potential complications are to be minimized. A cavalier approach to shunt placement by less experienced staff may result in breakdowns in technique and poor results.

SHUNT COMPLICATIONS

The most common complications of shunting are infection and dysfunction. Shunt infections most often result from colonization of the shunt hardware by skin organisms. *Staphylococcus aureus* and *Staphylococcus epidermidis* are the most common offenders. Typically, the child with shunt infection presents with low-grade fever, CSF pleocytosis, and evidence of shunt obstruction. It has been our practice to institute broad-spectrum antibiotic coverage at the first sign of a shunt infection. Once definitive cultures are obtained, the antibiotic coverage can be narrowed to cover the specific infective organism. Antibiotic therapy is continued with the shunt in place until the CSF is sterilized (i.e., until further cultures from the shunt remain negative). If antibiotic therapy does not sterilize CSF in 3 or 4 days or if the patient's clinical condition deteriorates, the infected shunt hardware is removed and ventriculostomy is performed. Once CSF is appropriately sterilized, all old hardware is removed and an entirely new shunt system is placed. Generally, all cases of shunt infection should be considered as potential ventriculitis and should be treated with antibiotics for three full weeks.

The second common complication of shunts is shunt obstruction. Proximal end obstructions secondary to obstruction of the catheter by choroid plexus or proteinaceous debris are all too common. This problem may be minimized by adequate positioning of the proximal end of the shunt away from choroid plexus or ventricular wall. Disconnections and distal end obstructions may also occur. In general, we believe that evaluation of the suspected shunt malfunction should include a plain radiographic shunt series, to evaluate for possible disconnections. In order to determine ventricular size CT examination of the head should be performed before sampling CSF from the shunt or depressing the shunt bulb. Shunt bulb dynamics can be assessed by determining the rate of depression and refill of the shunt bulb. In a patient with symptoms of shunt failure, however, a normal shunt pump should not be construed as excluding the possibility of shunt failure. In all such cases, further investigation is mandatory. We prefer the shunt tap as the ultimate test of shunt dynamics and function. Telemetric intracranial pressure–monitoring devices and Doppler flow studies carry much promise for noninvasive investigation of shunt patency in the future.

SUGGESTED READING

McLaurin RL, ed. Pediatric neurosurgery: Surgery of the developing nervous system. 2nd ed. San Diego: Grune & Stratton, 1989.
Scott RM, ed. Hydrocephalus. Baltimore: Williams & Wilkins, 1990.

PATIENT RESOURCE

The Spina Bifida Association of America, National Office
1700 Rockville Pike, Suite 540
Rockville, MD 20852
(301) 770-7222

NEONATAL BRAIN INJURY: PERIVENTRICULAR HEMORRHAGE AND HYPOXIC-ISCHEMIC ENCEPHALOPATHY

REBECCA N. ICHORD, M.D.

Hypoxic-ischemic and hemorrhagic brain injury remain among the most important challenges to neonatalogists who treat critically ill newborns. Periventricular hemorrhage (PVH) affects 25 to 30 percent of infants who at birth weigh less than 1500 g, and it is associated in many cases with the more serious sequelae of posthemorrhagic hydrocephalus (PHH) and periventricular leukomalacia (PVL). The risk of major handicap following PVH is increased only with higher grades of hemorrhage (Table 1), whereas PVL and PHH carry a very high risk of major handicap. The challenges in managing brain injury in premature infants include preventing PVH when possible, minimizing progression to higher grades, and managing PHH when it occurs.

In contrast to premature newborns, full-term newborns who suffer a cerebral hypoxic-ischemic event manifest more diffuse encephalopathy that is variable in duration and severity and frequently associated with seizures. The long-term outcome is related to the severity of the immediate postnatal encephalopathy, which may be graded as mild, moderate, or severe (Table 2). A high risk of major handicap is associated principally with severe encephalopathy. The challenges of managing hypoxic-ischemic encephalopathy (HIE) in the full-term newborn begin with diagnosis. Many other conditions may mimic HIE, including prenatal onset infection, brain dysgenesis, and perinatal infection. Aside from diagnosis, the challenges to neonatalogists include treating seizures and preventing postnatal progression of the injury as a consequence of the multiple organ dysfunction common in these infants.

PERIVENTRICULAR HEMORRHAGE

Management of PVH begins with detection. Because PVH and PVL are clinically silent in a majority of infants, infants at high risk are routinely examined with cranial ultrasonography. This includes an initial scan within 48 hours of birth for infants who weigh less than 2000 g at birth or are born at 32 weeks' gestational age or earlier. If the initial scan is abnormal, follow-up scans are obtained weekly until ventricular size, site and extent

Table 1 Radiologic and Pathologic Correlates of Periventricular Hemorrhagic and Ischemic Lesions in Premature Infants

Radiologic Findings	Pathologic Findings
Hemorrhagic lesions: Ultrasound Appearance (Computed tomography [CT] grade)	
Germinal matrix hemorrhage (I)	Subependymal hemorrhage
Small IVH (II)	Small IVH (<50% of ventricle), no ventricular dilatation
Large IVH (III)	Large IVH (>50% of ventricle), with ventricular dilatation
Intraparenchymal hemorrhage (IV)	Hemorrhagic infarction or extension of germinal matrix hemorrhage
Ischemic lesions: Ultrasound appearance	
Intraparenchymal echodensity (IPE), transient	Pathologic correlate of the ultrasound finding of transient IPE is uncertain
IPE, prolonged (>10 days)	Gliosis, microcalcification
Cystic degeneration of IPE:	Cystic periventricular leukomalacia
Unilateral vs. bilateral	
Focal vs. diffuse	
Late sequelae: MRI or CT appearance	
Porencephaly	Large cystic encephalomalacia
Ventriculomegaly, normal head circumference (HC)	White matter atrophy
Ventriculomegaly, excessive HC	Posthemorrhagic hydrocephalus
White matter abnormalities	Abnormal myelination
Delayed myelination	Delayed myelination

Table 2 Staging of Encephalopathy in Full-Term Infants

Variable	Stage I	Stage II	Stage III
Consciousness	Hyperalertness, irritability	Lethargy	Unresponsiveness
Neuromotor status	Normal tone, brisk deep tendon reflexes	Moderate tone abnormalities	Flaccid, no movement
Neonatal reflexes (suck, Moro)	Intact	Diminished	Absent
Autonomic status	Sympathetic predominance	Parasympathetic	Labile
Seizures	None	Common	Uncommon

of hemorrhage, and site and extent of periventricular ischemic lesions can be shown to be stable for 2 or 3 consecutive weeks. Repeat imaging is indicated if there is a clinical change, such as excessive increase in head circumference, unexplained drop in hematocrit, or new neurologic abnormalities.

Infants born weighing more than 2000 g or later than 32 weeks' gestation who develop neurologic signs or symptoms should undergo a thorough evaluation (see Hypoxic-Ischemic Encephalopathy). If neuroimaging reveals periventricular or intraventricular hemorrhage in an infant of this size or maturity, the evaluation should include a search for coagulation abnormalities and brain magnetic resonance imaging (MRI) to rule out a vascular anomaly as a cause for the hemorrhage.

Management of PVH in its acute stage consists of supportive measures aimed at optimizing cerebral physiologic homeostasis. Invasive intracranial monitoring is not employed in newborns because of unacceptable morbidity and no clear demonstration of benefit. Our approach incorporates efforts to avoid wide swings in blood pressure or cerebral perfusion by avoiding rapid intravascular volume shifts, minimizing extremes of ventilation and oxygenation, minimizing painful manipulations, and prompt recognition and treatment of pneumothorax and patent ductus arteriosus. Seizures may occur in the setting of acute PVH and should be treated in the same way as in term infants with hypoxic-ischemic injury (see subsequent discussion).

POSTHEMORRHAGIC HYDROCEPHALUS

Hydrocephalus is defined as progressive ventricular enlargement beyond the 97th percentile for gestational age, as shown by serial ultrasound examinations. It is viewed as a symptom of excessive intracranial pressure if it is accompanied by excessive growth of head circumference or by symptoms of lethargy, vomiting, apnea, or pupillary or vertical gaze abnormalities. The reported prevalence ranges from 10 to 25 percent of infants with PVH and increases with higher grades of hemorrhage. The natural history of hydrocephalus is one of spontaneous arrest or regression in 40 to 60 percent of cases and relentless progression in the remainder. Intermittent cerebrospinal fluid (CSF) drainage by lumbar or ventricular puncture can delay but not prevent the need for shunting procedures in infants with progressive, symptomatic hydrocephalus.

A practical approach to managing these infants incorporates the use of acetazolamide and furosemide; invasive CSF drainage is reserved for symptomatic infants who fail to respond to medical therapy and who are poor surgical candidates. Treatment is considered for infants with ventricular dilatation exceeding the 97th percentile for gestational age on two or more weekly cranial ultrasound examinations. A lumbar puncture prior to treatment that shows an opening pressure greater than 15 cm H_2O may be helpful to confirm that ultrasound findings or clinical symptoms (e.g., lethargy,

apnea, gaze abnormalities) could be attributed to elevated intracranial pressure. Knowledge of CSF protein content is also important in planning the optimal time for a permanent shunting procedure. Treatment with acetazolamide is begun at a dose of 25 mg per kilogram per day in three doses, along with furosemide, 1 mg per kilogram per day in two doses. Acetazolamide doses may be increased weekly if the response is unsatisfactory, in increments of 10 to 25 mg per kilogram per day, up to a maximum of 100 mg per kilogram per day. Electrolytes, acid-base status, and nutrition must be monitored, and if excessive metabolic acidosis occurs and is unresponsive to administration of supplemental bicarbonate (Bicitra or Polycitra), the dose may need to be reduced. Furosemide dose may be increased up to 2 mg per kilogram per day, with appropriate monitoring of serum potassium.

Intermittent or temporary CSF drainage may be necessary if progressive, clinically symptomatic hydrocephalus is unresponsive to medical therapy. Serial lumbar puncture, daily or every other day, removing enough CSF to lower opening pressure by half, is possible if the hydrocephalus is communicating and if the infant tolerates the procedure. Ventricular puncture or ventriculostomy may be necessary if the hydrocephalus is noncommunicating, and permanent shunting must be delayed because the infant is a poor surgical candidate (e.g., owing to size, poor nutrition, unstable lung disease, intra-abdominal complications, sepsis).

HYPOXIC-ISCHEMIC ENCEPHALOPATHY

There is general agreement that the diagnosis of perinatal hypoxic-ischemic brain injury should fulfill two kinds of criteria: (1) evidence of severely compromised fetal or neonatal perfusion or gas exchange, such as by intrapartum fetal heart rate abnormalities, depressed Apgar scores, acidosis, or multiorgan ischemic injury, and (2) acute neurologic dysfunction, evident within 24 hours of the HIE, evolving over 24 to 72 hours and resolving partially or completely in days to weeks. We monitor the severity of the encephalopathy using the clinical staging system described by Sarnat: stage I (mild), irritability and minor alterations in tone and behavior; stage II (moderate), depressed consciousness, pronounced tone abnormalities, loss of functional behaviors, and frequently seizures; and stage III (severe), unresponsiveness to noxious stimuli, global flaccid weakness, loss of neonatal reflexes, with or without seizures.

The management of an acute encephalopathy in a newborn should begin with a broad consideration of causes. As infants with brain maldevelopment are more vulnerable to perinatal complications, a search should be made for disorders of prenatal onset. Thus, the evaluation should include a careful review of the history for symptoms of gestational abnormalities such as pregnancy-induced hypertension, maternal infection, maternal toxin exposure, abnormal fetal movements, and intrauterine growth retardation. The infant should be carefully examined for signs of congenital malformations or defined genetic syndromes, cranial trauma, intrauterine infection, thromboembolic phenomena, and ongoing sepsis or major organ failure. For all infants with moderate or severe encephalopathy of suspected perinatal origin, we recommend neuroimaging and lumbar puncture within 24 to 48 hours of birth.

Cranial ultrasonography may be the most accessible and least risky neuroimaging modality for a critically ill infant, and ideally it should include Doppler evaluation of dural sinuses to rule out dural sinus thrombosis. Head CT should be performed within this time frame if there is a suspicion of extra-axial hemorrhage (subdural, subarachnoid) or stroke in utero, as these are more often missed by ultrasound. As the encephalopathy evolves, serial cranial ultrasonography may help document, with minimal risk to the infant, the course of cerebral edema or the evolution of subcortical white matter ischemic injury. By 7 to 14 days, head CT is helpful in defining the severity and distribution of hypoxic-ischemic changes. Brain MRI would be performed in this time frame in lieu of head CT if there is a suspicion of brain dysgenesis (such as migrational anomalies), which may predispose the fetus to perinatal maladaptation.

Lumbar puncture should be done as soon as the infant's cardiorespiratory status allows it to be accomplished with minimal risk. Opening pressure should be measured, if possible, and CSF sent for cell count, glucose, protein, and bacteriologic studies. If the fluid is bloody, it should be spun down immediately to look for xanthochromia, in order to distinguish between subarachnoid hemorrhage and traumatic puncture. If the encephalopathy is unexplained, delayed in onset, or out of proportion to the suspected hypoxic-ischemic event, additional CSF should be examined for elevated glycine level and for viral infection.

Further laboratory evaluation of the encephalopathic newborn should be done to detect and allow treatment of conditions that may mimic, or may accompany, hypoxia-ischemia. These include glucose, calcium, acid-base balance, Pao_2, $Paco_2$, sodium, blood urea nitrogen, and liver transaminase values, hematology profile, urine sediment and chemistry, urine toxicology, and bacterial cultures. We study all infants with poorly explained acute encephalopathy for inborn errors of metabolism; the workup includes studies of plasma lactate, ammonia, quantitative plasma amino acids, and urine for organic acids.

The rationale for treatment of HIE is based on clinical and experimental evidence that irreversible brain injury evolves over hours to days following an ischemic or hypoxic event. In experimental paradigms for HIE, the extent of recovery depends in part on restoration of adequate cerebral energy metabolism, recovery of ion homeostasis, and modifying excitatory neurotoxicity. "Brain resuscitation" in the newborn is a continually evolving concept, but in theory it should rest on several principles: (1) maintenance of adequate cerebral perfusion, (2) assurance of generous cerebral oxygen and glucose delivery, (3) restoration and main-

tenance of fluid and ion homeostasis, and (4) treatment of seizure activity without compromising cerebral perfusion. Very few controlled studies of these approaches have been reported, and results are mixed. We advocate an empiric approach based on these principles, with emphasis on maintaining the infant within a narrow range of optimal physiologic parameters: (1) maintaining normovolemia, (2) supporting mean arterial pressure and arterial glucose content toward the upper end of the range considered normal for age and gestation, and (3) controlling ventilation to provide high normal levels of Pao_2, while avoiding extremes of $Paco_2$. The value of steroids, osmotic agents, barbiturates, or hyperventilation in treating elevated intracranial pressure in newborns remains unproven.

NEONATAL SEIZURES

Seizures in newborns may be defined as paroxysmal behavioral events observable at the bedside (clinical seizures), or paroxysmal electrical events (electrographic seizures), which may not coincide. We use one of a variety of clinical descriptive classifications put forward to define suspected seizures (Table 3). Every effort is made utilizing electroencephalography (EEG) and clinical observation to distinguish whether clinical paroxysms, such as tonic extensor posturing, or subtle stereotypies (bicycling limb movements) represent true electrocortical events, intracranial pressure phenomena, or subcortical release phenomena with no epileptiform equivalent on EEG. Treatment with anticonvulsants is initiated if (1) there is strong clinical suspicion of seizures and the paroxysms have immediate adverse effects on the infant's cardiorespiratory status or (2) subtle, nonthreatening but recurrent clinical events occur in an infant with epileptiform EEG abnormalities. Standard 16-channel EEG is performed as soon as possible after the onset of suspected clinical seizures. The presence and severity of background abnormalities are noted, and they provide a useful objective means of serially monitoring the severity of acute encephalopathy. This may prove especially useful for infants who require neuromuscular-paralyzing agents to manage severe lung disease. The presence of epileptiform abnormalities on EEG of an infant suspected of having clinical seizures strongly supports our decision to use anticonvulsant

Table 3 Classification of Clinical Seizures in Neonates

Commonly associated with electrographic correlate:
  Focal clonic: Unifocal, multifocal, hemiconvulsive, axial
  Focal tonic: Eye deviation, asymmetric truncal
  Generalized myoclonic
  Apnea
Uncommonly associated with electrographic correlate:
  Generalized tonic: Flexor, extensor, mixed
  Multifocal myoclonic
  Subtle, or motor automatisms: Oral-buccal-lingual movements; pedaling, stepping, swimming movements

drugs. However, serial recordings may be necessary and should involve careful bedside correlation of clinical and electrical events by skilled observers. This provides a basis for determining which specific clinical events are most likely to be related to electrocortical events and perhaps more likely to respond to drug treatment.

For all types of neonatal seizures the efficacy of standard anticonvulsant drugs is poor. The more severe the underlying structural brain injury, the worse is the prognosis for immediate seizure control and for long-term outcome. Phenobarbital remains our drug of first choice and should be given in a loading dose of 20 mg per kilogram by slow IV infusion, with appropriate monitoring and adjustment of infusion rate in case of hypotension. Repeated boluses of 5 mg per kilogram at intervals of several hours for recurrence of seizures within 24 hours may be necessary, and doses should be titrated to achieve serum levels of 20 to 40 mg per liter while avoiding hypotension and exacerbation of myocardial depression. If seizures recur despite this regimen of phenobarbital loading, we often give a trial of benzodiazepine (diazepam, 0.2 mg per kilogram, or lorazepam, 0.05 to 0.1 mg per kilogram). If this appears effective, we may repeat it at 6 to 8 hour intervals, as needed for recurrence of seizure activity. If frequent repeated dosing of benzodiazepines over 24 to 48 hours, in addition to a previous high therapeutic loading dose of phenobarbital, appears necessary, we suggest adding phenytoin in a loading dose of 20 mg per kilogram by slow IV infusion. Additional 5 mg per kilogram boluses may be given as needed, titrating for seizure control or a serum level of 20 to 30 mg per liter.

The decision to continue anticonvulsants after loading doses achieve seizure control depends on several factors. If seizure control required two or more drugs, and if frequent seizures occurred over the course of 48 hours, and if the EEG remains strongly epileptiform after initial control of clinical seizures is attained, then an anticonvulsant is continued at a maintenance dose. Phenobarbital is preferable because when given orally its kinetics are more predictable than those of phenytoin. It is given at a dose of 3 to 4 mg per kilogram per day, titrating as needed to a blood level of 15 to 40 mg per liter, in order to minimize recurrence of clinical seizures while avoiding undesirable side effects (excessive sedation, irritability). The duration of maintenance anticonvulsant therapy is determined along similar lines. If the encephalopathy has shown considerable improvement and seizures have not recurred over the course of 1 to 2 weeks of maintenance anticonvulsant therapy, we recommend discontinuing the drug. Though such infants remain at high risk for eventual recurrence of seizures, for many it will be months, or perhaps years, before seizures recur. Whenever possible, it is preferable to spare the developing brain the side effects of anticonvulsants during the early months of life.

DISCHARGE PLANNING AND FOLLOW-UP CARE

Most infants who have survived moderate or severe neonatal encephalopathy from any cause require additional services upon discharge. Feeding problems are common; they may require merely patience and perseverance or nasogastric tube feeding. Infants often have altered behavioral regulation, leading to sleep disturbances and irritability, which heavily tax the coping resources of even the strongest families. Continued recovery, or the sequelae of permanent brain injury, often lead to delays in development from the earliest weeks of life. Parents are sensitive to the failure of their child to smile, vocalize, and attend to the environment. These early functional deficits may impair the attachment of parent to child, adding to parental anxiety and making a difficult care-giving situation even worse. Such infants and their families are usually referred to home care services immediately upon discharge, including a nurse to oversee nutrition and medical issues and a developmental therapist to help the parents adapt to the infant's functional deficits, particularly in feeding. Neurologic follow-up is usually scheduled within 4 to 6 weeks of discharge in order to address concerns regarding seizures and functional delays. This also affords parents an opportunity to review the underlying diagnoses and to discuss prognosis to the extent this is possible.

SUGGESTED READING

De Vries LS, Larroche J-C, Levene MI. Intracranial sequelae. In: Levene MI, Bennett MJ, Punt J, eds. Fetal and neonatal neurology and neurosurgery. New York: Churchill Livingstone, 1988:346–353.

Mizrahi EM, Kellaway P. Characterization and classification of neonatal seizures. Neurology 1987;37:1837–1844.

Sarnat HB, Sarnat MS. Neonatal encephalopathy following fetal distress. Arch Neurol 1976;33:696–705.

Volpe J. Hypoxic-ischemic encephalopathy: Clinical aspects. In: Volpe J, ed. Neurology of the newborn. Philadelphia: WB Saunders, 1987:236–280.

Volpe JJ. Intraventricular hemorrhage in the premature infant—current concepts. Part I. Ann Neurol 1989;25:3–11.

SYRINGOMYELIA

SETH M. ZEIDMAN, M.D.
RICHARD B. NORTH, M.D.
THOMAS B. DUCKER, M.D.

Ollivier d'Angers coined the term *syringomyelia* in 1827 to describe a dilated, cerebrospinal fluid (CSF)–filled cavity within the spinal cord. Syringomyelia has been defined as a cystic accumulation of fluid within the spinal cord, which may or may not communicate with the central canal. Dilatation of the central canal with its ependymal lining is termed *hydromyelia;* extension of the cyst into the spinal cord parenchyma constitutes *syringomyelia.* We consider syringomyelia and hydromyelia as a single clinical entity and treat patients with both conditions in like fashion.

PATHOPHYSIOLOGY

An understanding of the pathophysiology of syrinx formation is essential to rational therapeutic intervention, which should be tailored to the individual patient. Several theories regarding the pathogenesis of syringomyelia have been proposed.

Syringomyelia classically has been divided into two major categories:

1. *Communicating syringomyelia* is defined as primary dilatation of the central canal, nearly always associated with abnormalities of the foramen magnum. Syringomyelia in the setting of a type I Chiari malformation is the most familiar and frequent form of spinal cord cavitation seen by clinicians. It is rarely seen in conjunction with basilar arachnoiditis.
2. In *noncommunicating syringomyelia* the cavity arises in cord substance but is not in communication with the central canal or subarachnoid space. Syringomyelia may be secondary to spinal cord trauma, tumor, or arachnoiditis or of undetermined origin.

Post-traumatic syringomyelia may develop after minor spinal cord injury. It presents as a delayed, progressive neurologic deficit extending beyond the site of the injury.

DIAGNOSIS

The evaluation of patients suspected of having syringomyelia should begin with a comprehensive history and physical and neurologic examination. In addition to meticulous sensory and motor assessment, examinations of cranial nerve, cerebellar, and rectal function are essential elements of a complete evaluation. The clinical history is often the most important element in the diagnosis of syringomyelia. The presenting symptoms can be highly variable. Most patients' status gradually worsens over several years. Some patients report rapid declines in function punctuating clinical plateaus that last several years. The variable clinical course makes assessment of the efficacy of treatment particularly difficult. Patients can deteriorate at such a slow rate that they are unaware of any change until they become nonambulatory.

Syringomyelia may be asymptomatic, or it may present with widespread sensory loss and quadriparesis, with upper extremity atrophy and lower extremity spasticity. The classic presentation of a cervical syrinx includes upper extremity weakness and atrophy with a suspended and dissociated sensory loss beginning in the hands. Loss of sensation to pain and temperature in the involved dermatomes is due to destruction of pain fibers crossing anterior to the central canal. Numbness and pain are frequent presenting complaints. The sensory deficit is frequently asymmetric. As the disease progresses, involvement of the long motor and sensory pathways in the spinal cord is accompanied by lower motor neuron weakness of the upper extremities. Scoliosis is frequently present; rarely, neurogenic arthropathies develop in the later stages of the disease.

Recent studies indicate that the most common presentation of the onset of the disorder is pain in the anatomic distribution of the syrinx in conjunction with the subtle signs and symptoms of myelopathy. These are usually protracted but can occur acutely.

RADIOLOGIC STUDIES

Plain radiographs are helpful in identifying bony abnormalities associated with syringomyelia such as scoliosis, basilar invagination, Klippel-Feil anomaly, and occult spina bifida. They are an important part of the complete evaluation of the patient with syringomyelia. Flexion/extension views should be performed to exclude spinal instability.

Magnetic resonance imaging (MRI) defines anatomy in the sagittal and axial planes and is the diagnostic modality of choice for defining the anatomy of patients suspected of having syringomyelia. It is highly specific, sensitive, and noninvasive. Minimum views in the initial evaluation of syringomyelia should include T1-weighted sagittal and transverse views. T2-weighted and mixed-density images complement but do not replace the T1 scans. Imaging of the entire rostrocaudal extent of the syrinx is essential. MRI shows the low-signal cavity within the spinal cord and provides the transverse and rostrocaudal dimensions of the cavity, the extent of cerebellar tonsillar herniation, and the ventricular size. MRI generally provides all the information needed to plan the surgical approach. MRI with gadolinium enhancement is useful for differentiating syringomyelia from tumor cyst.

Computed tomography (CT) myelography is an

excellent tool for evaluating suspected syringomyelia. Intramedullary tumors commonly produce striking focal cord enlargement, frequently associated with almost complete block. In contrast, the enlargement produced by syringomyelia is diffuse and extends over many segments.

THERAPY

Diagnosis and therapy should be expeditious, because patients who progress beyond a certain level of disability are unlikely to achieve functional recovery. The most rational approach to surgical treatment addresses the underlying pathophysiologic disturbance.

Patients with a Chiari malformation in addition to syringomyelia should undergo suboccipital craniectomy and upper cervical laminectomies to decompress the foramen magnum. We favor intradural exploration and lysis of subarachnoid adhesions using the operating microscope. We attempt to achieve active CSF flow by lysis of subarachnoid adhesions but limit dissection around and between the tonsils because of the risk of devascularizing neural tissue. Once the intradural portion of the procedure is complete, the dura is closed with lyophilized cadaveric dural or fascial graft. Watertight dural closure is essential to prohibit entry of blood and extracellular fluid into the subarachnoid space, which can promote adhesions that limit free CSF circulation. In our experience, occlusion of the obex with tissue, Teflon, or other material increases the risk of morbidity without improving outcome over that of standard posterior fossa decompression with laminectomy and duroplasty.

For patients whose syringomyelia is associated with hydrocephalus, ventriculo-peritoneal shunting is the procedure of choice, especially if CSF pressure is increased. If symptoms do not improve, consideration should be given to direct shunting of the syrinx.

Patients resistant to other forms of therapy may benefit from establishment of a communication between the syrinx and the subarachnoid space. The opening into the syrinx is made in the thinnest portion of the spinal cord, usually the area of the dorsal root entry zone. Shunting from the syrinx to the pleural or peritoneal cavity has been successful, particularly in the presence of arachnoiditis. Some patients require both posterior fossa decompression and direct syrinx decompression via a shunting procedure.

RESULTS

Posterior fossa decompression is associated with significant morbidity and mortality. Postoperative hem-

orrhage, infection, and neurologic injury all are possible, though microneurosurgical technique, improved anesthesia, and perioperative management have markedly reduced the morbidity and mortality that previously were associated with this procedure. Postoperatively, initiation of feeding should be undertaken with caution, because patients are at high risk for aspiration. Additional risks include postoperative hydrocephalus, increased intracranial pressure, and aseptic meningitis. Results are difficult to assess in the immediate postoperative period because of the variable and chronic clinical course of syringomyelia.

Careful preoperative explanation of the potential benefits of operation is important to patient satisfaction. Patients are counseled that surgery rarely restores normal function. The operation should arrest the progression of weakness and muscle atrophy and prevent increased numbness. In our experience, most patients report postoperative improvement in functional abilities, although neurologic examination reveals no objective change. Patients with long-standing and severe neurologic deficits may have unrealistic expectations for postoperative recovery. Patients with mild neurologic deficits who undergo operation early in the disease process generally do well.

Assessing the results of treatment and comparing the efficacy of the various modalities available today is very difficult owing to the rarity of the condition, the variability and chronicity of the clinical course, and the relatively short follow-up. Patients must be followed for extended periods to determine the efficacy of any therapeutic intervention.

Advances in imaging technology have increased the number of patients identified with syringomyelia and the diagnostic accuracy of evaluating and following these patients. The optimal therapy for these complex lesions remains to be defined.

SUGGESTED READING

Batzdorf U. Syringomyelia: Current concepts in diagnosis and treatment. Baltimore: Williams & Wilkins, 1991.

Gamache FW, Ducker TB. Syringomyelia: A neurological and surgical spectrum. J Spin Dis 1989;3:293–298.

Matsumoto T. Surgical management of syringomyelia—current results. Surg Neurol 1989;32:258–265.

Vaquero J, Martinez R, Arias A. Syringomyelia-Chiari complex: Magnetic resonance imaging and clinical evaluation of surgical treatment. J Neurosurg 1990;73:64–68.

THE LEARNING-DISABLED CHILD (HYPERACTIVITY/ DYSLEXIA)

MARTHA BRIDGE DENCKLA, M.D.

DEFINITIONS

Hyperactivity is the shortened and commonly used term that represents the official DSM-III-R category, Attention Deficit Hyperactivity Disorder (ADHD). This symptom-complex, a diagnosis by history, is a polythetic diagnosis (i.e., no one item is necessary, no one item is sufficient). ADHD includes assorted items referable to observed inattentiveness, impulsivity, and hyperactivity. Any above-threshold total number of assorted items rated as "pretty much/very much" over a period of at least 6 months (6 of 14 items is enough for teenagers; 8 of 14 items is the elementary school threshold number) permits the diagnosis of ADHD. Thus, it is possible for a child to be diagnosed as having ADHD who exhibits little or no hyperactivity. A return to an amended version of the earlier DSM-III dichotomy between ADD (no H) and ADHD is probably for DSM-IV. The diagnosis of ADD vs. ADHD will remain polythetic, history based, and dependent upon the observer's relative experience with and tolerance for developmentally expected observable behaviors. No test or measurement is validated for use in the diagnosis of ADHD. Certain other diagnoses (e.g., pervasive developmental disorder) preclude the diagnosis of ADHD in the DSM-III-R algorithm, but comorbidities with oppositional-defiant or conduct disorder, with Tourette syndrome, with anxiety, and with depression are recognized and present additional complexities for the clinician. The comorbidity with one or more academic learning disabilities (LDs) (reading disability [RD] or "dyslexia" being the prototype) is commonly appreciated and is the combination most often seen by pediatricians and neurologists (not by psychiatrists).

Dyslexia (RD and reading/spelling disability; in older patients residual spelling/written language disability with documented *past* RD) simply means difficulty in acquisition and use of academic language skills (reading, spelling, mechanics of written language other than handwriting) that is unexpected on the basis of normal general development and measured aptitude. It is easier to make this definition into a sentence, however, than to make it into a clinical reality. In practice, it is not straightforward to decide what aspects of development (how many and to what degree) must be "normal," which measurement of aptitude is a valid measure thereof, and which tests of reading, spelling, and/or written language are valid representations of those skills. Furthermore, many exclusions (emotional problems, inadequate schooling, excessive absences or school changes) are theoretically invoked, but they are rarely taken into consideration when interpreting aptitude or achievement gaps. The concept of dyslexia, then, is that of unexpected failure in achieving literacy, where the word *unexpected* reflects the presence of adequate environmental, emotional, and intellectual endowment but some subtle imperfection existing in the neurocognitive status of the individual.

Dyslexia is a term used more often by the medical profession than by the educational establishment mandated by PL94-142 to educate appropriately those with *RD*. RD is the prototype LD. *Eligibility* for public school services is usually established by calculating a discrepancy between aptitude and achievement and declaring (with variability among local systems) what is "significant"; some systems also require a second eligibility criterion to be met in the documentation of a processing deficit (the educational term for a subtle neurocognitive impairment). Biomedically based research on dyslexia has reached a critical mass of consensus that phonology, a subdomain of language, is the locus of processing deficit (subtle neurocognitive impairment) relevant to dyslexia. Neither educational practice nor the psychiatric profession's DSM-III-R (or proposed DSM-IV) currently recognize this research consensus as official mechanism.

INTER-RELATIONSHIP OF HYPERACTIVITY (ADHD) AND DYSLEXIA (RD)

Upon first inspection of any official diagnostic classification (DSM-III-R, [International Classification of Disease edition 9, or ICD 9]), it would appear that these entities are of totally different types, since ADHD is an axis I (or psychopathologic) disorder in DSM-III-R, whereas all of the developmental disorders, dyslexia (RD) included, are on axis II (conceptualized as characterizations of the individual's intrinsic constitutional "equipment," as modeled on mental retardation). This conceptualization is challenged by the daily general experience of most clinicians who evaluate academic underachievers. Conners (whose name is identified with the evolution of rating scales for hyperactivity) questions the separability of ADHD and RD in theoretical, as well as clinical, reality. For 30 years, in fact, inspiring the term *minimal brain dysfunction,* the overlapping coexistence of hyperactivity and dyslexia has been acknowledged. Most referrals come with chief complaints of learning and behavior problems. Recent magnetic resonance imaging (MRI) studies reveal similar anterior (frontal) brain width anomalies in persons with supposedly pure RD and pure ADHD. There are pure cases of each, but the mixed cases far outnumber these except in facilities explicitly labeled "psychiatric" or "mental health" clinics, where oppositional-defiant conduct is the more prevalent comorbid disorder. From epidemiologic (not clinical) samples, it appears that 11 percent of ADHD children also have official LDs (mostly RDs), but far more than that underachieve in school; conversely, 33 percent of LD (mostly RD) children turn out to meet criteria for ADHD. The prevalence of LD/ADHD comorbidity in pediatrics or neurology clinics is closer to 80 percent. Even a subspecialist like myself, who has published on dyslexia and is known to be focused on LD, rarely sees a pure dyslexic. Clinically, the physician who gets an academic underachiever referral is facing much the same diagnostic disentanglement as the physician who is asked about an adult with mental deterioration, "Is this aphasia or is this dementia?" The mental status associated with pure aphasia is focally in the domain of linguistic impairment, and this is even more microscopic in developmental dyslexia. The mental status associated with many of the dementing illnesses and with pure ADHD is concentrated in the domain of executive function (attention, inhibition, organization) affiliated with "frontal" anatomy. Mixed cases give mixed mental status results.

DIAGNOSIS OF LD/ADHD

It follows from these facts that the physician who deals with cases of hyperactivity/dyslexia (i.e., ADHD/RD) must either perform or interpret data that add up to a detailed mental status examination as well as collect historical information from school and home. The diagnostic process involves concepts from psychiatry, developmental psychology, education, law, and sociology. To move from diagnosis to treatment, it is even more necessary to know the law and the community resources, because most of the means of treatment are not in the hands of physicians or medical institutions. The neurologic dysfunction involved is extremely subtle, so that diagnosis is time consuming, labor intensive, and intel-lectually challenging, while practice in this field is also the ultimate in community medicine. Diagnosis of *society* (its demands and resources) interacts with diagnosis of the brain's most uniquely human and variable attributes. Related to this complexity is the need to translate terms from one related field to another; for example, *learning disability* as a legal-bureaucratic eligibility as opposed to an intrinsic constitutional weakness of the central nervous system (the biomedical concept). Thus, the clinician may tell the patient (or the parent of the patient), "No, you do not have what the school system will consider a learning disability in terms of eligibility for accommodations or services," but "Yes, you do have the neurocognitive characteristics currently biomedically identified with a learning disability."

Assuming that the physician is *not* a subspecialist in behavioral or developmental behavioral neurology, his or her diagnostic role resides in (1) history taking (Table 1), including collection of appropriate rating scales; (2) assessment of the motor examination with special attention to developmental aspects thereof (see Table 2); (3) review of relevant records (Table 3); and (4) referral for those neuropsychoeducational tests not previously done and hence not part of the record review (so whatever is the remainder of Table 3). What the physician himself/herself does and what the referral pattern for further testing should be depend upon what is available in the physician's immediate community. The physician's position with respect to neuropsychology and psychoeducational testing is the same as to radiologic or laboratory testing: the physician cannot order what is not available. Ideally, the physician is trying to collect previously available or proactively ordered collection of laboratory data relevant to the biomedical and psychosocial interpretations that lead to treatment plans for LD/ADHD. As in any other diagnostic formulation, the physician looks for patterns or configurations of history, physical examination, and laboratory findings that are consistent with the established diagnostic prototype or sufficiently close to that prototype to warrant therapeutic trial on that assumption.

Prototypical pure dyslexic (RD) persons have all ratings (Conners, Children's Behavior Checklist of Achenbach, and Barkley) below threshold values for ADHD and have no problems as long as books are not involved in their lives. If there was any preschool worry about this child, it was in regard to speech and language, but the difficulty with reading was unexpected and out of

Table 1 Specific History Details Relevant to RD/ADHD

Family history: Ask about as many members of as many generations as possible of same or similar difficulties (see below); plus academic (e.g., reading, spelling, writing) underachievement

Personal history relevant to dyslexia (RD): Delayed speech, poor articulation, stuttering, dysgrammatism, mis-sequencing (sounds, words), word-finding difficulty, delay in learning color names

Personal history relevant to hyperactivity (ADHD): "Difficult" or "colicky" newborn, irritability or temper tantrums, sleep problems, intolerance of need to wait, intolerance of limits set, distractibility, impersistence, disorganization, forgetfulness, impulsivity, recklessness

Table 2 Neurodevelopmental Signs Relevant to LD/ADHD*

Age-inappropriate Motor Sign	Suggests Mental Correlate
Extraneous movements (also called associated, overflow)	Deficient inhibition
Choreiform movements	Subtle instability
Slowness of fingers or feet	Slowness
Mis-sequencing	Poor sequential organization
Impersistence	Impersistence

*Relevance is "neighborhood," frontal/prefrontal, striatal, possibly cerebellar.

proportion to any preschool concern. There are no other significant life problems except in reaction to the academic difficulties. There is often a family history of difficulty with reading, spelling, or learning a foreign language, not only in the immediate family but also in aunts and uncles (the mother's brothers should be asked about in particular). Testing reveals some linguistic inefficiency, *not always dramatic* unless the testing specifically probes the speech-sound system (with phonologic awareness/segmentation and symbol-sound non-meaningful code relationships, like reading or memorizing nonsense). Strong visual-spatial abilities are common among dyslexic (RD) persons.

ADHD is a diagnosis by history (interviews rated, e.g., by DSM-III-R criteria, CBCL, Conners, Barkley) and then refined or quantified in severity by assessment. Nothing found on assessment, however, has the power on its own to make or break the diagnosis. Nonetheless, signs of inadequate attention, inhibition, and organization as correlates on the neurodevelopmental (especially motor; see Table 3), and more directly on psychological, assessments enhance the physician's understanding and management of the case and, if there is controversy (e.g., between home and school), help to "break the tie." As with RD, family history is often positive, but it may be more subtle and multifarious.

Pure prototypes are rare in clinical practice, so mixtures of the two pictures given above and a mixed family history with RD, ADHD, and RD/ADHD members all in one family are common. The proportions of real-life difficulty due to the RD (linguistic) versus the ADHD (attentional-organizational) components of the school underachievement vary from case to case. Pseudo-ADHD is sometimes encountered, especially if the receptive linguistic deficit is quite severe but unsuspected; any child who is not able to learn may "tune out" and present as a "phenocopy" of inattentive and restless classroom behavior.

TREATMENT

While not unique to LD/ADHD, the pervasive clinical reality with respect to LD/ADHD is that three out of four (sometimes four out of five; see Table 4) treatment components are not directly under the control of the diagnostician or within the medical community and are not equally available to all patients. Educational therapies are never covered by medical insurance, and recently, speech/language therapies (except for illness- or injury-related deficits acquired at a specified postnatal time) are not usually covered. Public schools dispense remediation under formulas for eligibility that (see above) not only differ conceptually from biomedical diagnosis but also vary from place to place and from year to year. Even private schools that have smaller classes, and potentially greater flexibility, may choose to ignore the needs of LD/ADHD students or to exclude them; the pervasive powers of the physician may prevail upon, but still rely upon "the kindness of strangers."

The result of the limitations placed on the physician's ability to prescribe school conditions and individualized cognitive or academic tutoring is that the physician tends to emphasize medications and family-oriented mental health interventions, just because these are within the medical community's control. One of the most difficult decisions for the physician is how much to tell the patient or the family about the gap between the ideal and what is realistically available. A related decision is how much time does the physician devote to advocacy for each patient's publicly funded program or to encouraging families' advocacy? A major component of management of LD/ADHD cases is deciding, on a case-by-case basis, how much of this ideal and real, biomedical and sociological, complexity is communicated to the family.

Unequivocally to be communicated, however, is the advice to avoid time-consuming and costly offerings of

---

Table 3 "Laboratory" Data to Review or (if Not Available) to Order for Workup of LD/ADHD

1. Conventional laboratory tests only as history suggests (thyroid, metabolic, chromosomes, toxins, EEG)
2. Psychoeducational—IQ, academic achievement
   Psychoeducational—"processing" tests
   Report cards with scores and grades
   Teacher's notes and anecdotal descriptions
3. Parent and teacher rating scales and checklists (Conners, Barkley, Achenbach)
4. Neuropsychological profile (may make use of psychoeducational data as part of assessment), probing domains of:
   Attention
   Executive function ("frontal")
   Language*
   Visual perception
   Spatial ability
   Motor skills (praxis)
   Memory (verbal and visual)

*Screening level; age-inappropriate scores indicate referral for full speech/language evaluation.

Table 4 Treatment Components for Patients Whose Diagnosis Is LD or ADHD

1. School placement and academic therapy:
   General:
     Small classes (if severe, self-contained special class or school)
     Supportive (non-moralizing)
     Structured (explicitly organized)
     Stimulating (intrinsically motivating)
   Specific:
     Subject-matter (e.g., reading) tutoring
     Organizational tutoring
     Behavior modification
     Social skills training
2. Speech/language therapy, if indicated
3. Mental health intervention, if indicated:
   Cognitive-directive-skills-oriented
   Psychotherapy for depression/anxiety, other comorbidity
4. Parent training in behavior modification and cognitive accommodations for deficits
5. Pharmacotherapy:
   Psychostimulants
   Antidepressants
   Anxiolytics

unproven therapies. The physician can at least preserve the precious time of childhood (not a resource to be squandered) and the family's resources by steering patients *away* from generalized "neurologic tune-ups" like patterning, sensorimotor integration, or eye exercises (all offering prerequisite training); special lenses or overlays for reading that may be harmless but divert resources from tutoring; and special diets for regulation of activity and attention. A variety of therapies of a non-educational nature come and go; some are entrenched under the supervision of well-established paramedical specialties but remain unexamined in terms of efficacy. (Of course, to be fair, so is most education.) The physician should look into the specifics (locally) of some of the paramedical therapies and not be automatically or globally negative, because for some age groups (preschoolers) and some circumscribed developmental problems these approaches may be helpful in an adjunctive way. Generally, these assorted therapies are *not* to be recommended for the LD/ADHD conditions under consideration here, because other treatments are more pressing and frills are contraindicated. Furthermore, consideration should be given to the psychological side effects of too many therapies and of therapies that appear unrelated to the patient's day-to-day problems. The message, "I must be really defective or damaged," may be a side effect of well-intended, unproven exercises, especially if scheduling such therapy precludes a beloved extracurricular activity. The physician follows the principle *prima non nocere* by directing most patients and their families away from therapies other than those listed as options in Table 4.

In more proactive advising of patients and families, the ideal would be to team with someone trained in special education, as I have done for the past 15 years. The special educator works with the physician as a combination "nurse practitioner and social worker" who understands the "laboratory tests" (see Table 3) and knows the community resources (not only public and private schools but a "little black book" of tutors, speech/language therapists, and mental health resources). I strongly recommend that any physician who undertakes to care for LD/ADHD patients identify such a special educator as a colleague who either attends the interpreting-advising-feedback visit with the physician or subsequently holds a separate follow-through conference.

In the many cases when RD and ADHD coexist, there is also the problem of comorbidity with depression (of the reactive-to-failure type) and anxiety. The physician will lead in deciding whether intervention by a mental health professional is in the foreground of a treatment plan and whether mental health intervention is to be combined with psychostimulant medication. If so, referral to a psychiatrist (usually one trained in child psychiatry, even if the patient is an adult) is the most parsimonious recommendation. If no medication is to be prescribed there may be other, non-M.D. mental health providers who are more familiar with the needs of LD children (linguistic, organizational) or who work in settings where their counseling, educational therapy, and/or language therapy can be conveniently integrated. Absent a well-trained, developmentally oriented child psychiatrist, the physician may prescribe stimulant medication and opt for the "packaged" tutoring/mental health referral. In either case, the physician needs to know what type of mental health service is offered and whether it is appropriate for a patient who has neurodevelopmental deficits. If the available mental health professional does not recognize the terms in the report, it is not likely that the therapy offered will be customized for the RD/ADHD patient.

With the special educator (consultation in office or by phone) the physician needs to explore what school settings are available to the patient. If the patient is eligible for public school services, the physician needs to consider the level of services (self-contained all day is necessary for some patients; an hour of reading instruction in a resource room is enough for others) and make recommendations for regular classroom accommodations. I often advise bypass strategies: substituting oral reports for written work, reducing written homework loads, and use of a word processor (minimizing handwriting altogether) are among the most common accommodations for many of my RD/ADHD patients. This can occur even if students are not "coded" as eligible for services (some private schools are the most flexible), but the public school is more likely to implement accommodations for "coded" students. The physician's presence in a community over a period of years allows accumulation of experience, so that, at least for a goodly percentage of cases, the educators will heed advice (especially with respect to motor, attentional, and social skills) and develop bypass strategies or individualized approaches. The authority of the physician can be used to modify the written work–load, to make legitimate some alternative means of fulfilling assignments and taking examinations, and to set up gatekeeper systems that check homework and issue discreet extra reminders about assignments.

Probably the most important treatment delivered by the physician to the RD/ADHD patient, the family, the teachers, and anyone else involved is the interpretation of the context in which the RD/ADHD symptom complex is to be viewed. This interpretation starts by announcing that the patient is neither "bad" nor "dumb." It continues by tackling the next question, "Is this a neurologic problem?" I always explain that we infer from these patterns of skills and behaviors and their often familial clustering that the symptom complex is neurologic, in the sense of brains built differently; only rarely do I encounter a case in which the evidence constrains me to speak of neurologic injury, illness, or damage. I find that delivering the message that the patient's RD/ADHD weaknesses are neurologic, in the sense of "the brain you were born with," needs to be embedded in telling everyone involved all the strengths of that brain. That is why short evaluations are dangerous; even over the telephone, I may be quite certain about what is wrong, but I know I cannot deliver the part of the treatment that is perhaps of greatest value, the understanding of the patient's intrinsic brain characteristics, without knowing what is "right." This unusual aspect of the treatment, the emphasis on what is right as well as what is wrong, makes the complex diagnostic process a necessity and the physician's gift of articulate explanation the cornerstone of treatment. Whatever the short-term implications of the legalistic calculation of eligibility for services (emanating from the psychoeducational data collected/interpreted by the physician), in the long run, an understanding (by all persons concerned) of the patient's equipment, in as much detail as is feasible, carries the most weight prognostically. For example, I spend as much time exploring the possible talents of the patient (e.g., music, art, theater, sports, love of animals) as pushing for academic therapies or accommodations. A youngster who spends all free time running to tutors and psycho-therapists while struggling through each school day will run out of self-esteem and motivation. I see the most important role of the physician in putting academic achievement into a biologic context, emphasizing the many aspects of adaptive behavior that add up to a healthy, functional human being. Although I apportion a third of my recommendations to academic matters, a full third is directed toward a search for or reinforcement of other skills, and the final third toward interpersonal (social) adjustments. With respect to the impact of ADHD on interpersonal (social) aspects of life, it is my advice to tell patients, their parents, and their teachers that neurologically based weak control does not mean absolutely that the child can't help it; rather, I emphasize that more explicit structured teaching (which includes behavior modification) of appropriate social behaviors is needed where the brain is "weak." I explain that, just as you teach in an explicit, structured fashion *b/d* to a dyslexic, so do you teach *do/don't* to a child with ADHD. I also explain how the home and school environment must hold back, slow down on independence for ADHD youngsters, gradually weaning from supervision those for whom the position that they are old enough to do that without adults means giving them enough rope to hang themselves, whether this means failing to do necessary work on time or doing undesirable acts. I explain both "not doers" and "bad actors" among the ADHD population in terms of understanding forgetfulness, distractibility, and impulsivity on a brain basis and treating them in a preventive, *not* a punitive, frame of mind. Ironically, "de-moralizing" the ADHD issues prevents demoralization of ADHD-affected persons.

Explanations and interpretations are the most important treatments the physician dispenses for RD/ADHD.

PHARMACOTHERAPY

Despite all the research on catecholamines, treatment by means of psychoactive agents remains empirical and symptom-, rather than syndrome, oriented. The psychostimulants, in particular, are nonspecific adjunc-tive agents; they are *not* like thyroid hormone to the hypothyroid patient. Nor does a patient necessarily have to fulfill current syndrome criteria for ADHD in order for a stimulant to help the attention deficit, since symptomatic relief rather than syndrome cure is what is on offer. I explain to patients, parents, and teachers that stimulants are like the antipyretic or anti-inflammatory agents: Methylphenidate is the aspirin of the nervous system. Response to stimulant medication proves nothing about diagnosis (as is the case with most responses to aspirin). Long-term syndromic ADHD outcome is not stimulant related. Pure dyslexic persons who need to exert supranormal attention in order to persist in book-related work may also benefit from stimulant effects, just as nearly every workplace in this country tacitly acknowledges (through the availability of caffeine) the benefits of stimulants (in moderation) with respect to productivity.

Having explained the symptomatic, adjunctive (i.e., alone, without a program they won't do much), nonspecific nature of stimulants, I also explain the relatively benign nature of these short-acting (even in sustained-release forms) agents. Remarkably free of systemic side effects and with remarkably reversible side effects that are clearly in the line of direct behavioral observation, stimulants are the "why-not-try?" agents because the risk-benefit ratio is so favorable. I explain to teenagers (the most reluctant pill consumers, at least if those pills are prescribed) that pill forms of stimulants are but the more rigorously formulated cousins of the ubiquitous, less rigorously brewed, coffee and tea used by all in their society. The "de-medicalization" or "normalization" of the use of stimulants, by pointing out that the beverages share a pharmacology text chapter with methylphenidate and dextroamphetamine, also has a calming effect on parents and teachers.

I have fewer concerns about well-known side effects of stimulants (growth, eating, sleeping, tics, mood changes), most of which are easily managed, than about strictly psychological side effects like those of telling a child, "Take your pill that makes you behave like a good child." Besides being untrue, this message is harmful. Making a child feel like an out-of-control robot that is run by a good-child pill is a devastating side effect. The truer message is that the stimulant helps the control part of the brain. I tell little children that it helps them to put on their brakes faster. My point is this: The message delivered with the stimulant is as important as its pharmacology. I also explain that at present we do not know whether stimulants confer benefit with respect to proactive executive functions like planning, organization, or flexible strategy generating. We know best that stimulants confer benefit on sustained attention, efficiency of motor output (handwriting), and related productivity. In classrooms, the stimulants enhance availability for teaching but do not demonstrably raise final grades. Thus, over-reliance on pharmacotherapy is a side effect, since many aspects of RD/ADHD still require the other treatments listed in Table 4. Increasing focused and sustained attention and increasing output efficiency are still considerable benefits, however. Trials of stimulants should be custom cut to revolve around target periods with target activities on a basis that is a *per case* (or issue of the year, even within a case). There is no upper age limit for the use of stimulants and no rigid rules on timing or number of doses. A general approach is outlined in Table 5.

Comorbidities (increasingly prevalent with older patients) necessitate more specialized trials of other classes of catecholamine-enhancing agents; I refer to psychopharmacology experts, usually someone trained in psychiatry, when tricyclics or fluoxetine is under consideration, since the comorbidities in question (with the possible exception of tic disorder or Tourette's syndrome, although that, too, varies by locality) are within the psychiatric roster. Since I practice as a subspecialist in neurology, for uncomplicated cases I try to work with and through the pediatricians and family practice physicians who are the primary care providers, since the stimulants are likely long to be part of the patient's medical regimen and I prefer to keep such agents in the foreground of the patient's record. I start the trial by helping to select the target time or target activity, provide copies of rating scales and checklists for observing parents, spouses, or teachers, and maintain telephone contact for the trial period (2 to 3 weeks, see Table 5). A placebo week would be desirable, but availability of placebo can be (as it is for me) an impractical ideal. I remain "on reserve" to consult again and re-evaluate after an interval that ranges (as case needs dictate) from 6 months to 3 years.

There is no reason to prefer methylphenidate to dextroamphetamine as a starting choice, but by usual and customary standards it has become the first in line. The tic issue is under reinvestigation, and reconsideration of dextroamphetamine for ADHD with tic disorder as comorbid risk may reduce the need for tricyclic agents. I have not observed good results with pemoline, but it is considered a respectable third choice after both methylphenidate and dextroamphetamine fail. I find that most stimulant "failures" stem from unrealistic expectations of what the drugs can achieve, inadequacy of at least one of the other aspects of what should be a multifaceted program, or impatience with fine tuning the dose or dosing schedule to optimize benefits and minimize appetite and sleep disturbances. The concept that there is no correct dose or correct dose schedule is not easy to communicate to every family (or primary provider) and, like the rest of the treatment plan, requires much explanation and translation into layman's language.

In summary, the realities of managing cases of hyperactivity/dyslexia recall to the physician the meaning of the title doctor, which is derived from *docere*, to lead or teach.

SUGGESTED READING

Denckla MB, Rumsey JM. Developmental dyslexia. In: Ashbury AK, McKhann GM, McDonald WI, eds. Diseases of the nervous system: Clinical neurobiology. 2nd ed. Philadelphia: WB Saunders, 1992: 631.

Duane D, ed. [Special issue on learning disabilities.] Psychiatr Ann, 1991;21.

Voeller KKS, ed. Attention deficit hyperactivity disorder. J Child Neurol 1991;6(Suppl).

PATIENT RESOURCES

LDA
4156 Library Road
Pittsburgh, Pennsylvania 15234

CHADD
1859 North Pine Island Road
Suite 185
Plantation, Florida 33322

Orton Dyslexia
724 York Road
Towson, Maryland 21204

Table 5 Pharmacotherapy Choices

1. If simple, uncomplicated attention deficit, methylphenidate
2. If side effects or no benefit from 1, dextroamphetamine
3. If side effects or no benefit from 1 and 2 and/or patient resists use of "pills," caffeine (in a beverage)
4. If trials 1, 2, and 3 fail, see below
5. If depressed/obsessive-compulsive plus attention deficit, tricyclic (depressed, anxious) or fluoxetine (depressed, obsessive-compulsive)

Principles for trial of 1, 2, or 3 (psychostimulants):
  Start on a Saturday, so parents or spouse can observe, continue for week.
  Choose a "target activity" whereby improved attention and productivity can be seen:
    Week 1: 0.3 mg/kg/dose
    Week 2: 0.6 mg/kg/dose
  Collect rating scales, anecdotal narratives if effective dose is found for "target activity"; confer to decide number of doses per day (maximum of four) depending on patient's life's demands.
  "Drug holidays" as patient's life allows.

INFECTIOUS DISEASES (NONVIRAL)

BACTERIAL MENINGITIS

MARTIN G. TÄUBER, M.D.
JAY H. TUREEN, M.D.
MERLE A. SANDE, M.D.

In bacterial meningitis, as in few other infectious diseases, promptly establishing a presumptive diagnosis and instituting empiric therapy can be absolutely critical for the outcome. The diagnostic consideration of meningitis is obvious in patients who present with the classic symptom triad of fever, headache, and stiff neck. Other signs and symptoms that occur less frequently in meningitis include photophobia, vomiting, focal neurologic deficits, altered sensorium, and seizures. In patients with several of these signs and clinical evidence of meningeal irritation (meningismus, Brudzinski's and Kernig's signs), meningitis is by far the most likely diagnosis, and the immediate goals should be identifying the pathogen, initiating age-appropriate empiric therapy, and determining the level of supportive care necessary for the patient. Bacterial meningitis, however, can be present when the clinical diagnosis is not obvious. This is particularly true at the extremes of age, in infants and in elders. In children younger than 2 years of age with bacterial meningitis, signs of meningeal inflammation are frequently absent, and the most common clinical presentations include only fever and alteration of level of consciousness (irritability, lethargy), which are present in more than 90 percent of patients. Similarly, in elderly patients fever may be minimal, headache may not be a prominent complaint, signs of meningeal irritation may be difficult to elicit, and not infrequently changes of mental status are the only signs that bring the patient to medical attention.

MENINGEAL PATHOGENS

The age of the patient, other patient characteristics, and some clinical signs allow the examiner to make an educated guess of the organisms that most likely are responsible for an individual case of bacterial meningitis. The patient's age is of primary importance (Table 1). Three types of pathogens (*Streptococcus agalactiae* [group B streptococcus], gram-negative enteric organisms *[Escherichia coli, Klebsiella pneumoniae]*, and *Listeria monocytogenes*) cause most cases of bacterial meningitis in neonates. In children aged 2 months to approximately 4 years, *Haemophilus influenzae* is the most common organism, followed by *Streptococcus pneumoniae* and *Neisseria meningitidis*. Since the recent introduction and routine use of potent conjugate *Haemophilus* vaccines, *Haemophilus* meningitis will decrease in frequency while the other pathogens will become relatively more important. In older children and adults, *N. meningitidis* and *S. pneumoniae* are responsible for the bulk of the cases. The characteristic petechial or purpuric skin rash of *N. meningitidis* sets this organism

Table 1 Pathogens of Bacterial Meningitis and Their Age-Related Relative Frequency (USA, 1986)

Organism	Overall Frequency (%)	Age-Related (%)				
		0–1 mo	*1 mo-4 yr*	*5–29 yr*	*30–59 yr*	*60+ yr*
H. influenzae	45	5	70	10	5	3
S. pneumoniae	18	2	15	20	40	50
N. meningitidis	14	1	10	40	10	2
Group B streptococci	6	48	2	1	3	3
Others*	17	44	3	29	42	42

*Includes *L. monocytogenes*, *E. coli*, other Enterobacteriaceae, *P. aeruginosa*, *S. aureus*.
Adapted from Wenger JD, Hightower AW, Facklam RR, Group BMS et al. J Infect Dis 1990; 162:1316; with permission from The University of Chicago.

apart from other meningeal pathogens. Furthermore, meningococcus is the only meningeal pathogen that leads to small epidemic clusters in the United States and causes catastrophic epidemics in many other parts of the world. In addition to newborns, pregnant women, alcoholics, diabetics, and patients who take corticosteroids or are immunosuppressed, are prone to meningitis caused by *L. monocytogenes*. Parameningeal infections such as otitis media or sinusitis may lead to meningitis, usually caused by *H. influenzae* or *S. pneumoniae*. These two organisms, (and occasionally *Staphylococcus aureus*), are also responsible for most cases of meningitis where a cerebrospinal fluid (CSF) leak (from a basal skull fracture) may lead to recurrent episodes of bacterial meningitis. Depending on the location, dermal sinuses that communicate with the central nervous system, may lead to meningitis due to skin organisms (*Streptococcus pyogenes*, gram-negative bacilli) or organisms in the oropharynx. Meningitis following neurosurgical procedures or penetrating head trauma tends to be caused by organisms that do not play an important role in other cases of meningitis, particularly gram-negative bacilli and *S. aureus*.

DIAGNOSIS

The diagnosis of bacterial meningitis is established by examination of CSF. Before one performs a lumbar puncture (LP), two questions have to be answered. First, is the disease progressing so rapidly or is it so far advanced that even a short delay in antibiotic therapy could adversely affect outcome? In light of the grim prognosis for patients who suffer from advanced, rapidly progressive meningitis, we recommend institution of therapy without delay and postponement of an attempt to obtain CSF until therapy has been started. One or two blood samples for culture should be obtained before administering the first antibiotic dose. In patients who are stable and are unlikely to be adversely affected if antibiotics are not administered immediately, LP is first performed. The second question to be answered before performing the LP is whether the patient is at risk for cerebral herniation as a consequence of the removal of CSF and whether, therefore, computed tomography (CT) should be performed before LP. In general, we feel that LP is safe, unless a patient has clear clinical signs of increased intracranial pressure: impaired mental status, focal neurologic signs, or papilledema. Seizures in a patient with suspected meningitis, in the absence of other signs of increased intracranial pressure, does not deter us from performing LP without prior head CT. If performing a head CT first is deemed safer, antibiotic therapy should be instituted after blood is taken for culture, and the patient should be watched closely while in the scanning room and waiting in a hallway for the examination.

During LP, CSF pressure should always be recorded, since increased intracranial pressure often predicts meningeal inflammation. The CSF should be immedi-

ately examined by the physician performing the LP, rather than being sent to the laboratory, as valuable information can be obtained within only a few minutes. A Gram stain examination of uncentrifuged (in the case of turbid CSF) or centrifuged CSF can be rapidly performed and reveals whether white blood cells are present, what type of white blood cell is predominant, and whether organisms are present. Gram stain examination should be repeated in the microbiology laboratory, where an experienced technician has the time to carefully search the slide for rare organisms. Additional tests to be performed routinely by the laboratory include CSF glucose and protein concentrations and, most important, cultures for bacteria and fungi. Many laboratories offer other tests based on the detection of bacterial antigens by immunochemical methods, such as counterimmunoelectrophoresis (CIE) or latex particle agglutination (LPA). These tests can be particularly helpful in patients who have partially treated bacterial meningitis (i.e., the patient who presents while taking oral antibiotics), and in that setting either a CIE or LPA should be requested routinely.

EMPIRIC ANTIBIOTIC THERAPY

Empiric antibiotic therapy generally must be given before the causative organism can be definitively identified. Empiric therapy is selected to cover the likely pathogens, a task that is not too difficult in meningitis because of the limited number of usual pathogens. In order to be effective, antibiotics must produce a bactericidal effect in the CSF, the site of infection. This is an area of impaired host defenses, and antibiotics that have only bacteriostatic effect often result in treatment failure. Table 2 summarizes our choices for empiric therapy in different patient populations, designed to cover all likely pathogens. Doses of antibiotics recommended in the therapy of meningitis are listed in Tables 4 and 5. It is recommended that antibiotics be admin-

Table 2 Empiric Antibiotic Therapy of Bacterial Meningitis

Patient Group	Antibiotic
Neonates	Ampicillin plus aminoglycoside or ampicillin plus cefotaxime
Infants (1–3 mo)	Ampicillin plus cefotaxime
Children (3 mo–6 yr)	Third-generation cephalosporin
Older children, adults (no specific risk factors)	Penicillin G or third-generation cephalosporin
Immunocompromised patients	Third-generation cephalosporin plus ampicillin (plus aminoglycoside)
Neurosurgery, head trauma patients	Third-generation cephalosporin plus nafcillin (plus aminoglycoside)
Chronic CSF fistula	Third-generation cephalosporin plus nafcillin

Third-generation cephalosporins: cefotaxime, ceftriaxone, ceftizoxime.

istered intravenously by bolus infusion in relatively large doses. Large doses are needed because only a small fraction of the serum concentration (between 3 and 15 percent for most beta-lactam antibiotics) penetrates into the CSF and because only antibiotic concentrations that exceed the minimal bactericidal concentration (MBC) manyfold are rapidly bactericidal in the CSF against meningeal pathogens.

We would base empiric therapy primarily on the age of the patient, with modifications if there are definitive findings on Gram stain examination or unusual risk factors in the patient (see Table 2). If two regimens seem appropriate, it is safer to choose the one with broader coverage, as it can be usually modified within 24 to 48 hours when definitive identification is provided by the laboratory. An important factor that affects the choice of empiric antibiotic therapy is the emergence of organisms that exhibit altered resistance to antibiotics. For example, pneumococci that are relatively resistant (minimal inhibitory concentration [MIC] 0.1 to 1.0 µg per milliliter) or very resistant (MIC $>$ 1.0 µg per milliliter) to penicillin, have been described since 1978. In geographic areas such as the San Francisco Bay area, where the highly resistant strains continue to be very uncommon, penicillin remains a valid empiric choice for patients who are most likely to have either pneumococcal or meningococcal meningitis. However; patients who have recently traveled to certain parts of the world (e.g., Spain, Southern Africa) may have acquired a resistant strain, and in that situation, a third-generation cephalosporin would be more appropriate while awaiting sensitivity results. If the patient is also at risk for infection with *L. monocytogenes*, ampicillin should be added. For patients at risk for infections caused by

difficult to treat gram-negative bacilli that are very likely resistant to many beta-lactam drugs, we consider it safe to include an aminoglycoside in the initial empiric therapy regimen until the organism has been identified and its sensitivities are known (see Table 2).

DEFINITIVE ANTIBIOTIC THERAPY

Once the causative organism has been identified by culture and sensitivity, therapy can and should be adjusted to provide optimal but narrow coverage. In many cases, there are several equivalent choices, and Table 3 lists some of them. Tables 4 and 5 list the dosages used for pediatric and adult patients for the antibiotics most commonly used to treat meningitis. We treat meningitis for a total of 7 days if the disease is caused by *H. influenzae* or *N. meningitidis,* for 10 to 14 days when any of the other common organisms, including pneumococci, are responsible, and for 21 days for neonatal meningitis.

ADJUNCTIVE THERAPY WITH DEXAMETHASONE

Several recent clinical trials have indicated that adjunctive therapy with dexamethasone, 0.15 mg per kilogram IV every 6 hours for 4 days, improves the neurologic and audiologic outcome of patients with bacterial meningitis. This has been shown most clearly for children with *H. influenzae* meningitis; data on children with pneumococcal and meningococcal meningitis and for adults with bacterial meningitis are more limited. It should also be noted that both experimental and clinical data suggest that the maximal benefit of dexamethasone is achieved when the drug is given either shortly before or at the same time as the first antibiotic dose. This is probably related to the fact that corticosteroids reduce the release of proinflammatory cytokines that are stimulated by bacterial products liberated from the pathogen by the bactericidal action of antibiotics.

Based on the available data, we recommend giving

Table 3 Antibiotic Therapy for Specific Bacterial Pathogens

Organism	Antibiotics*
H. influenzae	Third-generation cephalosporin, ampicillin (if sensitive), chloramphenicol†
S. pneumoniae	Penicillin G, third-generation cephalosporin Chloramphenicol†
Reduced penicillin-sensitive	Third-generation cephalosporin
Penicillin-resistant	Third-generation cephalosporin or vancomycin
N. meningitidis	Penicillin G, chloramphenicol†
S. agalactiae	Penicillin G or ampicillin
L. monocytogenes	Ampicillin (plus aminoglycoside) or trimethoprim-sulfamethoxazole
Enterobacteriaceae	Third-generation cephalosporin with or without aminoglycoside
P. aeruginosa	Ceftazidime plus aminoglycoside or fluoroquinolone (e.g., ciprofloxacin)
S. aureus	Nafcillin

*Third-generation cephalosporins: cefotaxime, ceftriaxone, ceftizoxime.
†For penicillin-allergic patients.

Table 4 Dosage of Antibiotics Commonly Used in the Therapy of Bacterial Meningitis

Antibiotic	Dose and Dosing Interval	
	Children (>1 mo)	Adults
Penicillin G	50,000 U/kg q4h	3–4 M U q4h
Ampicillin	75–100 mg/kg q6h	2 g q4h
Cefotaxime	50 mg/kg q6h	2–3 g q6h
Ceftriaxone	50 mg/kg q12h	2–3 g qd
Ceftizoxime	50 mg/kg q6h	4 g q8h
Nafcillin	50 mg/kg q6h	1.5 g q4h
Chloramphenicol	25 mg/kg q6h	1.5 g q6h
Vancomycin	10 mg/kg q6h	0.5 g q6h
Trimethoprim-sulfamethoxazole	5/25 mg/kg q6h	5/25 mg/kg q6h

Table 5 Dosage of Antibiotics for Neonates Commonly Used in the Therapy of Bacterial Meningitis

Drug (mg/kg)	Infants Aged <1 Week		Infants Aged >1 Week	
	Birth Weight <2000 g	Birth Weight >2000 g	Birth Weight <2000 g	Birth Weight >2000 g
Penicillin G	50,000 U q12h	50,000 U q8h	50,000 U q8h	50,000 U q6h
Ampicillin	50 q12h	50 q8h	50 q8h	50 q6h
Nafcillin	50 q12h	50 q8h	50 q8h	50 q6h
Piperacillin	75 q12h	75 q8h	75 q8h or q12h	75 q6h
Mezlocillin	75 q12h	75 q8h	75 q8h or q12h	75 q6h
Cefotaxime	50 q12h	50 q8h	50 q8h	50 q6h
Ceftazidime	50 q12h	50 q8h	50 q8h	50 q6h
Vancomycin*	10 q12h	10 q12h	15 q8h	15 q8h
Tobramycin*	2 q12h	2 q12h	2 q8h	2 q8h
Gentamicin*	2.5 q12h	2.5 q12h	2.5 q8h	2.5 q8h

*Optimal dose should be established by monitoring peak and trough serum levels.

dexamethasone to all children over 6 weeks of age with bacterial meningitis, beginning, if possible, 10 to 15 minutes before the first antibiotic dose. Use of dexamethasone in newborns has not been fully evaluated, although studies are currently in progress. Dexamethasone therapy should not be restricted to children with severe disease, because hearing loss is also prevented in children who have relatively mild disease. In adult patients, we restrict the use of dexamethasone to patients who exhibit clinical evidence of impaired central nervous system physiology with altered mental status, high CSF pressure on LP, signs of brain edema on CT, impairment of hearing, or rapidly progressive disease with large bacterial load in CSF as evidenced by many organisms on Gram stain. When instituting dexamethasone therapy, it is important to confirm the bacterial cause of meningitis. If this cannot be achieved within 24 to 48 hours, we consider it safer to stop the anti-inflammatory drug and to reassess the appropriateness of the chosen antimicrobial therapy. At present, there is no evidence that treatment with dexamethasone for 1 to 2 days has any adverse effect on outcome in viral meningitis.

Based on the clinical studies available, the risk of serious side effects of dexamethasone at the recommended dose seems relatively small. The only major side effect noted in the first study from the Dallas group included two patients with acute gastrointestinal bleeding that required transfusions, and two additional children had heme-positive stools. In subsequent studies, the frequency of occult blood in the stool was no different for children treated with antibiotics alone or antibiotics plus dexamethasone. Nevertheless, it is recommended that patients who are given dexamethasone be closely monitored for any evidence of gastrointestinal blood loss.

SUPPORTIVE CARE

For critically ill patients with bacterial meningitis, aspects of supportive care can become extremely impor-

tant and may mandate early admission to a critical care unit. These patients are frequently neurologically depressed and prone to seizures, and they may need intubation for airway protection or assisted ventilation. In addition, children may have complex requirements for fluid supplementation. The syndrome of inappropriate secretion of antidiuretic hormone (SIADH) occurs in some children with meningitis, and when present prevents normal fluid excretion, leading to fluid overload if intravenous fluids are not restricted. Conversely, some patients with meningitis are dehydrated at the time of admission and need volume expansion to restore normal circulating volume. We recommend that a careful clinical assessment of fluid status be made at admission, fluid deficits be repleted, and patients monitored for SIADH (serum and urine electrolytes and osmolality) every 6 hours during the first 48 hours of hospitalization. If SIADH is not present, maintenance fluids should be given; however, if SIADH is present (as evidenced by falling serum sodium value and reduced urine output with urine sodium concentration >50 mEq per liter), fluids should be reduced to two-thirds maintenance volume until the SIADH has resolved, usually within 1 or 2 days. Fluid administration is such an important consideration in patients with meningitis for two reasons: first, fluid disturbances are common in meningitis, owing to fever, poor intake, vomiting, bacteremia, and possibly SIADH, and second, complex disturbances in intracranial physiology in this disease may be directly influenced by fluid status. Many patients with meningitis have an impairment of cerebrovascular autoregulation, which renders cerebral blood flow dependent on blood pressure. In this setting, the combination of systemic hypotension and intracranial hypertension can result in a dangerous reduction in cerebral perfusion pressure (the difference between mean arterial blood pressure and intracranial pressure), leading to cerebral ischemia. Conversely, experimental data indicate that increasing cerebral blood flow resulting from increased systemic blood pressure can potentiate intracranial hypertension. We recommend that for critically ill patients with meningitis (rapidly deteriorating neurologic status, coma) strong consideration be given to intracranial pressure monitoring and that the cerebral perfusion pressure be maintained at 50 to 70 mm Hg in children with meningitis, and above 80 mm Hg in adults.

In addition to these supportive measures, we attempt to actively reduce intracranial pressure in some patients with meningitis. While there is minimal controlled experience in reduction of intracranial pressure in meningitis, we employ measures that have been shown to be efficacious in other forms of intracranial disease: hyperventilation (with arterial pressure for carbon dioxide to 25 to 30 mm Hg), dexamethasone (if not already part of therapy), CSF removal if an intraventricular catheter is in place for intracranial pressure monitoring, and possibly intravenous mannitol, 0.25 g per kilogram.

SHORT- AND LONG-TERM FOLLOW-UP

If a patient responds clinically to institution of therapy, we do not repeat LP or recommend an end-of treatment LP. If however, there are doubts about the adequacy of therapy in a critically ill patient or about the accuracy of the initial diagnosis, we have a low threshold for repeating LP. Pediatric patients not infrequently develop a secondary fever after an initial response to therapy. This is most commonly due to infected intravenous lines, secondary infections that require drainage (septic arthritis, purulent pericarditis, pleural or intracranial empyema) or drug fever. Sterile subdural effusions, which develop in approximately one-third of children with meningitis, usually do not require drainage unless symptoms or signs of intracranial hypertension are present. Obstructive hydrocephalus usually manifests within the first few weeks after infection and should be treated with ventriculoperitoneal shunting. Neurologic sequelae, including hearing impairment, cranial nerve palsies, and motor deficits, can improve for several months after the acute illness, and appropriate, individually tailored supportive therapy should be arranged for patients who are left with sequelae from the disease.

SUGGESTED READING

Klein JO, Feigin RD, McCracken GH Jr. Report of the task force on diagnosis and management of meningitis. Pediatrics 1986; 78: 959–979.
Täuber MG, Sande MA. General principles of therapy of pyogenic meningitis. Infect Dis Clin North Am 1990; 4:661–676.
Tunkel AR, Wispelwey B, Scheld WM. Bacterial meningitis: Recent advances in pathophysiology and treatment. Ann Intern Med 1990; 112:610–623.

BRAIN ABSCESS AND PARAMENINGEAL INFECTIONS

J. DOUGLAS MANN, M.D.

Brain abscess and parameningeal infections are uncommon but potentially lethal and disabling clinical problems that are often difficult to diagnose in their early, and most treatable, stages. The magnitude of the problem is increasing as the incidence of immune deficiency disorders, intravenous street drug use, and penetrating head wounds increases. Effective treatment requires knowledge of the early clinical presentations, available diagnostic studies, and treatment modalities. In this chapter I review diagnostic and management options for patients with brain abscess, subdural empyema, and cranial and spinal epidural abscess.

BRAIN ABSCESS

Brain abscess is a focal infection of brain parenchyma, usually without accompanying meningitis or parameningeal infection. Lesions are encapsulated and have a central core of necrotic material and pus. Untreated, bacterial abscesses produce major disability and death by destroying brain tissue and by the effects of increased intracranial pressure (ICP). Despite major advances in diagnostic techniques, neurosurgical methods, and antibiotics, the mortality rate associated with brain abscess is 30 percent. More than 50 percent of survivors suffer neurologic sequelae.

Etiology

Table 1 lists the infections and predisposing conditions commonly associated with brain abscess and the organisms most likely to be causative. In 20 percent of cases, a source of infections is never discovered. Pulmonary infections account for 15 percent, ear infection 15 percent, sinusitis 20 percent, periodontal infection 15 percent, neurosurgical procedures 5 percent; the remainder have miscellaneous causes such as head trauma, retropharyngeal infection, IV drug abuse, endocarditis, and abdominal/pelvic infection.

In 75 percent of cases, the abscess is solitary. Multiple abscesses occur in the setting of hematogenous spread from distant sites. Half the cases are the result of infection by a single organism; the remainder have two or more pathogens.

Table 1 Infections and Predisposing Conditions Associated with Brain Abscess plus Common Pathogens

Predisposing Condition	Likely Pathogens
Chronic ear infection	Gram-negative aerobes, *Proteus*, *Pseudomonas*, *Klebsiella*, *Escherichia*, *Bacteroides fragilis*, anaerobes
Sinus or mastoid infection	*Staphylococcus aureus*, streptococci, *B. fragilis*, *Haemophilus*
Periodontal infection (dental procedures)	Mixed flora, streptococci
Pulmonary infection (bronchiectasis, lung abscess, cystic fibrosis)	Mixed flora, *B. fragilis*, streptococci, *Nocardia*
Penetrating head wound, neurosurgical procedure	*Staphylococcus pyrogenes*, *S. aureus*, streptococci, *Enterobacter*
Endocarditis	Mixed flora, *S. aureus*
Abdominal or pelvic infection	Mixed flora, gram-negative bacilli, *Pseudomonas*
Immunodeficiency	*Nocardia*, *Toxoplasma gondii*, *Aspergillus*, *Candida*
Diabetes mellitus	*Rhizopus*
IV use of street drugs	Mixed flora, *Staphylococcus epidermidis*
Unknown	*S. aureus*, aerobic or anaerobic streptococci, *B. fragilis*, *Enterobacter*

When a local pericranial infection is the cause, the abscess is often solitary and found in a part of the brain near the site of primary infection. Hence, frontal lobe lesions are seen with maxillary sinusitis, whereas mastoid or ear infections lead to temporal or cerebellar infection. Once an abscess is located, a careful examination of contiguous structures is mandatory in all patients.

Clinical Features

Patients with brain abscess present with generalized or focal headache (prevalence 75 percent), nausea and vomiting (50 percent), seizures (30 percent), and altered mental status (50 percent). Nuchal rigidity is observed in 30 percent of patients at presentation, whereas fever, often low-grade, is present in only 50 percent. Given the size of many of the lesions and the extent of associated cerebral edema, the percentage with focal neurologic findings is surprisingly small (less than 50 percent in some series). Fewer than 25 percent have papilledema at presentation. Duration of symptoms is highly variable, from hours to many weeks. Most patients are symptomatic less than 2 weeks and report a progressive course.

Diagnosis

The diagnosis is suspected on the basis of these history and examination findings, especially when they are associated with any of the predisposing conditions listed in Table 1. The progression of the illness is often more impressive than any individual sign or symptom. The clinician should not be put off by absence of fever or of an elevated white blood cell count. Human immunodeficiency virus (HIV)–infected patients who have any of the combination of symptoms and signs described above are investigated for brain abscess.

Routine laboratory studies usually yield limited specific information. The leukocyte count and differential cell count are abnormal in fewer than half the cases, and the erythrocyte sedimentation rate was less than 40 in 70 percent of patients in one series.

Lumbar puncture (LP) is hazardous and when brain abscess is suspected should not be performed before imaging. This is particularly important when there are focal findings on examination. Abscesses of even modest size often have large areas of surrounding edema associated with brain displacement; this makes the risk of herniation following LP extreme. The usefulness of information obtained from LP is limited, because the protein, glucose, and cells are often normal or nonspecifically changed and cerebrospinal fluid (CSF) cultures grow a pathogen less than 10 percent of the time. LP can be performed when imaging demonstrates no mass effect and normal CSF spaces and there is no clinical evidence of spinal cord involvement.

The study of choice is magnetic resonance imaging (MRI) or computed tomography (CT) of the head, with and without contrast enhancement in either case. Both methods have advantages. CT scanning is usually readily available, requires minimal patient co-operation, takes considerably less time than MRI, and is tolerated better by acutely ill patients. Sinuses and mastoids can be imaged at the same time. While ring enhancement is easily detected by CT, specificity in distinguishing abscess from tumor or stroke is less than for MRI. MRI is more useful than CT in establishing a diagnosis of abscess because it is more sensitive in distinguishing between cerebritis (focal infection without capsule formation) and abscess; it provides greater detail in terms of capsule uniformity, and it gives a clearer definition of the central regions of the lesion and the degree of surrounding edema. MRI provides information in multiple viewing planes and is more sensitive in picking up multiple abscesses, especially small satellite lesions. It is superior to CT in detecting abscesses adjacent to bone, which can be particularly important with posterior fossa lesions. MRI is most useful for following the evolution of the lesions during therapy. Beneficial effects of therapy are correlated with a reduction in the hypointense T2-weighted signal of the abscess capsule. This finding is both more specific and evident earlier than any changes that can be seen with CT. For patients who in response to antibiotics show no improvement or sudden worsening, MRI is the study of choice to document possible causes, such as abscess rupture into the ventricles.

Therapy

When imaging yields a diagnosis of probable brain abscess, a chest radiograph, electrocardiogram (ECG), and blood cultures are obtained, as cardiac and pulmonary sources account for 20 percent of cases. Cardiac ultrasonography is indicated in patients who exhibit no obvious source of infection and in those with abnormalities on the cardiac examination, chest radiograph, or ECG. Thorough assessment of the sinuses, teeth, and ears is mandatory, including cultures if infection is detected. HIV status is determined in all patients.

Major management issues center on (1) choice, timing, and duration of antibiotics; (2) timing and type of neurosurgical intervention; (3) treatment of ICP; (4) use of anticonvulsants; and (5) use of imaging in follow-up.

Antibiotics

Intravenous antibiotics should be given as early as possible in the treatment of brain abscess and perimeningeal infection. If there is a strong suspicion of intercurrent meningitis, therapy is begun immediately and is not delayed until neuroimaging of the brain or biopsy is performed. The initial choice of antibiotics (Table 2) for bacterial abscess depends on the probable organism, based on the source of the abscess; Gram stain characteristics and culture results in material obtained at surgery; antibiotic sensitivity of the organisms; central nervous system (CNS) and abscess penetration characteristics of the drugs; and host factors such as drug allergy and immunocompetence. Streptococci are isolated from 40 percent of all bacterial abscesses. Anaerobes are found in more than 30 percent, often as part of a mixed infection. Commonly encountered anaerobes include *Bacteroides,* streptococci, and *Fusobacterium* organisms. Aerobic gram-negative organisms coming from otic, pelvic or abdominal, and head trauma sites commonly include *Proteus, Pseudomonas, Klebsiella,* and *Escherichia coli,* whereas gram-positive aerobes usually include streptococci or staphylococci.

In some patients it is not possible to obtain abscess material, and 20 percent of cultures of pus obtained directly from lesions fail to grow organisms because of

Table 2 Antibiotics Dosing Schedules Useful in the Treatment of Brain Abscess and Parameningeal Infections of Adults*

Antibiotic	IV Dosage†
Penicillin G	4 million units, q4h
Nafcillin	2 g, q4h
Vancomycin	1 g, q8h
Metronidazole	500 mg, q6h
Chloramphenicol	1.5 g, q6h
Ceftriaxone	4 g, q12h
Ceftazidime	6 g, q6h
Cefotaxine	6 g, q4h
Gentamicin	1.5 mg/kg, q8h
For suspected *T. gondii* abscess:	
Sulfadiazine	4 g, q6h
Pyrimethamine	75 mg, q8h‡

*Dosing for infants, children, and adults who weigh less than 60 kg must be done on a per kilogram basis according to published guidelines. Adjustments in doses must also be made if renal function is impaired.
†Standard IV adult dosage
‡Folinic acid must be administered concurrently, 10 mg per day.

prior use of antibiotics or unreliable laboratory technique. Thus, empiric therapy may be necessary.

When the organism cannot be identified, a combination of penicillin G plus an agent active against B. fragilis is given. Penicillin G is active against gram-positive organisms and many anaerobes such as *Bacteroides* and streptococci, the major exception being B. fragilis. Metronidazole is given as the second antibiotic for its bactericidal action against B. fragilis. It is preferred over chloramphenicol, which is bacteriostatic for that organism. Metronidazole exhibits excellent abscess penetration that is not influenced by the presence of steroids. It is not inactivated by abscess pus, and it does not interfere with the action of penicillin.

Vancomycin should be used if the patient is allergic to penicillin or if a methicillin-resistant strain is isolated. Nafcillin should be used instead of penicillin when staphylococcus is strongly suspected, especially in the setting of trauma or post surgical abscess.

Addition of a third-generation cephalosporin (ceftazidime, ceftriaxone, or ceftaxine) or trimethoprim-sulfamethoxazole is indicated when gram-negative bacteria are isolated or seen on Gram staining.

An alternative starting regimen to penicillin-metronidazole is a third-generation cephalosporin plus metronidazole. This combination is more effective in the setting of penicillin-resistant anaerobes or chloramphenicol-resistant gram-negative aerobes.

Amphotericin B (AMB) is the drug of choice for most fungal abscesses. 5-Flucytosine is an oral agent effective against some strains of *Candida* and *Cryptococcus* organisms and may be useful as an adjunct to AMB. Ketoconazole and miconazole penetrate the CNS poorly. Fluconazole and itraconazole are new oral agents that may prove effective against CNS fungal infections.

Local instillation of antibiotics into the abscess at

the time of surgical drainage is a controversial practice.

IV antibiotics are continued 4 to 8 weeks. MRI is used to follow resolution of the lesions. Guidelines for the use of oral antibiotics in the late stages of therapy are not available. If the patient is improved and stable over the last 2 weeks of IV therapy there is probably no need to continue oral medication. Evidence for a relapse after antibiotic therapy has been discontinued is an indication for a thorough workup, including repeat cultures and a return to IV medications. The relapse rate is less than 10 percent.

Surgical Intervention

Surgical options include biopsy of the lesion, abscess drainage, and abscess extirpation. Of these, biopsy and drainage are clearly the most useful in early management. Extirpation is a major procedure and limited to accessible lesions that do not respond adequately to more conservative measures such as drainage and antibiotics. Abscess drainage using stereotaxic techniques with CT guidance is relatively safe and clearly improves the outcome when combined with appropriate antibiotic therapy. The technique is particularly useful when there are multiple abscesses and when repeat drainage is needed. Critically ill patients tolerate this procedure better than extirpation.

Surgical procedures are not needed when the diagnosis is clearly cerebritis. In a stable or improving patient with cerebritis, MRI repeated at weekly intervals can be used to determine response to antibiotic therapy and the need for biopsy or drainage.

Intracranial Pressure Management

Steroids can improve a patient's clinical status dramatically by reducing brain edema and ICP. The effect is often rapid, with benefits noted within the first day. Dexamethasone, 4 mg every 6 hours, is given after a 20 mg loading dose and continued until control of ICP has been achieved. It is then tapered off over 4 to 6 days. Steroids can complicate management by reducing antibiotic entry into the abscess, reducing ring enhancement on CT or MRI, and retarding capsule development around the abscess. These effects are superseded when ICP is a life-threatening problem. The need for steroids is usually limited to a few days, and they do not promote the spread of infection when used as suggested here.

Obtunded patients with brain edema and shifted intracranial contents are managed in an intensive care unit with ICP monitoring. Mechanical ventilation to PCO_2 of less than 30 torr is helpful in controlling ICP. Mannitol in IV doses of 0.5 to 1.5 mg per kilogram as a 20 percent solution given over 30 minutes can be administered every 3 to 4 hours, as needed, in the first few days. The major goals include reducing resting ICP to less than 250 mm H_2O and preventing the development of A waves or plateau waves, with their attendant fall in cerebral perfusion pressure and the increased risk of herniation.

Anticonvulsant Therapy

A generalized seizure can raise ICP dramatically in patients whose pressure-buffering systems are all but exhausted. Prophylactic anticonvulsants are used in most patients early in therapy. They are always used when there is a history of seizures and in patients with increased ICP or shifted intracranial contents. In adults, 1 g of phenytoin is given IV over 20 minutes, followed by a daily maintenance dose of 100 mg every 8 hours, PO or IV, adjusting to achieve therapeutic blood levels.

If there are no seizures during the first 3 weeks and the edema subsides with effective abscess therapy, phenytoin is tapered off over the next 3 weeks. If seizures occur at any time, daily anticonvulsants sufficient to maintain therapeutic blood levels are given for at least a year. Unfortunately, seizures are a common sequela (20 to 70 percent), and many patients develop epilepsy more than 2 years after the acute event.

Additional Considerations

Brain abscess is a predisposing factor in the development of inappropriate secretion of antidiuretic hormone (ADH). Owing to hyponatremia, this can be a major cause of poorly controlled seizures, even with therapeutic anticonvulsant levels. Intracranial hypertension is also more difficult to manage. Daily serum electrolyte values are obtained during the first week to screen for this problem and to determine the need for fluid restriction.

Patients often are confined to bed for extended periods; obtundity and neurologic deficits can result. Subcutaneous heparin, scrupulous nursing care, and daily physical therapy are needed to reduce the risks of bed confinement.

While the degree of neurologic impairment depends in large part on the amount and location of tissue destruction, the long-term prognosis is critically dependent on starting a quality rehabilitation program early in recovery. Such a program includes a neurologically sophisticated approach that reflects awareness of the plasticity of the nervous system and the behavioral consequences of CNS damage.

SUBDURAL EMPYEMA

Subdural empyema is an infection in the subdural space, between the dura and the arachnoid, usually overlying the cerebral hemispheres. Spread of infection from contiguous sources, especially acute sinusitis or ear infection, is the most common cause. Head trauma, osteomyelitis, and meningitis in children are other known associations. Hematogenous seeding of a preexisting subdural hematoma occurs rarely.

Etiology

The organisms most often cultured are similar to those for brain abscess: staphylococci in association with head trauma or neurosurgical procedures; gram-negative aerobes, and aerobic and anaerobic strepto-cocci with ear infection; *Bacteroides,* mixed strepto-cocci, and gram-negative aerobes from sinus sources; and *Haemophilus influenzae* in children with meningitis.

Clinical Features

Subdural empyema is a neurologic emergency. Patients are acutely and severely ill with fever, headache, nausea and vomiting, obtundity, nuchal rigidity, focal seizures, multiple neurologic deficits, and intracranial hypertension. They often demonstrate rapid clinical deterioration. Involvement of cranial nerves III and VI along with bradycardia suggests intracranial hyperten-sion with impending transtentorial herniation.

Diagnosis

MRI of the head with and without contrast is the study of choice. Coronal views are particularly valuable for posterior fossa lesions. CT with and without contrast is the alternative study and should be used with bone windows in addition to MRI when there is a suspicion of fracture. Arteriography is useful for ruling out mycotic aneurysm suggested by subarachnoid blood on MRI or CT, or the finding of an isolated third nerve palsy, with or without pupillary involvement. Plain films and bone scan are not helpful. Lumbar puncture is contraindi-cated.

Therapy

Management is directed toward eliminating the causative infective agents in both the subdural abscess and in the primary source of infection, reducing intra-cranial pressure, and controlling seizures.

Surgical drainage of the abscess at the earliest opportunity is essential for successful treatment. Place-ment of multiple burr holes or craniotomy is necessary in virtually all cases, particularly with posterior fossa or multiloculated lesions. Pus must be stained and carefully cultured for anaerobes in addition to aerobic organisms, fungi, and *Mycobacterium tuberculosis.* Material from otic or sinus sources of infection needs to be cultured separately. Infections of mixed flora are common in the primary sources, and recurrence is likely if they are not adequately treated.

Intravenous antibiotic therapy should be directed against staphylococci, streptococci, *B. fragilis,* gram-negative aerobes, and *H. influenzae.* Treatment should include (1) nafcillin, 2 g every 4 hours (vancomycin, 1 g every 8 hours if the patient is allergic to penicillin); (2) ceftriaxone, 4 g every 12 hours or ceftazidime, 6 g every 6 hours; and (3) metronidazole, 500 mg every 6 hours. Final adjustment of antibiotics follows receipt of culture and Gram stain results. Antibiotic therapy is continued 4 weeks and without surgical drainage will be ineffective.

The same considerations that govern management

of ICP and seizures in brain abscess apply in sub-dural empyema. Increased ICP is almost invariably present.

Seizure disorder (prevalence 20 to 40 percent) and hemiparesis (up to 40 percent) are the two most common sequelae in survivors. Coma on admission is associated with a 60 percent mortality rate in some series and may be the best predictor of poor outcome.

CRANIAL EPIDURAL ABSCESS

Cranial epidural abscess is a localized infection between the dura and the skull. The common predis-posing factors are similar to those for subdural empyema: spread of infection from contiguous sources such as sinus, orbit, mastoid, or ear; neurosurgical procedures; epidural intracranial pressure monitoring; head trauma with skull fracture. The abscess grows by dissecting the dura away from the inner table of the skull. Hence the infection is usually sharply circumscribed and slow growing.

Etiology

Pathogens include *S. aureus* and *S. epidermidis* from head trauma or neurosurgical procedures. Other organ-isms commonly encountered include hemolytic and microaerophilic streptococci, *H. influenzae* and gram-negative aerobes, *B. fragilis* and other anaerobes, and *Rhizopus* (mucormycosis).

Clinical Features

Unlike that of subdural empyema, the course may be indolent and the patient may have few symptoms other than localized tenderness over the abscess, dull head-ache, and low-grade fever. A developing epidural abscess may be missed when attention is focused on the antecedent head trauma or on treatment of the localized sinus or ear infection. Facial pain and edema may occur when there is infection of the bone. Cranial nerve paresis is seen when the abscess involves sites of cranial nerve penetration of the dura. An example is petrous tip involvement producing Gradenigo's syndrome, deficits referable to cranial nerves V and VI with severe pain. In advanced cases, patients develop focal or generalized seizures, mental status changes, nuchal rigidity, focal neurologic deficits, and increased ICP. Spread of the inflammatory process can lead to dural sinus or cortical vein thrombosis with rapidly developing cerebral edema, seizures, and cortical venous infarction. Rupture of the infection through a thinned or necrotic dura leads to subdural empyema or meningitis and rapid clinical deterioration.

Diagnosis

The diagnosis is made with contrast-enhanced multiplanar MRI supplemented as needed by cranial CT with contrast and bone windows. If an epidural lesion is found, additional views of the sinuses, mastoids, and orbits should be obtained. Skull films and bone scan usually add little information. Lumbar puncture is hazardous and does not increase the accuracy of diagnosis.

Therapy

Surgical drainage and decompression are indicated. Craniectomy is necessary if the bone is infected. Dural débridement is usually all that is needed, though dural excision and grafting may be required. Any communication between a sinus cavity and the epidural space is closed. Material obtained at surgery is cultured for bacteria, fungi, and mycobacteria and stained. Antibiotic therapy is adjusted according to the results. Initial antibiotic therapy is the same as for subdural empyema and should be directed toward treating *S. aureus,* aerobic streptococci, and anaerobes.

SPINAL EPIDURAL ABSCESS

Infection of the spinal epidural space is a neurologic emergency. Delay in recognition or treatment leads to irreversible, devastating neurologic deficits. The spinal epidural space lies between the spinal dura and the inner walls of the spinal canal. It is an area of low tissue pressure and is normally filled with fat and an extensive venous plexus. The space is widest in its posterior portions and in the thoracic area and is narrowest in the low cervical plexus outflow area. Infections are most common in the thoracic segments and cause intense local pain, nerve root irritation with referred pain distally, weakness, and spinal cord compression. The abscess may extend many levels above or below the area of greatest tenderness, at times involving the entire spinal epidural space.

Etiology

Causes include direct extension from local or contiguous sources, including vertebral body osteomyelitis (prevalence 10 percent), retropharyngeal infection (rare), perinephric or psoas abscesses (10 percent), and infections in the retroperitoneal or retromediastinal areas (8 percent). Hematogenous spread occurs from pulmonary (6 percent), skin (21 percent), or pelvic or abdominal (10 percent) sites of infection. Iatrogenic causes include back surgery, placement of epidermal catheters for anesthesia or pain control, dorsal column stimulator implantation, and lumbar puncture (5 percent). Intravenous drug abuse is increasingly noted as a cause (5 percent).

The most common infectious agent is *S. aureus* (62 percent), which, along with other gram-positive cocci such as streptococci, accounts for 75 percent of all cases. Gram-negative aerobes account for most of the remainder; *M. tuberculosis* and fungi are rare causes.

Clinical Features

Clinical features progress through four phases whose total duration ranges from hours to weeks. Localized back pain with paraspinous muscle spasm and exquisite tenderness of the spinous processes is often the earliest clinical picture. Pain may be lateralized to either side of the back and is very sensitive to palpation or even slight body movement. The next phase involves nerve root irritation and referred pain distally to extremities, abdomen, or thorax. Referred pain can include abdominal and thoracic viscera, confounding identification of the problem. Focal or regional motor weakness results from ventral root involvement. The third phase includes progressive weakness and sensory loss secondary to spinal cord compression. The sensory loss often has an ascending pattern of progression. Bowel and bladder impairment are prominent. Untreated, the syndrome progresses to paralysis with profound sensory loss secondary to spinal cord edema and necrosis. In chronic cases, the syndrome resembles spinal cord neoplasm. In acute cases, it can mimic demyelinating transverse myelitis. Fever is present in about half the cases, and the leukocyte count is frequently normal. Patients seek medical attention because of the severe back pain and not necessarily because of symptoms of infection.

Diagnosis

MRI of the spine is the diagnostic study of choice. The entire length of the cord can be imaged in multiple planes along with surrounding bones, cartilage, and soft tissues. MRI is particularly useful when searching for osteomyelitis or extension of infection into the epidural space from a local source. Cord compression is easily identified, as is the extent of the infection. Myelography with CT is the alternative study of choice. Spine radiography or CT is indicated when there has been trauma.

If myelography is performed, care must be taken not to introduce infection into the spinal subarachnoid space with the lumbar puncture needle as it passes through an infected epidural space. Pain and the pattern of neurologic deficits can guide avoidance of infected areas. A C1-2 puncture is performed when the pain and other neurologic findings are referable to the lumbar or thoracic areas. Advancing the needle into the epidural space and withdrawing the stylet can result in identification of localized accumulations of pus before the dura is punctured.

Therapy

When spinal epidermal abscess is considered, the neurosurgical team is notified as early as possible in the workup. Surgical drainage of the abscess and spinal cord decompression are done immediately. The effectiveness of steroids in reducing cord compression secondary to abscess is unproven. Material obtained at surgery is cultured for aerobic and anaerobic bacteria, fungi, and tuberculosis. Gram and acid-fast stain findings are sometimes diagnostic and can prompt early, aggressive treatment for gram-negative organisms before culture results are available.

Antibiotic coverage is initially directed against staphylococci, streptococci, and gram-negative aerobes. Nafcillin, 2 g every 4 hours, is combined with either gentamicin, 1.5 mg per kilogram every 8 hours after a loading dose of 2.0 mg per kilogram, or a third-generation cephalosporin. Antibiotics are adjusted according to sensitivities obtained from cultures. Vancomycin is substituted for nafcillin if there is a history of penicillin allergy or if resistant organisms are cultured. Antibiotics are continued 4 weeks after drainage (6 to 8 weeks if osteomyelitis is the source of the infection). Prognosis depends on early treatment and is poor if paraparesis or paralysis is present longer than 48 hours. The outcome tends to be worse when the abscess is in the cervical region. Recovery is complete in 40 percent of cases when the spinal cord findings are minimal at the time of presentation.

SUGGESTED READING

Chun CH, Johnson JD, Hofstetter M, Raff MJ. Brain abscess: A study of 45 consecutive cases. Medicine 1986;65:415–431.
Lasker BR, Harter DH. Cervical epidural abscess. Neurology 1987; 37:1747–1753.
Saez-Llorens XJ, Umana MA, Odio CM, et al. Brain abscess in infants and children. Pediatr Infect Dis J 1989;8:449–458.
Sandhu FS, Dillon WP. Spinal epidural abscess: Evaluation with contrast-enhanced MR imaging. Am J Roentgenol 1992;158: 405–411.
Silverberg AL, DiNubile MJ. Subdural empyema and cranial epidural abscess. Med Clin North Am 1985;69:361–374.
Wispelwey B, Dacey RG, Scheld WM. Brain abscess. In: Scheld WM, Whitley RJ, Durack DT, eds. Infections of the central nervous system. New York: Raven Press, 1991:457–486.

TUBERCULOUS MENINGITIS

THOMAS MOENCH, M.D.

Tuberculous meningitis (TBM) usually results from rupture into the subarachnoid space of an adjacent tuberculous focus. Because of the lack of effective host defense at this site, morbidity and mortality rates are high unless prompt diagnosis and chemotherapy follow. Thus, TBM is a highly lethal but also very treatable disease that has become more frequent owing to the general rise in tuberculosis and the increased incidence of meningeal disease seen in patients infected intercurrently with tuberculosis and human immunodeficiency virus (HIV).

TBM classically presents with a subacute, nonspecific prodrome of fever, malaise, and headache, followed by meningismus, cranial nerve palsies, and progressive obtundity and paralysis. Clues to the diagnosis include a history of tuberculosis contact, concurrent extrameningeal disease evident on chest radiographs or elsewhere, or a positive purified protein derivative (PPD) of tuberculin test (present in 50 to 75 percent of cases). Blood studies are usually not helpful, although hyponatremia or an elevated alkaline phosphatase value supports the diagnosis. Most important is the examination of the cerebrospinal fluid (CSF), which typically shows lymphocytic pleocytosis, elevated protein, and depressed glucose. Early in the disease, the cells may be predominantly neutrophils and the glucose is normal in almost one-fifth of cases, but both generally shift toward the classical pattern on repeated studies.

The most important principle in diagnosis is repeated examination of CSF for mycobacteria. At least four specimens of 10 to 20 ml each should be centrifuged and the pellets examined by fluorochrome stain and cultured.

DRUG THERAPY

The availability of antituberculosis drugs has dramatically improved the outcome of TBM. The newer, highly bactericidal multiple-drug regimens have not been compared with earlier regimens or with each other in controlled trials. A strong rationale can nevertheless be constructed for their use in light of their success in rapid sterilization and cure with short-course regimens for pulmonary tuberculosis, and from knowledge of their ability to penetrate into the CSF.

It cannot be overemphasized that antituberculosis therapy must be initiated when TBM is suspected, not delayed until microbiologic proof has been obtained. At best, only a third of initial CSF acid-fast bacillus smears are positive, and even brief delay often results in increased mortality or residual deficits. Empiric antituberculosis therapy does not significantly reduce the yield of subsequent smears and cultures obtained expeditiously (within 1 week). The most important drugs for treatment of TBM are shown in Table 1 and are discussed in detail in the text.

Isoniazid

Isoniazid (INH) continues to be the cornerstone of treatment for tuberculosis in all its forms. It is bactericidal and penetrates into CSF extremely well (producing

Table 1 Drugs for Tuberculous Meningitis

Drug	Dose (mg/kg/day)	Route	Toxicity	Monitoring
Isoniazid (INH)	10 (max. 300 mg)	PO or per NG (IM available)*	Hepatitis, neuropathy, seizures, increased dilantin level	Alanine aminotransferase (ALT) weekly as inpatient then by clinical symptoms Monitor dilantin level
Rifampin (RIF)	Child: 15 Adult: 10 (max. mg/day)	PO or NG (IV available)†	Hepatitis, increased drug metabolism (steroids, warfarin)	Monitor ALT as for INH
Pyrazinamide (PZA)	25 (max. 2.5 g)	PO or per NG	Hyperuricemia, gout, rash	Uric acid
Streptomycin (STM)	Child: 30 Adult: 15 (max. 1 g)	IM	Vestibular, cochlear, rash	Test gait, monthly audiometry
Ethambutol (EMB)	25 for 2 months, then 15	PO or per NG	Optic neuritis Rash	Monthly visual acuity and red-green with large doses
Dexamethasone	Child: 0.3 Adult: 16 mg/day	IM or PO		

*PO or NG are preferred, but IM is available when PO or NG are not practical.
†PO or NG are preferred, but IV is available when PO or NG are not practical.

40 percent of the serum level with uninflamed meninges, 100 percent of serum level with meningeal inflammation). Many authorities have recommended increased doses (10 to 15 mg per kilogram per day) of INH for the initial phases of treatment of TBM. However, I recommend conventional doses of 10 mg per kilogram per day for children and a maximum dose of 300 mg per day. It is clear that some of the toxicity of INH is dose related; particularly, the synergistic hepatotoxicity of INH and rifampin appears to be exacerbated by larger doses of INH. To avoid potential neurologic toxicity (seizures, peripheral neuropathy) of INH it should be given with pyridoxine, 50 mg per day (adults).

Rifampin

Rifampin (RIF) has revolutionized the therapy of pulmonary tuberculosis, speeding cure of the disease and allowing much shorter treatment courses when it is given in combination with INH (with or without other drugs). It appears also to enhance the cure rate of TBM and to allow shorter-term therapy, though admittedly the studies showing this are fewer, smaller, and less definitive than those for pulmonary disease. Its penetration into the CSF is poor without inflammation but rises to 20 percent of the serum value with meningeal inflammation, resulting in bactericidal CSF levels. Rifampin should be a part of all regimens for TBM that is due to sensitive organisms.

Pyrazinamide

Like RIF, pyrazinamide (PZA) has been found to be a potent drug whose rapid bactericidal action has allowed further reduction of the duration of therapy for pulmonary disease. It has a unique ability to act on slowly metabolizing populations of bacteria. PZA is especially

attractive for TBM owing to its excellent CSF penetration (equal to that of INH).

Streptomycin

Streptomycin (STM) is useful mainly as an additional drug in the context of suspected or proven drug resistance or as a substitute when other drugs are not tolerated. Although it fails to enter the CSF unless there is meningeal inflammation, it enters well enough to achieve therapeutic concentrations when inflammation is present. It can be argued that STM might accelerate mycobacterial killing in TBM and thus would be useful routinely as a fourth drug. I, however, advise against routine use of STM because of its toxicity (auditory, vestibular, renal) and the uncertainty of its additional benefit.

Ethambutol

Like STM, ethambutol (EMB) is useful mainly as an additional resource against resistant organisms or in case of drug intolerance. Although previously it was used as a first line agent in TBM, it is now clear that EMB is a "weak drug" that adds little to the sterilizing ability of INH, RIF, PZA, or STM in the treatment of pulmonary tuberculosis.

Recommended Regimen

I recommend a regimen consisting of INH (with pyridoxine), RIF, and PZA. When drug resistance is suspected, STM should be added until sensitivities are known. If STM is relatively contraindicated (age over 50 years, renal insufficiency), EMB may be substituted for it. Drug resistance should be suspected if the patient has previously undergone treatment for tuberculosis, is an immigrant from a developing country, or is in contact with other patients who have drug-resistant infection.

Duration of Therapy

Several studies suggest that TBM may be treated with rapidly sterilizing multiple-drug regimens for periods as short as 9 months. This would be expected to be the case, as the number of organisms in TBM is generally small. Moreover, most other forms of extrapulmonary tuberculosis have been shown to be reliably treated with 9 month regimens. I favor a 12 month course for TBM: INH, RIF, and PZA for the first 2 months, each given daily, followed by 10 additional months of INH and RIF given daily or twice weekly. (If twice weekly therapy is chosen [to increase compliance by use of supervised therapy], the adult dose at each visit is 900 mg INH and 600 mg RIF.) I believe this more prolonged (12 month) therapy is justified for TBM owing to the graver consequences of a CNS relapse and because the number of TBM patients treated to date with regimens of 9 months or shorter is relatively small.

Drug Toxicity

The most important and most frequent toxicity, to the liver, is due to combined use of INH and RIF. Patients should have baseline liver chemistry studies and weekly ALT determinations during the inpatient phase of therapy. Mild elevations (<5 times normal) of ALT are common and inconsequential, but at or above this point both INH and RIF should be stopped. During this period, PZA should be continued and EMB and STM added. Once the ALT is normal, INH should be reinstituted with continued twice weekly ALT monitoring. Most often, INH is tolerated as long as RIF is not reintroduced. In this case, therapy can be completed with INH, PZA, STM, and EMB. PZA and STM are stopped at 2 months, and INH/EMB are continued to complete 18 months. If ALT rises at reintroduction of INH, the INH is again withdrawn, the ALT value allowed to fall to normal, RIF reintroduced with monitoring, and therapy completed with RIF, PZA, STM, and EMB (again, PZA and STM for 2 months only, and therapy extended to 18 months).

PZA is not usually hepatotoxic at the dose and duration recommended. It frequently elevates the uric acid value and less commonly causes gout: with the former effect it should be continued, but with the latter discontinued.

Corticosteroids

Corticosteroids should be used in all cases of TBM. Evidence of corticosteroid efficacy has continued to accumulate and now includes a prospective controlled trial. Steroids reduce brain edema and inhibit the inflammatory response, which contributes to cranial nerve and vascular damage and compromise normal CSF flow. Theoretical arguments against their use have been disproven. Steroids do not delay elimination of TB organisms: antituberculosis drugs are very effective in eliminating sensitive mycobacteria, even in the most severely immunocompromised persons, including those taking steroids in large doses. Moreover, although it has been hypothesized that reduction of meningeal inflammation by steroids might reduce the penetration of drugs that require inflammation for adequate entry (RIF, STM, EMB), recent work has demonstrated that INH, PZA, RIF, and STM levels in the CSF were not reduced by steroid treatment of TBM.

I recommend therapy with dexamethasone, 16 mg per day for adults and 0.3 mg per kilogram per day for children who weigh less than 40 kg, given IM for all patients whose diagnosis is definitely or very probably TBM. This dose is continued 3 weeks and then tapered off to zero in 4 mg decrements (adults) every 5 days. Toxicity with this large-dose but brief corticosteroid therapy is minimal.

In most cases it is prudent to withhold steroid therapy when the diagnosis of TBM is in substantial doubt. Here, it is most important to avoid obscuring the results of a therapeutic trial of antituberculosis therapy. Response to such a therapeutic trial will determine decisions regarding further therapy for presumed TBM or the continuation of diagnostic efforts.

MANAGEMENT OF COMPLICATIONS

Increased Intracranial Pressure

Increased intracranial pressure, and resulting hydrocephalus, is a common complication of TBM and contributes to mortality and residual deficits. Prompt and effective management can much reduce morbidity. Computed tomography (CT) has markedly improved our ability to detect these problems at an early stage; CT should be done routinely in patients with TBM on presentation and repeated with any substantial clinical deterioration.

Increased intracranial pressure may present early (within 2 weeks of presentation). Mild cases can be managed with repeated lumbar puncture, acetazolamide, 30 mg per kilogram per day in three doses, to reduce CSF production, and institution of antituberculosis drugs and steroids. If such purely medical therapy fails to promptly relieve signs and symptoms of increased intracranial pressure, or in more severe cases, a ventricular drain should be placed. If after 2 weeks' therapy the drain is still required, it should be changed to a permanent ventriculoperitoneal shunt.

When increased intracranial pressure presents late (after several weeks' antituberculosis drugs and steroids), it is highly unlikely to respond to temporary measures. A ventriculoperitoneal shunt should be placed without delay.

Modern shunting hardware and techniques have

reduced complications of these procedures. Moreover, the fact that shunts often need to be placed in patients with active CNS mycobacterial infection does not result in mycobacterial infection of the hardware, or systemic spread of the infection to the peritoneum, so long as the patient is receiving effective antituberculosis therapy.

Tuberculomas

Tuberculomas presenting as symptomatic space-occupying lesions are uncommon in developed countries. However, with the advent of CT it is found that small, asymptomatic, parenchymal lesions can be detected in 10 to 28 percent of patients who have TBM. These lesions are generally very responsive to medical therapy. Surgical therapy not only is unnecessary but often leads to increased deficits.

Occasionally, tuberculomas present late, after weeks or even a few months of antituberculosis therapy. This is probably due to release of antigens from killed organisms and to the restoration of the delayed-type hypersensitivity that may have been "damped" by the extent of illness and debilitation at presentation. The inflammation, edema, and mass effect that can accompany this process can generate new and life-threatening deficits. Immunosuppressive therapy (steroids) is effective in most cases. Dexamethasone, 16 mg per day for adults or 0.3 mg per kilogram for children, should be given for 4 weeks, then slowly tapered off, using the clinical response as an indication of the appropriate rate. Antituberculosis therapy should be continued and generally not altered. This complication is rarely caused by ineffective antimicrobial therapy but rather by a counterproductive host immune response.

SPECIAL CASES

HIV Infection

The acquired immunodeficiency syndrome (AIDS) epidemic has resulted in increased rates of tuberculosis worldwide. Moreover, though only 2 percent of tuberculosis cases among HIV-negative patients are complicated by meningitis, for HIV-infected patients with tuberculosis the risk of TBM is 10 percent. The presentation of TBM is very similar in HIV-infected patients and in other patients, although HIV-infected patients are less likely to have an elevated spinal fluid protein value. The response to therapy in HIV-infected patients is likewise similar to that in uninfected patients. Tuberculosis is prominent among the causes of meningitis in HIV-infected patients, particularly among those with high rates of both HIV and TB infection (IV drug users, Haitian immigrants, homeless persons). Like other patients, HIV-infected patients frequently have active extrameningeal tuberculosis as a clue to the nature of their CNS process.

Failure to Improve

In patients with a confirmed diagnosis of TBM, failure to improve usually results from advanced disease before institution of therapy. The possibility of hydrocephalus or mass effect from tuberculoma should be sought by CT. If steroids have not yet been instituted, they should be added. One should also consider the possibility of drug resistance, and a four-drug regimen should be employed while awaiting sensitivity data.

When a patient with an unconfirmed case fails to improve, in addition to the above considerations the possibility of an alternative diagnosis must be reconsidered. Further diagnostic tests should be considered, including biopsy of relevant extracranial sites of known abnormalities (e.g., pulmonary lesions evident on chest x-ray) as well as meningeal and brain biopsy.

Unconfirmed Cases That Improve in Response to Antituberculosis Treatment

It is important to realize that a substantial percentage of cases of TBM (even in autopsy-confirmed series) are never confirmed by smear or culture (between 10 and 50 percent, depending on how vigorously the diagnosis is pursued). Thus, it is often appropriate to complete antituberculosis therapy begun empirically if the clinical suspicion of TBM was high and the response was convincing, even without microbiologic confirmation. Often an initially negative PPD test result becomes positive as the patient improves, after about 3 weeks' therapy, lending strong support to the original clinical suspicion. Repeated chest radiographs may show evolution to a miliary pattern. Likewise, serial spinal taps often show evolution of the picture and strengthen the case for TBM (shift to lymphocyte predominance over 1 to 2 weeks and progressive drop in glucose value).

SUGGESTED READING

Bullock MRR, Van Dellen JR. The role of cerebrospinal fluid shunting in tuberculous meningitis. Neurology 1982; 18:274–277.

Girgis NI, et al. Dexamethasone adjunctive treatment for tuberculous meningitis. Pediatr Infect Dis J 1991; 10:179–183.

Kaojarern S, et al. Effect of steroids on cerebrospinal fluid penetration of antituberculous drugs in tuberculous meningitis. Clin Pharmacol Ther 1991; 49:6–12.

Molavi A, LeFrock J. Tuberculous meningitis. Med Clin North Am 1985; 69:315–331.

Visudhiphan P, Chiemchanya S. Hydrocephalus in tuberculous meningitis in children: Treatment with acetazolamide and repeated lumbar puncture. J Pediatr 1979; 95:657–660.

CEREBRAL CYSTICERCOSIS IN NORTH AMERICAN CHILDREN

WENDY G. MITCHELL, M.D.

Cerebral cysticercosis occurs when the larvae of *Taenia solium* lodge in the tissues of the central nervous system. Many people mistakenly believe that cysticercosis is contracted by consumption of undercooked pork. While consumption of pork carrying *T. solium* larvae is the route of acquisition of the intestinal tapeworm, cysticercosis is caused by fecal-oral transmission of the ova shed by the intestinal (or adult) parasite. A household or community contact (i.e., food preparer) may carry the *T. solium* tapeworm. Autoinfection, though possible, is rarely documented. Nearly all cases of cerebral cysticercosis in children in Los Angeles have occurred in Hispanics, but some are clearly acquired within the United States by children who have never lived or traveled in Latin America. Most children infected without leaving the United States have adult household contacts who have recently arrived from or traveled to Latin America. A few cases have been seen in recent immigrants from Southeast Asia. A few non-Hispanic children whom we have seen with cysticercosis have had prolonged exposure by household contact with recent immigrants from Latin America, who usually work as housekeepers or in child care. A few patients, including some who have never eaten pork, have no travel history or household contact with recent arrivals from Latin America, but this is clearly the exception.

Severe parasitism with multiple active cysts is common in Third World countries but is very unusual in children in developed countries. Repeated reinfection is common in underdeveloped countries, while children seen in the United States often had a limited period of exposure.

Several forms of cerebral cysticercosis are recognized. The most common form seen is actively inflamed lesions, representing one or several dying organisms and the resultant tissue reaction. It is important to realize that this presentation indicates that the larva has died, and the inflammation is the brain's response to the released antigens of the resorbing organism. Inactive lesions, with residual gliosis and calcification at the site of a resorbed cyst, may coexist with acute inflammatory cysticercosis or be seen alone. Patients with inactive disease may present with seizures, or abnormalities may be found incidentally on scans done for other reasons. Single calcified lesions raise suspicion of cysticercosis, but the diagnosis cannot be proven in most cases. Acute encephalitic cysticercosis may mimic "aseptic meningitis" or viral encephalitis clinically. Intraventricular or subarachnoid (racemose) cysticercosis presents when free-floating cysts block cerebrospinal fluid (CSF) pathways, causing acute or intermittent hydrocephalus.

Active uninflamed cysts (single or multiple) are rarely seen in children in the United States, but are a common presentation in Latin America. These cysts contain living larvae. Cysts may cause mass effect or seizures. It is this form of cysticercosis that is commonly treated with antiparasitic agents (praziquantel or albendazole). Several forms may coexist in one person, although we have never seen racemose (intraventricular) and parenchymal cysticercosis in the same individual.

Although all clinical types of cerebral cysticercosis may occur in North American children, single enhancing cysts account for at least 90 percent of cases. The child usually presents with seizures, sometimes preceded by headache for a few days. Seizures may be partial simple, partial complex, or generalized. Postictal hemiparesis is common, but persistent focal neurologic abnormalities are rare. In urban emergency rooms, contrast-enhanced computed tomography (CT) is often performed immediately, and the presumptive diagnosis is made on the basis of a typical clinical presentation and neuroradiologic findings. More invasive and expensive testing, such as lumbar puncture, magnetic resonance imaging (MRI), or lesion biopsy is reserved for the child whose clinical or radiographic presentation is atypical. In children with radiographically typical enhancing lesions, MRI may show more detail but usually adds nothing to the diagnosis and is an unnecessary expense. Previously recommended "screening" tests such as soft tissue radiographs for calcified cysts are generally unnecessary, have a low yield, and do not alter treatment.

Intraventricular or subarachnoid cysticercosis is rare in children but is potentially rapidly lethal. Of more than 100 cases of cerebral cysticercosis documented in the last 10 years at Children's Hospital, Los Angeles, only three were intraventricular. One child presented in a moribund condition after less than 12 hours' symptoms of headache and vomiting. He collapsed at school and died shortly after arrival. On postmortem examination he was found to have a free-floating cyst blocking the foramen of Monroe. The other two presented with acute obstructive hydrocephalus, and did well after undergoing shunting and cyst extraction.

Cysticercosis may be an incidental finding on neuroimaging in an asymptomatic child or in one who has another neurologic disease. We have found both acutely inflamed lesions and calcified lesions in patients imaged for head trauma, and followed an asymptomatic but radiographically typical enhancing lesion in a child undergoing serial neuroimaging procedures for a brain tumor.

Serum and CSF antibody titers to cysticercosis have not generally been helpful, although a new method was recently developed at Centers for Disease Control by Wilson and her colleagues. Older methods relied upon enzyme-linked immunosorbent assay (ELISA), which had very low sensitivity. A newer method uses enzyme-linked immunoelectrotransfer blot (EITB) and is somewhat more sensitive, though it still cannot detect antibodies in some patients with inactive (calcified) disease or a single enhancing lesion. Sensitivity for intraventricular cysts, which pose greater diagnostic problems, is probably too low for the test to be definitive. This method is more sensitive for serum than CSF.

THERAPY

Diagnosis of cysticercosis in a child with a single inflamed cyst rests on a typical clinical presentation and CT, and, more importantly, on a typical pattern of resolution of the lesion. Thus, diagnosis and treatment are inextricably intertwined, both based on watchful waiting. An algorithm for management of the single enhancing lesion is illustrated in Figure 1. Definitive diagnosis may not be possible without following the child for 6 to 8 weeks, and performing at least one follow-up CT scan. The initial CT image may look quite alarming, but the discrepancy between the findings on CT and on clinical examination is generally quite striking. While CT shows an enhancing lesion, often surrounded by substantial areas of edema, the child looks strikingly well, particularly after recovering from immediate effects of seizures and administered anticonvulsants. In the absence of persistent focal deficits on neurologic examination or any signs of increased intracranial pressure, we feel that it is prudent to watch the child closely and treat only with anticonvulsants (generally phenobarbital, carbamazepine, or phenytoin). We ask the parents to watch the child closely for any symptoms of increasing brain edema. We have not used either corticosteroids or antiparasitic agents such as praziquantel. The child generally is seen again in a few weeks, and repeat CT is scheduled 6 to 10 weeks after presentation. By the first follow-up CT scan, more than half show shrinkage of the enhancing ring, conversion of the enhancing ring to a nodule, or complete resolution of the lesion. A few show no change, although edema is generally reduced. If the lesion has not resolved or become calcified, scans are repeated at approximately 2 month intervals. All lesions are resolved or calcified by 6 months after presentation. Prognosis is excellent. We generally continue anticonvulsant therapy for 18 to 24 months, then gradually taper the dose. About 60 percent remain seizure free off anticonvulsants after 2 years' treatment. The patients who have recurrent seizures are treated for another 2 to 3 years, then if they are seizure free the dose is tapered again. Long-term remission of epilepsy is about the same as for any child with secondary epilepsy. Recurrent enhancing cysts have been seen months or years later in a few individuals, presumably due to reinfection.

Several patients with single lesions who were initially thought possibly to have cysticercosis had atypical CT findings. Atypical lesions had either larger enhancing rings, unusual positions (such as in basal ganglia or deep white matter), or incomplete or irregular rings. When follow-up scans showed unresolved or enlarging lesions, brain biopsy or another diagnostic test was performed. Lesions included low-grade gliomas, sterile abscess, and other granulomatous diseases. In no case did the delay cause injury to the patient. The differential diagnosis also included other infections, particularly tuberculoma, toxoplasmosis, and fungal abscess, other tumors, and sarcoidosis.

The child with multiple enhancing lesions, particularly two or more acutely inflamed lesions, presents less of a diagnostic problem, as titers are quite likely to be positive. If CT shows typical lesions and the child

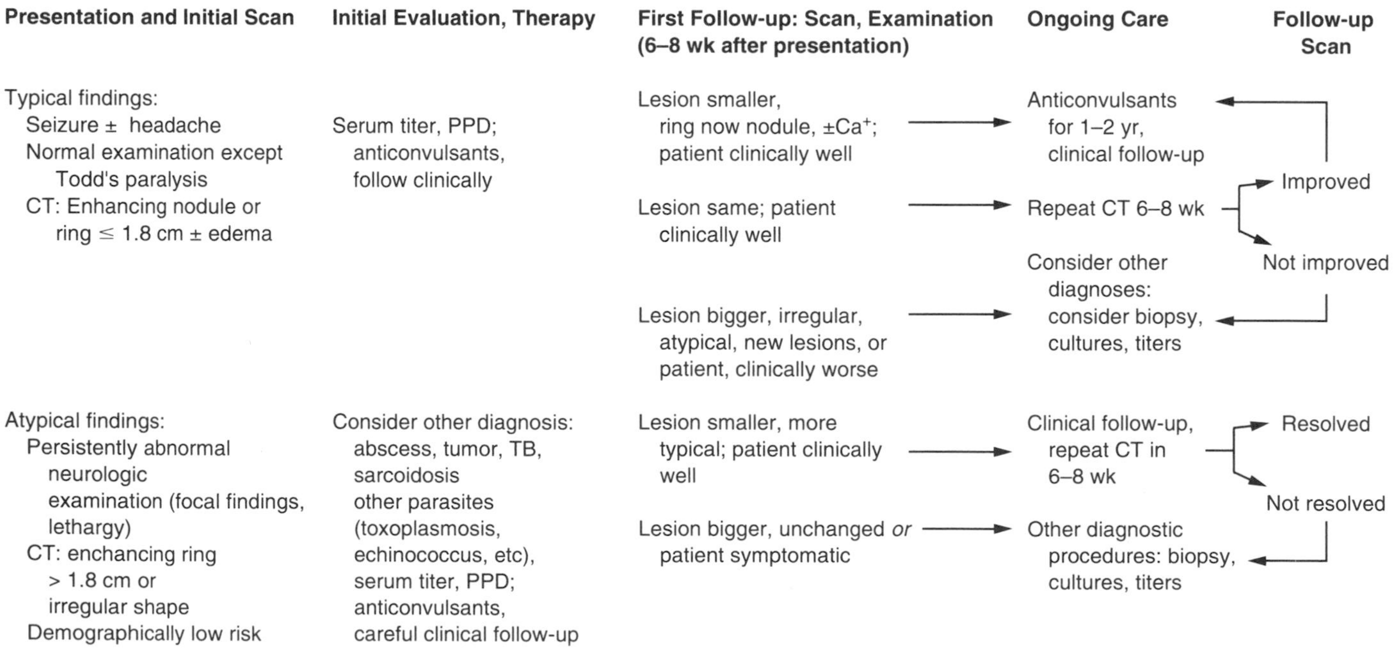

Presentation and Initial Scan	Initial Evaluation, Therapy	First Follow-up: Scan, Examination (6–8 wk after presentation)	Ongoing Care	Follow-up Scan

Typical findings:
  Seizure ± headache
  Normal examination except
    Todd's paralysis
  CT: Enhancing nodule or
    ring ≤ 1.8 cm ± edema
	Serum titer, PPD;
	anticonvulsants,
	follow clinically
		Lesion smaller,
		  ring now nodule, ±Ca+;
		  patient clinically well →
		
		Lesion same; patient
		  clinically well →
		
		Lesion bigger, irregular,
		  atypical, new lesions, or
		  patient, clinically worse →
			Anticonvulsants
			  for 1–2 yr,
			  clinical follow-up
			
			Repeat CT 6–8 wk
			
			Consider other
			  diagnoses:
			  consider biopsy,
			  cultures, titers
				← Improved
				
				Not improved

Atypical findings:
  Persistently abnormal
    neurologic
    examination (focal findings,
    lethargy)
  CT: enchancing ring
    > 1.8 cm or
    irregular shape
  Demographically low risk
	Consider other diagnosis:
	  abscess, tumor, TB,
	  sarcoidosis
	  other parasites
	  (toxoplasmosis,
	  echinococcus, etc),
	  serum titer, PPD;
	  anticonvulsants,
	  careful clinical follow-up
		Lesion smaller, more
		  typical; patient clinically →
		  well
		
		Lesion bigger, unchanged or →
		  patient symptomatic
			Clinical follow-up,
			  repeat CT in
			  6–8 wk
			
			Other diagnostic
			  procedures: biopsy,
			  cultures, titers
				← Resolved
				
				Not resolved

Figure 1. An algorithm for management of a single enhancing lesion of cysticercosis.

appears well, treatment and follow-up are the same as if the child had a single lesion.

The acute encephalitic form of cysticercosis generally presents with seizures, fever, signs of meningeal irritation, and numerous small enhancing nodules scattered throughout the cerebral parenchyma on CT. CSF pleocytosis is present, and titers are positive in both blood and CSF, even by the less sensitive ELISA methods. Anticonvulsants are the only treatment generally needed. We have followed four children who presented with this form of cysticercosis. Long-term prognosis is good. Even with multiple calcified inactive lesions, patients with this presentation have generally experienced complete recovery and remission of their epilepsy.

Intraventricular cysticercosis is an acute neurosurgical emergency. The cyst may move freely and intermittently blocks CSF pathways, causing acute obstructive hydrocephalus. Ventriculoperitoneal shunt or ventriculostomy is mandatory. After initial decompression, neurosurgical extraction of the cyst by an open or stereotactic procedure may be performed. As there is some concern that other intraventricular cysts may be present, some neurosurgeons leave a ventriculoperitoneal shunt in place even after successful extraction of an apparently single cyst. Racemose cysticercosis has not been found to respond to antiparasitic agents.

Active, uninflamed cysts, either single or multiple, are responsive to praziquantel. The child should be treated if the cyst is symptomatic (i.e., causing mass effect or seizures). Praziquantel will kill the larva which results in inflammation and edema and clinical symptoms similar to those of a spontaneously inflamed cyst. Praziquantel is generally used at a dose of 50 mg per kilogram per day, given for 14 days. Headaches and irritability are to be expected, owing to the edema produced around the dying organism. Corticosteroids (dexamethasone or prednisone) may be needed for all or part of the course, particularly if there are multiple lesions, but they are not recommended for prophylaxis or for children who have minimal symptoms. Anticonvulsants are generally used whether or not praziquantel is prescribed. Albendazole, 15 mg per kilogram per day for a month, is as efficacious as praziquantel but is not available in the United States.

There is no strong indication for treating asymptomatic uninflamed cysts found incidentally on CT. Occasionally, when lack of definitive diagnosis of cysticercosis complicates management, we have treated an otherwise asymptomatic nonenhancing cyst to avoid more invasive procedures such as biopsy. The typical response of the lesion to praziquantel confirms the diagnosis.

SUPPORTIVE SERVICES

Parents and older children need substantial reassurance and support. Most immigrant Latin American parents have heard of cysticercosis and may know other family members who have had it. More acculturated second-generation families, however, may not be familiar with the illness. Parents and children feel substantial anxiety at the thought of "worms" in the brain, and need reassurance that the organism is quite tiny and likely to disappear completely. Recently, a bright, academically gifted adolescent came to us several months after diagnosis of cysticercosis with substantial new academic and behavioral problems, initially thought to be due to his anticonvulsants. Only after a prolonged interview and substantial guesswork did we discover that he thought that his brain harbored something akin to a large earthworm. He was too terrified to discuss his fears either with his family or at previous clinic visits. After detailed explanation of cysticercosis, including showing him his own CT scans and demonstrating the shrinkage and resolution of the cyst, his fears abated and behavior returned to normal.

When an affected child has not recently lived or traveled in Latin America, the source of the infection is some concern. We assume that a family member or other household contact harbors a tapeworm, or at least harbored one in the past. However, the interval between acquisition of the larva and clinical presentation may be as long as several years. The Los Angeles County Health Department has been helpful in collecting fecal specimens from family members for examination for ova and parasites. Many of our patients come from families who have no source of regular medical care or health insurance; testing for *T. solium* must be done by a public agency. Though a variety of other parasites have been found, we have found only one adult carrier of *T. solium*.

SUGGESTED READING

Mitchell WG, Crawford TO. Intraparenchymal cerebral cysticercosis in children: Diagnosis and treatment. Pediatrics 1988; 82:76–82.

Sotelo J, Escobedo F, Penagos P. Albendazole vs. praziquantel for therapy of neurocysticercosis. Arch Neurol 1988; 45:5532–5534.

Wilson M, Bryan RT, Fried JA, et al. Clinical evaluation of the cysticercosis enzyme-linked immunoelectrotransfer blot in patients with neurocysticercosis. J Infect Dis 1991; 164:1007–1009.

NEUROSYPHILIS

JONATHAN D. GLASS, M.D.

For physicians practicing in the United States during the early 20th century, syphilis was a major public health problem. Gradually, owing to public health initiatives and the introduction of antibiotics, syphilis became a relative rarity from the mid-1950s to the 1980s; the incidence of primary and secondary syphilis dropped from 75 cases per 100,000 in 1947 to a low of four cases per 100,000 in 1955. Since 1985, however, the incidence of syphilis has risen dramatically, reaching 20 cases per 100,000 in 1990. This resurgence of syphilis as a widespread health problem is due to several societal factors, including a decline in socioeconomic and education levels and, for a large proportion of the population, difficulty gaining access to health care. Syphilis in all of its forms is now regularly encountered by both primary practitioners and neurologists, and its spread within the human immunodeficiency virus (HIV)–infected population has resulted in new challenges in both diagnosis and treatment. As we approach a new century, Sir William Osler's statement of 100 years ago again rings true: "He who knows syphilis, knows medicine."

DIAGNOSIS

The first challenge in the therapy of neurosyphilis is in making the diagnosis. A correct diagnosis requires a high degree of suspicion coupled with specific clinical findings that are supported by laboratory data. A full description of the clinical syndromes associated with the invasion of the nervous system by *Treponema pallidum* is beyond the scope of this chapter; however, Table 1 lists common manifestations of neurosyphilis according to the stage of disease.

Serology

Serologic tests for syphilis remain the most helpful aids to diagnosis, but their interpretation can at times be confusing. Serologic tests of blood and cerebrospinal fluid (CSF) fall into two classes, nontreponemal and treponemal. The nontreponemal tests, such as the Venereal Disease Research Laboratory (VDRL) and rapid plasma reagin (RPR), detect a patient's response to cardiolipin-lecithin-cholesterol antigens. Although such antibodies are produced during infection with *T. pallidum*, false positive results can be seen in a variety of other conditions (Table 2). The treponemal tests detect antibodies directed specifically against treponemal antigens, and include the fluorescent treponemal antibody–absorption test (FTA-ABS) and the microhemagglutination assay for *T. pallidum* (MHA-TP). Treponemal tests are much more specific and thus give fewer false

Table 1 Neurologic Manifestations of Syphilis by Stage

Stage	Manifestation
Primary	None
Secondary	Syphilitic meningitis, cerebrovascular syphilis, optic neuritis, otitis
Tertiary	Pachymeningitis, cerebral and spinal gummas, general paresis (dementia), optic atrophy, tabes dorsalis

positive results; however, since they remain positive even after the disease has been successfully neutralized, they are less useful than the nontreponemal tests for diagnosing active syphilis. The two types of serologic tests are used in conjunction with one another. The nontreponemal tests are most often used for screening patients for syphilis and, because reactivity is proportionate to the burden of disease, for monitoring therapeutic efficacy. Because the more specific treponemal tests are not quantitative and give results that frequently remain positive after successful treatment, they are not used to monitor disease activity but rather to exclude false positives from the group of patients with reactive nontreponemal tests.

Cerebrospinal Fluid

The cerebrospinal fluid (CSF) must be examined from all patients who have a positive serum FTA-ABS and whose past antibiotic therapy cannot be confirmed as adequate. (A negative serum FTA-ABS rules out all forms of syphilis, including neurosyphilis.) The CSF should also be examined if a patient was previously treated but has a serum VDRL or RPR titer higher than post-treatment levels or has a clinical syndrome consistent with neurosyphilis. Any patient being treated for neurosyphilis must have a lumbar puncture before antibiotic treatment begins.

Spinal fluid should be examined for white blood cells, protein, and VDRL reactivity. (CSF-RPR test is not recommended.) Active neurosyphilis is almost always associated with an abnormal spinal fluid. (An exception may be the HIV-infected patient, see below.) In patients with syphilitic meningitis or meningovascular syphilis, mononuclear pleocytosis and elevated protein are the rule, and the CSF-VDRL is reactive in more than 90 percent of cases. Patients with tertiary forms of neurosyphilis are less likely to show abnormalities in all three of these CSF parameters (white blood cells, protein, and VDRL reactivity), but patients with active disease, such as general paresis, always exhibit some CSF abnormality. In end-stage disease (tabes dorsalis), however, the CSF may return to normal, apparently representing burnt out neurosyphilis that is no longer responsive to therapy.

Some controversy persists about the categorization and treatment of the patient who has abnormal CSF but is neurologically asymptomatic. These patients are more

Table 2 Potential Causes of False Positive Serologic Tests for Syphilis

Type of Test	Infectious Causes	Noninfectious Causes
Reaginic or nontreponemal tests (RPR, VDRL)		
Bacterial	Pneumococcal pneumonia, scarlet fever, leprosy, lymphogranuloma venereum, relapsing fever, bacterial endocarditis, malaria, rickettsial disease, psittacosis, leptospirosis, chancroid, tuberculosis, *mycoplasma* pneumonia, trypanosomiasis	Pregnancy, chronic liver disease, advanced cancer, intravenous drug use, multiple myeloma, advanced age, connective-tissue disease, multiple blood transfusions
Viral	Vaccinia (vaccination), chickenpox, HIV, measles, infectious mononucleosis, mumps, viral hepatitis	
Treponemal tests (FTA-ABS, MHA-TP)	Lyme disease, leprosy, malaria, infectious mononucleosis, relapsing fever, leptospirosis	Systemic lupus erythematosus

From Hook EW III, Marra CM. Acquired syphilis in adults. New Engl J Med 1992; 326:1060–1069; with permission.

likely to develop symptomatic neurosyphilis than those without CSF abnormalities and should be considered candidates for treatment. A patient in whom neurosyphilis is suspected but whose CSF-VDRL is nonreactive may benefit from a CSF FTA-ABS. A positive result is not useful because of frequent contamination of the CSF with serum, but a negative test rules out the diagnosis of neurosyphilis.

THE HIV-INFECTED PATIENT

A substantial number of cases of neurosyphilis are now being encountered in the HIV-infected population. Co-infection with HIV and syphilis most likely occurs because populations who are at high risk for HIV are also at high risk for syphilis. Primary infection with syphilis has also been implicated in increased risk for HIV transmission. For several reasons, neurosyphilis is more difficult to diagnose in persons also infected with HIV than in persons infected with syphilis alone. First, intercurrent infection with HIV and *T. pallidum* apparently alters both the clinical course and the laboratory characteristics of neurosyphilis. Several HIV-infected patients have recently been reported who have unusual (or unique) CNS manifestations of syphilis, such as spinal involvement or necrotizing brain lesions (quaternary syphilis). Also, the normal time course for progression from primary syphilis infection to tertiary complications in patients with HIV may be reduced from decades to just a few years, perhaps because of the immunosuppressive effects of HIV. Second, the clinical abnormalities seen with HIV, including meningitis, vascular disease, and dementia, can mimic those of neurosyphilis. Thus, patients infected with HIV alone may also show persistent CSF pleocytosis or elevations in CSF protein, or may show no CSF abnormalities in the presence of demonstrable infection with *T. pallidum;* either scenario creates confusion when the diagnosis of neurosyphilis is being considered. Finally, in HIV-infected persons blood and CSF serologic tests may give false negative results for syphilis. Paradoxically, some HIV-infected patients who have biopsy-proven secondary syphilis have been found to have nonreactive serum VDRL and FTA-ABS tests. The CSF-VDRL may also be nonreactive in HIV-infected patients with active neurosyphilis.

Because HIV can coexist with neurosyphilis, all patients with neurosyphilis should be tested for HIV infection. Similarly, if a patient with HIV infection has a neurologic illness, neurosyphilis should be considered a strong possibility. Further, patients who are infected with HIV and syphilis and who have neurologic abnormalities should probably be treated for neurosyphilis even if the CSF test results are normal.

THERAPY

Adequate treatment of neurosyphilis requires that treponemicidal concentrations of antibiotics be introduced into the CSF for a sustained period of time. Penicillin remains the antibiotic of choice; no large studies have demonstrated comparable efficacy for any other antibiotic. All patients with the diagnosis of neurosyphilis should receive intravenous therapy with aqueous crystalline penicillin G, 4 million units every 4 hours, for 14 days. Intravenous therapy with penicillin should always be started in hospital, because some patients with a large systemic burden of *T. pallidum* can experience a Jarisch-Herxheimer reaction (fever, rigors, leukocytosis). This can usually be managed with acetaminophen. Intravenous therapy services in the home have obviated hospitalization for the complete course. Patients with asymptomatic neurosyphilis (who have CSF abnormalities but no clinical neurologic disease) should receive the same course of treatment.

Pharmacologic studies have determined that the recommended course of benzathine penicillin, 2.4 million units weekly for 3 weeks, if injected into muscle, will not produce treponemicidal levels of the drug in the CSF. Because *T. pallidum* has been isolated from the

CSF of some patients treated with benzathine penicillin, it would seem prudent to risk overtreating rather than undertreating any single patient with neurosyphilis. This argument is even more germane to the HIV-infected patient, whose neurosyphilis may take a more aggressive course.

A substantial number of patients with "penicillin allergy" turn out to have negative skin tests, and can in fact safely be given penicillin. Thus, any patient with a history of penicillin allergy should first undergo skin testing to confirm an allergic response. Patients with true penicillin allergy can then be treated with other antibiotic regimens, though none has been proven to provide a long-term cure. The currently suggested alternatives are oral tetracycline, 500 mg four times per day; or doxycycline, 100 mg twice a day for 30 days; or intramuscular ceftriaxone, 1 g daily for 14 days. Tetracyclines should not be given to pregnant patients.

FOLLOW-UP

It is mandatory that all patients with suspected neurosyphilis undergo lumbar puncture before beginning treatment. The CSF must then be re-examined after antibiotic therapy, so that comparisons can be made of cell counts, protein levels, and VDRL titer. CSF pleocytosis should decline following effective therapy; an elevation in cell count would warrant consideration of further antibiotic treatment. Thereafter, the CSF should be examined at 3 to 6 month intervals for a steady decline in all three parameters. No good data exist on when a patient's CSF should normalize, but a rule of thumb is that cell count and protein levels should return to normal by 1 year and that the CSF-VDRL titer should resolve in conjunction with the serum titer. A rebound in CSF abnormalities (in the absence of some other explanation) heralds either recrudescence or reinfection, and thus necessitates another full course of antibiotic treatment.

Patients co-infected with HIV and syphilis may show persistent CSF pleocytosis or elevations in protein unrelated to neurosyphilis; in these patients, CSF-VDRL may be the most useful barometer of disease activity. A few patients, however, may also be nonreactive for CSF-VDRL; in such cases, clinical assessment of disease activity becomes the gold standard.

The resolution of clinical symptoms and signs depends on the degree of structural damage to the nervous system incurred during the course of infection. In patients with tertiary forms, treatment with penicillin can be expected only to halt progression of disease, not to reverse the dementia, myelopathy, or blindness.

SUGGESTED READING

Davis LE, Schmitt JW. Clinical significance of cerebrospinal fluid tests for neurosyphilis. Ann Neurol 1989; 25:50–55.
Hook EW III, Marra CM. Acquired syphilis in adults. N Engl J Med 1992; 326:1060–1069.
Simon RP. Neurosyphilis. Arch Neurol 1985; 42:606–613.

LYME DISEASE

PATRICIA K. COYLE, M.D.

Lyme disease (Lyme borreliosis) accounts for almost 90 percent of vector-borne infections in the United States. It is due to a spirochete, *Borrelia burgdorferi*, which is inoculated into humans by the bite of an infected *Ixodes* tick. These poppyseed-sized ticks are endemic in Europe and parts of North America. European Lyme disease differs somewhat from the North American infection. In Europe neurologic involvement is typically lymphocytic meningoradiculitis (Bannwarth's syndrome) associated with marked cerebrospinal fluid (CSF) changes. In North America this syndrome is unusual, and CSF abnormalities are much less striking. This probably reflects antigenic differences in *B. burgdorferi* strains isolated from the two areas.

Lyme disease is endemic in the Northeast coastal states (particularly New York), the upper midwest (Minnesota and Wisconsin), and the Pacific coast. It produces a systemic infection that may involve multiple organ systems, including the skin, joints, heart, and eyes, as well as the peripheral (PNS) and central (CNS) nervous systems. The only pathognomonic marker is the occurrence of erythema migrans (EM), an expanding circular skin lesion at the site of the tick bite. Spirochetes may then disseminate from this skin lesion into blood and spread to multiple organs. If the host's immune system fails to eradicate organisms, a persistent chronic infection results. Infection with *B. burgdorferi* may be asymptomatic, or may produce disease early or late. Neurologic involvement occurs in as many as 40 percent of symptomatic infections. Neurologic Lyme disease (neuroborreliosis) manifests as any of a variety of PNS and CNS syndromes (Table 1).

DIAGNOSIS

The Centers for Disease Control and Prevention (CDC) use a very strict case definition for diagnosis. They require a patient to have documented EM or to

Table 1 Neurologic Syndromes Associated With
Lyme Disease

CNS syndromes
  Headache with or without meningismus/constitutional features
  "Aseptic" meningitis
  Meningoencephalomyelitis
  Encephalopathy
PNS syndromes
  Cranial nerve (Bell's) palsy
  Radiculoneuropathy (includes radiculitis, mononeuritis,
    plexopathy, polyneuropathy, carpal tunnel syndrome)
  Myalgia/myositis
Postinfectious syndromes
  Persistent fatigue, malaise
  Persistent headache
  Persistent encephalopathy
  Persistent myalgias (fibromyalgia syndrome)/arthralgias

have a characteristic late disease feature (neurologic, rheumatic, or cardiac) with laboratory confirmation (positive culture, anti–*B. burgdorferi* antibodies in serum or CSF, or rising titer of antibodies). This CDC definition is useful for epidemiologic purposes, but it fails to diagnose a number of infected patients. EM does not occur in a significant number of patients. Culture of *B. burgdorferi* is extremely difficult, and some patients who receive early antibiotics will not make detectable amounts of free antibodies. I consider the current diagnosis of Lyme disease to be a clinical one. I use laboratory data to support my clinical suspicion, but I never use negative results to deny treatment to suspicious cases. Certainly the occurrence of EM establishes a diagnosis of Lyme disease. Unfortunately, only 60 to 80 percent of patients note the rash. Tick bite or tick exposure preceding onset of neurologic disease is suggestive, but fewer than half of neurologic Lyme disease patients report such a history. Residence in or travel to an endemic region, extraneural involvement, and a suggestive neurologic syndrome are all helpful clues. Because it is not practical to try to culture or stain for *B. burgdorferi* in clinical samples, laboratory tests rely on the host's immune response. The most frequently used laboratory test for Lyme disease is detection of anti–*B. burgdorferi* antibodies. Several important caveats must be kept in mind. First, specific antibodies document exposure but not necessarily active infection. Second, about 5 percent of neurologic patients are seronegative. Third, antibody testing is not standardized and there is interlaboratory variation. Both false positive and false negative results occur.

I carry out CSF examination in all suspected cases of neurologic Lyme disease. Abnormalities such as mononuclear and plasma cell pleocytosis, and intrathecal anti–*B. burgdorferi* antibody production, are helpful when present. However, CSF may be normal in neurologic Lyme patients. I frequently use ancillary (neuroimaging and nerve conduction) tests to help document neurologic involvement. There are a number of exciting research tests for Lyme disease. These include detection of *B. burgdorferi* antigens and nucleic acids (polymerase chain reaction) in CSF, the lymphocyte stimulation test using *B. burgdorferi* antigens, and detection of *B. burgdorferi*–specific immune complexes. Unfortunately, these assays are not routinely available, but it is likely that some of them will become useful diagnostic tests in the future.

THERAPY

Currently there is no consensus on the optimal treatment regimen for Lyme disease. The choice of antibiotics and, in particular, the duration of treatment vary among physicians practicing in different regions. The antibiotics most commonly used to treat Lyme disease are listed in Table 2. Some have been examined in controlled trials; others are being used empirically. My general approach is to treat early and aggressively with antibiotics that penetrate tissue sites well and provide sustained therapeutic levels. My drug choice is based on the type of involvement and clinical severity.

Erythema Migrans

I treat EM with 30 days' oral therapy with doxycycline, or amoxicillin with or without probenecid. I prefer to treat for a month rather than 2 weeks. Doxycycline is a semisynthetic oxytetracycline. I do not use it in children younger than 9 years because it discolors teeth. I instruct my patients not to take it on an empty stomach and warn them that they may experience skin photosensitivity reactions. I recommend the use of sun blocks. I tell them not to take it simultaneously with antacids, calcium, or iron medications, because metal ions can inactivate doxycycline. Sometimes patients initially tolerate only twice daily dosing but after several days can go to a thrice daily schedule. Amoxicillin is an ampicillin analogue. When I use amoxicillin, I generally add probenecid to increase drug half-life, though rashes are more common when the two drugs are used together. Recent data suggest that amoxicillin alone works as well as the combination therapy.

I have had excellent results with doxycycline and amoxicillin and have not needed to go to other agents. I have no personal experience with the combination of amoxicillin and a beta-lactamase inhibitor for Lyme disease. I never use erythromycin, oral penicillin, or tetracycline, because these drugs are not as effective as my first-line choices.

Several new oral antibiotics are being used to treat Lyme disease. Azithromycin is a macrolide that has been reported to be effective for uncomplicated EM when used for 5 to 7 days; however, EM patients with constitutional symptoms did better with 3 weeks of amoxicillin. It is possible that a longer course of azithromycin would have been as effective in these patients, but this was not assessed. In a patient who is allergic to penicillins, cephalosporins, and tetracyclines, I use azithromycin rather than erythromycin. Clarithromycin is another new macrolide that is being used to

Table 2 Antibiotics Used to Treat Lyme Disease

Drug	Dose	Comments
Oral (up to 30 days)		
Amoxicillin (Amoxil, Polymox, Wymox) ± probenecid	500–1,000 mg t.i.d. ± 500 mg t.i.d. probenecid Child: 50 mg/kg/day (to 1–2 g) ± 40 mg/kg probenecid (not used under age 2)	Gastrointestinal (GI) problems, hypersensitivity reactions (increased with probenecid)
Doxycycline (Vibramycin)	100 mg t.i.d. (not used under age 9)	Photosensitivity, GI problems, discoloration of developing teeth, not used in pregnancy
Azithromycin (Zithromax)	500 mg/day	Not given with meals or antacids, GI problems, duration of therapy unclear
Cefuroxime axetil (Ceftin)	500 mg b.i.d. Child: 125–250 mg b.i.d.	GI problems, bitter taste, hypersensitivity reactions
Amoxicillin/Clavulanate (Augmentin)	500 mg t.i.d. Child: 40 mg/kg/day in three doses	GI problems, hypersensitivity reactions
Clarithromycin (Biaxin)	500 mg b.i.d.	GI problems, not used in pregnancy
Cefixime (Suprax)	800 mg/day Child: 8 mg/kg/day	GI problems, hypersensitivity reactions
Parenteral (at least 2 wks)		
Ceftriaxone (Rocefin)	2 g/day Child: 75–100 mg/kg/day (max. 2 g)	Hypersensitivity reactions, GI problems, cholelithiasis
Penicillin G	20–24 mU/day, q4h schedule Child: 0.3-0.5 mU/kg/day	Hypersensitivity reactions
Cefotaxime (Claforan)	2 g t.i.d. Child: 120–200 mg/kg/day, q6h schedule	GI problems, hypersensitivity reactions
Chloramphenicol (Chloromycetin)	250–1,000 mg q6h	Blood dyscrasias
Ampicillin (Polycillin, Omnipen)	3 g q6h Child: 300–400 mg/kg/day, q4–6h schedule	Hypersensitivity reactions

treat some Lyme patients. I have no personal experience with it, and I am not aware of any data to suggest it is superior to azithromycin for Lyme disease. Cefuroxime axetil, a second-generation cephalosporin, has also been reported to be effective for EM. The major side effect is drug-related diarrhea. I recommend taking the medication with food to enhance drug absorption. Cefixime is an oral third-generation cephalosporin that is being used to treat Lyme disease, but I have no personal experience with it. In Europe, oral roxithromycin and co-trimoxazole have been used successfully to treat late Lyme infections. Such late and more severe infections normally are treated with parenteral antibiotics. In another recent European study, combined oral therapy with doxycycline and a fluoroquinolone (ciprofloxacin or perfloxacin) for 4 to 6 weeks was reported to give better results than monotherapy. The possibility of using extended or combination oral treatment in place of parenteral treatment is intriguing, but I consider it unproven at the present time.

Neurologic Syndromes

The only neurologic syndromes that I treat with oral antibiotics are isolated Bell's palsy and mild chronic polyneuropathy (which manifests as intermittent pares-

thesias). I treat for 30 days. In both cases I screen CSF to make sure it is entirely normal. If it is not, I use parenteral antibiotics. I also use parenteral antibiotics in patients with normal CSF if they have significant constitutional symptoms (fever, headache, stiff neck). My drug of choice is IV ceftriaxone. This has been shown to be superior to IV penicillin for Lyme disease. I give ceftriaxone once a day, and most of my patients are treated by home infusion. When patients give a history of penicillin allergy I investigate them for ceftriaxone allergy before starting treatment, since 5 to 17 percent of penicillin-allergic patients also are allergic to ceftriaxone. I frequently admit these patients to the hospital for close observation while they receive their first one or two doses. The major side effect of ceftriaxone is diarrhea, and, particularly in children, cholelithiasis. Diarrhea is treated symptomatically, but in rare instances *Clostridium difficile* colitis may develop. These patients have watery stools and cramping. Stool should be cultured for toxin, and the patient can be started on metronidazole, 250 mg PO four times a day, or vancomycin, 125 mg PO four times a day. In patients with a history of gastrointestinal problems, I add active culture yogurt or acidophilus to their daily diet. A Jarisch-Herxheimer–like reaction occurs in 10 to 20 percent of parenterally treated patients, generally within 24 to 48 hours of starting treatment. I treat this reaction symptomatically with antipyretics and anti-inflammatory agents but do not stop the antibiotic. Fever several days into therapy should not be attributed to a Herxheimer reaction. I treat with ceftriaxone for a minimum of 2 weeks, and in long-standing infections with more severe CNS involvement I extend treatment up to 4 to 6 weeks.

Alternative parenteral drugs include penicillin G; however, data from studies in vitro and in vivo suggest that penicillin is not an optimal drug to treat *B. burgdorferi* infection. Although penicillin has been quite effective against European Lyme disease, treatment failures have been documented, particularly in North American patients. Cefotaxime, another third-generation cephalosporin, has also been used in Lyme disease, with generally good results. The dosing schedule (three times daily) is not as convenient as that for ceftriaxone. Doxycycline can be given IV rather than PO. Finally, chloramphenicol is a potential agent for patients who cannot take cephalosporin or penicillin. This is based on one well-documented case in the literature in which a patient failed to respond to large doses of ceftriaxone and penicillin therapy but finally responded to chloramphenicol. Ampicillin has been used to treat some Lyme patients, but the results are anecdotal. I have never needed to resort to this particular antibiotic.

In pregnant patients I prefer to use parenteral therapy with ceftriaxone. With regard to corticosteroids, my basic policy is to avoid using them in neurologic Lyme patients. For example, I do not use prednisone for Bell's palsy secondary to Lyme disease. My reason is the suggestive data that indicate corticosteroids enhance treatment failure. The one exception may be combined use of antibiotics and steroids for severe Lyme cardiac cases.

Postinfectious Lyme Syndrome

Following treatment, particularly in infections beyond the local (EM) stage, it is not unusual for patients to experience prolonged complaints of fatigue, headache, joint pain, muscle aches, or mild memory/concentration problems. This has been referred to as the postinfectious Lyme syndrome. I warn patients that these minor problems may continue for months, but I also reassure them that they should gradually improve over time. I treat them symptomatically. Fatigue may respond to drug treatment with amantadine, pemoline, or Prozac. These patients should also be questioned about sleep disturbances. I treat persistent headaches with tricyclic antidepressants, nonsteroidal anti-inflammatory agents, or behavioral modification and muscle relaxation techniques. I treat chronic joint and muscle pains with graded exercise programs, tricyclics, nonsteroidal anti-inflammatory agents, or dietary 3-*n* fatty acid supplementation. I evaluate cognitive problems with formal neuropsychological testing, to provide objective documentation of deficits as well as to obtain a quantitative baseline. I refer some patients for cognitive retraining or behavioral modification. I treat others with CNS stimulants or tricyclics.

Response to Therapy

I monitor therapeutic response clinically, but I also document whether there is improvement in laboratory abnormalities. Clinical improvement is generally noted within days of starting antibiotics in patients who present in the early disseminated stage (meningitis or radiculitis). Patients with facial nerve palsy may not improve any more rapidly than those with idiopathic Bell's palsy. In the late persistent stage (encephalomyelitis, encephalopathy, polyneuropathy) improvement is more gradual and extends over months.

I always obtain baseline CSF values for neurologic Lyme patients. In patients with encephalopathy I get baseline cognitive function tests. In patients with neuropathy I get baseline neurophysiologic tests. If results are abnormal, these baseline tests are repeated 3 to 6 months after treatment to document improvement. Nonspecific magnetic resonance imaging (MRI) abnormalities, which are found in about 25 percent of patients, may or may not improve. If baseline CSF is abnormal, I like to repeat a lumbar puncture within 3 months of treatment.

I have found treatment relapse or failure to be unusual after an adequate course of ceftriaxone. There are a few such patients, however. I first try to determine whether I am dealing with a postinfectious syndrome rather than active infection. I do not hesitate to repeat studies, including CSF examination. If CSF is abnormal or there are objective new findings, I generally repeat a longer course of ceftriaxone. In certain cases it may be useful to monitor CSF levels and if the CSF level is subtherapeutic to boost the daily ceftriaxone dose to 4 g. When patients fail to respond to ceftriaxone despite good CSF levels, I go to an alternative parenteral drug. Doxycycline can be given IV, and this parenteral route results in higher serum and CSF drug levels than the oral route. Pulsed large-dose treatment with cefotaxime has been reported to work in a few refractory cases. This involves a cycle of treatment for 1 or 2 days, followed by no treatment for 6 days. This cycle is repeated six to ten times. Another alternative is an extended period (2 to 3 months) of oral therapy with a different agent. I find refractory or relapsing cases to be exceptional.

Asymptomatic Patients

I am frequently asked what I do with the asymptomatic seropositive patient. First, I convince myself that the antibody reaction is not a false positive one. I repeat a titer in several weeks, and request a Western blot. If seropositivity is genuine and if there is no history of antibiotic treatment, I treat for 30 days with an oral agent.

PREVENTION

Almost all cases of Lyme disease are due to the bite of an infected tick. Preventive measures include avoidance of tick-infested areas; the use of clothing barriers, repellents, and acaricides; and early tick removal from the bite site.

Ticks feed during warm weather. Humans are most likely to be bitten by nymphal ticks, which feed in late spring and early summer. Adult ticks, which feed mostly in fall and winter and occasionally in early spring, are much less likely to bite humans. Therefore spring and summer are the times of year when people are at greatest risk to contract Lyme disease. Ticks infest wooded as well as shrubby and brushy areas and are least likely to be found in the interior of well-maintained lawns. Areas inhabited by deer could well be Lyme endemic. People need to be particularly alert to their risk when they are in wooded and shrubbed areas, though infected ticks have even been found in urban parks in Baltimore and Philadelphia. Wearing protective clothing minimizes skin exposure sites. This includes wearing a hat and long-sleeved shirt and long pants, tucking the pants into socks, and wearing light-colored clothing. After coming in from the outdoors careful inspection of body parts for tiny attached ticks is in order. In particular, a child's scalp should be examined. A quick shower may facilitate body inspection. Some commercially available insecticides are active against tick vectors, and spraying infested areas has been proposed. Repellents are also available that can be applied to clothing, though they must be applied anew on every outing. Early tick removal is a critical factor. An infected tick does not transmit *B. burgdorferi* until it has been feeding longer than 24 hours. Ticks removed before 24 hours are not likely to cause Lyme disease. The best removal technique involves gentle traction with tweezers to lift the tick in one piece, including its mouth parts. The tick should be saved for later identification.

Prophylactic antibiotic treatment of a tick bite is controversial as a preventive measure. Several studies have found no benefit to prophylactic treatment, and I do not use it. I do check acute- and convalescent phase serum samples for anti–*B. burgdorferi* antibodies and treat patients who are antibody positive. Clearly, patients are at higher risk for Lyme disease if the deer tick is from a highly endemic region, is engorged, and has likely been attached for several days. In such cases there may be a case for treatment. One problem with empiric treatment is the possibility of creating a seronegative patient whose status will be difficult to interpret in the future.

The ultimate preventive measure for Lyme disease would be an effective and safe vaccine. A dog vaccine is already licensed for use in a number of states. It appears to be safe and to offer some degree of protection, although annual booster doses are recommended. Vaccines are being evaluated in several animal models of Lyme disease, and recently vaccination using a specific *B. burgdorferi* protein called OspA was found to be protective in mice. It is likely that within the next few years a vaccine will be available to test in humans.

SUGGESTED READING

Coyle PK, ed. Lyme disease. St. Louis: Mosby–Year Book, 1993.
Dattwyler RJ, Halperin JJ, Volkman DJ, Luft BJ. Treatment of late Lyme borreliosis — randomised comparison of ceftriaxone and penicillin. Lancet 1988;1:1191–1194.
Philipson A. Antibiotic treatment in Lyme borreliosis. Scand J Infect Dis 1991;S77:145–150.
Rahn DW, Malawista SE. Lyme disease: Recommendations for diagnosis and treatment. Ann Intern Med 1991;114:472–481.

PATIENT RESOURCES

The following private organizations offer information, literature, and educational materials on Lyme disease.

American Lyme Disease Foundation, Inc.
Royal Executive Park
3 International Drive
Rye Brook, NY 10573
(914) 934-9155

Lyme Borreliosis Foundation, Inc.
Box 462
Tolland, CT 06084
(203) 871-2900

Lyme Disease Coalition of New Jersey, Inc.
Box 1437
Jackson, NJ 08527
(908) 363-4070

Lyme Disease Resource Center
Box 9510
Santa Rosa, CA 95405
(707) 575-5133

VIRAL INFECTIONS

CONGENITAL VIRAL INFECTIONS

ALAN R. SEAY, M.D.

The prevalence of congenital and perinatal viral infections among newborn infants is estimated to be 1 to 2 percent. Cytomegalovirus (CMV) infections account for the majority of cases, whereas the other viruses mentioned in this review account for the remainder. All viruses that infect fetuses and newborns can produce a wide variety of clinical conditions, ranging from asymptomatic, subclinical infections to florid, multiple organ, systemic illnesses resembling bacterial sepsis. Although some viruses produce a diagnostically distinctive clinical syndrome, serologic testing and viral cultures are necessary to ensure a virus-specific diagnosis. Infections with herpes simplex virus (HSV) and some with varicella-zoster virus (VZV) are the only congenital viral infections for which specific antiviral chemotherapy has been shown to be effective in reducing morbidity and mortality. The long-term effectiveness of treating infants with perinatally acquired human immunodeficiency virus (HIV) infections is not fully known, but it is being investigated intensively. For the majority of infants with congenital-perinatal infection, supportive management, passive immunization, and isolation from other susceptible neonates are the mainstays of management.

HUMAN IMMUNODEFICIENCY VIRUS

During the past decade, the number of cases of perinatally acquired HIV infection reported annually in the United States has risen from 8 in 1982 to nearly 800 in 1991. This dramatic increase has paralleled the increasing incidence of HIV infections in women of childbearing age. A variety of epidemiologic data suggest that the prevalence of HIV seropositive women of childbearing age in the United States is about 0.15 percent (1.5 in 1000). Based on current projections of birth rates and estimating a 30 percent risk that an HIV seropositive pregnant woman will transmit HIV to her child, calculations indicate that approximately 4000 new cases of perinatally acquired HIV will occur in the United States in 1993. Of the infants who acquire HIV perinatally, 10 to 15 percent become symptomatic within the first few months of life, and most of these die within the first year of life. Of infants who develop acquired immunodeficiency syndrome (AIDS), 50 percent do so by age 1 year and more than 80 percent by 3 years. The cause of death for many children with AIDS is a secondary opportunistic infection such as CMV or *Pneumocystis carinii* that frequently involves the central nervous system.

Antiviral Therapy

Zidovudine (azidothymidine or AZT) has been useful in suppressing clinical symptoms and prolonging survival in older children, adolescents, and adults with AIDS. Although the efficacy and risks of this agent for perinatally acquired HIV infections in young infants and children has not been fully evaluated, symptomatic children are treated with doses of 180 mg per square meter of body surface given orally every 6 hours (720 mg per square meter per day). Children treated for AIDS are enrolled in specific treatment protocols and followed carefully in a specifically designed, multidisciplinary pediatric AIDS clinic.

The therapeutic role in perinatally acquired HIV infections for dideoxyinosine, dideoxycytidine, other antiretroviral drugs, and immunomodulating agents, such as IV gamma globulin, is not known but is being investigated at a number of centers.

Whether perinatal HIV infections can be prevented by treating HIV-infected women during pregnancy has not been determined. Little is known about benefits and risks of exposing a fetus to zidovudine or other antiretroviral agents. For newborns of HIV-infected women, sequential clinical examinations and laboratory monitoring of immune function, HIV-specific antibodies, and HIV antigens may be required for 2 to 3 years before the child's true HIV infection status is known with certainty. Recent studies have shown that testing infants for HIV-specific immunoglobulin A (IgA) antibodies, instead of IgG antibodies, leads to an earlier specific diagnosis with very low rates of false positive and false negative results. With an early accurate diagnosis, decisions concerning use of antiretroviral drugs can be made more confidently for individual patients. Zidovudine prophylaxis is given to neonates and infants at high risk of acquiring HIV and is continued until the true status of HIV infection can be ascertained.

Supportive Management

For children with perinatally acquired HIV infections, secondary bacterial, fungal, parasitic, and viral infections develop and are frequently responsible for the patient's pain and discomfort, multiple medical problems, and death. Supportive measures include encouraging adequate nutrition and fluid intake and treating secondary infections aggressively. An attempt is made to prevent exposure to potentially lethal viral infections such as chickenpox, and when HIV-infected children are exposed to VZV passive immunization with 1.25 ml (125 U) of varicella-zoster immune globulin (VZIG) is indicated.

HERPES SIMPLEX VIRUS

HSV, types 1 and 2, may affect neonates by causing localized infections of skin, mucous membranes, and eyes; central nervous system infections; and disseminated infections. Approximately 70 percent of localized HSV infections progress to involve the central nervous system or become disseminated if they are not treated promptly at the onset of initial symptoms.

Antiviral Therapy

During the past few years both vidarabine and acyclovir (acycloguanosine) have been shown to be effective and safe for treatment of neonatal HSV infections. Both drugs markedly lower the mortality rate and improve the outcome of survivors of neonatal HSV infections if they are started within 3 to 5 days after appearance of the earliest symptoms and signs. In comparison with vidarabine, acyclovir produces fewer adverse reactions and improves survival and long-term outcome. Acyclovir is now considered the drug of choice for treatment of neonatal HSV infections.

Infants strongly suspected or known to have any form of neonatal HSV infection are started on acyclovir, 10 mg per kilogram every 8 hours (30 mg per kilogram per day). The total calculated dose is dissolved in dextrose-saline solution to a maximum concentration of 5 mg per milliliter. Each dose is infused intravenously over an hour, and the drug therapy continues 14 days. During acyclovir therapy, infants are monitored frequently for possible drug-induced anemia, leukopenia, thrombocytopenia, hepatocellular enzyme elevation, and elevations of serum concentrations of BUN and creatinine.

An alternative to acyclovir for systemic therapy is vidarabine. This drug is given in a single daily dose of 30 mg per kilogram. Each dose is solubilized in dextrose-saline solution to a maximum concentration of 0.5 mg per milliliter and infused IV over 12 to 18 hours for 14 days. Large volumes of fluids are coadministered to ensure solubilization. Adverse reactions include vomiting, lethargy, tremor, myoclonus, and fluid overload. Patients are monitored for drug-induced bone marrow suppression and elevated hepatocellular enzyme values.

Herpetic keratoconjunctivitis is treated with topical 1 percent trifluorothymidine or 3 percent vidarabine ophthalmic ointment administered every 4 to 6 hours for 2 to 3 weeks. Infections of deep structures or chambers of the eye are treated with parenteral acyclovir, as described above.

Supportive Therapy

HSV infections can cause a variety of physiologic disturbances in neonates, including respiratory distress, acidosis, hypoglycemia, electrolyte dearangements, jaundice, disseminated intravascular coagulopathy (DIC), seizures, and cerebral edema. These medical complications may be severe, and they require specific evaluation and early intervention.

Acute HSV infections may result in permanently impaired vision and hearing, seizures, and a chronic encephalopathy with cognitive deficits, motor deficits, or both. These complications require consultations with appropriate specialists and educators to ensure that the child receives appropriate support services and therapy and achieves the highest level of function possible.

CYTOMEGALOVIRUS

Congenital CMV infections occur in approximately 1 percent of all newborns in the United States. Fortunately, 90 percent of the infections are subclinical and do not cause any short-term or long-term symptoms or impairments. Only 1 percent of congenital CMV infections cause symptomatic neurologic illness.

Antiviral Therapy

At present there is no effective antiviral agent for the treatment of congenital CMV.

Supportive Therapy

Babies with disseminated CMV infection require aggressive supportive measures to manage secondary complications such as hypoglycemia, jaundice, DIC, sepsis, hydrocephalus, cataracts, chorioretinitis, and seizures. Some of the neonates who appear to have asymptomatic congenital CMV infection during subsequent follow-up evaluations are found to have sensorineural hearing loss, speech delay, and mild cognitive deficits. These children benefit from speech and hearing therapy and special educational assistance.

Congenital CMV infections may play a role in the causation of infantile spasms in some patients. Adrenocorticotropic hormone therapy for infantile spasms is avoided in infants that are known to be excreting CMV because of the potential risk of inducing a fulminant CMV infection.

Many physicians and parents express concern about the risk for susceptible pregnant women, often health care and day care personnel, of acquiring primary CMV infection from a baby who is excreting CMV. When CMV excretion from an infant is documented, simple contact isolation procedures provide effective protection against CMV. Although any pregnant woman should minimize or completely avoid direct contact with an infant excreting CMV, strict and elaborate isolation of these infants is not warranted.

Chronic, congenital CMV infection, unlike acute, postnatally acquired CMV infection, does not interfere with the infant's immunocompetence nor does it increase complication rates due to other commonly acquired childhood infections. Special measures are not necessary to prevent babies with congenital CMV infection from acquiring other infections, and these infants should receive all routinely recommended immunizations later in infancy.

VARICELLA-ZOSTER VIRUS

Antiviral Therapy

A newborn whose mother develops VZV infection during the last 5 days of pregnancy or within the first 2 days after delivery should receive VZIG, 1.25 ml (125 U) IM, to provide passive protection against VZV. Similarly, newborns exposed to VZV whose mother is not immune to VZV or whose immune status is not known should receive passive protection with VZIG within 4 days of exposure.

Neonates with congenital or perinatally acquired VZV infection are treated with acyclovir, 30 mg per kilogram per day. The drug is used in the same way as for HSV infections.

Supportive Therapy

Though rare, congenital VZV infections may cause a variety of complications involving the eye, skin, peripheral nervous system, and central nervous system. Ophthalmologic and neuroradiologic evaluations, and occasionally electromyography and nerve conduction studies, are needed to assess the full extent of the deficits caused by congenital VZV. Future involvement of physical therapists, occupational therapists, ophthalmologists, and plastic surgeons may be needed to manage secondary complications of congenital VZV.

RUBELLA VIRUS

Antiviral Therapy

Rubella virus causes disseminated, persistent infection in the fetus, and congenitally infected infants may excrete virus and be contagious for many months after birth. No specific antiviral therapy is available that eradicates active rubella infection in the fetus or newborn, improves their congenital defects, or beneficially alters their postnatal course.

A few adolescents and adults with stigmata of congenital rubella infection have developed a slowly progressive neurologic disorder associated with panencephalitis and persistent central nervous system infection with rubella virus. Isoprinosine and amantadine each have been given to several patients with progressive rubella panencephalitis, but neither drug altered progression of disease. Active immunization of all susceptible women and girls before they become pregnant continues to be the only specific way to prevent the occurrence and disastrous consequences of congenital rubella virus infection.

Supportive Therapy

Because neonates with congenital rubella virus infections can develop an acute, life-threatening, multisystemic illness, vigorous supportive measures may be needed to treat acid-base disorders, hypoglycemia, hypocalcemia, hemorrhagic diathesis, jaundice, hepatitis, glaucoma, heart disease, pulmonary hypertension, and seizures. Consultations with ophthalmologists, cardiologists, speech and hearing pathologists, and psychologists may be needed to adequately manage the child's glaucoma, cataracts, chorioretinitis, hearing loss, and cognitive deficits. The incidence of endocrinopathies, including diabetes mellitus, growth hormone deficiency, and hypothyroidism, is higher than expected in adolescents and young adults who had congenital rubella infections. Long-term clinical follow-up and periodic laboratory testing are needed to detect and appropriately manage these complications as early as possible.

Infants who excrete rubella virus should be isolated from other infants in the nursery. Female health care workers should determine whether they are susceptible to rubella infection by having the level of antirubella antibodies in their serum measured. Pregnant women with a low level of antirubella antibodies should avoid exposure to infants who are excreting rubella virus and should not be given live, attenuated rubella vaccine. Any susceptible pregnant woman exposed inadvertently to an infant excreting rubella should have acute- and convalescent-phase serum antibody titers measured to determine whether she acquired an acute infection. If an antibody rise confirms acute rubella infection, the decision to continue or to terminate the pregnancy can be made based on the stage of pregnancy and the theoretical risks to the fetus.

After discharge from the hospital, contact isolation procedures at home for infants excreting rubella need not be elaborate, but susceptible pregnant women should not be exposed to these infants. Periodic cultures of nasopharynx and urine can be used to determine when the infant is no longer excreting virus.

Because congenital rubella infection confers lifelong

immunity against rubella, rubella vaccination is not necessary later in childhood. The child should receive all other commonly recommended childhood immunizations.

ENTEROVIRUSES

Antiviral Therapy

Although rare reports document intrauterine infection with poliovirus, coxsackievirus, and echovirus, the majority of neonates infected by enteroviruses acquire infection either intrapartum or perinatally via horizontal transmission. Neonatal coxsackievirus and echovirus infections often occur as epidemics in nurseries and may cause severe, systemic illness that is clinically indistinguishable from bacterial sepsis or disseminated HSV infection. Approximately 50 percent of infected neonates develop evidence of meningoencephalitis, and the mortality rate may reach or exceed 50 percent. Once infection is established, no specific antiviral therapy is available. Recent studies of an echovirus-11 nursery epidemic, however, showed that spread of infection could be prevented by passive immunization of exposed infants with human immunoglobulin that contained specific antibodies to echovirus-11.

Supportive Therapy

Myocarditis, congestive heart failure, hepatitis, encephalitis, cerebral edema, seizures, and paralysis can complicate neonatal enteroviral infections. Antiarrhythmia drugs, digitalis, and antiepileptic medications may be required to control these complications. Mannitol and hyperventilation are used to control increased intracranial pressure associated with cerebral edema, but corticosteroid therapy is not recommended because of the potential risk of precipitating fulminant, generalized infection. Long-term respirator care may be necessary for those rare newborns who develop severe generalized muscle weakness that impairs respiratory functions.

After the neonatal period, infants with enteroviral infections should receive all routinely recommended immunizations. Because neonatal poliovirus infection will result in specific immunity only to the one strain of poliovirus with which the infant is infected, trivalent poliovirus vaccine should be given as part of the vaccination schedule.

OTHER VIRUSES

Measles virus, western equine encephalitis virus, Venezuelan equine encephalitis virus, lymphocytic choriomeningitis virus, and parvovirus 19 are rare causes of congenital/perinatal infections. These viruses can cause skin lesions, encephalitis, or paralysis. Specific antiviral therapy is not available for any of these infections. Infected infants are managed by instituting isolation procedures and providing general supportive care. Occasionally, passive immunization with human immunoglobulin containing high levels of virus-specific antibodies may be useful in preventing exposed neonates from acquiring clinical infections and preventing spread to other susceptible neonates and infants in the family or nursery.

SUGGESTED READING

Connor E, McSherry G. Antiviral treatment of human immunodeficiency virus infection in children. Semin Pediatr Infect Dis 1991; 2:285–300.
Edelson PJ, ed. Childhood AIDS. Pediatr Clin North Am 1991; 38:1–199.
Hanshaw JB, Dudgeon JA, Marshall WC. Viral diseases of the fetus and newborn. Philadelphia: WB Saunders, 1985.
Pizzo PA, Wilfert CM. Pediatric AIDS. Baltimore: Williams & Wilkins, 1991.
Whitley RJ. Therapy of herpes simplex virus infections of the central nervous system: Neonatal herpes and herpes simplex encephalitis. Semin Pediatr Infect Dis 1991; 2:263–269.

PATIENT AND PARENT RESOURCES

Literature
Frank I, Brownstone D. The parent's desk reference. New York: Prentice Hall, 1991.

Fulton GB, Metress E, Price JH. AIDS: Resource materials for school personnel. J School Health 1987;57:14–18.

Moore C. A reader's guide for parents of children with mental, physical, or emotional disabilities. 3rd ed. Rockville, Md: Woodbine House, 1990.

Associations
Children's Hospital of St. Paul
Biomedical Research Institute
Cytomegalovirus Program
345 North Smith Avenue
St. Paul, MN 55102
(612)298-8835

National AIDS Information Clearinghouse
1600 Research Blvd.
Rockville, MD 20850
(800)458-5231

Pediatric AIDS Project
National Center for Family-Centered Care
Association for the Care of Children's Health
3615 Wisconsin Avenue, N.W.
Washington, DC 20016
(202)244-1801

Public Health Service
AIDS Hotline
(800)342-AIDS

VIRAL ENCEPHALITIS

HELENE RUBEIZ, M.D.
RAYMOND P. ROOS, M.D.

Increased attention has been focused on the viral encephalitides as a group since the emergence of a new encephalitis agent, human immunodeficiency virus type 1 (HIV-1, discussed in the chapter *Neurologic Diseases Associated with Human Immunodeficiency Virus Type 1 Infection*). In addition, the correct diagnosis of viral encephalitis and identification of the particular pathogen involved have assumed new importance because of the advent and continuing promise of new antiviral therapy and because of the potential for developing new molecular diagnostic tools.

DIAGNOSIS

Encephalitis is characterized by headache, fever, meningeal signs, and, in contrast to meningitis, the presence of signs of central nervous system (CNS) parenchymal dysfunction. The latter signs are usually manifest as disturbances in the state of consciousness, seizures, and focal neurologic signs. Most viruses produce a clinically indistinguishable diffuse encephalitis syndrome. In contrast, herpes simplex virus type 1 (HSV-1) produces a focal encephalitis (see below). Less commonly, arboviruses, Epstein-Barr virus (EBV), cytomegalovirus (CMV), echovirus, mumps virus, and lymphocytic choriomeningitis virus (LCMV) can also localize to a specific area of the brain and produce focal signs.

The diagnosis of viral encephalitis can be aided by careful examination of epidemiologic and clinical information, and laboratory test results. One should always determine the patient's place of residence, travel history, exposure to insects or animal bites, contact with sick family members, and immunization history. A history of a dog bite, for example, clearly raises the possibility of rabies, whereas exposure to mouse droppings or a pet hamster may suggest infection with LCMV. The particular time of the year may also provide clues to the pathogenic virus. For example, arboviral encephalitis, which is spread in most cases by mosquitoes, occurs in the United States during the summer or early fall. Enteroviruses similarly peak in these seasons, whereas mumps predominates in the spring. Other diseases, such as herpes simplex virus type 1 encephalitis (HSVE), occur in any season.

Additional clues to a particular viral pathogen may be obtained from examining the symptoms or physical findings that accompany the encephalitis. A skin rash may be associated with infections caused by arboviruses, certain enteroviruses, LCMV, EBV, and measles virus. Parotitis suggests mumps virus or perhaps an enterovirus. Retinitis is seen with CMV. A tick bite may precede some of the arbovirus infections. Jaundice can be seen with CMV and EBV infection. Arthritis suggests the possibility of arboviruses or LCMV.

Laboratory studies are important in confirming the inflammatory nature of the CNS disease. The cerebrospinal fluid (CSF) generally contains 10 to 1,000 mononuclear cells per cubic millimeter but usually fewer than 300 cells per cubic millimeter. About 75 percent of patients have a polymorphonuclear response early that changes to a mononuclear response after about 48 hours. Fewer than 5 percent of patients have acellular CSF, especially early in the disease course. There is generally normal or elevated opening pressure, mildly elevated CSF protein, and an elevated ratio of CSF to serum immunoglobulin G (IgG). CSF oligoclonal bands are frequently present, though they may be obscured because of the diffusely increased IgG from blood-brain barrier damage. CSF sugar is generally normal, although an abnormally low level is not infrequent in mumps virus or LCMV infection. The CSF should always be sent for viral, bacterial (including tuberculosis), and fungal culture, Gram stain, acid-fast stain, cryptococcal antigen, and Lyme and syphilis serologic tests. Feces, urine, and throat washings should also be collected for virus isolation. Serum collected on admission and a few weeks later should be tested for antibodies to a battery of neurotropic viruses to identify a fourfold rise in titer indicating a recent infection. CSF and serum antibody levels should be obtained to determine whether there is evidence of intrathecal synthesis; intrathecal synthesis may be difficult to detect in the face of generalized blood-brain barrier damage.

Although the cell counts, CSF IgG, oligoclonal bands, and negative bacterial cultures are important in supporting the presence of a nonbacterial, inflammatory CNS disease, the tests for antibody titer and virus isolation are generally of little help in the treatment of the acute encephalitis, for a variety of reasons. (1) Attempts to isolate virus from the CSF are usually unsuccessful. (2) Isolations of virus from non-neural tissue must be interpreted with caution, since passenger viruses unrelated to the CNS infection may be present. (3) The fourfold elevation of antibody titer appears in convalescent serum and so is of little value early in the course of the disease. (4) The presence of a fourfold elevation in antiviral antibody titer may be misleading, as the elevation may be secondary to unrelated intercurrent infections; in addition, a reactivation of HSV from fever may produce a misleading rise in antibody titer to this virus. Despite the limitations (and expense) involved in many of these tests, they provide important public health information; however, increasing financial pressures related to hospitalization costs and the development of new molecular diagnostic assays, such as the use of the polymerase chain reaction (PCR), may decrease the frequency of some of this testing.

It is generally advisable to obtain an emergent computed tomography (CT) study prior to the lumbar puncture (LP) if there are signs of focal neurologic dysfunction or increased intracranial pressure. CT and magnetic resonance imaging (MRI) are generally im-

137

portant in supporting the presence of an inflammatory CNS disease and differentiating other processes. The electroencephalogram (EEG) is usually abnormal in encephalitis, reflecting the parenchymal involvement; epileptiform activity is sometimes seen. Characteristic EEG findings may be seen in HSVE (see below).

We generally repeat the LP in 24 to 48 hours if the patient does not improve clinically or if there was an initial polymorphonuclear response. If the patient does improve, we avoid a repeat LP since the CSF findings can be confusing; for example, there may be an increase in the number of CSF white cells despite clinical improvement. In addition, it is a mistake to wait for acellular CSF, because the CSF pleocytosis can last 1 or 2 months.

Appropriate tests should be performed to rule out other processes that may masquerade as viral encephalitis: bacterial abscess, parameningeal infections, Lyme disease, fungal meningoencephalitis, tuberculoma, sarcoidosis, lues, vasculitis, subdural hematoma, toxic encephalopathy, and cerebral infarction. Viral encephalitis should be differentiated from postinfectious encephalomyelitis (PIE), a white matter–demyelinating process thought to be a result of an autoimmune response rather than direct viral destruction. PIE is usually seen days or weeks after an exanthematous viral infection. Measles is the most likely antecedent cause of PIE worldwide; in the United States, PIE is most frequently associated with flu-like illness or varicella.

HERPES SIMPLEX VIRUS TYPE 1 ENCEPHALITIS

HSVE is of special importance because it carries a significant mortality rate, is the most frequent cause of sporadic encephalitis in the United States (accounting for perhaps 10 percent of all viral encephalitides), and because there is effective antiviral therapy. Its distinctive pathology and selective involvement of the inferior frontal and medial temporal lobes leads to a characteristic focal encephalitis syndrome. The usual clinical manifestations include fever, headache, and behavioral abnormalities. A disturbed state of consciousness, with lethargy and obtundation is not infrequent. Seizures are common, frequently focal in character. Focal signs occur in more than 75 percent of patients with hemiparesis, aphasia, memory loss, visual field defects, and cranial nerve dysfunction.

The CSF in HSVE patients has abnormalities similar to those seen with other encephalitides, except for an occasional increase in red cells. CSF white cells generally number between 50 and 500 per cubic millimeter with an elevated protein value generally below 200 mg per 100 ml. Virus is rarely isolated from the CSF. Serologic testing is of limited value, since anti–HSV-1 antibody usually is not elevated early in the disease and because it may rise secondary to reactivation of virus unrelated to the encephalitis. The EEG may confirm the temporal lobe localization of the disease, with periodic sharp activity arising from one or both temporal regions superimposed on a slow, low-amplitude background; at

times, one sees a burst suppression pattern. CT scan may be normal or may show areas of low attenuation and localized edema in the temporal lobes; areas of hemorrhage are occasionally present; contrast enhancement may be seen after the first week. MRI may be abnormal despite a normal CT scan, attesting to its superior sensitivity. MRI usually shows evidence of increased brain water content and breakdown of the blood-brain barrier on T2-weighted spin-echo technique with increased signal intensity in the frontotemporal and insular regions and the cingulate gyrus.

Treatment of Suspected HSVE

The presence of fever and headache with behavioral abnormalities and focal signs or seizures should suggest the possibility of HSVE. Any patient with a syndrome suggesting HSVE should have an emergent imaging study. An LP should be performed unless there are clinical signs or imaging evidence of significant brain edema; brain biopsy should be considered in these latter cases to substantiate the diagnosis. If there is no or minimal evidence of increased intracranial pressure, an LP should be obtained and acyclovir should be given at a dosage of 10 mg per kilogram every 8 hours for 14 days. The dose of acyclovir should be adjusted for patients with renal dysfunction. Administration of the drug should not be delayed, since the efficacy of treatment depends on the duration of disease prior to therapy (as well as the patient's age and level of consciousness). Because treatment is most effective if begun early in the disease course, physicians should have a low threshold for starting acyclovir, even in atypical cases.

There has been a great deal of discussion of the role of brain biopsy in HSVE. The reasons for considering a biopsy are at least partly due to difficulties in making a secure diagnosis of HSVE: the virus is rarely isolated from the CSF; anti-HSV antibodies rise late during the disease, and this elevation may be misleading. Investigators have also stressed the importance of a brain biopsy in ruling out other treatable focal processes that clinically resemble HSVE. One must be skeptical of these latter studies recommending a brain biopsy in presumed HSVE cases for two reasons. Some of the studies did not include an evaluation of the patient by a neurologist; more importantly, no MRIs were performed in the evaluation of the presumed HSVE cases because the studies were conducted in the pre-MRI era. For these reasons, a new study is needed that includes both a neurologist's evaluation and MRI to rationally guide us regarding the need for a brain biopsy.

Our present approach (Figure 1) toward putative HSVE cases with a typical clinical picture and confirmatory supportive laboratory studies (including an MRI that shows bilateral temporal lobe abnormalities) is to treat with acyclovir and not to perform brain biopsy; if these patients continue to deteriorate or begin to display atypical clinical findings or confusing laboratory study results when retested, a biopsy should be considered. In more questionable cases in which there is a suspicion of

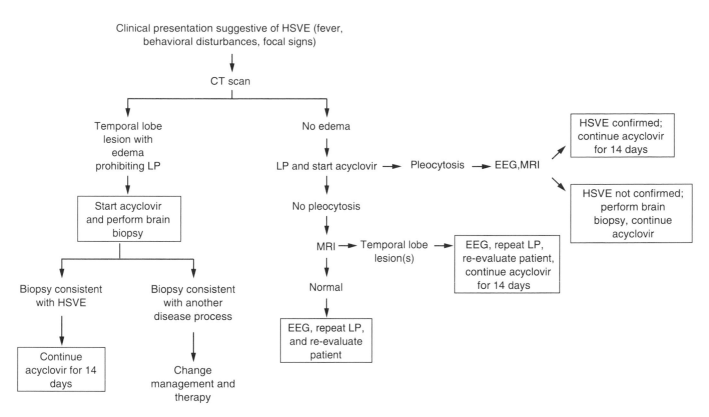

Figure 1 Evaluation of suspected HSVE.

an alternative disease process, we treat with acyclovir and proceed with brain biopsy. If increased intracranial pressure contraindicates an LP, a brain biopsy is obtained with aggressive treatment of the increased intracranial pressure (see below). One hopes that better diagnostic techniques, such as the identification of HSV genome in the CSF by use of the PCR, will provide a sensitive and reliable approach to these patients and make discussions of brain biopsy unnecessary.

If brain biopsy is indicated, a craniotomy should be performed. The region sampled should be an area with maximal involvement as demonstrated on the MRI; critical functional regions should be avoided if possible. The brain tissue should be cultured for HSV (as well as other infectious agents) and also processed for immunohistochemistry and histopathology. Brain biopsy is generally a safe procedure in the hands of an experienced neurosurgeon.

At times patients with definite HSVE have shown clinical deterioration after acyclovir treatment because of a relapse of the encephalitis. In such cases, imaging studies should be repeated to look for evidence of an alternative CNS disease process. If none is found, we suspect a relapse and treat with larger doses of acyclovir, 15 mg per kilogram every 8 hours, for a longer course, 21 days, although there are no conclusive data on its effectiveness. PCR studies of CSF from treated and relapsed cases will hopefully clarify the appropriate management of these patients.

GENERAL SUPPORTIVE CARE

There is at present relatively little specific antiviral treatment for acute viral encephalitis, aside from acyclovir for HSVE. This disappointing situation may change: the advent of HIV encephalitis has been a major stimulus in the development of antiviral drugs. In addition, the identification of a number of virus receptors on cells and a better understanding of the details of viral replication and expression may allow the generation of novel molecular approaches to antiviral therapy. Unfortunately, we are presently left with general supportive care in most patients with viral encephalitis.

General supportive measures should include proper fluid and nutritional management, monitoring of electrolytes and renal function, and skilled nursing care. Patients do not generally require quarantine unless a viral exanthem is present. Precautions should be taken when handling body fluids and stools. If the patient has a decreased level of consciousness or poorly controlled seizures, admission to the intensive care unit is indicated. Intubation and mechanical ventilation should be employed if the respiratory system is compromised. Anticonvulsants should be reserved for patients with clinical seizures. At times, the behavioral abnormalities associated with HSVE resemble seizures despite the absence of clear-cut seizure discharges on the electroencephalogram; in these cases, it is advisable to maintain the patient on therapeutic doses of the appropriate anticonvulsant.

The presence of increased intracranial pressure should be appropriately treated. Patients should be intubated and given controlled hyperventilation. Fluids should be restricted and mannitol administered with maintenance of the serum osmolarity between 300 and 310 mOsm per liter. Although the use of steroids in acute CNS viral infections is controversial, we treat with intravenous dexamethasone, 0.6 mg per kilogram, followed by 0.2 mg per kilogram every 6 hours.

SUGGESTED READING

Schroth G, Gawehn J, Thron A, et al. Early diagnosis of herpes simplex encephalitis by MRI. Neurology 1987; 37:179–183.

VanLandingham KE, Marsteller HB, Ross GW, et al. Relapse of herpes simplex encephalitis after conventional acyclovir therapy. JAMA 1988; 259:1051–1053.
Whitley RJ. Herpes simplex virus infections of the central nervous system: A review. Am J Med 1988; 85(Suppl 2):61–67.
Whitley RJ. Viral encephalitis. N Engl J Med 1990; 323:242–250.
Whitley RJ, Alford CA, Hirsch MS, et al. Vidarabine versus acyclovir therapy in herpes simplex encephalitis. N Engl J Med 1986; 314:144–149.

PATIENT RESOURCE

Further information about epidemics or disease outbreaks can be obtained from the Centers for Disease Control in Atlanta, Georgia (404) 332-4555. Their publication *Morbidity and Mortality Weekly Report* is a valuable resource, providing updates regarding disease prevalence and geographic distribution.

HERPES ZOSTER

J. RICHARD BARINGER, M.D.

Herpes zoster, commonly referred to as *shingles,* has been recognized for decades. The condition is so well-known and so stereotyped in its presentation that the diagnosis is often made by relatives or friends before the patient consults a physician. Though the disease is common at any age, its frequency is especially high in the seventh and eighth decades, and for these patients it may present particularly distressing problems in the form of a severe and persistent postherpetic neuralgia that is resistant to treatment.

Much has been learned about the disease in recent years through the application of sophisticated tissue culture and virologic techniques for detection of latent virus. It is clear that zoster arises because of the colonization of human sensory ganglia by varicella-zoster virus, the virus that causes chickenpox. Apparently, at the time of the acute infection in childhood, the virus succeeds in colonizing numerous sensory ganglia, most notably the trigeminal and thoracic ganglia. The virus remains latent in sensory ganglia, presumably in the neurons, for decades, erupting later, either spontaneously or when the host's cell-mediated immunity is impaired. In this respect, the virus is similar to herpes simplex virus, which commonly colonizes either the trigeminal or sacral ganglia and can cause recurrent lip or genital lesions.

The clinical manifestations of herpes zoster are relatively stereotypical, although the condition may occasionally cause diagnostic confusion when pain occurs before the rash appears. Typically, zoster presents as a segmental radicular pain in one or another division of the trigeminal zone or in one of the cervical or thoracic dermatomes. The pain is sharp or lancinating and quite severe and is associated with prominent dysesthesias, and often with diminished sensibility in the affected dermatome. Despite the sensory loss, the affected segment is exquisitely sensitive to tactile stimulation. Usually within one to a few days, the diagnosis becomes evident because of the appearance of vesicles on an erythematous base in the distribution of the pain. Vesicles increase in size, become pustular, crust, and slowly heal, frequently leaving a zone of hypalgesia as the residuum of the infection. Dissemination of lesions beyond the zone of radicular involvement is seen occasionally in elderly patients but is most often a problem in immunocompromised persons. Dissemination commonly occurs in patients affected by cancer, leukemia, Hodgkin's disease, or acquired immunodeficiency syndrome (AIDS) or in patients who are profoundly immunosuppressed for organ transplantation.

Occasionally, the condition can be confused with cutaneous herpes simplex. Herpes simplex lesions tend to be much more restricted (i.e., to only a small area of the skin), commonly are recurrent in the same area, are usually far less painful than zoster lesions, and do not produce hypesthesia in the involved segment. The two viruses can be distinguished by culture of the vesicle fluid; herpes simplex virus is usually quite easy to propagate in tissue culture, whereas varicella-zoster virus, because of its cell association, is more difficult.

COMPLICATIONS

The complications of varicella-zoster infections can be quite severe and uncomfortable for the patient. Ocular involvement by the virus is common in patients who have zoster involving the first division of the fifth cranial nerve. The virus can cause ulcerations of the eyelids, conjunctivitis, keratitis, and uveitis. Prompt referral to a qualified ophthalmologist is important in the care of patients with ophthalmic zoster.

A variety of complications of zoster relate specifically to its effect on the nervous system. The most severe and prevalent of these is postherpetic neuralgia, a prolongation of the zosteriform pain well after the lesions heal. The neuralgia may persist months or even years in some cases. Postherpetic neuralgia is much more common after age 50 years. The dysesthetic, lancinating pain is exacerbated by the lightest touch of clothing or other tactile stimuli on the affected zone. It tends to be particularly severe at night and may result in marked incapacity. Although commonly treated by narcotics, the pain usually is not relieved by these medications, and they carry with them the risk of habituation and addiction. For reasons that are unknown, the pain is particularly severe in the elderly, and it is often compounded by profound frustration and depression.

Occasionally, patients with zoster may experience focal weakness in the motor segments corresponding to the segmental sensory disturbance. This is presumably due to spread of the virus and/or the inflammatory process into the anterior horn of the spinal cord. The prognosis for recovery from the motor involvement is usually good. Rarely, patients experience symptoms and signs pointing to a myelopathy, again thought to be the result of progression of the virus and the inflammatory response centrally into the spinal cord.

Rarely, elderly patients or those who are immunocompromised experience generalized encephalitis characterized by confusion, obtundation, seizures, and coma. This appears to be more frequent as a consequence of zoster in the ophthalmic division than in other dermatomes, but it has occasionally been seen with zoster in the thoracic region. Encephalitis is frequently attended by spinal fluid pleocytosis with elevated protein levels.

Finally, it has recently been recognized that a few patients with ophthalmic division zoster may suffer strokes in the hemisphere ipsilateral to the zoster, often several days or weeks after the zoster lesion. Zoster virus antigen has been demonstrated in thrombosed cerebral vessels in several of these cases, and it is presumed that the virus has the capability of infecting the vessel wall, resulting in focal thrombosis and infarction in the territory of the involved vessel.

TREATMENT OF ACUTE HERPES ZOSTER

The treatment of herpes zoster is still controversial, despite the fact that hundreds of articles have been written on the subject and that antiviral drugs, notably acyclovir (Zovirax), are readily available.

Acyclovir is an effective antiviral agent, both in tissue culture and in vivo. In vitro, it is less effective against varicella-zoster virus than against herpes simplex virus. The efficacy of acyclovir has been most convincingly demonstrated for immunocompromised patients who are affected with disseminated zoster. In these cases, IV administration of acyclovir, 5 mg per kilogram every 8 hours for 5 days, produces more rapid clearing of lesions than placebo. Thus, it is clear that for patients with disseminated zoster IV acyclovir is the treatment of choice.

What to do for immunocompetent patients with herpes zoster is less clear. Since these patients usually are not hospitalized, the use of intravenous medication is usually not considered necessary. It has been shown that oral acyclovir in very large doses of 800 mg taken five times daily diminishes the rate of new lesion formation and results in more rapid progression of the vesicles to crusting, together with a reduction in pain. The evidence that acyclovir diminishes the frequency or the severity of postherpetic neuralgia is, at best, tenuous. While the rationale for the use of the drug seems quite appropriate, and its effect in immunocompromised patients with disseminated zoster seems incontrovertible, the difference that it makes in patients with zoster who are not immunocompromised is less easily demonstrated. This might result from the fact that the antiviral effect of acyclovir is more evident in patients who lack an immune response, whereas in immunocompetent patients the majority of the effective defense against zoster is the patient's own immune system and the antiviral drug plays a lesser role. It is my practice to treat patients with acyclovir who (1) are elderly, (2) have ophthalmic zoster, or (3) have particularly severe pain. Because children and young adults with zoster often have a salutary course no matter what is done, the need to treat them with acyclovir is less compelling. On the other hand, for elderly persons with ophthalmic zoster and a great deal of pain I have occasionally initiated treatment in the hospital with intravenous acyclovir, hoping to maximize the antiviral effect early, and switched them to oral acyclovir as soon as the acute pain and illness were under control.

The second therapeutic dilemma that confronts the physician caring for a patient with herpes zoster concerns the use of systemic corticosteroids. There have been a number of controlled clinical trials (reviewed by Huff) to study the efficacy of systemically administered corticosteroid preparations for the treatment of herpes zoster. The rationale that has been put forth for their use is that the acute ganglionitis that takes place with herpes zoster is an inflammatory process that might, in and of itself, be responsible for the pain and postherpetic neuralgia, and that suppression of this process might ameliorate these symptoms. Against this idea is the fact that postherpetic neuralgia is quite frequent in patients with AIDS who develop zoster. While there are a few small and well-controlled series that demonstrate reduction of postherpetic neuralgia pain at 3 to 4 months in patients treated with steroids, other series have failed to demonstrate any benefit. A recent meta-analysis of four trials of systemic corticosteroid in patients with herpes zoster suggested that steroids were effective in reducing postherpetic neuralgia at 6 to 12 weeks, but the efficacy against postherpetic neuralgia at later times was uncertain. A large multicenter blinded study comparing steroids alone, acyclovir alone, and acyclovir with steroids is currently in progress, so that more information concerning this topic may be available shortly.

My current practice is to treat all patients over 50 years of age with oral acyclovir, 800 mg five times daily for 5 to 7 days, based on the fact that this therapy is rational, is proven to be efficacious in immunocompromised hosts, and results in more rapid clearing of the virus-induced skin lesions with immediate reduction in pain that is superior to that produced by placebo. I strongly urge the use of acyclovir for ocular zoster in elderly patients, because of its demonstrated benefit in this condition and the hope that the uncommon but extremely serious complications of encephalitis or stroke might be averted in this group of patients. I do not think it unreasonable to admit a seriously ill patient to a hospital to initiate the antiviral treatment with intravenous acyclovir. Because there is some indication that systemic steroids appear to decrease the degree of pain as far out as 6 to 12 weeks, if the patient is elderly (at higher risk for developing postherpetic neuralgia) and does not have contraindications to use of steroids (hypertension, ulcers, diabetes), I administer prednisone in doses beginning at 60 mg daily, tapering off rapidly over a period of 2 to 3 weeks, in the hope that the combination of the antiviral agent and the anti-inflammatory effect of the prednisone would effect more rapid resolution of the patient's symptoms. I consider the use of prednisone in this circumstance discretionary, because the evidence for its efficacy is at the moment controversial and the possibility of unanticipated complications in the elderly is real. Because acyclovir is efficacious, safe, and well-tolerated, I would not administer prednisone in the absence of the antiviral compound.

TREATMENT OF POSTHERPETIC NEURALGIA

There are a number of treatments for postherpetic neuralgia, most of which have not benefited from carefully controlled trials. In the hands of many neurologists, amitriptyline seems to have a beneficial effect, both because of its efficacy in diminishing pain and because of its antidepressant effect. Its tendency to produce dry mouth, constipation, somnolence, and confusion in elderly patients often limits its utility. A number of patients seem to respond favorably to carbamazepine in doses from 600 to 1200 mg daily, and treatment with this medication is worthy of trial in patients with refractory pain. Phenytoin may be used as an alternative, but in my experience it has been less helpful than carbamazepine. The use of capsaicin cream has recently become popular for decreasing postherpetic neuralgia. Again, the evidence for its efficacy is controversial, but aside from the possibility of inducing some burning with too frequent application, the side effects of the topical medications seem minimal. The patient needs to be reassured that, in the great majority of cases the severity of postherpetic neuralgia will diminish over time.

Acyclovir appears at this time to be the cornerstone of rational therapy for zoster. Its benefits are particularly well-demonstrated for disseminated zoster in immunocompromised hosts and for more rapid resolution of ophthalmic zoster, and, with less confidence for more rapid resolution of cutaneous zoster lesions. Though it appears to reduce the acute pain of zoster, its efficacy in the treatment of postherpetic neuralgia still leaves much to be desired. For this reason, the ongoing trials comparing acyclovir, acyclovir and corticosteroids, and corticosteroids alone may provide very useful information on the best way to prospectively manage these patients.

SUGGESTED READING

Carmichael JK. Treatment of herpes zoster and postherpetic neuralgia. AFD Practical Therapeutics 1991; 44:203–210.
Huff JC. Herpes zoster. Curr Probl Dermatol 1988; 1:8–40.
Huff JC, Bean B, Balfour HH, et al. Therapy of herpes zoster with oral acyclovir. Am J Med 1988; 85(Suppl 2A):84–89.
Lycka BAS. Postherpetic neuralgia and systemic steroid therapy: Efficacy and safety. Pharmacol Ther 1990; 29:523–527.
Portenoy RK, Duma C, Foley KM. Acute herpetic and postherpetic neuralgia: Clinical review and current management. Ann Neurol 1986; 20:651–664.
Wood MJ, Ogan PH, McKendrick MW, et al. Efficacy of oral acyclovir treatment of acute herpes zoster. Am J Med 1988; 85(Suppl 2A):79–83.

RABIES

THIRAVAT HEMACHUDHA, M.D.
HENRY WILDE, M.D., F.A.C.P.

Rabies is a neurotropic viral infection that can be acquired by all mammals, though different species have different levels of susceptibility. Rabies is enzootic in most of the world, except in island populations (e.g., Japan, Britain, Hawaii, Australia, New Zealand). In the developing countries of Asia, Africa, and South America, canine rabies predominates; wildlife populations (e.g., raccoons, foxes, skunks, bats) are the major reservoirs in North America and Europe, where countries have enforced quarantine and canine immunization regulations. Although rabies among wildlife represents a more distant risk to humans, it remains a continuous public health hazard owing to the potential for incidental transmissions to domestic animals and thence to humans. The very many unvaccinated dogs and cats that live in close contact with humans present a grave risk to the poor population of the world. The World Health Organization (WHO) reports at least 50,000 human deaths from rabies every year, and virtually all are due to dog and cat bites. The disease is thought to be under-reported and represents an economic burden in many parts of the world where adequate postexposure treatment is neither affordable nor readily available. The increase in worldwide tourism and movements of refugees and economic migrants mandates that general physicians and consultant neurologists acquire basic knowledge of rabies even if their own region is rabies free. A more detailed discussion of the virology, epidemiology, pathophysiology, and clinical features of veterinary and human rabies can be found in several recent monographs. In this chapter we address practitioners in developed and mostly rabies-free countries where postexposure treatment decisions are based on epidemiologic data and exposure to wildlife or domestic animals that have contact with wildlife and bats. The same physician will, however, have to be prepared to advise persons who intend to travel to canine rabies–endemic regions, or give advice or reassurance to those exposed abroad. We present a management and problem-solving outline for North American and European clinicians who may encounter an occasional rabies exposure.

ANIMAL RABIES

Dogs and to a lesser extent cats are the animals most often responsible for human rabies exposure. The biting animal may show classic symptoms of rabies and is then described as suffering from "furious hydrophobia." A rabid animal, however, may be docile, partly paralyzed, and indeed may behave quite normally. An experienced veterinarian often can detect subtle signs that suggest rabies in such an animal. Dogs can recover from rabies and may, though rarely, continue to secrete viable virus in their saliva. The behavior of the biting animal (e.g., provoked or unprovoked attack) in a region where canine rabies is endemic should not be emphasized in making postexposure treatment decisions. Several treatment failures have been attributed to delay in initiating vaccination while an animal that appeared relatively normal was being observed. Canine rabies vaccine failures also are not uncommon in canine rabies–endemic regions. Whether the biting dog or cat has been absolutely restricted from contact with other dogs or wildlife and whether it has been reliably and repeatedly vaccinated should carry more weight in treatment decisions than the animal's behavior. Modifications of this "not to observe biting dogs or cats before start of treatment" recommendation would be indicated in a rabies-free or low-risk area. Treatment may be discontinued if the responsible dog or cat remains healthy throughout an observation period of at least 10 days. Whenever possible, killing of a biting animal and immediate brain examination by fluorescent microscopy may be an alternative to determine whether postexposure treatment should be initiated. Often, however, this is not possible, as in Buddhist countries, where there is religious and cultural opposition to killing.

Any bite by a wild mammal in any part of the world where there is wildlife or canine endemic or epizootic rabies is a potential exposure and requires immediate institution of postexposure therapy. If there is adequate laboratory and field experience to indicate that there is no infection in the species involved, local health authorities may be justified in refraining from recommending specific antirabies treatment.

THE NATURE OF THE WOUND

The risk of rabies increases with the severity of wounds. The virus can be introduced through cuts, puncture wounds, mucous membranes, and aerosol inhalation. Head, face, neck, and hand injuries carry the highest risk and usually are associated with a shorter incubation period. However, any transdermal wound at any site can cause death from rabies. This means that it is the severity of the wound (transdermal or superficial) and not the location that determines the rabies risk.

POSTEXPOSURE PROPHYLAXIS

Wound Care

Immediate and thorough cleansing of wounds with soap and water is an effective measure for rabies prevention. This should be carried out and repeated even if the patient does not present immediately. It is followed by treatment with substances of proven lethal effect on rabies, such as 70 percent ethanol or a solution of iodine. Soap should be flushed from the wounds before a viricidal drug is applied, lest it neutralize the drug's activity. The public should be educated in simple local wound treatment and warned against using procedures that may cause further contamination. Suturing the wound should be avoided; however, if it is necessary it should be done after thorough infiltration of the wounds with rabies immune globulin. Tetanus prophylaxis and antibiotics should be given as indicated for any trauma.

Vaccination

Brain Tissue–Derived Vaccines

The WHO Committee on Rabies discourages use of brain tissue–derived vaccine as of 1992. The vast majority of postexposure treatments in canine rabies–endemic poor countries, however, still utilize Semple (SV) or suckling mouse brain (SMB) rabies vaccines. The potency of these products is uncertain, and they have unacceptable side effects.

Tissue Culture and Purified Duck Embryo Rabies Vaccines

In North America, human diploid cell rabies vaccine (HDCV) has been the product of choice and is widely available. Other equally safe and effective vaccines used worldwide, considerably less expensive and interchangeable with HDCV, are (1) purified vero cell rabies vaccine (PVRV), (2) purified chick embryo cell vaccine (PCEC), and (3) purified duck embryo vaccine (PDEV) (not to be confused with the old duck embryo vaccine, which was much less potent and had unacceptable side effects).

Any of these vaccines is given using the following proven intramuscular (IM) schedule:

One dose of vaccine is injected into the deltoid region or anterolateral thigh muscle of children on days 0, 3, 7, 14, and 30. Rabies vaccine should never be injected into the gluteal region. A second abbreviated schedule using two IM doses on day 0, and one each on days 7 and 21 is being advocated in Europe, but it has been shown that this regimen results in significant suppression of the antibody response if given with rabies immunoglobulin (RIG), and we discourage its use.

Tissue culture and duck embryo vaccines are expensive and not affordable in most poor countries. WHO has therefore accepted the proven reduced-dose, multiple-site intradermal administration of these vaccines. Vaccination using an intradermal schedule of PVRV, PCEC, and HDCV has been widely practiced in Thailand for more than 7 years. This method is recommended only for clinics whose staff is experienced in intradermal administration and that treat enough patients so that the remaining reconstituted vaccine is used up within 1 or 2 days. This intradermal postexposure schedule consists of 0.1 ml vaccine injected at two sites on days 0, 3, and 7 and at one site on days 30 and 90. Antibody titers with this regimen are equal to those with the conventional IM schedule and resist antibody suppression from RIG.

Rabies Immunoglobulin

RIG should be given with the first dose of vaccine for all category III exposures (Table 1), even if the patient presents after considerable delay. The WHO does, however, recommend that it not be given longer than 7 days when a vaccine schedule alone was started without

Table 1 Guide for Postexposure Rabies Treatment*†

Category	Type of Contact‡	Recommended Treatment
I	Touching or feeding animal, licking over intact skin.	None if reliable case history is available.
II	Minor bites on uncovered skin, licks over broken skin, minor scratches or abrasions with no bleeding	Administer vaccine immediately.§ Stop treatment if animal (only dog or cat) remains healthy throughout observation period of 10 days or if animal is killed and found to be negative for rabies by fluorescent antibody test (FAT).
III	Single or multiple transdermal bites or scratches, licks over mucosa	Administer rabies immunoglobulin and vaccine immediately. Stop treatment if animal (only dog or cat) remains healthy throughout observation period of 10 days or if animal is killed and found to be negative for rabies by FAT.

*In any case where a reliable history cannot be obtained (e.g., small child, mentally retarded person) and there is the possibility that mucous membrane or trivial undetectable exposure may have occurred, immediate treatment should be considered.

†Since prolonged incubation periods have been noted, exposed persons who present for evaluation and treatment even months after having been bitten should be dealt with in the same manner as if the exposure had occurred recently.

‡Contact with a suspected or confirmed rabid domestic or wild animal or animal unavailable for observation. Exposure to rodents, rabbits, and hares seldom if ever requires specific antirabies treatment.

§If an apparently healthy dog or cat in or from a low-risk area is placed in observation, the situation may warrant delaying initiation of treatment.

RIG on day 0 in order to prevent interference with the active immune response. Two kinds of rabies antibody preparations may be used: human rabies immunoglobulin (HRIG) and equine rabies immunoglobulin (ERIG). The sensitivity of the patient to ERIG should be determined before it is used. As much as possible of the recommended dose (20 IU per kilogram body weight of HRIG or 40 IU per kilogram body weight of ERIG) should be infiltrated in and around the wounds, if this is anatomically feasible. The remainder should be administered IM (into the gluteal region) in a single dose and followed by a complete course of vaccine. It has been shown that even infected wounds can be safely injected after proper cleansing and antibiotic administration.

In rabies-endemic areas, it is not uncommon to see patients with multiple severe wounds where the calculated RIG dose is not adequate for infiltration of all sites. It has been our practice to dilute the RIG with normal saline to an appropriate amount so that all wounds can be infiltrated. There is as yet no scientific basis for this practice, but we knew one patient who received a potent tissue culture vaccine and RIG without delay and the calculated RIG dose was not adequate to infiltrate all wounds. The patient succumbed to rabies encephalitis within a month.

HRIG is available in some countries but is very expensive and in limited supply. It has virtually no side effects and is the RIG product of choice.

Early crude preparations of ERIG had a poor reputation owing to a high rate of anaphylaxis and serum sickness–like reactions. However, some of the highly purified European products now available produce reactions in as few as 1 percent, are more readily available than HRIG in developing countries, and cost only a fraction of the price. A skin test has to be performed first by injecting 0.1 ml of a 1:10 dilution of the ERIG intradermally and observing the site for at least 15 minutes, as outlined in the package insert. In the event that HRIG is not available and the skin reaction to ERIG is positive, ERIG may still be used but only with suitable precautions and in a facility that is able to manage anaphylaxis.

PRE-EXPOSURE IMMUNIZATION

Pre-exposure immunization should be offered to persons at high risk of exposure, such as laboratory staff who work with rabies virus, veterinarians, animal handlers, wildlife officers, cave explorers, and others who live in or travel to areas where rabies is endemic. The primary immunization schedule consists of three intramuscular (one full dose) or intradermal (0.1 ml) injections on days 0, 7, and 28. A few days' variation is acceptable. The WHO Rabies Advisory Committee recommends the following schedules for boosters:

1. Persons who work with live rabies virus should have their serum tested for rabies virus–neutral-

izing antibodies every 6 months. A booster dose should be administered when the titer falls below 0.5 IU per milliliter. In practice, many laboratories where rabies titer determinations may not be available may elect to give a booster dose every 6 months.
2. Persons at continued risk of rabies exposure (but less than those in category 1), such as veterinarians and tourists to rabies-endemic regions, should ideally have serum samples tested annually to ensure that the antibody titer is above 0.5 IU per milliliter.

In practice, tourists and expatriate residents in endemic regions are often advised to obtain rabies vaccine booster doses every 3 years. Along with this, such persons must be made aware of the necessity of getting additional boosters on days 0 and 3 if they suffer a possible rabies exposure.

POSTEXPOSURE TREATMENT OF PREVIOUSLY VACCINATED PERSONS

1. Persons with reliable history of full pre- or postexposure treatment with a tissue culture or PDEV should be given only two booster doses, either IM or intradermal, on days 0 and 3 without rabies immunoglobulin, regardless of how much time has elapsed since the previous vaccination series.
2. Persons with a history of pre- or postexposure treatment that utilized brain tissue–derived vaccine (Semple or SMB) of unproven potency should receive a complete postexposure course, including RIG if indicated (category III exposure).

ADVERSE REACTIONS

Vaccines

Modern tissue vaccine and PDEV may produce mild local and rare mild systemic reactions. These can usually be managed with antihistamines, analgesics, and reassurance. Serum sickness–like reactions have been reported in persons who received several booster doses as part of continuing pre-exposure prophylaxis.

Rabies Immunoglobulin

HRIG carries virtually no risk but may cause local pain at injection sites. ERIG carries a small but definite risk of anaphylaxis and serum sickness–like reactions. Almost all of the latter appear 1 week after ERIG administration and resolve within 1 week, and symptoms are usually controllable with reassurance, antihistamines, and nonsteroidal anti-inflammatory agents. Corticosteroids should not be given in this setting, since they interfere with the active immune response.

TREATMENT OF CLINICAL RABIES

No intervention is known that will save patients who have developed symptoms of rabies. Various immuno-modulators and antiviral agents and intensive care have been tried without success. Sedation and good nursing care should be emphasized. Persons who care for rabies patients should receive appropriate prophylaxis, de-pending on the degree of exposure to infected saliva and body fluids.

SUGGESTED READING

Hemachudha T. Rabies. In: Vinken PJ, Bruyn GW, Klawans HL, McKendall RR, eds. Viral disease. Handbook of clinical neurology. Vol. 56. Amsterdam: Elsevier, 1989:383–404.
WHO Expert Committee on Rabies. 8th report. Geneva: World Health Organization, 1992.
Wilde H, Chutivongse S, Tepsumethanon W, et al. Rabies in Thailand: 1990. Rev Infect Dis 1991; 13:644–652.

NEUROLOGIC DISEASES ASSOCIATED WITH HUMAN IMMUNODEFICIENCY VIRUS TYPE 1 INFECTION

JUSTIN C. McARTHUR, M.B., B.S., M.P.H.

The nervous system is involved frequently during HIV-1 infection, sometimes before immunodeficiency becomes advanced. About 40 percent of patients with acquired immunodeficiency syndrome (AIDS) or symptomatic HIV infection (AIDS-related complex [ARC]) develop a neurologic syndrome, and 10 percent of all patients with AIDS initially present with nervous system complaints. About half the neurologic manifestations are due to direct or indirect effects of HIV-1 on the nervous system and half result as opportunistic or secondary complications of the immune deficiency induced by HIV-1. The pathogenic mechanisms of the HIV-1–related neurologic disorders are incompletely understood, but treatment is available for most of them, particularly if they are recognized early.

HIV-1–RELATED NEUROLOGIC DISORDERS

Some of these disorders occur early in the incubation period of HIV-1 infection, before any constitutional symptoms develop. Others typically occur in patients with symptomatic HIV infection (ARC) or after an AIDS-defining illness. The timing of these specific disorders, the differences in course, and the pathologic differences suggest that different pathogenic mechanisms underlie them.

HIV-1–Related Meningitis

One or two percent of recently infected persons develop acute aseptic meningitis, with headache, meningismus, cranial neuropathies, and occasionally transient encephalopathy. This disorder appears to represent the initial response of the central nervous system (CNS) to viral invasion and there is intrathecal synthesis of antibody to HIV-1. As many as 30 percent of HIV-1 carriers have a more indolent variant of HIV-1–related meningitis with chronic pleocytosis and headaches. Typically, the acute symptoms of HIV-1–related meningitis are self-limited, require only symptomatic treatment with analgesics and antipyretics, and resolve within a few weeks. Serologic testing for HIV-1 (and probably human T-cell lymphotropic virus I [HTLV-1]) should be added to the evaluation of patients with aseptic meningitis or chronic pleocytosis. It is uncertain whether the development of symptomatic meningitis or the detection of silent cerebrospinal fluid (CSF) abnormalities is predictive of subsequent progressive neurologic involvement.

HIV-1 Dementia

After the development of AIDS, 15 to 20 percent of patients develop signs of progressive subcortical dementia. This syndrome was added to the list of AIDS-defining illnesses in 1987 (Table 1). Also termed HIV-1 encephalopathy, AIDS-dementia complex, and subacute encephalitis, the mental dulling, intellectual impairment, and memory loss initially can be mistaken for depression or other psychiatric syndromes. The disorder occurs in all groups at risk for HIV-1 infection, including children. The prevalence in *healthy* HIV-1 carriers is very low. Based on current evidence, there is no justification for policies of employment disability based solely on HIV-1 serologic testing. In the early stages of dementia, the clinical features are nonspecific and stringent criteria

Table 1 Major Neurologic Complications of HIV-1 Infection

HIV-1–Related Disorders	Opportunistic Processes
Acute aseptic meningitis	Cryptococcal meningitis*
Chronic pleocytosis	Toxoplasmosis*
HIV-1 dementia*	Cytomegalovirus (CMV) retinitis or encephalitis*
Vacuolar myelopathy	Other opportunistic CNS infections*
Predominantly sensory neuropathy	CMV or herpesvirus group radiculitis
Inflammatory demyelinating polyneuropathy	Progressive multifocal leukoencephalopathy*
Mononeuritis multiplex	Primary CNS lymphoma*
Myopathy	Systemic lymphoma*
Toxic effects of antiretroviral drugs	Neurosyphilis

*AIDS = defining diseases

should be used to avoid overdiagnosis of this condition (Table 2). Neuropsychological testing with simple bedside tests of psychomotor speed (Grooved Pegboard, Trailmaking Test) or memory are particularly sensitive for early HIV dementia, but premorbid factors, including age, education, and substance use, must be considered in interpreting neuropsychological performance. Diagnostic precision is important not only for therapeutic reasons, and because this disorder defines a case of AIDS, but also because the diagnosis carries serious prognostic and legal implications. Serial assessments are important for confirming progressive deterioration and excluding other potentially reversible causes of encephalopathy (see Table 2 and Figure 1). Cranial MRI and CSF analysis should be performed in most patients, along with a simple neuropsychological test battery. The Mini Mental Status Examination is, unfortunately, not a sensitive instrument for detection or for monitoring of neurocognitive status.

The pathogenesis of HIV-1 dementia is unclear, for, although there is evidence of brain infection with HIV-1, the amount of productive virus is relatively small. Frequently, there is discordance between the clinical findings and the relatively minor neuropathologic changes observed. It is likely that indirect mechanisms of neural cell dysfunction or damage are important, perhaps mediated by neurotoxic viral proteins or through the effects of cytokines released from activated or HIV-infected macrophages. The mainstay of treatment currently is the use of an antiretroviral agent to block reverse transcriptase, an enzyme critical for the productive phase of the life cycle of HIV-1. Initially HIV dementia should be treated with zidovudine (Retrovir), beginning with 500 to 1000 mg daily. Because dementia frequently develops after other AIDS-defining illnesses in patients who have already used zidovudine for prolonged periods, an alternative agent is didanosine (Videx), given in doses of 150 to 300 mg twice daily, based on weight. Principal side effects of zidovudine are anemia and neutropenia, which can be attenuated by dose reduction or the use of erythropoietin (Epogen) or growth factors such as granulocyte macrophage colony stimulating factor

Table 2 Criteria for Diagnosis of HIV-1–Related Dementia

HIV-1 seropositivity (Western blot confirmation)
History of *progressive* cognitive or behavioral decline
Nonfocal or diffuse CNS signs on neurologic examination
Deterioration on *serial* neuropsychological tests in at least two areas, including frontal lobe, motor speed, and nonverbal memory
Absence of major affective disorder or active substance abuse
Absence of metabolic derangement (e.g., hypoxia, sepsis)
Absence of CNS opportunistic infections or neoplasms:
  CT or MRI shows normal picture or atrophy or white matter rarefaction
  CSF tests negative for VDRL and cryptococcal antigen

Key: CT = computed tomography; MRI = magnetic resonance imaging.

(GMCSF) or granulocyte colony stimulating factor (GCSF) (Neupogen) to stimulate bone marrow production. Other side effects include dose-related toxic myopathy, gastrointestinal upset, and, in the first few weeks of treatment, headache. Adverse effects of didanosine include pancreatitis and dose-related toxic sensory neuropathy. A third nucleoside analogue, dideoxycytidine (Hivid) has been licensed for combination use with zidovudine, but little information is available on its efficacy in treating dementia. With zidovudine, previously untreated patients with a mild or moderate degree of HIV-1 dementia often show improvement within a few weeks, particularly in memory and psychomotor speed. Unfortunately, the clinical benefits are usually limited to a few months and the disorder then progresses again. The efficacy of didanosine in reversing the dementia is unproven, and CSF penetration of this agent is less than that of zidovudine. Patients with far advanced dementia rarely improve with antiretroviral therapies and they survive only a few months. Symptomatic treatment is an important adjunct to antiretroviral treatment. Patients with mild or moderate dementia and marked apathy may respond to small doses of methylphenidate (Ritalin), starting with 5 mg twice a day, although there is a risk of seizures. If marked depressive symptoms are present, tricyclic antidepressants can be tried in 25 to 50 percent of the usual dose. Because patients with HIV dementia are extremely susceptible to the adverse effects of psychoactive drugs, hypnotics and anxiolytics should be avoided or used only in reduced doses.

With patients with progressive dementia, medicolegal issues—arranging for a durable power of attorney, completion of a living will, and dispersal of assets—must be discussed early, before the dementia becomes too severe. Testamentary capacity should be carefully documented.

HIV-1–Associated Myelopathies

As many as 20 percent of patients with AIDS are affected with a noninflammatory vacuolar myelopathy that manifests itself as progressive spastic paraparesis and sensory ataxia and is often accompanied by progressive dementia. Patients with HIV-1 infection may be intercurrently infected with HTLV-I, a retrovirus that also causes a progressive myelopathy, which can be excluded by serologic testing. As with HIV-1 dementia, the pathogenic mechanisms have not been fully elucidated. The effects of cytokines released by activated macrophages or toxic and metabolic factors may be important. The diagnostic approach should exclude structural or compressive lesions and correctable nutritional deficiencies such as vitamin B_{12}. A sensory level and localized back pain or percussion tenderness are unusual. If these features are present, MRI of the spine or myelography should be performed to exclude extrinsic cord compression from epidural abscess or tumor. Mild elevation of the protein value and pleocytosis (5 to 20 leukocytes) are common, and a more inflammatory CSF profile should prompt a search for herpesvirus group infection (which produces ascending myelitis) or neurosyphilis. I have not found zidovudine or other antiretroviral therapies to be useful in reversing the myelopathy, which usually progresses inexorably. Important strategies include the use of antispasticity agents such as lioresal (Baclofen) and rehabilitation with provision of assistive devices.

Peripheral Nerve Disorders Associated with HIV-1 Infection

Sensory Neuropathy

Some 30 percent of patients with frank AIDS develop a neuropathy characterized by painful sensory symptoms in the feet. Most develop this neuropathy late in the course of HIV-1 infection, usually in association with systemic opportunistic infections. This disorder can usually be recognized by the characteristic complaints of dysesthesias and contact hypersensitivity in the feet associated with reduced or absent ankle reflexes and elevated vibratory thresholds and hyperalgesia. Electrophysiologic studies are helpful but not essential for diagnosis. They usually reveal a neuropathy that affects both sensory and motor fibers and is suggestive of dying-back axonopathy. Nerve biopsy usually is not necessary in the clinical setting.

Consideration should be given to nutritional and toxic causes of sensory neuropathy such as alcohol, diabetes, pyridoxine excess, vitamin B_{12} deficiency, and the use of neurotoxic antiretroviral agents such as didanosine and dideoxycytidine. Occasionally, symptoms stabilize with zidovudine; however, more often there is no dramatic response to antiretroviral therapy. Treatment is aimed at symptomatic relief with pain-modifying tricyclic antidepressants such as amitriptyline (Elavil) or nortriptyline (Pamelor). Treatment begins with a small dose (e.g., nortriptyline, 10 mg twice a day), which is increased slowly, as tolerated. Neither carbamazepine nor phenytoin, nor, indeed, topical agents such as capsaicin (Zostrix-HP) have proved useful. For constant burning dysesthesias, high-concentration (30 percent) lidocaine cream may provide transient relief.

Inflammatory Demyelinating Polyneuropathies

A number of possibly immune-mediated phenomena have been described in association with HIV-1 infection, including inflammatory demyelinating polyneuropathies (IDPs). In contrast to HIV-related sensory neuropathy, IDP typically occurs at a relatively early stage of HIV-1 infection, before immunodeficiency develops. Typically, there is profound motor weakness, which sometimes develops acutely as Guillain-Barré syndrome (GBS) and in association with CSF pleocytosis. More often, IDPs present as a chronic, sometimes relapsing process. The recognition of this association between HIV-1 and IDP means that a careful search for risk factors for HIV-1 infection and serologic testing should be made when any patient presents with IDP. Plasmapheresis is the treatment of choice, because it is less likely than corticosteroids to cause additional immunosuppression. In GBS, a course of five plasma exchanges is given. With chronic IDP an induction course is followed by maintenance exchanges as needed. When plasmapheresis is impractical, immunoglobulin G (IgG) or short courses of corticosteroids are generally tolerated well and do not trigger opportunistic infections. For chronic IDP, I use a 5 day course of immunoglobulin, 0.8 g per kilogram IV. IgA deficiency must be ruled out to prevent an anaphylactic reaction to the IV immunoglobulin.

Cytomegalovirus and Other Herpesvirus Radiculitides

CMV can cause a progressive radiculopathy involving lumbar and sacral roots. Clues to recognizing this entity include advanced immunodeficiency with CD4 count below 100, CMV infection elsewhere—retinitis, viremia, and subacute radiculopathy developing over 1 to 4 weeks. Usually, there is polymorphonuclear pleocytosis, and CMV can often be isolated by culture from the CSF. An acyclovir analogue, ganciclovir (Cytovene), can reverse the radiculopathy if treatment is started before paralysis is complete. Cytovene is initially given at a dose of 10 mg per kilogram per day in two doses for 14 days, followed by daily IV infusion of 5 mg per kilogram as maintenance. The principal side effect is neutropenia.

Five to ten percent of patients with HIV-1 infection develop herpes zoster radiculitis. Dermatomal herpes zoster does not require specific treatment unless multiple cervical or lumbar dermatomes are involved. Here, the potential exists for severe myeloradiculitis with permanent motor deficits, and IV acyclovir (Zovirax, 30 mg per kilogram per day), should be used. The development of postherpetic neuralgia may require pain-modifying agents such as amitriptyline (Elavil) or carbamazepine (Tegretol). After the vesicles have completely healed, topical capsaicin (Zostrix) can reduce the neuralgic pains if applied for at least 2 weeks.

Myopathies

Polymyositis is an uncommon complication of HIV-1 infection that sometimes responds to immunomodulatory agents such as corticosteroids or IV immunoglobulin. Because of the potential for infectious complications with steroids and the expense of IV immunoglobulin, use of these agents should be restricted to patients with function-limiting weakness, greatly elevated serum creatine phosphokinase (CPK), and biopsy evidence of myofiber necrosis and inflammatory infiltrates. A toxic myopathy can develop after prolonged use of zidovudine, after 6 to 12 months of treatment with more than 500 mg per day. The clinical features of toxic myopathy are indistinguishable from those of polymyositis. If a zidovudine drug holiday of 2 to 4 weeks is accompanied by clinical improvement in myalgias and a drop in CPK, I assume that it was a toxic myopathy and reduce the dose of zidovudine or switch to an alternative antiretroviral such as didanosine.

OPPORTUNISTIC PROCESSES

Opportunistic infections and neoplasms of the CNS are common in association with HIV-1 infection, reflecting the underlying immunodeficiency produced by infection and lysis of CD4 lymphocytes by HIV-1. Usually opportunistic infections do not develop until the CD4 count is below 200. Patients may have multiple concurrent opportunistic processes, or opportunistic processes may coexist with HIV-1–related neurologic disorders. An AIDS patient who develops an opportunistic infection will need lifelong maintenance therapy.

Intracranial Focal Lesions

A variety of disorders can cause intracranial focal lesions, including toxoplasmosis, primary CNS lymphoma, progressive multifocal leukoencephalopathy (PML), cryptococcosis, and other bacterial and fungal infections. Multiple intercurrent opportunistic processes may coexist. Because specific treatment is available for many of these complications, early detection and accurate diagnosis are critical. Figure 1 shows a management approach based on magnetic resonance appearance, and

Figure 2 represents an approach based on the empiric toxoplasmosis therapy.

Cryptococcal Meningitis

Cryptococcus neoformans, a ubiquitous yeast, produces CNS infection in about 10 percent of patients with AIDS, and in some it may be the first recognized manifestation of HIV infection. The most common presentation is headache, meningismus, altered mentation, cranial neuropathies, fever, and vomiting. This constellation of symptoms can mimic bacterial meningitis, cerebral toxoplasmosis, other opportunistic processes and, when more indolent, HIV-1 dementia. Cryptococcomas can form in the brain, expanding Virchow-Robin spaces and producing mass lesions. They are usually located in basal ganglia and are not enhancing. The CSF usually has *normal* cellular and protein constituents; however, cryptococcal antigen is always detectable and fungal cultures always grow the organism. An induction course with amphotericin B, 0.6 mg per kilogram per day, is recommended to administer a total of 1 g. For severe cryptococcal meningitis, a second antifungal agent, flucytosine (Ancobon), should be added, although it can cause diarrhea and myelosuppression. During successful treatment, both serum and CSF cryptococcal antigen titers can be expected to fall by at least four dilutions and fungal cultures become negative. The CSF should be re-examined at the end of induction therapy or if there is recrudescence of symptoms. Persistently positive fungal cultures imply failure or relapse. The cryptococcal antigen titer can remain positive, and this does not imply treatment failure. Suppressive treatment with fluconazole (Diflucan), 200 mg daily, is necessary for lifelong maintenance. The median survival time after diagnosis with cryptococcal meningitis is about 9 months, and relapse occurs in about 60 percent of cases.

Cytomegalovirus Encephalitis and Retinitis

CMV can cause infection of the retina, producing vision loss in as many as 20 percent of patients with AIDS. CMV also produces an encephalitis that can be difficult to distinguish from HIV dementia. CMV encephalitis often presents as a subacute decline in memory and cognition over 2 to 4 weeks, with periventricular changes on magnetic resonance images and hyponatremia from intercurrent CMV adrenalitis. Ganciclovir (Cytovene) is a useful suppressive agent for CMV retinitis but so far has not proven effective for treatment of encephalitis, possibly because of delays in recognizing CMV encephalitis. Foscarnet is an alternative antiviral agent that is used after ganciclovir fails. It causes nephrotoxicity and electrolyte abnormalities and is administered by prolonged IV infusion.

Cerebral Toxoplasmosis

Infection with *Toxoplasma gondii,* an obligate intracellular protozoan, causes necrotic abscesses that are

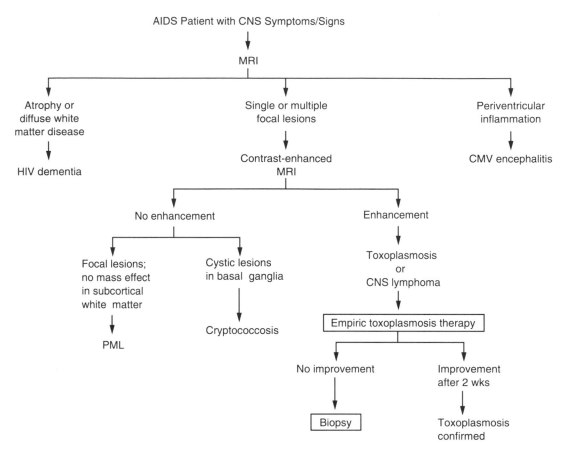

Figure 1 Use of MRI in evaluation of CNS symptoms and signs in AIDS. Key: CMV, cytomegalovirus; CNS, central nervous system; CT, computed tomography; PML, progressive multifocal leukoencephalopathy. (Modified from Olsen WL. MRI of the brain in patients with AIDS. MRI Decisions 1991; 5:19–28; with permission. © 1991, Physicians World Communications Group. All rights reserved.)

often multifocal and scattered throughout the cerebral hemispheres, though they have a predilection for the basal ganglia. Toxoplasmosis occurs in 5 to 10 percent of patients with AIDS, typically presenting with fever, altered mentation, seizures, and focal neurologic signs that develop subacutely over a few days. Imaging studies demonstrate multiple contrast-enhancing mass "ring" lesions, but the radiologic appearances are not specific for toxoplasmosis and can be mimicked by lymphoma or other causes of abscess. Serologic testing of blood or CSF is not diagnostic, because as many as 15 percent of patients with proven toxoplasmosis have indetectable *Toxoplasma* IgG. However, because most patients with toxoplasmosis have detectable anti-*Toxoplasma* IgG, a negative titer in a patient with an intracranial mass lesion should suggest an alternative diagnosis. Prompt institution of antimicrobial therapy with pyrimethamine (Daraprim), 150 mg load then 75 mg daily, with sulfadiazine, 1.5 mg four times daily (or clindamycin [Cleocin], 900 mg four times a day for sulfa-allergic patients) leads to clinical and radiologic improvement in about 80 percent of patients within 1 to 4 weeks. Corticosteroids should be restricted to patients with large lesions and mass effect. Lifelong suppressive therapy with pyrimethamine, 50 mg daily,

and clindamycin 300 mg BID, is necessary. Relapse occurs in about 10 percent and is usually linked to noncompliance with maintenance therapy.

Primary Central Nervous System Lymphoma

About 4 percent of patients with AIDS develop primary CNS lymphoma. The lymphoma, often multicentric and of B-cell origin, behaves aggressively. The typical presentation is slowly progressive neurologic deterioration with encephalopathy, focal signs, and seizures leading to death within 3 months. Because the radiologic appearance cannot be reliably distinguished from that of toxoplasmosis, biopsy is often necessary. CSF cytologic examination is rarely diagnostic, and lumbar puncture may be contraindicated because of mass effect or the risk of herniation. The lymphoma is radiosensitive and responds to whole-brain radiation with neurologic stabilization; however, because of progression of systemic HIV disease, survival time is short (median of 3 to 6 months after radiation). Because of the difficulty in distinguishing toxoplasmosis from lymphoma on clinical or radiologic grounds, empiric anti-*Toxoplasma* therapy is usually initiated for most patients with an intracranial mass lesion, particularly if it is

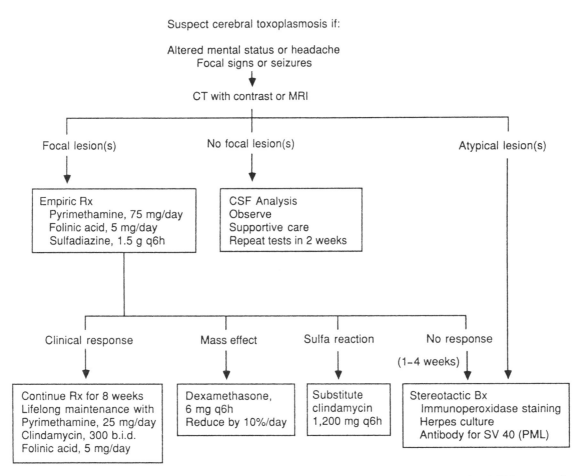

Suspect cerebral toxoplasmosis if:

Altered mental status or headache
Focal signs or seizures

↓

CT with contrast or MRI

| Focal lesion(s) | No focal lesion(s) | Atypical lesion(s) |

Empiric Rx
  Pyrimethamine, 75 mg/day
  Folinic acid, 5 mg/day
  Sulfadiazine, 1.5 g q6h

CSF Analysis
Observe
Supportive care
Repeat tests in 2 weeks

Clinical response — Mass effect — Sulfa reaction — No response (1–4 weeks)

Continue Rx for 8 weeks
Lifelong maintenance with
Pyrimethamine, 25 mg/day
Clindamycin, 300 b.i.d.
Folinic acid, 5 mg/day

Dexamethasone,
6 mg q6h
Reduce by 10%/day

Substitute
clindamycin
1,200 mg q6h

Stereotactic Bx
  Immunoperoxidase staining
  Herpes culture
  Antibody for SV 40 (PML)

Figure 2 Management of intracranial focal lesions. Key: CT, computed tomography; MRI, magnetic resonance imaging; PML, progressive multifocal leukoencephalopathy.

enhancing (see Figure 2). The indications for biopsy are listed in Table 3.

Progressive Multifocal Leukoencephalopathy

PML develops in as many as 4 percent of patients with AIDS, typically with progressive accumulation of focal neurologic deficits. Diagnosis is usually made from the typical clinical course and from imaging studies that demonstrate multiple asymmetric areas in the subcortical white matter (involving U fibers) without mass effect or prominent enhancement. Biopsy may be necessary to differentiate PML from cerebral toxoplasmosis, other opportunistic infections, or CNS lymphoma (see Figure 1). Immunostaining with antibody to SV 40 or JC virus is necessary for definitive pathologic diagnosis. The neurologic disorder usually progresses inexorably to death over weeks, or at most a few months. Interferon-alpha and cytosine arabinoside are two experimental therapies that may slow the course of progression but that have not been tested in controlled trials.

Neurosyphilis

While it is not strictly an opportunistic infection, the course of syphilis may be accelerated by the disturbance

Table 3 Indications for Brain Biopsy in AIDS

Failed empiric antitoxoplasmosis therapy
Accessible lesion, no coagulopathy
Karnovsky function scale > 70 (i.e., independent)
No immediate life-threatening systemic disease
Radiation therapy acceptable to patient

in cellular immunity that attends HIV-1 infection. The clinical features of neurosyphilis may be modified and the time course from primary to tertiary syphilis shortened. There are reports of false negative serologic test results for patients with biopsy-proven syphilis, though in general syphilis serologic tests are reliable. Because of poor CSF penetration, benzathine penicillin is inadequate for the treatment of neurosyphilis. In a neurologically normal HIV-1 carrier with a history of *treated* syphilis who is serofast (rapid plasma reagin ≤ 1:8 consistently), I do not advocate additional penicillin therapy or routine lumbar puncture. When neurologic symptoms are present, however, even if they are not typical of neurosyphilis, the CSF should be examined. If the CSF Venereal Disease Research Laboratory (VDRL) test result is positive or serum rapid plasma reagin is high (>1:16) and clinical features are suggestive of neurosyphilis, I have a low threshold for treatment

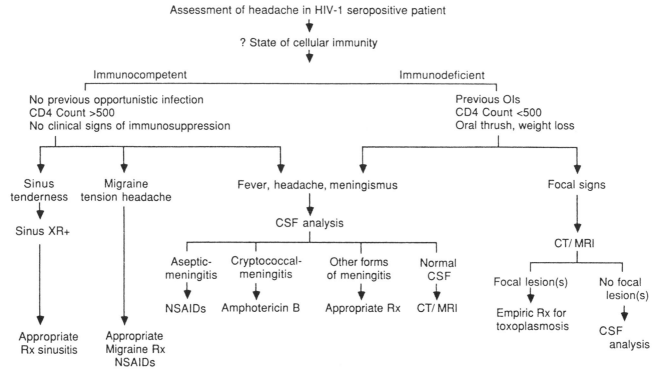

Figure 3 Assessment of headache in the HIV-1 seropositive patient. Key: CSF, cerebrospinal fluid; CT, computed tomography; MRI, magnetic resonance imaging; NSAIDs, nonsteroidal anti-inflammatory drugs.

with IV penicillin, 24 mU for 10 days, or procaine penicillin, 2.4 mU with probenecid for 10 days, followed by re-examination of the CSF 2 months after therapy.

THE WORRIED WELL

Given that an estimated 1 million Americans are already infected with HIV-1, the burden placed on neurologists for assessment of HIV-1 carriers with symptoms such as headache likely will increase. Usually, knowledge of the systemic stage of HIV-1 disease and immune status are the most helpful information, and an approach for evaluation of headache can be followed as in Figure 3. Other neurologic symptoms, including memory complaints or neuropathic symptoms, may require neurologic evaluation, but for most healthy HIV-1 carriers with normal CD4 counts, reassurance can usually be given that serious neurologic complications are unusual at this early stage of infection. Neurodiagnostic studies should be limited, and lumbar puncture particularly is rarely useful at this stage because of the high frequency of silent HIV-1–related CSF abnormalities.

SUGGESTED READING

Bartlett JG. 1992–1993 Recommendations for the medical care of persons with HIV infection. A guide to HIV care from the AIDS Care Program of The Johns Hopkins Medical Institutions. Critical Care America, 1992. [Available from AIDS Care Program, The Johns Hopkins Medical Institutions, 1830 Building, Suite 7400, Baltimore, Maryland 21287]

Kieburtz K, ed. Neurology of HIV infection. Semin Neurol 1992; 12.

Rosenblum ML, Levy RM, Bredesen DE. AIDS and the nervous system. New York: Raven Press, 1988.

PATIENT AND PHYSICIAN RESOURCES

AIDS Bibliography. National Library of Medicine (three on-line data bases: AIDSLINE, AIDSDRUGS, AIDSTRIALS; for free information packet call (800)638-8480).

AIDS Clinical Trials Information Service. [National clearinghouse for treatment trials.]
Box 6421
Rockville, MD 20850
(800)TrialsA
FAX: (301)738-6616
TTY/TDD:(800)243-7012

AIDS Experimental Treatment Directory, published by AmFAR, 1515 Broadway, 36th floor, New York, NY 10036, (212)719-0033.

AIDS Resources, regional: 24 hour National AIDS Hotline (800)342-AIDS. Spanish speakers (800)342-SIDA, from 8:00 A.M. to 2:00 A.M. (EST).

AIDS Treatment News [twice monthly newsletter]
(800)Treat12

Treatment Issues. [Newsletter of experimental AIDS therapies published ten times annually by Gay Men's Health Crisis (GMHC) (212)337-3541.]

OTHER INFLAMMATORY DISEASES AND DEMYELINATING DISEASES

OPTIC NEURITIS

SHIRLEY H. WRAY, M.D., Ph.D., F.R.C.P.

Optic neuritis is a manifestation of multiple sclerosis (MS). In 56 to 72 percent of adult patients with isolated optic neuritis, brain magnetic resonance imaging (MRI) shows multifocal, high-signal intensity, white matter lesions that suggest the diagnosis of MS.

The initial attack of optic neuritis, characterized by sudden vision loss, ipsilateral eye pain, and dyschromatopsia, is unilateral in 70 percent of adult cases and bilateral in 30 percent. In my patient population, the incidence of optic neuritis in adult women exceeds that in men by a ratio of 1.8:1.

The prognosis for the recovery of "Snellen acuity" following an initial attack of optic neuritis is good. Between 65 and 80 percent of patients regain 20/30 vision or better. Of these, 45 percent recover rapidly within the first 4 months, 35 percent recover normal or nearly normal acuity at 1 year, and 20 percent fail to make any significant improvement.

THERAPY

There is no specific treatment for optic neuritis, and evidence that any of the following treatments influences outcome is unconvincing: retrobulbar injection of triamcinolone, prednisone by mouth, or daily IM or SC injections of corticotropin for 30 days.

In a 1977 controlled, single-blind trial, 31 optic neuritis patients were treated with a single retrobulbar injection of triamcinolone within the first 2 weeks of vision loss. Thirty untreated patients served as controls. The results showed a trend toward more rapid recovery of vision in the treated group but no significant difference from the controls in visual acuity, color vision, or visual fields for the first 6 months after treatment. The researchers concluded that routine use of corticosteroids is not justified in unilateral optic neuritis when vision in the other eye is good. Shortening the period of visual disability in bilateral disease, or in unilateral disease when vision in the other eye is poor, was considered a justifiable indication for steroid therapy.

The effect of pulsed IV 6-methylprednisolone (6-MP) therapy on MS was reported in a 1980 study. Intravenous (IV) 6-MP produced fast clinical improvement from acute relapse, but it made no lasting difference in the course of the disease.

A short course of large doses of IV 6-MP produced similar rapid clinical improvement in 12 consecutive patients (nine women, three men) with optic neuritis studied in 1988. Within 7 to 90 days of onset, each received 6-MP, 500 or 250 mg IV, every 6 hours for 3 to 7 days. The initial visual acuity ranged from no light perception to 20/30. Visual acuity was followed daily, and visual fields were charted on admission and every other day. After 3 to 7 days of 6-MP treatment the drug was abruptly discontinued and either therapy was stopped or rapidly tapering oral doses of corticosteroid were administered. After treatment, visual acuity and visual fields were followed weekly for 1 month, monthly for 3 months, and subsequently every 3 months. There was no untreated control group in this study. The authors concluded that patients with optic neuritis may benefit from intravenous methylprednisolone.

Subsequent to this study, and in order to re-evaluate the documented visual outcome, Wall matched 26 untreated optic neuritis control cases examined over 6 months to the 12 6-MP–treated cases and reported no significant difference in the final visual acuity between the treated patients and an untreated group, regardless of whether the Snellen fraction ($t = -0.94$; degree of freedom $= 38$; $P = 0.36$ [two-tailed]) or the log MAR ($t = -1.20$; degree of freedom $= 38$; $P = 0.24$ [two-tailed]) acuity was used.

This comparison did not establish that treatment of optic neuritis with IV 6-MP does not work, only that current data fail to show any long-term benefit if visual acuity is used as the final measurement. Caution is warranted, however, since IV 6-MP treatment has potentially serious side effects, including psychological disturbance, hypertension, hyperglycemia and, more rarely, anaphylactic reactions, seizures, and sudden death.

A report of a possible harmful late effect of 6-MP therapy in optic neuritis supports this cautionary note.

Twenty-six optic neuritis patients from southern Israel were studied. Six patients were treated with 6-MP, 1,000 mg IV for 8 hours on 3 consecutive days, and no oral steroid was administered subsequently. Fourteen patients were treated with prednisone, 1 mg per kilogram daily PO for 10 days, and then tapered off during a period of 3 to 5 weeks. Six patients were left untreated. Improved vision, measured as an improvement in visual acuity of at least one line on the Snellen chart, the number of recurrent attacks of optic neuritis, and conversion to MS were all recorded.

The results showed that 6-MP therapy improved vision faster (mean = 8 days) than prednisone (mean = 32 days) or no treatment (mean = 40 days). All 6-MP–treated cases improved and so did 12 of 14 prednisone-treated cases. Only 3 of the 6 untreated patients improved spontaneously.

Overall, 30 percent (8 of 26) of patients had one or more recurrent attacks of optic neuritis. The recurrent rate was higher in the 6-MP–treated group (4 of 6) compared with the prednisone group (2 of 14) and the untreated cases (2 of 6).

The conversion to MS was also significantly higher in the 6-MP–treated group (5 of 6) than in the prednisone group (1 of 4) or the untreated cases (0 of 6). In the 6-MP–treated patients, MS was diagnosed clinically within 7 to 18 months of the first attack of optic neuritis. The observation of a high rate of recurrent optic neuritis and apparently increased conversion to MS in the 6-MP group is both surprising and disturbing, even though the patient population was extremely small.

The need for a much larger, and thus statistically more predictive, sample has now been addressed by a multicenter randomized, controlled trial of corticosteroids for treatment of acute optic neuritis. Four hundred fifty-seven patients were randomly assigned to receive (1) oral prednisone (Deltasone), 1 mg per kilogram of body weight per day for 14 days, (2) methylprednisolone (Solu-Medrol), 250 mg IV every 6 hours for 3 days, followed by oral prednisone (Deltasone), 1 mg per kilogram per day (rounded to the nearest 10 mg) for 11 days, or (3) oral placebo for 14 days. Each treatment period was followed by a short course of oral prednisone, which was then tapered off. Visual function was assessed over a 6-month follow-up period.

The trial was designed to answer the following questions: Does treatment with either oral prednisone or IV methylprednisolone improve vision outcome after acute optic neuritis? Does either treatment speed recovery of vision? What are the complications of treatment in relation to its efficacy?

The results showed that IV methylprednisolone followed by oral prednisone speeds recovery of vision loss due to optic neuritis and results in only slightly better vision at 6 months. Oral prednisone alone, as prescribed in this study, provided no benefit in terms of either the rate of recovery or the outcome at 6 months, and the investigators concluded that this drug is ineffective for optic neuritis.

Surprisingly, prednisone was found to increase the risk of new episodes of optic neuritis. The data showed that 20 patients (13 percent) in the IV methylprednisolone group, 42 (27 percent) in the oral prednisone group, and 24 (15 percent) in the placebo group had at least one new episode of optic neuritis (in either eye) during the 6 to 24 months' follow-up. Relative risk for oral prednisone versus placebo was 1.79 (95 percent confidence interval, 1.08 to 2.95). The results of this therapeutic trial are applicable to the care of most patients who suffer an acute unilateral attack of optic neuritis. The message is clear: *Do not prescribe prednisone.*

The question remains, however, whether IV methylprednisolone is the drug of choice for acute unilateral optic neuritis. In the trial, methylprednisolone compared with placebo was found to be beneficial during the first 15 days of vision loss to speed vision recovery. When the risk of serious side effects associated with large IV doses of methylprednisolone, the inconvenience of hospitalization to the patient, and the expense are all considered, however, it is clear that this therapy is not justified, except perhaps for the exceptional patient who requires the rapid return of stereoscopic vision essential to job skills (e.g., seamstress, dentist).

I consider IV methylprednisolone the drug of choice currently to treat (1) optic neuritis in the only good eye (contralateral visual acuity 20/60 or worse), or (2) bilateral simultaneous optic neuritis (visual acuity 20/60 or worse in both eyes).

The following regimen produced onset of vision recovery in all the patients I have treated with IV methylprednisolone: 1 g methylprednisolone IV in 1,000 ml dextrose-saline daily for 3 days, 500 mg of methylprednisolone IV in 500 ml of dextrose-saline IV daily for 3 days, followed by 250 mg methylprednisolone IV in 250 cc of dextrose-saline for 3 days. Vision recovery was associated with shrinkage of a scotoma or complete resolution of a central field defect. No patient had any serious side effects. Insomnia was the only disturbing symptom.

In the multicenter trial, reversal of visual field defects was reported to be slightly better in the methylprednisolone group ($P = 0.001$) than in the placebo group. These data, and my own experience, make large doses of IV methylprednisolone the treatment of choice for *selected* cases of optic neuritis.

DOCTOR-PATIENT RELATIONSHIP

There is no question that essentially untreatable conditions place a special burden on the doctor-patient relationship, and optic neuritis, with its painful promise of MS, is no exception. If the physician cannot treat the patient, the patient's needs and fears become part of the condition itself; and the patient's need to hope, the fear of being unable to cope, the doctor's wish to reassure on the one hand and to tell it the way it is on the other, all contribute their own weight to the burden. The physician, facing each patient's different individual concerns, must try to tell the diagnostic truth in such a way that patients are left to feel that it is possible for them to be in control of the changes that will occur in their lives. Over the years, I have never ceased to be amazed by the resolve of so many of my patients to do just this and to resume, as much as they possibly can, the activities that were important to them before they fell ill. I have been even more amazed at the gratitude so many of them feel after being able to do so.

SUGGESTED READING

Beck RW, Cleary PA, Anderson MM, et al. A randomized controlled trial of corticosteroids in the treatment of acute optic neuritis. N Engl J Med 1992; 326:581.

Dowling PC, Bosch VV, Cook SD. Possible beneficial effect of high dose intravenous steroid therapy in acute demyelinating disease and transverse myelitis. Neurology (NY) 1980; 30:33.

Herishanu YO, Badarna S, Sarov B, et al. A possible harmful late effect of methylprednisolone therapy on a time cluster of optic neuritis. Acta Neurol Scand 1989; 80:569.

Spoor TC, Rickwell DL. Treatment of optic neuritis with intravenous megadose corticosteroids. A consecutive series. Ophthalmology 1988; 95:131.

Wall M. Megadose corticosteroids for optic neuritis. Ophthalmology 1988; 95:1006.

Wray SH. Optic neuritis. In: Albert DM, Jakobiec FA, eds. The principles and practice of ophthalmology. The Harvard system. Philadelphia: WB Saunders, in press.

POSTINFECTIOUS ENCEPHALOMYELITIS AND TRANSVERSE MYELITIS

WILLIAM R. TYOR, M.D.

Postinfectious encephalomyelitis or acute disseminated encephalomyelitis affects persons of all ages, though it is less common in the first decade of life. It typically follows an infection such as measles, rubella, chicken pox, or another exanthem, or vaccination. It may begin with seizures, headache, and fever, and over days involves multifocal areas of brain stem, spinal cord, and optic nerves, as part of a uniphasic illness. Patients may develop hemiplegia, paraplegia, sensory deficits, ataxia, and optic neuritis. The diagnosis is clinical, and frequently there is moderate leukocytosis, accelerated sedimentation rate, slowing on electroencephalography (EEG), and cerebrospinal fluid findings consistent with aseptic meningitis. Magnetic resonance imaging (MRI) of the brain is helpful and on T2-weighted images demonstrates areas of increased intensity in white matter.

Transverse myelitis has a similar age distribution to postinfectious encephalomyelitis, and about 30 to 40 percent of patients have a history of antecedent infection within days to weeks of the myelitis. Transverse myelitis can be caused directly by a number of infectious agents, including syphilis, *Borrelia burgdorferi,* herpesviruses, human immunodeficiency virus type 1, and human T cell lymphoma virus type 1, and is also seen in association with multiple sclerosis. For the purposes of this discussion, I confine the use of the term to idiopathic, postinfectious, or postvaccinal transverse myelitis. Usu-

ally the initial manifestations are weakness in the legs, sensory disturbance and sensory level, back pain, and sphincter dysfunction. It is paramount to rule out other causes of myelopathy, such as neoplastic, vascular, or infectious ones. Spine radiography and computed tomography (CT) with and without contrast medium, or, if available, MRI with and without gadolinium should be obtained as soon as possible. Following spine imaging, cerebrospinal fluid analysis should be performed to rule out an infectious or neoplastic cause and immunoglobulin G (IgG) index and oligoclonal bands should be measured. Other testing, such as MRI of the brain and serum analysis, should be based on the clinical suspicion of the causes, including multiple sclerosis, vitamin B_{12} deficiency, infection, cancer, connective tissue disorders, and others. Investigations to date strongly support the hypothesis that postinfectious encephalomyelitis and transverse myelitis are autoimmune diseases, lending support to studies that suggest immunosuppressive therapy is beneficial.

THERAPY DIRECTED AT THE DISEASE PROCESS

Once a diagnosis of postinfectious encephalomyelitis or transverse myelitis has been established, corticosteroid treatment should be considered. No controlled clinical trial has been performed and both diseases may spontaneously remit. Because of (1) the likelihood that postinfectious encephalomyelitis and transverse myelitis are autoimmune diseases, (2) their similarities with multiple sclerosis, and (3) reports of beneficial effects of corticosteroid treatment, I recommend such treatment. Methylprednisolone, 15 mg per kilogram (1 g), is administered intravenously in 500 ml of normal saline solution over 2 hours, once a day for 3 days (Table 1). This is followed by prednisone, 1 mg per kilogram (60 to 80 mg) taken orally for 7 days and then tapered by 10 mg

Table 1 Routine Therapy and Prophylaxis of Complications in Postinfectious Encephalomyelitis and Transverse Myelitis

---

Direct therapy
  Methylprednisolone, 1 g in 500 ml normal saline IV over 2 hours daily for 3 days, followed by prednisone, 60-80 mg PO daily for 7 days, followed by a rapid taper over 2 weeks.
  Antacids, potassium
  Monitor potassium and glucose

Prophylaxis of complications
  If bedridden: Physical therapy for passive range of motion.
    Frequent turning, protective pads, and egg-crate mattress
    Anti-thromboembolic device (TED) hose, heparin (5000 units SC q12h) if not contraindicated.
    Respiratory care to prevent atelectasis and pneumonia
    Monitor urinary function
    Psyllium tablets daily to aid bowel motility

For patients who are stable or improving
  Physical and occupational therapy
  Psychological support/treatment

---

every 3 days. The most frequent side effects of steroid therapy include mood alterations, insomnia, fluid retention, potassium loss, elevated blood pressure, acne, hyperglycemia, and gastrointestinal complications. Rarely, patients who receive large doses of corticosteroids develop avascular necrosis of the hip. Whenever possible, a tuberculin skin test and control for anergy should be applied before corticosteroid therapy begins and a chest radiograph obtained to rule out pulmonary evidence of active or quiescent tuberculosis. Prophylaxis of patients receiving steroids with antacids and appropriate oral intake of potassium-rich foods is advisable, as well as monitoring serum potassium and glucose levels.

TREATMENT OF COMPLICATIONS

In severe cases it may be necessary to give prolonged intravenous corticosteroid therapy, and if there is evidence of significant central nervous system edema, efforts to reduce the edema such as administration of mannitol, reverse Trendelenberg position, and hyperventilation may be necessary. Surgical intervention for the placement of intracranial pressure monitoring and decompression may be indicated.

Seizures may also complicate postinfectious encephalomyelitis and should be treated with anticonvulsants such as phenytoin, carbamazepine, and phenobarbitol. Phenytoin is most commonly used and has the advantage over carbamazepine of intravenous administration if necessary. The initial dose is 10 to 15 mg per kilogram, to be given no faster than 50 mg per minute to avoid cardiac dysrhythmias. Patients are typically maintained on 300 mg per day, provided therapeutic levels are attained.

Proper care of the bedridden patient is critical to prevent complications such as decubitus ulcers, thrombophlebitis, contractures, and peripheral nerve compression. A physical therapist should be involved early for passive range of motion procedures; splinting should be provided to prevent contractures; and protective pads are applied to the elbows and heels to prevent decubitus ulcers. An egg-crate mattress or air mattress should be used, the patient should be turned frequently (at least every 2 hours), and the skin should be kept clean. For prophylaxis of deep venous thrombosis TED hose should be applied and heparin, 5000 units subcutaneously every 12 hours, may be used unless hemorrhagic lesions are noted on brain imaging or the patient is known to have another potential source of bleeding. Pneumatic calf compression is a good alternative if heparin is contraindicated.

For patients with dysphagia it may only be necessary to puree or liquefy their diet, but if there is any significant risk of aspiration a feeding tube should be placed. Jejunal placement of the tip of the feeding tube may be necessary, slow drip administration of isotonic products (Osmolite or Isocal) rather than bolus feedings are preferable, and the head of the bed should be elevated. Patients receiving total enteral nutrition may require 1500 to 3000 kcal per day.

Respiratory care is also crucial because patients with postinfectious encephalomyelitis and transverse myelitis are frequently bedridden and may develop atelectasis and pneumonia. Respiratory therapy and good pulmonary toilet should be instituted. Patients with postinfectious encephalomyelitis or cervical myelitis may develop paralysis of the respiratory muscles, and pulmonary function should be monitored. If they are able, forced vital capacities should be performed twice daily or more frequently. Alternatively, oximetry, if available, may be used for continuous monitoring.

Bladder dysfunction is common in transverse myelitis and may be encountered in postinfectious encephalomyelitis as well. Urgency, frequency, and incontinence are frequent symptoms in patients with hypotonic or spastic bladder. Monitoring frequency and volume of urination over 48 hours, followed by determination of postvoiding residual, should help assess whether the bladder is spastic or hypotonic. Residual urine less than 150 ml suggests normal or spastic function, and a greater residual suggests a hypotonic bladder. Hypotonic bladder can be treated by having the patient employ a Credé technique of bladder massage: pressure is applied downward to the lower abdomen while bearing down and it may also be useful for men to sit while applying this technique. The urine should be acidified by daily intake of ascorbic acid, 500 to 1000 mg, to help prevent infection. If this method fails, oxybutenin, 2.5 to 5.0 mg PO twice or thrice daily, may be helpful and may also be used in conjunction with intermittent catheterization. The patient can be taught self-catheterization, to be performed every 4 to 6 hours. If these measures are unsuccessful in achieving a postvoiding residual less than 150 ml, I refer patients to a urologist experienced in assessing and treating neurogenic bladder. This is because the bladder may be spastic, dysynergic, or hypotonic, and assessment with urodynamics will enable you and the urologist to determine if a different medication should be tried or whether eventually an indwelling catheter should be placed.

Constipation is also common, though other causes should be considered, including constipation secondary to medications or metabolic abnormalities. Psyllium tablets or dioctyl sulfosuccinate can be given daily. If this is unsuccessful, enemas should be administered or, if necessary, manual extraction performed. Laxatives and suppositories should be avoided, but they may be necessary. Mild agents such as prune juice and magnesium hydroxide (milk of magnesia) may be helpful, but occasionally I resort to bisacodyl (Dulcolax) or glycerin suppositories, mineral oil, or even magnesium sulfate or sorbitol.

Pain and spasticity also occur in association with postinfectious encephalomyelitis and transverse myelitis. For spasticity, baclofen may be effective, 5 to 10 mg PO at bedtime initially, and then increasing every 3 days to twice or thrice daily dosing until symptoms and signs improve or until the patient has significant side effects that preclude effective treatment. Alternatively, diazepam, initially at 2 mg per day PO, can be used as an adjunct to baclofen or alone. Both medications can be increased significantly, if tolerated, and I have used as much as 120 mg per day of baclofen alone and as much as 80 mg per day of diazepam alone. The most common side effects of diazepam and baclofen are drowsiness and weakness. I reserve dantrolene sodium for severe refractory cases because of its potential liver toxicity. Intrathecal administration of baclofen or diazepam should be reserved for severe cases of spasticity that are refractory to all the aforementioned medications.

Dysesthetic pain often responds to tricyclic agents like amitriptyline. I start at 25 mg PO at bedtime and observe for 4 weeks before increasing the dose. If the patient is not significantly relieved, I increase by 25 mg every 5 days until there is relief of pain, the patient experiences side effects, or the total daily dose is 200 mg. The most common side effects of amitriptyline are drowsiness, dry mouth and eyes, and urinary retention. Carbamazepine or phenytoin is also used for dysesthetic pain. Carbamazepine is given initially, 200 mg PO at bedtime and after 5 days the dose is increased to twice a day and then after another 5 days to three times daily dosing. The physician may titrate to high–therapeutic range blood levels before assuming medication failure. Drowsiness, blurred vision, and ataxia may also limit use

of carbamazepine, and blood counts and liver enzymes should be monitored before and 1 month after initiation of therapy.

Once the patient is stable or improving, more extensive physical, occupational, and, if necessary, speech and swallowing therapy should be instituted. The patients may perform active resistance exercises in addition to passive range of motion. The patient may need to learn transfer techniques and adaptive measures for daily living. Orthotic devices, canes, or walkers may be necessary. Social services and vocational rehabilitation should be utilized as needed. Occupational therapists may also assess the need for alterations at home or at work. It may be necessary to train family members in care techniques or to provide home health care givers.

Most patients recover to some extent, and as many as a third of those who develop transverse myelitis recover fully. A significant percentage of patients, however, have residual deficits and require not only many of the therapeutic and supportive modalities mentioned above but also psychological support, and possibly treatment. Amitriptyline, as described above, or another antidepressant may be used, and often consultation with a psychiatrist or psychologist is beneficial. Patients and their families may also derive some support from speaking with other patients and their families who have suffered from postinfectious encephalomyelitis, transverse myelitis, or some other chronic debilitating disease such as multiple sclerosis. Although technically these patients do not suffer from multiple sclerosis, sometimes it is beneficial for them to meet other patients through the local chapter of the National Multiple Sclerosis Society.

SUGGESTED READING

Cohen JA, Lisak RP. Acute disseminated encephalomyelitis. In: Aarli JA, Behan WM, Behan PO, eds. Clinical Neuroimmunology. New York: Blackwell, 1987:192.

Dowling PC, Bosch VV, Cook SD. Possible beneficial effects of high-dose intravenous steroid therapy in acute demyelinating disease and transverse myelitis. Neurology 1980; 30:33–36.

Lipton HL, Teasdall RD. Acute transverse myelopathy in adults. Arch Neurol 1973; 28:252–257.

Ropper AH, Poskanzer DC. The prognosis of acute and subacute transverse myelopathy based on early signs and symptoms. Ann Neurol 1978; 4:51–59.

MULTIPLE SCLEROSIS

RICHARD A. RUDICK, M.D.

In an era of increasing reliance on sophisticated brain imaging and chemical and electrical tests, the neurologist must steadfastly remember that the diagnosis of multiple sclerosis (MS) is based on *clinical* features *supplemented* by laboratory findings, rather than the converse. I have seen dozens of patients who learned of a diagnosis of MS through a magnetic resonance imaging (MRI) report. Some of these people had MS, but some did not. A basic diagnostic requirement is the presence of multiple areas of clinically evident central nervous system (CNS) demyelination spread over time in the absence of an alternative diagnosis that presents in that fashion. The history and neurologic examination are of primary importance in establishing the diagnosis, whereas adjunctive laboratory tests play a major role in confirming the diagnosis and eliminating alternative diagnostic possibilities. It is often necessary to observe the patient over time, frequently with repeated clinical and laboratory testing, to determine with confidence whether or not MS is present.

Errors in MS diagnosis are of two types. The first is diagnosing MS in patients with no definable neurologic disease. It is extremely common for a person to "acquire" a diagnosis of MS because of nonspecific neurologic symptoms such as weakness, fatigue, or tingling, at times supplemented by minimal signal changes on MRI. I have followed dozens of such patients for years, becoming less and less convinced of the diagnosis as the years passed. In some cases, psychologically-based somatization emerges as a significant cause. I have taken the diagnosis away in many of these cases, often with surprisingly positive results. The second type of error is in patients who clearly have neurologic disease but have an alternative diagnosis such as neurosarcoidosis, or systemic lupus erythematosus (Table 1). I have listed a number of "red flags" of possible diagnostic error that can be considered in each new MS patient (Table 2). These red flags have been very helpful in my experience.

My practice is to discuss the diagnosis with the patient in an open, honest fashion. After the first visit, I often make the following statement, "I think that you have a condition called multiple sclerosis, but before I can be certain we need to conduct some testing." When the diagnosis has been confirmed I indicate to the patient, "You have an illness called multiple sclerosis, and I would like to answer your immediate questions and then arrange a time to sit down with you and your family to discuss it in some detail." When the diagnosis is in doubt, I discuss that just as directly, saying, "I think that there is a possibility that you have multiple sclerosis, but I can't be sure about it." I then explain the basis for the uncertainty (e.g., not enough evidence, concern about a

Table 1 Conditions Commonly Misdiagnosed as Multiple Sclerosis

Vascular diseases
  Small-vessel disease
  Vasculitis

Structural lesions
  Craniocervical junction
  Posterior fossa
  Spinal cord

Degenerative diseases
  Motor system disease
  Spinocerebellar degeneration

Other conditions
  Cobalamin deficiency
  Sjögren's syndrome
  Sarcoidosis
  Human T-cell lymphotropic virus-I infection
  Nonspecific MRI abnormalities

Table 2 Red Flags in the Diagnosis of Multiple Sclerosis

Absence of oculomotor or optic nerve findings
Absence of a clinical remission
Syndrome that could be explained by localized disease
Absence of sensory or bladder involvement
Absence of CSF abnormalities

tumor) and make a plan to follow the problem. This is usually a relief to patients, many of whom have seen other neurologists who "didn't tell me anything."

It is important to realize that there are significant implications of an MS diagnosis and they are all bad. An individual may find that he can no longer get medical insurance or a promotion at work, and the disease may restrict various educational, vocational, or family options. This can also be discussed directly with a patient, indicating that it is better not to make a diagnosis that could be premature or in error.

COMPREHENSIVE CARE

Comprehensive care for patients with MS extends beyond neurologic diagnosis and pharmacotherapy. Needed services include support and information over time, physical therapy, occupational therapy, psychological assessment and intervention, help with various social services, and attention to family, vocational, and insurance concerns. An interdisciplinary approach is more effective in addressing many of the problems that cannot be managed by an isolated neurologist. At the Cleveland Clinic Foundation's Mellen Center for Multiple Sclerosis Treatment and Research, neurologists function as members of a *treatment team* consisting of occupational and physical therapists, social workers, psychologists, nurses, and neurologists. I frequently refer patients to the *nurse* for educational sessions with patients and families, particularly when the diagnosis is new but also for specific issues during the course of therapy. The nurse also evaluates and manages bowel and bladder symptoms and skin care and is an important liaison between neurologist, treatment team, and patient. I refer to the *physical therapist* for strengthening and stretching programs if a patient exhibits spasticity, gait ataxia, or weakness; for walking aids; and for a fitness program as part of a wellness program. I refer to the *occupational therapist* for adapted equipment, including wheelchair specifications and adapted computers; for environmental assessments, including satisfactory activity configurations; and for assessment and therapy of arm ataxia. I refer to a *social worker* for family assessments, insurance, and vocational concerns, and to assist with community resources. I refer to a *psychologist* for evaluation and treatment of emotional distress and coping problems, and to assess cognitive and memory function. Additionally, I occasionally refer to *dietitians, speech therapists, urologists, ophthalmologists, neurosurgeons, plastic surgeons,* and *orthotists.* At any point in time, one or two members of the treatment team may be very active while others are quiescent. As time passes, needs change and different team members can be called upon to assist.

EDUCATION AND COMMONLY ASKED QUESTIONS

Most patients ask certain questions, particularly early after a new diagnosis. In my opinion, it is important to provide reading material for the patient and his family *as well as* an opportunity to discuss some of what they read and their concerns. Some of the more helpful references for patient education are listed at the end of this chapter.

What will happen to me? Patients need to know that MS is inherently unpredictable. I emphasize that there is a spectrum of severity, just as with every other chronic medical disease. Patients are often surprised and relieved to learn that a significant proportion of patients (about a third) remain unimpaired for many years. When favorable prognostic signs are present (e.g., predominance of sensory symptoms, paucity of cerebellar or pyramidal deficits), I point these out to patients while acknowledging that there are no precise predictors for individual patients. When a patient is disabled or significantly distressed by anticipatory anxiety about the possibility of disease progression, I refer for psychological assessment. Usually, such persons have had a pattern of similar emotional responses to perceived threats.

How can I control my illness? Most patients believe that certain types of behavior worsen or improve their illness. Their beliefs are unpredictable and often surprising. I encourage patients to openly discuss what they think will improve or worsen their MS. At times it is possible to redirect a patient's need for control by focusing on healthy living that can be managed in a positive way. For example, patients can frequently regain a sense of control by instituting a fitness program or improving their diet.

When should I call you? Patients want access to their neurologist but don't know when to call. I advise the patient to call when he feels it *may* be necessary. Most patients learn over time when it is necessary to call. I limit patients who call inappropriately. I also find it useful to see patients every 6 or 12 months, depending on disease severity, even when there are no new problems. This allows me to follow the status of neurologic impairment. It also decreases the number of phone calls, since patients often "save" their concerns for the appointment.

Will my children get this? I inform patients directly that the lifetime risk to a child of an MS mother is 3 to 5 percent. This is 30 to 50 times greater than for the general population but still represents a small risk. This is readily explained to MS patients. The risk to a child of an MS father appears much smaller, for reasons that are unclear.

Can I have a baby? Pregnancy has a predictable effect on the pattern of MS, in that symptoms usually improve during pregnancy but worsen during the first 12 weeks postpartum. There is no evidence that the overall course of MS, including the eventual degree of disability, changes significantly as a result of one or more pregnancies. Therefore, I advise women with mild to moderate disability to plan pregnancies on the basis of issues other than MS. It appears that breast feeding has little if any effect on the frequency, timing, or severity of postpartum exacerbations.

SYMPTOM PHARMACOTHERAPY

Spasticity

Spasticity is characterized by increased muscle tone, hyperreflexia, and limb spasms, usually accompanied by weakness and loss of dexterity. Patients complain of stiffness, spasms, pain, and immobility. Lower limb flexion or extension spasms occur spontaneously or may be precipitated by attempts at volitional movement, position changes, or sensory stimuli. The gamma-aminobutyric acid (GABA) agonist baclofen is the drug of choice for symptomatic spasticity in MS. I start with 5 to 10 mg three times per day and intermittently increase the dose to achieve a therapeutic response or to limit side effects. I instruct the patient to gradually increase the dose with weekly adjustments of 10 mg per 24 hours. I ask the patient to phone at 4-week intervals to report the effects of the drug and any side effects. Most patients respond optimally to doses in the 40 to 60 mg per day range, although an occasional patient benefits from doses as large as 400 mg per day. The principal limitations of baclofen are confusion and sedation, principally in cognitively impaired patients, or increased muscle weakness, particularly in patients who depend on extensor spasticity for ambulation. These problems can be minimized by starting with very small doses and by very slowly adding increments. The patient should be cautioned against abrupt baclofen withdrawal, as confusional states or seizures may occur.

For patients with nocturnal spasms, particularly with sleep disturbance, I use diazepam as an antispastic drug. I start with 5 mg at bedtime, increasing if needed. For patients with recurrent flexor or extensor spasms during the day, I start with 2 mg two or three times per day, with gradual increments. Rarely is it necessary to exceed 5 mg three times per day, but some patients require as much as 20 mg three times per day for very severe flexor spasms. Patients may experience troublesome dizziness, drowsiness, distractability, and confusion. Diazepam appears to be more effective when used in combination with baclofen, since benzodiazepines can potentiate the GABA-ergic effects of baclofen. The addition of 0.5 to 1 mg of diazepam twice per day, which is usually not associated with sedation, may be effective in a patient taking baclofen.

Dantrolene is an effective alternative for patients who do not respond well to baclofen or diazepam or cannot tolerate the central effects of these drugs. Dantrolene prevents activation of myofibril contraction and thereby consistently results in muscle weakness in addition to having an antispastic effect. Therefore, it is most useful in nonambulatory patients. The drug should be used cautiously in patients with myocardial disease. Dantrolene is instituted at 25 mg daily and gradually increased to a maximum dose of 100 mg four times per day. The smallest effective dose should be used, since the drug can cause toxic hepatitis. Asymptomatic transaminasemia has been reported to precede the onset of toxic hepatitis, so I monitor transaminase levels before and during dantrolene therapy. I measure transaminase levels weekly for 4 weeks, then monthly. Diarrhea is the principal minor side effect.

Recent experience suggests a role for intrathecal baclofen in patients with intractable spasticity of spinal origin who do not respond to or cannot tolerate oral antispastic drugs. Continuous intrathecal infusion of baclofen, 200 to 800 μg per day, effectively relieves spasticity in my experience. I am not yet certain how best to select patients for intrathecal baclofen, but it appears to be particularly useful for those who are still ambulatory but are significantly impaired owing to spasticity.

Depression and Emotional Distress

Depression occurs commonly at certain times during the course of MS, usually in response to a perceived loss or threat. Depression is also a common reaction when the disease is first diagnosed, when symptoms become persistent rather than occasional, and when patients experience vision loss or no longer can walk independently. Depression should be treated aggressively, because it has a significant negative impact on quality of life, social relationships, and job performance. I have a low threshold for exploring emotional issues, for referring to a psychiatrist or psychologist, and for a trial of a tricyclic antidepressant. For patients with associated anxiety and insomnia I prefer amitriptyline. For patients

with concurrent bladder symptoms I often use imipramine, because of its alpha-adrenergic properties. For older patients or those with memory impairment, I prefer a drug with less anticholinergic properties, such as desipramine or nortriptyline.

Emotional lability is less common than depression in MS patients, but it can be equally disabling. MS patients can experience a disconnection between internal and external mood states, presumably owing to CNS demyelination. Patients may exhibit pathologic laughing and weeping, with severe uncontrollable paroxysms of inappropriate laughing or weeping unrelated to external events. This may respond to small doses of amitriptyline (e.g., 25 to 75 mg per day).

Cognitive dysfunction is more common in MS than is generally appreciated, probably because the changes are often mild and selective. Cognitive dysfunction should be suspected when there is poor work performance or family disintegration or when compliance with medical or rehabilitative therapies is poor, even when cognitive function appears good to casual observation. Neuropsychological assessment is required to define the presence and type of cognitive impairment. Tests should include sensitive measures of complex attention and information processing, learning and recent memory, and concept formation or problem solving. There is no known effective drug therapy, although patients can often learn compensatory strategies and may benefit from cognitive rehabilitation.

Ataxia

Cerebellar ataxia, one of the most disabling of all MS problems, is also one of the least responsive to pharmacotherapy. Despite reports of effectiveness, I have not found isoniazid to be useful or well-tolerated. Similarly, I have most often been disappointed with the results of various other drugs I have tried, including baclofen, carbamazepine, clonazepam, propranolol, choline, lecithin, meprobamate, and mysoline. In my experience, clonazepam works best. I start with 0.5 mg at bedtime and increase gradually to an end point of sedation or effective control of cerebellar tremor. Rarely is it advisable to increase the clonazepam dosage greater than 2 mg four times a day. We have treated approximately 10 patients with severe, persistent and disabling tremor with stereotactic ventral lateral thalamotomy. In almost all, the intensity of tremor was diminished, and in a few cases patients made functional gains. Overall, however, this technique cannot be recommended because of the frequent occurrence of contralateral hemiparesis and progression of MS.

Spasms and Seizures

Dystonic spasms, or tonic seizures, consist of brief, recurrent, painful posturing of one or more extremities, not associated with altered consciousness or urinary incontinence. These spasms are exquisitely sensitive to carbamazepine. It may not be necessary to achieve anticonvulsant blood levels. I start at 200 mg twice per day, which usually controls these spasms. In my experience, other anticonvulsants are less effective.

Seizures occur in approximately 5 percent of MS patients and usually take the form of a single tonic-clonic motor seizure, generalizing from a focal origin. Generalized motor seizures in MS can be readily controlled with phenytoin, assuming an adequate phenytoin blood level. Alternatively, carbamazepine can be used, but with carbamazepine MS patients are often bothered by increased axial instability.

Fatigue

Fatigue in MS is usually described as a feeling of disabling exhaustion that comes on with exertion, particularly late in the day. It is necessary to rule out depression or a sleep disorder as the cause of fatigue. Bladder dysfunction is a common but uncommonly recognized cause of fatigue in MS; patients may wake on numerous occasions because of nocturia. The proper treatment in this instance is directed at bladder dysfunction. For disabling fatigue not caused by depression or sleep dysfunction, I start with amantadine, 100 mg twice per day. This is taken on awakening and again around noon, to avoid insomnia. Pemoline, 37.5 mg in the morning, is effective for some patients who have not responded to amantadine.

Heat Sensitivity

MS symptoms worsen or recur in the heat, and increased ambient temperature may lead to exhaustion or exertion-induced transient neurologic dysfunction. This arises from conduction failure in partially demyelinated CNS fibers. I recommend cool showers or air conditioning in the summer for heat-sensitive MS patients. Dramatic deterioration can be observed in a febrile MS patient, frequently in association with a urinary tract infection. Therefore, fever is aggressively treated and specific infections are treated with appropriate antibiotics.

Pain Syndromes

Pain syndromes are common in MS patients. *Facial pain* may take the form of typical trigeminal neuralgia or atypical facial pain. Both are due to disease in the pontine tegmentum. I use carbamazepine as the first drug for paroxysmal facial pain in MS patients. I have frequently found it necessary to gradually increase the dose until patients experience limiting toxicity. For patients who do not respond to or cannot tolerate carbamazepine, amitriptyline, phenytoin, or baclofen monotherapy are alternatives. If these are ineffective, patients may respond to the combination of perphenazine and amitriptyline (e.g., Triavil). Therapy is started at 2 mg perphenazine and 25 mg amitriptyline twice a day, with gradual weekly increments to a maximum of 12 mg perphenazine and 150 mg amitriptyline. Side effects

from perphenazine can be serious and include drug-induced parkinsonism, tardive dyskinesia, hepatitis, and the neuroleptic-malignant syndrome. When medical treatment fails, percutaneous trigeminal rhizotomy may result in relief.

Paroxysmal limb paresthesias present as brief tic-like pain, or less often burning dysesthesia lasting up to 1 minute. Treatment is similar to drug therapy for trigeminal neuralgia.

Chronic limb dysesthesia, commonly described as burning, tingling, or a crawling sensation, is often associated with progressive myelopathy, Lhermitte's phenomenon, or transverse myelitis. Many patients find tricyclic antidepressants effective, but the response rate is only 20 to 40 percent in my experience. Anticonvulsant drugs such as phenytoin may be tried, but I have not found it very effective. A transcutaneous electronic nerve stimulation unit and cognitive behavior therapy may be useful for patients who fail to respond to other measures.

Chronic back pain is extremely common and in most cases is due to mechanical stress caused by ataxia and weakness. In the absence of disc disease, pain rarely radiates below the knees. Therapy initially involves nonsteroidal anti-inflammatory drugs and physical therapy to improve posture and restore strength to abdominal and paraspinal muscles. Occasionally, prescription of a proper walking aid, ankle-foot orthosis, or proper seating in a wheelchair may be helpful. Leg pain, especially if it is radicular, extending below the knee to the ankle, should be investigated to exclude a herniated disc.

Pulmonary Dysfunction

Pulmonary dysfunction is not commonly recognized in MS but is common in nonambulatory patients. Patients do not complain of dyspnea, because oxygenation is maintained. Pulmonary function testing in the nonambulatory patient usually documents a pattern of restrictive pulmonary dysfunction, often with markedly impaired maximal expiratory pressures. I strongly discourage patients from cigarette smoking and recommend influenza and pneumococcal vaccination for nonambulatory MS patients. It is important to recognize that nonambulatory patients are at high risk of aspiration pneumonia, particularly with a fever. Pulmonary therapy has not been evaluated, but it may be useful for severely affected MS patients.

DISEASE PHARMACOTHERAPY

Steroids in Multiple Sclerosis Patients

More rapid recovery from attacks with corticotropin compared with placebo was documented in a multicenter trial in the mid-1960s. Since then, even though the relative value of adrenal corticosteroids has not been rigorously investigated, they have largely supplanted corticotropin in the treatment of MS attacks. Recent evidence suggests that large-dose pulses of IV methylprednisolone (MP) may have a more rapid onset of action and better efficacy than corticotropin or other steroid preparations. I use short courses of steroids for acute exacerbations. There is no evidence that long-term corticosteroid therapy slows or halts the progression of MS; this issue is currently the subject of a randomized clinical trial. Until additional evidence is forthcoming, steroids should be reserved for acute exacerbations. Furthermore, excessive or injudicious use of steroids should be avoided by restricting use to documented exacerbations of functional significance. For example, I treat patients with new leg weakness, loss of hand dexterity, or obvious visual deterioration, but I avoid using steroids for symptom fluctuations when there is no clear deterioration on the neurologic examination and no significant functional consequence. Physicians and patients are well aware of the gradual loss of steroid responsiveness with repeated steroid courses as the disease progresses. Patients typically reach a stage of steroid unresponsiveness. It is unclear whether this can be delayed or prevented by restricting use of steroids, but it appears prudent to do so.

For significant attacks, I use IV MP, administered in an outpatient setting. MP, 500 mg, is given IV daily for 3 days. Complete blood count and electrolytes are checked on days 1 and 3, and vital signs are monitored daily. Patients are treated with cimetidine or ranitidine as ulcer prophylaxis during the time they are taking steroids. Following the third MP infusion, prednisone, 60 mg, is administered in a single morning dose for 3 days, followed by tapering of the drug over the next 15 days in 10 mg decrements every 3 days. If clear deterioration occurs during the steroid taper, prednisone is tapered more slowly. In rare instances, patients may become "steroid dependent," in that they may be unable to withdraw from corticosteroids without exhibiting unequivocal clinical deterioration. Very slow tapering of steroids and conversion to alternate-day steroids can be tried. Long-acting oral steroids (e.g., dexamethasone) and divided doses are discouraged, because blood levels of exogenous steroids in the early morning hours suppress the normal endogenous surge of adrenocorticotropic hormone. This may result in adrenal atrophy within the 3 week treatment course.

This protocol has been tolerated well in my experience. Roughly 25 percent of patients have reported significant insomnia, which can be treated effectively with short-acting hypnotics. I have encountered significant depression on only one occasion, and that patient experienced recurrent severe depression that was unequivocally linked to MP treatment. Prophylaxis with lithium for a subsequent course of steroids totally abrogated depression in that patient. Patients commonly experience salt and fluid retention, which is managed by salt restriction, elastic stockings, and leg elevation. I never use diuretics, because of the risk of electrolyte derangements, particularly severe hypokalemia. Osteoporosis is a significant concern, particularly in a postmenopausal, immobile woman who repeatedly must take a course of steroid. Such patients are at increased risk for pathologic fractures. They should be treated with estrogen replacement, calcium, vitamin D, and physical therapy for mobilization. Caution should be used in the patient with known heart disease because of the possibility of congestive failure. Hypokalemia usually is not a problem in the absence of an independent cause of potassium wasting. Oral potassium should be administered to patients with heart disease or concurrent diuretic therapy and electrolytes are monitored carefully during therapy.

Immune Suppression in Multiple Sclerosis Patients

Most clinical trials of generalized immune suppression have found negative results or at best only modest efficacy. It is my opinion that immune suppression should be restricted to centers, generally within the context of a controlled clinical trial.

SUGGESTED READING

Rudick RA. Helping patients live with multiple sclerosis: What primary care physicians can do. Postgrad Med 1990; 88:197–207.

Rudick RA, Birk KA. Multiple sclerosis and pregnancy. In: Goldstein PJ, Stern BJ, ed. Neurologic disorders of pregnancy. 2nd rev ed. Mount Kisco, NY: Futura, 1992.

Rudick RA, Goodkin DE, eds. Treatment of multiple sclerosis: Trial design, results, and future perspectives. London: Springer-Verlag, 1992.

Rudick RA, Goodkin DE, Ransohoff RM. Pharmacotherapy of multiple sclerosis: Current status. Cleveland Clin J Med 1992; 59:267–277.

Rudick RA, Schiffer RB, Schwetz K, Herndon RM. Multiple sclerosis: The problem of misdiagnosis. Arch Neurol 1986; 43:578–584.

Shapiro RT. Symptom management in multiple sclerosis. New York: Demos, 1987.

Shapiro RT, ed. Multiple sclerosis. A rehabilitation approach to management. New York: Demos, 1991.

PATIENT RESOURCES

Associations

The Center for Independent Living is an advocacy organization that provides information and referral. It provides names of local organizations whose purpose is to help disabled persons maintain independence in the community.

The Health Insurance Association of America is a trade association and information resource for the American health insurance industry. It provides valuable educational services for the public.

National Multiple Sclerosis Society
733 3rd Avenue
New York, New York 10017-3288
(212) 986-3240.

National Multiple Sclerosis Society Information Resource Center offers information on a wide range of topics related to diagnosis, treatment, and research in MS. (800) LEARN MS.

National Multiple Sclerosis Society. Local Chapters offer information and referral; education; counseling; advocacy for services; and equipment assistance. Local numbers are available in area telephone directories or by calling the National MS Society at (212) 986-3240.

National Organization of Social Security Claimants' Representatives.
19 East Central Avenue
Pearl River, New York 10965
(914) 735-8812
A national organization of attorneys who will help with applications
and appeals of Social Security disability benefit denials.

Literature
Durgin RW, Lindsay N. The physically disabled traveler's guide.
Toledo, Ohio: Resource Directories, 1986.

Lechtenberg R. Multiple sclerosis fact book. Philadelphia: FA Davis,
1988.

Scheinberg LS, Holland NJ, eds. Multiple sclerosis: A guide for
patients and their families. New York: Raven Press, 1987.

Shuman R, Schwartz J. Understanding multiple sclerosis: A new
handbook for families. New York: Scribners, 1988.

Sibley WA, and the International Federation of Multiple Sclerosis
Societies, eds. Therapeutic claims in multiple sclerosis. New York:
Demos, 1988.

Strong M. Mainstay. For the well spouse of the chronically ill. Boston:
Little, Brown, 1988.

NEUROSARCOIDOSIS

JOEL C. MORGENLANDER, M.D.

Sarcoidosis is a multiple-system inflammatory granulomatous disease that frequently (prevalence 5 to 10 percent) has neurologic complications. In patients with previously diagnosed sarcoidosis, the occurrence of neurologic complications is more readily attributed to their underlying sarcoid; however, half of patients afflicted with neurosarcoidosis present with neurologic manifestations. Seventy-five percent of the patients who develop neurologic symptoms do so within the first 2 years of their diagnosis of sarcoid. For two-thirds of the patients the course is monophasic; one-third have a relapsing and remitting or progressive course. Most commonly, patients are between age 20 and 40 years, although children and older persons can be affected. In the United States, blacks are affected more often than whites, and there is no sex predominance.

NEUROLOGIC MANIFESTATIONS

The most common neurologic manifestation of sarcoidosis is cranial neuropathy, which occurs in approximately 50 percent of patients. The most frequent cranial neuropathy is a facial nerve palsy. This can be unilateral, bilateral, recurrent, or sequential. Other commonly involved cranial nerves include II, V, VIII, IX, and X. Aseptic meningitis occurs in 22 percent of all sarcoid patients and in 7 percent leads to either communicating or noncommunicating hydrocephalus. Parenchymal disease occurs in 48 percent of patients and most commonly results in hypothalamic dysfunction, but it may be manifested as an encephalopathy or vasculopathy, intracranial mass, myelopathy, headache, or stroke. Seizures result from parenchymal disease in 5 to 22 percent. Seizures may carry a poor prognosis because of the implied parenchymal damage, and these patients may have a more progressive course. Peripheral nerves

are affected in 17 percent of patients. Chronic sarcoidosis most often produces a predominantly sensorimotor axonal neuropathy, whereas acute sarcoid may cause a mononeuropathy, mononeuropathy multiplex, pure sensory neuropathy, Guillain-Barré syndrome, or cauda equina syndrome. There is overlap. Myopathy, seen in 15 percent, may be asymptomatic, nodular, acute, or chronic. Often the patient does not complain of proximal weakness but may have elevated muscle enzyme values or an abnormal muscle biopsy result.

Thus, there is a wide range of presentations of neurosarcoidosis. In a patient without known sarcoidosis these presentations need to be differentiated from other specific causes. For example, with multiple cranial neuropathies, diagnoses such as neurosyphilis, tuberculosis, carcinomatous meningitis, isolated angiitis of the central nervous system (CNS), and Lyme disease would need to be entertained. Periventricular parenchymal disease may result from multiple sclerosis, Sjögren's syndrome, systemic lupus erythematosus, or Behçet's syndrome. With optic neuropathy, one must consider multiple sclerosis, neurosyphilis, tuberculosis, Behçet's syndrome, and toxoplasmosis. A myopathy may suggest polymyositis and may be differentiated only by biopsy specimen demonstrating nonconsenting granulomas. Differential diagnosis of neuropathy would depend on the specific type of presentation. Finally, human immunodeficiency virus (HIV) infection may also present with many of the manifestations seen in neurosarcoidosis.

Recurrent neurosarcoidosis most often involves the area previously involved.

DIAGNOSTIC APPROACH

The diagnostic approach to a patient without known sarcoidosis is based on the possibility that the neurologic symptoms are due to sarcoidosis and investigating sites that are most commonly abnormal in systemic sarcoidosis (Table 1). General physical examination may demonstrate specific locations of abnormality that are accessible to biopsy. Frequently involved are the lung, lymph nodes, skin, and eyes. The chest film is abnormal in 80 to 90 percent, and lung biopsy can be performed

Table 1 Core Evaluation for Neurosarcoidosis

Physical examination
Chest radiograph
Serum calcium value
Serum angiotensin-converting enzyme level
Ophthalmologic consult (including slit-lamp examination)
Brain MRI with contrast, spinal cord MRI for appropriate
    symptoms
CSF examination: IgG index and oligoclonal bands
Creatine kinase level and electromyography for appropriate
    symptoms
Biopsy of involved tissue: skin, lymph node, conjunctiva, lacrimal
    gland, lung

bronchoscopically. Bronchoalveolar lavage may show increased T lymphocytes and increased T4-T8 ratio, nonspecific findings but suggestive of sarcoidosis. The Kveim-Siltzbach test is positive in 98 percent of patients with active sarcoid, but antigen is not commonly available in the United States. Gallium scintigraphy, sensitive but not specific, may demonstrate typical sites of involvement accessible to biopsy.

Elevation of serum angiotensin-converting enzyme (ACE) level is not specific for sarcoid but can be found in 40 to 90 percent of patients. Other disorders that may increase the serum ACE include diabetes mellitus, cirrhosis, hyperthyroidism, Gaucher's disease, and other pulmonary conditions such as tuberculosis and lung cancer. These disorders are often recognized clinically, so confusion in the evaluation of neurologic disease is rare. In sarcoid, the serum ACE level may follow the clinical activity of disease. ACE levels are higher in children. Alternately, if a patient is taking an ACE inhibitor, the level could be artificially low.

It is possible for the serum ACE level to be normal while the cerebrospinal fluid ACE level is elevated. Normally it is 30 times higher in serum than in cerebrospinal fluid (CSF). If the blood-brain barrier is compromised, as in inflammatory conditions such as meningitis or immune conditions such as multiple sclerosis or Guillain-Barré syndrome, the CSF level will rise. In sarcoidosis, it is theorized that CNS ACE is produced by macrophages in the CNS. The CSF ACE level may decrease with treatment of the underlying disorder. It is unlikely in routine cases that a CSF ACE level will help in diagnosis.

Owing to the inflammatory reaction, the immunoglobulin G (IgG) index can be elevated in sarcoidosis, and rarely oligoclonal bands are present. Usually the increase in IgG is polyclonal, and oligoclonal bands are absent, a differentiating point from multiple sclerosis. Frequently cerebrospinal fluid exhibits pleocytosis, predominantly of lymphocytes. Total protein is often elevated, and, rarely, glucose is decreased.

Neuroradiologic imaging is helpful for diagnosis. Magnetic resonance imaging (MRI) is more sensitive than computed tomography (CT) for identifying sarcoid-related abnormalities. Without the use of enhancement, periventricular lesions appear identical to those of multiple sclerosis. With the use of enhancement (gado-

pentetate dimeglumine) leptomeningeal abnormality typical of sarcoidosis can be demonstrated. Lesions involving the dura, hypothalamus, pituitary, and gray matter also help to separate the MRI findings from those of multiple sclerosis. CT can show hydrocephalus or enhancing hemispheric abnormality, but MRI is more sensitive, especially in periventricular and hypothalamic areas.

Visual, somatosensory, and brain stem evoked potential studies can be abnormal in the absence of clinical disease. Nerve conduction studies can show subclinical peripheral nerve involvement, which may help to differentiate neurosarcoidosis from central disorders.

In patients with sarcoidosis, separating sarcoid from steroid myopathy can be difficult. In either granulomas can be evident on muscle biopsy. Diminishing strength during steroid dose tapering, elevated muscle enzyme levels, and electromyography (EMG) demonstrating diffuse increase in spontaneous activity are all clues to the diagnosis of active sarcoid myopathy. A diagnostic trial of prednisone in larger doses may be necessary.

Ocular abnormalities are found in 25 to 50 percent of patients with sarcoidosis. A slit-lamp examination is useful for detecting uveitis, iridocyclitis, or keratoconjunctivitis. Conjunctiva or lacrimal gland is accessible for biopsy when either structure is clinically involved. Blind biopsy has a low yield. Optic atrophy secondary to external compression of the optic nerve, papilledema, and granulomas of the optic nerve may be evident.

It is difficult to distinguish sarcoid optic neuropathy from demyelinating optic neuritis. Atypical findings for demyelinating optic neuritis include progressive vision loss over 2 weeks and visual fields that show extensive field loss. The typical pattern seen in demyelinating optic neuritis is of a central scotoma with peripheral field constriction without progressive loss over an extended period.

To confirm the diagnosis of sarcoidosis a biopsy showing noncaseating granuloma or a positive Kveim test is recommended.

THERAPY

There has not been a randomized double-blind clinical trial of any specific therapy. Also, the rate of spontaneous remissions of clinical symptoms is high.

Symptomatic meningitic, parenchymal, peripheral nerve, or muscle disease is initially treated with prednisone. Patients with a single cranial neuropathy may start with 40 to 60 mg per day, whereas patients with significant parenchymal disease or myopathy start with 60 to 80 mg per day. The initial dose is maintained for 1 month, and perhaps longer, depending on clinical response. Weaning to an alternate-day regimen is done by reducing the alternate-day dose 10 mg weekly. Subsequent weaning by 10 mg is done monthly or bimonthly until the dose is 30 mg every other day, then further weaning is by 5 mg monthly. The rapidity of the weaning depends on clinical response and the neurologic manifestations treated. Single cranial or peripheral nerve abnormalities would be treated with more rapid weaning than more significant disease. Hydrocephalus due to parenchymal and meningeal disease should be treated with steroids first; if there is no response the patient will need a shunt. A mass of the CNS should be treated initially with steroids. If response is poor, a stereotaxic biopsy should be obtained. Approximately 90 percent of symptoms improve with steroid therapy.

For recurrent symptoms, the steroid dose is usually doubled or increased to the original starting dose, depending on severity of symptoms. Taper is once again initiated, although at a slower rate. For significant disability, hospitalization for 5 days' treatment with intravenous methylprednisolone, 500 mg every 6 hours may be necessary.

For patients with seizures, steroids should be used in conjunction with antiepileptic drugs. There is no interference with absorption or effectiveness.

For resistant cerebral, spinal, or ocular disease, localized radiation therapy may be of additional benefit. Other immunosuppressive agents, including cyclosporine, methotrexate, azathioprine, and chlorambucil, can be of use in severely affected patients who do not respond to large daily doses of prednisone. These therapies must be used with caution, owing to side effects.

Complications of long-term steroid use, such as CNS infection and myopathy, must be considered in the differential diagnosis when new symptoms arise in the treated patient with neurosarcoidosis.

Multisystem involvement in patients with sarcoidosis requires consultation with other physicians, including internists, pulmonologists, endocrinologists, and ophthalmologists. Rehabilitation is indicated for any patient who has a significant sensory or motor deficit or when cognitive effects inhibit normal activities of daily living.

SUGGESTED READING

Graham E, James DG. Neurosarcoidosis. Sarcoidosis 1988; 5:125–131.

Lieberman J. Enzymes in sarcoidosis. Clin Lab Med 1989; 9:745–755.

Schweisfurth H, Schiöberg-Schiegnitz S, Kuhn W, Parusel B. Angiotensin I converting enzyme in cerebrospinal fluid of patients with neurologic diseases. Klin Wochenschr 1987; 65:955–958.

Sherman JL, Stern BJ. Sarcoidosis of the CNS: Comparison of unenhanced and enhanced MR images. AJNR 1990; 11:915–923.

Stern BJ. Neurosarcoidosis. Neurol Chron 1992; 2:1–6.

PATIENT RESOURCE

National Sarcoidosis Foundation
Box 22868
Newark, New Jersey 07101
Telephone: (800) 223-6429

CEREBROVASCULAR DISEASES

TRANSIENT ISCHEMIC ATTACKS

CONSTANCE J. MEYD, M.D., M.S.

A transient ischemic attack (TIA) is a reversible focal neurologic deficit referable to a vascular distribution that lasts less than 24 hours. This clinical definition does not predict abnormalities of structure or function as seen on imaging studies — brain computed tomography (CT) or magnetic resonance imaging (MRI) — or electroencephalography (EEG), though most patients' studies are negative. A deficit that lasts longer than 24 hours but not weeks has been termed a reversible ischemic neurologic deficit (RIND), a term that has not been particularly useful in clinical decision making, and it is generally regarded as a minor stroke even when CT or MRI findings are negative. Most TIAs last several minutes and consist principally of negative symptoms (i.e., loss of function, such as weakness, heaviness, numbness, aphasia, diplopia, or visual field deficits). Positive phenomena such as scintillating scotoma and involuntary movements more likely represent migraine or seizure, both important diagnoses to exclude. TIAs are predictive of increased stroke risk and should be considered a neurologic emergency to be evaluated promptly. Two basic questions need to be addressed for any patient with TIAs: what is the vascular territory and what is the mechanism? The importance of vascular territory relates to prompt surgical intervention in patients with high-grade carotid disease and to the use of heparin in patients with threatened basilar occlusion.

MECHANISM

In the majority of cases, the mechanism of TIAs is embolism, either artery-to-artery (atherothrombotic disease) or cardiogenic. Atherothrombotic disease is secondary to underlying atherosclerotic plaque, a diffuse process with a predilection for large extracranial vessels. The carotid bifurcation, distal vertebrals, and takeoffs of the great vessels at the aortic arch are the most common sites of disease, becoming nidi for platelet-fibrin aggre-gates, which then fragment and embolize to distal intracranial branches. Occasionally, the intracranial vessels are primarily involved, with the carotid siphon, middle cerebral artery, and the basilar artery the most frequent sites of disease. Intracranial disease occurs with greatest frequency in black males and should also be suspected in patients who have no extracranial disease and no cardiac source.

The most common cardiac conditions that result in brain embolism are chronic atrial fibrillation, valve disease, and recent myocardial infarction.

When a vascular or cardiac source is not found, less frequent causes such as vasculitis, dissection, spasm, and hypercoagulable conditions should be considered, though in at least a third of cases no source is found. Historical features are not helpful in separating vascular from cardiac causes but are useful in diagnosing migraine, seizure, syncope, and hypoglycemia, all important mimics of TIA. The examination should be tailored to detecting retinal emboli, carotid and supraclavicular bruits, blood pressure difference between arms, and subtle residual neurologic signs (Table 1). The physician often must use a series of clues to localize the process; for example, a right retinal embolus in a patient with ill-defined left arm symptoms clearly predicts right carotid disease.

VASCULAR LOCALIZATION

Symptoms of anterior circulation ischemia include monocular visual obscuration (amaurosis fugax), mono- and hemiparesis, sensory loss in one or both extremities on one side, aphasia, and occasionally field deficits. The only absolute is amaurosis, as the retinal artery is the first major intracranial branch of the internal carotid artery. The classic description is an altitudinal loss, often incomplete and likened to looking through lace or cobwebs in the upper or lower half of the visual field. Complete monocular blackout of vision also occurs. Unfortunately, many patients do not cover each eye in turn and have ill-defined obscurations that defy clinical localization. The clinical impression of amaurosis may be completely reversed by detection of occipital infarction on scan. Language deficits almost always result from middle cerebral artery ischemia. Perhaps most problem-

Table 1 Physical Examination for Suspected Transient Ischemic Attacks

Finding	Significance
Blood pressure, both arms	Difference reflects proximal arch disease; clue to subclavian steal syndrome
Pulse	Irregularity suggests atrial fibrillation
Auscultation of carotid arteries and supraclavicular fossa	Bruits correlate with atherosclerotic disease
Palpation of superficial temporal, facial, and occipital arteries	Differences side to side suggest collateral flow secondary to atherosclerotic disease
Fundoscopic examination	Changes secondary to hypertension and diabetes suggest systemic disease; retinal emboli suggest carotid bifurcation disease

atic is intermittent weakness in an extremity, often described as "heaviness" or "numbness." Alone, this is not localizing and could involve anterior (cortical or deep) or posterior circulation. In the absence of amaurosis or a language deficit the extremity weakness should be considered sufficient cause to screen the anterior circulation with a noninvasive study, either duplex or magnetic resonance angiography (MRA).

Posterior circulation symptoms include field deficits, diplopia, ataxia, vertigo, hemiparesis, crossed motor and sensory symptoms (face on one side, limbs on the other). Dysarthria and dysphagia are not localizing except by the company they keep; both indicate oral-pharyngeal weakness secondary to a lesion anywhere in the corticospinal or peripheral pathways. Dysarthria in conjunction with aphasia or amaurosis is anterior disease, whereas dysarthria with diplopia is posterior disease. Vertigo alone is rarely secondary to cerebrovascular disease, however with ataxia and hemisensory signs medullary ischemia would be likely.

DIAGNOSTIC STUDIES

The initial laboratory data help to exclude systemic disease (diabetes, hepatic, renal, connective tissue) as a cause of symptoms, and the extent of laboratory testing depends on the clinical certainty of the diagnosis. A reasonable screen for all patients includes complete blood count, prothrombin time, partial thromboplastin time, erythrocyte sedimentation rate, serum test for syphilis, chemistry panel, urinalysis, and electrocardiography (ECG).

Vascular localization and mechanism are subject to confirmation with diagnostic studies. Duplex scanning of the carotid arteries is an excellent screen for carotid bifurcation disease, the most frequent site of atherosclerotic plaque. A completely normal scan or insignificant disease (less than 30 percent stenosis) virtually rules out

the extracranial carotid as the source of TIA symptoms. Disease in the 30 to 99 percent range should be confirmed with intra-arterial angiography. The indirect tests, oculopneumoplethysography (OPG) and supraorbital Doppler (SOD) ultrasonography, detect hemodynamically significant bifurcation disease and can be used as adjuncts to duplex or MRA.

MRA is a promising noninvasive technique for visualizing the extra- and intracranial circulation; however, resolution for definition of carotid bifurcation disease remains to be further validated against conventional angiography. For patients without an extracranial source of symptoms, the intracranial circulation can be non-invasively studied with MRA or transcranial Doppler (TCD). The latter study measures velocities in the major intracranial branches and ophthalmic arteries, providing an indirect flow measurement. Used alone or in conjunction with MRA, TCD is very useful for evaluating middle cerebral artery and basilar disease. Intra-arterial angiography remains the gold standard for evaluating structural lesions. The extent of the study should be tailored to the clinical presentation, but in general, both carotids and a vertebral should be studied. An aortic arch study is usually reserved for cases of suspected proximal disease as evidenced by vessel-specific symptoms in the absence of carotid bifurcation disease or with posterior symptoms and blood pressure difference between arms. The extent of carotid bifurcation disease has been standardized by the North American Symptomatic Carotid Endarterectomy (NASCET) and Asymptomatic Carotid Atherosclerosis Study (ACAS) groups. The percentage of stenosis is calculated from the formula

$$\text{Stenosis } (\%) = 1 - \frac{\text{MRL}}{\text{DRL}} \times 100$$

where the MRL is the minimal residual lumen measured at the narrowest portion and the DRL is the distal residual lumen measured distal to the stenosis at a point where the walls of the internal carotid artery have become parallel. When the DRL is diminished secondary to poststenotic flow reduction, the calculation is spurious and the extent of stenosis is deemed to exceed 95 percent.

A cardiac evaluation is indicated for all TIA patients—cardiac history, examination, and ECG—as coronary artery disease is common in patients with cerebrovascular disease. When the mechanism of TIA is probably cardioembolic further studies are usually done: transthoracic echocardiography or transesophageal echocardiography for valve and chamber abnormalities and Holter monitoring to detect arrhythmias.

A brain imaging study, either CT or MRI, detects silent and previously symptomatic infarctions, and occasionally detects unsuspected hemorrhage, subdural hematoma, or tumor. Electroencephalography is useful when the diagnosis is in doubt (a study positive for focal abnormality in the region of clinical interest may clinch the diagnosis) or when seizure is suspected.

TREATMENT

Atherothrombotic Disease

For patients with greater than 70 percent carotid stenosis and hemispheric or ocular TIAs prompt carotid endarterectomy (CEA) is indicated. If the disease is preocclusive (MRL <1 mm) intravenous heparin is given until surgery can be performed. For 30 to 69 percent stenosis, medical therapy (antiplatelet) versus surgery (endarterectomy) is still being evaluated in the NASCET Study. For patients who cannot or will not be NASCET subjects, the decision to treat medically or surgically depends on physician preference and patient risk factors. A reasonable choice would be antiplatelet therapy as a first attempt, reserving carotid endarterectomy for patients whose TIAs persist or who are young, at low surgical risk, and have greater than 50 percent disease. Preoperative cardiac consultation is recommended. Patients with less than 30 percent stenosis have not been shown to benefit from surgery and should be treated medically with antiplatelet drugs.

Antiplatelet therapy includes aspirin or ticlopidine. The recommended dose of aspirin has varied widely. A reasonable starting dose is 325 mg daily as an enteric coated tablet. If symptoms recur, adjusting the dosage to 650 mg twice daily remains an option. For patients who fail aspirin therapy or who are aspirin intolerant, ticlopidine is started, 250 mg twice daily. There is no dose titration. This drug is much more complicated to monitor: blood counts and neutrophil counts are required every 2 weeks, because neutropenia is a rare but potentially fatal side effect. Other limiting side effects are rash and diarrhea, the latter characterized by numerous stools rather than ones of a different consistency. Dipyridamole is not effective and is no longer used for TIA.

Anticoagulation with warfarin sodium (Coumadin) is reserved for nonoperative high-grade stenosis cases or those in whom antiplatelet therapy fails.

For patients with posterior circulation TIAs, the most threatening situation is impending basilar occlusion from atherosclerotic disease, which often manifests as crescendo TIAs. These patients are best managed on intravenous heparin, with careful attention to maintaining adequate blood pressure. They should be cared for at bed rest in an intensive care unit until their condition is stable and can be switched to Coumadin and can slowly increase their activity. These patients should undergo prompt cerebral angiography as noninvasive studies can only rule in, not rule out, significant basilar disease. If significant basilar stenosis is present the coumadin should be continued indefinitely. If it is not present, then coumadin can be continued for 3 to 6 months, at which time aspirin can be started.

Attention to risk factor management is indicated for all cases: smoking cessation and control of hypertension, diabetes, and hyperlipidemia. Many patients benefit from a frank discussion of the contribution of these factors to progression of atherosclerotic disease.

Cardiogenic Embolus

Patients whose source of brain embolus is chronic atrial fibrillation or rheumatic valvular disease should be treated with Coumadin on a long-term basis. In general, these patients should be admitted and placed on an intravenous heparin regimen, to protect them from further clot formation until Coumadin is therapeutic. A modest level of anticoagulation (1.3 to 1.5 times control) appears to protect against stroke.

Patients who recently suffered a myocardial infarction are anticoagulated acutely and maintained on coumadin at least 6 weeks. If an akinetic segment is detected on ECG, long-term Coumadin therapy is indicated; otherwise patients can then switch to aspirin.

Patients with both carotid atherosclerotic disease and a potential cardiac source are common. If the ipsilateral carotid disease is 70 percent or greater, CEA should be considered in the context of the increased risk of the cardiac condition. This is not a well-defined area. At one end of the spectrum are patients with chronic atrial fibrillation who can undergo operation without a major increase in risk. In contrast, the patient with a recent myocardial infarction and high-grade symptomatic disease should be managed medically with heparin, and then Coumadin. CEA could be considered at 4 to 6 months.

SUGGESTED READING

North American Symptomatic Carotid Endarterectomy Trial Collaborators. Beneficial effect of carotid endarterectomy in symptomatic patients with high-grade carotid stenosis. N Engl J Med 1991; 325:445–453.

ACUTE ISCHEMIC STROKE

STEPHEN M. OPPENHEIMER, M.B., M.R.C.P.,
FRCPC, F.A.C.T.

The past 5 years have seen an explosive increase in the understanding of the metabolic and parenchymal effects of stroke. The concept of therapeutic cytoprotection (the protection of prejudiced tissue at risk of death following ischemic insult) has burgeoned. Cytoprotective agents show considerable promise in studies in vitro and in animals, especially when administered before or immediately after experimental arterial occlusion, but controlled human clinical trials of these agents have demonstrated limited benefit. Despite this, I anticipate that the current fervor of research will produce effective cytoprotective therapies within the next few years.

In this chapter I outline a personal view of the medical management of the acute ischemic stroke and its complications, together with a consideration of new therapies of cytoprotection, reperfusion, and secondary prevention. An algorithm is offered in Figure 1 for the suggested investigation and management of the ischemic stroke victim.

PATHOPHYSIOLOGY

Therapeutic nihilism stems from the erroneous concept that after arterial occlusion all cerebral tissue within the considered distribution immediately becomes defunct. In the early 1980s, evidence accumulated that experimental occlusion of either the middle cerebral or carotid artery produces a central core of tissue that immediately dies but is surrounded by viable but functionally inert tissue (the penumbra). The blood supply to this region is substantially reduced but is not as poor as in the infarct core. If penumbral blood supply is restored, function may be recovered. Cerebral tissue also possesses variable ability to resist ischemia, dying only if

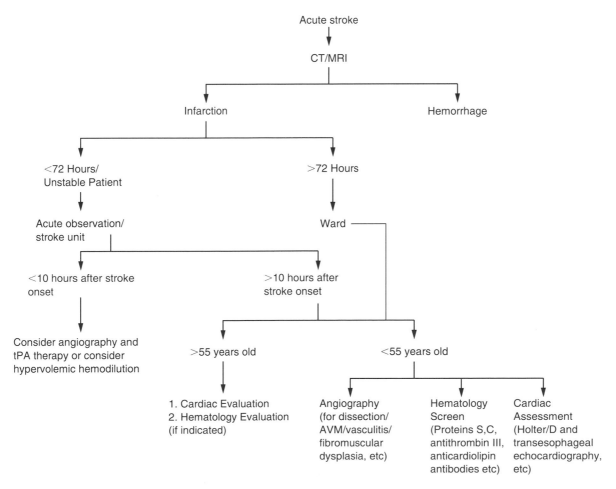

Figure 1 Suggested approach to investigation and management of the ischemic stroke victim. Key: tPA = tissue plasminogen activator; AVM = arteriovenous malformation.

this is prolonged. Therefore, a temporal window exists following an ischemic insult during which tissue remains viable. There are regional differences in the duration of the temporal window.

Recent positron emission tomography (PET), single photon emission computed tomography (SPECT), and magnetic resonance (MR) spectroscopy studies indicate the existence of the ischemic penumbra following stroke in humans. The interventions discussed below are aimed at increasing the viability of the ischemic penumbra and restoring it to normal function.

MEDICAL MANAGEMENT (FIGURE 2)

Blood Glucose

The blood glucose level is elevated in nearly a quarter of all stroke patients admitted to hospital. In some patients (especially those with mild elevation), this represents a response to stress. Others are known diabetics. However, a significant percentage of patients (6 percent) are previously undiagnosed diabetics (identified by elevated glycosylated HbA_{1c} levels) who have a markedly elevated random blood glucose level (>10 mM per liter). The prognosis for these patients during the first week and for those with known diabetes is poor. Mortality and infarct size are increased. Animal studies have shown that chronic or transiently elevated blood sugar is similarly disadvantageous in experimental stroke. I would therefore suggest instituting intravenous insulin therapy on a graded scale when blood glucose is at least 10 mmol per liter, in an attempt to protect the ischemic penumbra, which is poised on a metabolic knife edge. The optimal blood glucose range should lie between 6 and 9 mM per liter. In addition, it is probably unwise to administer intravenous glucose during the acute phase of stroke.

Hypoglycemia may present with either transient or permanent focal neurologic deficits. Most frequently, this is due to unbalanced exogenous insulin administration; less commonly, it is the presenting feature of medical rareties such as insulinoma or retroperitoneal sarcoma. Management obviously involves the administration of glucose and treatment of the underlying condition.

Blood Pressure

Approximately 80 percent of stroke patients are hypertensive on admission. In part, this reflects the primacy of hypertension as a stroke risk factor, but also the possible effects of the stroke itself on central autonomic control. Under normal circumstances cerebral autoregulation ensures that cerebral blood flow remains constant over a wide range of mean arterial pressure. Following stroke, the ability to autoregulate is lost in the environs of the infarct. Elevated blood pressure therefore poses a theoretical risk for bland stroke transformation into a hemorrhagic infarct. Yet convincing clinical confirmation of this circumstance is lacking. Conversely, lowering the mean arterial pressure to a level where cerebral blood supply is compromised might encourage stroke extension. The precise level at which blood pressure therapy should be instituted remains controversial. It is recommended that it begin at a higher range, generally with a mean arterial pressure of 130 to 140 mm Hg for patients with a history of hypertension. Treatment should be instituted with intravenous rapidly metabolized agents (such as sodium nitroprusside or labetalol), so that the dose can be titrated against the blood pressure value with little hangover effect. It should be remembered that hypertensive patients show arterial changes and that they appear to autoregulate at higher levels than their normotensive counterparts. Consequently, the lower blood pressure that such patients may be able to sustain without stroke extension may be less than that in normotensive patients.

Periods of hypotension may also occur after stroke and may be due to cardiac arrhythmias or a central effect

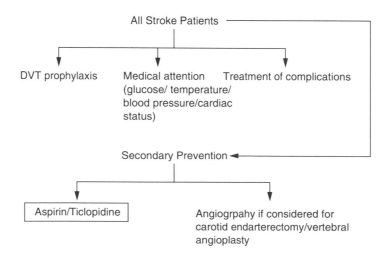

Figure 2 Medical management of stroke patients.

of the stroke on autonomic function. These have not received the attention they deserve, possibly because monitoring of intra-arterial pressure in stroke patients is an exception rather than the rule that it should be. Such hypotensive periods may lead to decreased blood supply to the penumbra and stroke extension. Consequently, patients should be monitored intensively for cardiac arrhythmias and hypotensive episodes over the first 3 days after stroke onset. These should be treated with appropriate antiarrhythmic agents; hypotensive medication should be abandoned if associated with such periods, and, if necessary, inotropes administered.

Body Temperature

Recently, attention has been focused on the role of body temperature and stroke prognosis. This follows the observation that the cytoprotective effects of the NMDA receptor antagonist MK 801 may be explicable in part by the 2° or 3°C hypothermia that the agent induces. Previously, Hindfelt showed that 44 percent of stroke patients were hyperthermic on admission. This was generally attributed to coincident infection (respiratory or urinary tract) or deep vein thrombosis rather than to the stroke itself. It was, however, shown that outcome at 3 months (as assessed by mortality and stroke score performance) was significantly worse with even slight increases of temperature (1°C). Recent animal studies have shown that a 2° or 3°C fall in body temperature may reduce infarct volume by 80 to 100 percent. Hyperthermia in these animal models is associated with alterations in blood-brain barrier permeability, intracerebral acidosis, impaired cerebral energy metabolism, and with changes in the release of excitotoxic amino acids. These deleterious effects can be overcome by cooling. It is prudent, therefore, to investigate fever vigorously in acute stroke patients and to treat underlying infections as soon as possible. The addition of an antipyretic agent such as aspirin should be considered. Trials are currently under way to investigate the clinical benefit of hypothermia in acute stroke.

Prophylaxis of Deep Vein Thrombosis

Deep vein thrombosis contributes to adverse stroke outcome by causing low-grade fever, and also by pulmonary embolism, which can be either catastrophic or insidious (in which case it can result in progressive hypoxia). Deep vein thrombosis is detected in 53 percent of paretic legs following stroke, 9 percent of such patients in Warlow's study developed pulmonary embolism. There appears to be no correlation with age, obesity, days spent in bed, or the severity of motor impairment. Prophylaxis with antiembolism stockings is prudent for all ischemic stroke patients, as is low-dose heparin therapy (5,000 units twice daily), except for those with mass effect from hemorrhagic transformation.

REPERFUSION TECHNIQUES

Reperfusion of ischemic tissue represents a logical approach to the treatment of stroke; however, there are certain conceptual caveats. First, reperfusion of such tissue could generate free radicals and exacerbate ischemic damage. Second, hemorrhage might ensue from the re-establishment of blood flow through vessels distal to the occlusion that themselves may be injured by ischemia. Third, it is not clear how long tissue remains viable and is salvageable by such methods. Finally, ischemic capillary damage can produce endothelial swelling, which compounds the thrombotic occlusion (no-reflow phenomenon). Reperfusion techniques would not be expected to overcome this circumstance. This said, two methods are currently available: hemodilution and thrombolytic therapy. Hemodilution may be either isovolemic (when a volume of blood is withdrawn equal to that of the diluting agent) or hypervolemic. The aim is to lower the hematocrit value and thereby decrease plasma viscosity (there is a linear relationship between the two), thus encouraging flow. However, blood shows nonlinear rheologic properties, and the precise effect in the cerebral capillaries is unclear. Other postulated mechanisms include cardiac output augmentation and the effect of reduced blood oxygen-carrying capacity producing cerebral vasodilatation and thereby increased blood flow in the ischemic penumbra. Two agents are currently used: dextran 40 and pentastarch. The latter has several theoretical advantages over dextran, including no anaphylactic reactions, kidney complications, or accumulation in the body. Neither isovolemic nor hypervolemic hemodilution has proven an unmitigated success in the treatment of ischemic stroke. This may be because few studies have investigated rapid lowering of the hematocrit within hours of stroke onset. Available data favor hypervolemic techniques with rapid dilution (within 12 to 24 hours) achieving a hematocrit value of 30 to 35 percent. Hypervolemic hemodilution is contraindicated in patients with congestive cardiac failure or renal failure.

Thrombolytic therapy has been advocated as another reperfusion technique. The earliest methods used parenteral intravenous streptokinase, with unacceptable hemorrhagic side effects. More recently, infusions of urokinase or streptokinase locally to the thrombosed vessel have been employed, as have local or parenteral infusions of tissue plasminogen activator (tPA). The former agents degrade fibrinogen and factors V and VIII, whereas the latter activates plasminogen, which itself is fibrinolytic. Theoretical disadvantages of the technique involve dissolution of the clot with distal embolization and hemorrhagic transformation of a bland infarct. The latter has proven to be a concern in several trials and may occur in 10 to 30 percent of cases. Although there have been many thrombolytic trials, consensus is difficult to achieve. This is because many of the studies involved small numbers of patients and different regimens of different thrombolytic agents administe ed at various times after the stroke. On balance, thrombolysis may prove of benefit in strokes of small to medium size (where the risk of hemorrhagic transformation is reduced) if instituted within 6 to 10 hours of stroke onset and in the posterior circulation, where there is a profuse collateral blood supply. Currently, a much-needed double-blind randomized trial is taking place evaluating the role of tPA, 0.9 mg per kilogram IV over 60 minutes, against a placebo. The regimen for local urokinase therapy as used at The Johns Hopkins Hospital employs an infusion of 250,000 units over 30 minutes followed by further infusion of 250,000 to 750,000 units over 4 hours. This is followed by systemic heparin therapy to prevent rethrombosis of the vessel.

CYTOPROTECTION

An alternative approach to salvaging the ischemic penumbra would be to administer agents that protect cells in this region. The concept of excitotoxicity implies that accumulation of neurotransmitters in inordinate amounts may actually damage cells on which they play a primarily informational role. This has been described for glutamate acting through NMDA or AMPA-Kainate receptors. Efficacy of glutamate antagonists in vitro has been promising, as have animal studies in which the agent is administered before stroke induction. When they are administered after experimental stroke, however, the results have, in general, been disappointing. As yet, there are no commercially available glutamate antagonists for use in humans.

An alternative approach would be to antagonize the intracellular effects of excitotoxins. Experimental evidence suggests that the lethal effects of glutamate are exerted through accumulation of intracellular calcium, which in turn activates proteases and other destructive enzymes. Calcium channel blockers have been used for many years for control of hypertension. Many do not cross the blood-brain barrier, although nimodipine is successful in this respect and has some specificity for the alpha subunit of brain voltage–operated L calcium channels. A small double-blind controlled trial suggested that some clinical efficacy could be expected with nimodipine, 30 mg every 6 hours for 4 weeks after stroke, though benefit was confined to moderately and severely affected patients. Systemic effects on blood pressure have proven to be more of a theoretical disadvantage.

MANAGEMENT OF THE COMPLICATIONS OF ACUTE ISCHEMIC STROKE

Hemorrhagic transformation occurs in 30 percent of all ischemic strokes and in 70 percent of those presumed to be of cardioembolic origin. However, only 17 percent of such patients show signs of neurologic deterioration, and this is more frequent with strokes of large volume that show mass effect. In deteriorating patients reduction of intracranial pressure is warranted with mannitol or furosemide or both; hematoma evacuation may be

contemplated, especially for cerebellar infarction, where the compactness of the posterior fossa ensures that increases of volume compromise the brain stem.

The precise incidence of cerebral edema after infarction is unclear. Autopsy studies suggest 90 percent in this selected population, whereas CT studies have produced lower figures—around 40 percent. Only when the lesion produces mass effect do such patients demonstrate evidence of neurologic deterioration. Treatment with mannitol and/or furosemide is the mainstay of therapy. Steroids have not been shown to be beneficial.

Seizures occur in 10 percent of ischemic strokes, 33 percent within the first 2 weeks. Their presence does not adversely affect prognosis, and they are generally easily controlled with monotherapy.

THE DETERIORATING STROKE

Stroke progression occurs in 20 to 40 percent of patients admitted in the acute stage. Several studies indicate that it is more common following vertebrobasilar than hemispheric infarction. Progression may occur at any time but is most frequent within the first week. Likewise, progression appears more commonly following large vessel occlusion than lacunar infarction. Deterioration seems especially likely with cerebellar infarction. Understandably, the prognosis worsens if the stroke progresses: mortality is 27 percent compared to 5 percent for patients who became stable within 24 hours of admission.

The pathogenesis of progression is unclear. In some cases it is undoubtedly due to extension of thrombosis by accretion in situ with subsequent blockage of perforating vessels in the brain stem or vital collateral vessels in the hemisphere. Distal embolization of friable clot may also be a mechanism. Progression of a stenotic lesion to complete occlusion may also occur with subsequent deterioration. All of these mechanisms have been observed in angiographic investigations of deteriorating patients, but such studies have involved small numbers and their representative nature is questionable. Other causes of deterioration include the accumulation of cerebral edema and hemorrhagic conversion, both when associated with mass effect. In view of the precarious existence of the penumbra, however, it seems reasonable to assume that in some situations deterioration may relate to the patient's general medical condition. In the first instance it is suggested that a search be made for contributing metabolic and physiologic derangements: disorders of blood sugar, cardiac output, blood pressure, and cardiac rhythm. These should be corrected, as discussed above. Infections should be treated and pyrexia brought under control. Dehydration, which can be associated with increased plasma viscosity, can also result in stroke progression and should be treated. Hypoxia, which may result from infection but also commonly from silent pulmonary embolism, should be sought and treated. Hyponatremia may occur in 10 percent of infarctions; the cause may be related to inappropriate antidiuretic hormone (ADH) secretion and can be associated with stroke progression. In this case, fluid restriction is required. Recently, some cases of hyponatremia have been associated with increased secretion of atrial natriuretic factor (ANF), in which case patients are likely to be dehydrated. Therefore, the investigation of hyponatremia should include measurements of plasma and urine osmolality, to distinguish this syndrome from that of inappropriate ADH secretion. Clearly, patients with hyponatremia due to ANF increases should be rehydrated.

While metabolic factors are being sought, intracerebral causes of deterioration should also be investigated. These include hemorrhage, increasing cerebral edema with mass effect, and hydrocephalus due to acqueduct stenosis secondary to brain stem edema. In addition, further embolization from a cardiac cause should be considered. Edema can be treated with mannitol and furosemide; hematomas can be evacuated if measures to reduce intracranial pressure fail. Hydrocephalus may be treated with shunting. The deteriorating cerebellar infarct should be referred for posterior fossa decompression.

If none of these factors is operant and deterioration seems likely to be caused by thrombus propagation, the conventional therapy has involved anticoagulation with heparin, although there are no convincing studies of its benefit in progressing cerebral infarction. When instituted, with the PTT ratio kept between 1.5 and 2, hemorrhagic complications appear minimal. Other measures that should be contemplated include angiography and administration of local thrombolytic therapy to the appropriate vessel in an attempt to produce reperfusion. No controlled trials of this therapy have yet been conducted. Hypervolemic hemoperfusion may also be considered in this circumstance.

STROKE IN PREGNANCY

The investigation and management of pregnant stroke patients requires some consideration. The incidence of ischemic infarction is 13 times greater during pregnancy than in a matched nonpregnant population. Arterial occlusion is the commonest cause of this event; venous thrombosis accounts for about 20 percent of strokes during pregnancy. Arterial infarction is most common in the second and third trimesters and in the first week postpartum, whereas venous occlusion occurs within the first four weeks after delivery. The cause of arterial infarction is not dissimilar from that of young strokes, the principal causes being cardiac. Infective endocarditis in the setting of pre-existing cardiac valve lesions usually involves *Streptococcus viridans.* Following delivery, infection with enterococci is likely. Treatment involves the identification of the causative organism and the institution of appropriate antibiotic therapy. Pregnancy may also encourage recrudescence of rheumatic heart disease with the attendant complications of

infective endocarditis, atrial fibrillation, and cerebral embolism. Such patients, like those with pre-existing nonvalvular cardiac lesions such as mitral valve prolapse, should be treated with penicillin prophylaxis. Atrial fibrillation in pregnancy, whether spontaneous or associated with rheumatic fever, should be managed with heparin. If it occurs de novo, heparin therapy followed by cardioversion should be attempted. If cardioversion is unsuccessful, subcutaneous heparin therapy may be instituted for the duration of the pregnancy. Warfarin has teratogenic potential.

A specific cardiomyopathy of pregnancy has been identified that is more common in older, multiparous black patients. The risk of cardiac embolization is increased in this condition, especially if there is congestive cardiac failure or mural thrombus formation. These instances, and the situation where stroke has already occurred in the presence of a cardiomyopathy, require treatment with heparin, as indicated.

Paradoxical embolism through a patent foramen ovale is also more common in pregnant women. This relates to the frequency of deep vein thrombosis in pregnancy. When it is discovered, intravenous heparin therapy is necessary, as is generally the case when stroke in pregnancy identified with a cardiac cause has already occurred.

Cerebral venous occlusion occurs most commonly in the second or third week post partum. In the past, common etiologic factors included sepsis, but in most cases a direct cause is not identifiable. Venous occlusion may be due to changes in coagulability during pregnancy that affect both clotting factors and platelets. The condition presents with headache and progressive neurologic deficits, frequently involving the legs bilaterally and the proximal parts of the arms. Focal or generalized seizures are common, as are impaired consciousness and papilledema. The clinical presentation is suspicious for the condition, which may be confirmed by angiography and MR imaging. The condition is often fatal (25 percent). Treatment involves maintenance of adequate hydration and control of seizures and of raised intracranial pressures if present. Anticoagulation is a controversial issue, but it could be considered if hemorrhagic infarction is not present. Recently, therapy with tPA has been considered, although controlled trials have not yet been conducted.

SECONDARY PREVENTION

Although in this chapter I focused on the management of the acute stroke, due thought should still be given at this stage to the secondary prevention of recurrences. This is important for patient counseling. The recently completed North American Symptomatic Carotid Endarterectomy Trial (NASCET) suggests that the risk of stroke recurrence is proportional to the *number* of risk factors. Consequently, risk factor identification and treatment are paramount. In addition, stroke recurrence in men has been shown to be significantly reduced by aspirin therapy, using a regimen of 325 mg four times per day. The precise dose of aspirin required for this effect is somewhat controversial; several European trials make claims for smaller doses. I usually start patients younger than 65 years on larger doses, provided they do not have symptoms of peptic ulcer. In the older population, the dose is amended, starting with 325 mg twice a day and increasing if no gastrointestinal symptoms occur. Recently, a new anti-platelet agent (ticlopidine) has become available; the standard dose is 250 mg twice a day with meals. This medication antagonizes adenosine diphosphate–induced platelet aggregation and may be somewhat more effective than aspirin in reducing stroke recurrence, at least for the first year after the initial event. There is a risk of reversible neutropenia, which is usually apparent within the first 3 months of therapy. It is suggested that blood tests be performed every 2 weeks for the first 3 months of therapy to identify this complication. The medication may be of use for patients who are intolerant of aspirin or who continue to have transient ischemic events despite aspirin therapy. It has proven benefit for women, an effect yet to be convincingly shown for aspirin.

The results of the NASCET have shown significant reduction of stroke recurrence following carotid endarterectomy performed within 3 months of the randomizing event. This benefit was proven in patients with high-grade carotid stenosis (70 percent or more). Therefore, patients who have recovered well from their stroke within the 3 month period and who are considered to have had a nondisabling stroke may benefit from the procedure. Owing to changes in cerebral autoregulation after stroke, it is not advisable to operate on patients with large infarcts for at least 4 to 6 weeks after the event. Those with smaller, non-disabling strokes may be considered for surgery at 2 to 3 weeks.

FUTURE THERAPEUTIC AVENUES

Research into new stroke therapies is advancing by leaps and bounds. It is likely we will see the development of thromboxane and platelet-activating factor antagonists and superoxide dismutase analogues and superoxide scavengers, as well as other novel agents that have been of benefit in animal stroke models. Therapeutic trials are under way with heparinoids and are being mooted for the 21-aminosteroids.

SUGGESTED READING

Barnett HJM, Hachinski VC, eds. Cerebral ischemia: Treatment and prevention. Neurol Clin 1992; 10.
Barnett HJM, Stein BM, Mohr JP, Yatsu F, eds. Stroke: Pathophysiology, diagnosis and management. New York: Churchill Livingstone, 1986.
Hachinski VC, Norris JW. The acute stroke. Philadelphia: FA Davis, 1985.
Oppenheimer SM, Hachinski VC. The complications of acute stroke. Lancet 1992; 339:721–724.

PATIENT RESOURCE

American Heart Association, National Center
7320 Greenville Avenue
Dallas, Texas 75231
(Local chapters in all states offer patient information and advice.)

EMBOLI OF CARDIAC ORIGIN

STEVEN J. KITTNER, M.D., M.P.H.
MARY W. HAWKE, M.D.

Cardioembolic stroke accounts for approximately 15 percent of all cerebral infarctions and about 25 percent of cerebral infarctions among young adults. The importance of the diagnosis of cardiogenic embolism lies in its implications for patient care. Unfortunately, for several reasons the diagnosis may not be straightforward. First,

Supported by a grant-in-aid from the American Heart Association and with funds contributed in part by the AHA Maryland Affiliate, Inc. Dr. Kittner was also supported by a Clinical Investigator Development Award (KO8-NS01319) and a Stroke Center grant (P01-N516332) from the National Institute of Neurological Disorders and Stroke.

while certain features of the history, neurologic examination, and neuroimaging studies may suggest the presence or absence of a cardiogenic mechanism, none of these features is sensitive or specific enough to be used in isolation. Second, a cardiac source of embolism frequently coexists with other potential causes of stroke such as extracranial carotid disease. Third, cardiac conditions differ both in the strength of association with stroke and in the evidence for a cardioembolic mechanism. The index of suspicion that a given stroke has a cardiac embolic mechanism may be based on three considerations: (1) Are the history, neurologic examination, and neuroimaging studies suggestive of a cardioembolic mechanism? (2) What is the evidence for other stroke mechanisms such as atherosclerosis or small vessel disease? (3) What is the likelihood that the patient's cardiac condition served as the source of embolism?

Certain clinical features can help raise or lower the index of suspicion for a cardioembolic mechanism (Table 1). Younger patient age, especially in the absence

Table 1 Stroke Characteristics Relevant to the Diagnosis of Cardiogenic Brain Embolism

Increase index of suspicion
  History
    Age < 55 years
    Systemic embolism
    Abrupt onset
  Examination
    Diminished level of consciousness at onset
    Cortical deficits (visual field abnormalities, neglect, aphasia)
  Neuroimaging studies
    Cortical infarct in multiple vascular territories
    Large infarction, including deep, large infarction
    Hemorrhagic infarction
  Angiography
    Major or branch vessel occlusion without significant proximal atherosclerosis
    Normal arteriography

Decrease index of suspicion
  Examination
    Pure motor hemiparesis
  Neuroimaging studies
    Deep, small infarct
  Angiography or noninvasive neurovascular studies
    Evidence for significant proximal atherosclerosis

Table 2 Cardiac and Other* Sources of Cerebral Embolism

Probable	Possible
Arrhythmias	Valvular abnormalities
Atrial fibrillation	Mitral valve prolapse
Sick sinus syndrome	Mitral annular calcification
Valvular abnormalities	Calcific aortic stenosis
Prosthetic valve	
Mitral stenosis	Myocardial abnormalities
Infective endocarditis	Atrial septal aneurysm
Marantic endocarditis	Right-to-left shunt without evidence of venous source of embolism
Myocardial abnormalities	Focal left ventricular akinesis or hypokinesis
Left ventricular global hypokinesis	
Ventricular aneurysm (dyskinesis)	Aortic plaque
Left atrial thrombus	
Left ventricular thrombus	
Myocardial infarction within 3 mo	
Cardiac tumor (myxoma)	
Right to left shunt with evidence of venous source of embolism	
Aortic plaque with mobile thrombus	

*Carotid and vertebrobasilar sources of artery-to-artery embolism are not considered in this classification

of factors that predispose to stroke, should increase the index of suspicion for a cardioembolic source. In addition, there are features of the stroke history, examination, and neuroimaging studies that bear on the likelihood of cardioembolic stroke mechanism. A history of systemic embolism, though rare, strongly suggests an embolic source proximal to the carotid and vertebral arteries. Abrupt onset is a more common but less specific feature of embolic stroke. Diminished level of consciousness at onset, either by history or on examination, is more common in patients with a cardiac source of embolism. Cortical signs such as aphasia or visual field deficit, particularly Wernicke's aphasia and isolated homonymous hemianopia, are also more common in patients with a cardiac source of embolism. Evidence of involvement of cortical structures in more than one vascular distribution, though infrequent, similarly suggests a proximal embolic source. Large infarctions, including deep, large infarction and hemorrhagic infarction, are also neuroimaging correlates of cardioembolic stroke. Failure to demonstrate atherosclerosis by angiography, and to a lesser extent by noninvasive studies, increases the likelihood of a cardioembolic stroke mechanism. Conversely, pure motor hemiparesis and deep, small infarcts are less common in patients with an embolic source. For carotid distribution transient ischemia attacks (TIAs), symptom duration of an hour or longer should heighten suspicion of a cardioembolic mechanism. It should be emphasized that none of these features is sufficiently sensitive and specific to establish or exclude the diagnosis of cardioembolic stroke, though they may be used as corroborating evidence.

It is useful for evaluation and management to divide cardiac sources of embolism into a probable and a possible category (Table 2). Most cardiac conditions in the "probable cardiac source of embolism" category cause stasis of blood and increased likelihood of thrombus formation. The evidence supporting their association with embolic stroke is compelling. Cardiac conditions in the possible category are common in the general population or their link with stroke is tenuous. For these conditions, judgments about a cardiogenic stroke mechanism depend heavily on the strength of corroborating evidence.

EVALUATION

We proceed with the same cardiac evaluation, regardless of whether it is prompted by a TIA or a completed stroke (Fig. 1). In addition to a complete cardiac and vascular physical examination, cardiac evaluation includes an electrocardiogram (ECG), transthoracic ECG, subsequent transesophageal ECG in selected cases, and Holter monitoring only if there is historical evidence to suggest atrial fibrillation or sick sinus syndrome. ECG may reveal atrial fibrillation or recent myocardial infarction. Transthoracic echocardiogram (TTE) is performed to look for dilated cardiomyopathy, cardiac wall motion abnormalities, ventricular and atrial thrombi, and conditions such as mitral stenosis or atrial myxoma. Contrast echocardiogram using bolus injections of agitated blood or saline is used to detect atrial septal defects or patent foramen ovale. In addition, TTE is frequently important in guiding the management of

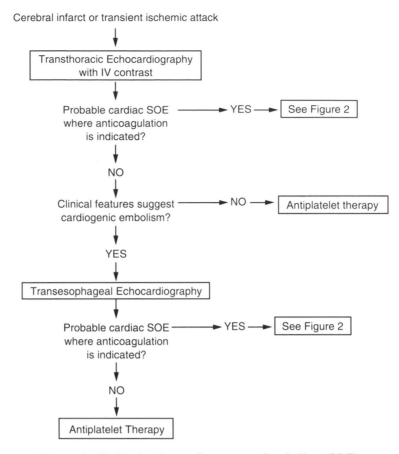

Figure 1 Evaluation for cardiac source of embolism (SOE).

the underlying cardiac disease when a probable cardio-embolic source is known to exist.

Transesophageal echocardiogram (TEE) is recommended when the TTE findings are normal and there is a high index of suspicion for a cardioembolic mechanism. TEE is more sensitive for detecting some potential cardiac sources of embolism that would alter management, including atrial septal defects, left atrial thrombi or myxomas, and mitral valve vegetations.

THERAPY

In this section we discuss management issues related to secondary prevention (prevention of recurrent stroke or TIA) rather than primary prevention (prevention of first stroke or TIA). Clinical trials for secondary prevention of cardioembolic stroke have not yet been reported. Therefore, the guidelines presented are based on observational studies and clinical judgment and should not be considered rigid prescriptions.

Patients with *probable* cardiac sources of emboli such as persistent atrial fibrillation, sick sinus syndrome, mitral stenosis, mechanical valves, dilated cardiomyopathy, left atrial or ventricular thrombi, and recent myocardial infarction are optimally treated with anticoagulation. Normal sinus rhythm should be restored in

patients with atrial fibrillation whenever possible, and patients with sick sinus syndrome should be evaluated to determine if a permanent pacemaker is warranted. Similarly, cardiac consultation should be sought for patients with mitral stenosis to determine if mitral valve replacement is warranted. In most cases, anticoagulation should be long term. Exceptions include (1) recent myocardial infarction (3 to 6 months anticoagulation), (2) normal sinus rhythm after atrial fibrillation (6 to 12 weeks), and (3) sick sinus syndrome (individualize).

Patients with a probable cardiac source of emboli who are not candidates for anticoagulation and those with a possible cardiac source of emboli such as mitral valve prolapse, mitral annular calcification, calcific aortic stenosis, atrial septal aneurysm, and focal left ventricular hypokinesis should be treated with antiplatelet agents. Appropriate therapy for complex atherosclerotic plaques of the ascending aorta or arch has not yet been determined, but we treat such patients with antiplatelet agents unless overlying mobile thrombi are visualized. If mobile thrombi are visualized on TEE we empirically recommend anticoagulation for 6 to 12 weeks, followed by antiplatelet agents.

Management is based on the principles of minimizing both the risk of infarct recurrence and the risk of comparatively serious complications from anticoagulation, such as intracranial bleeding or life-threatening

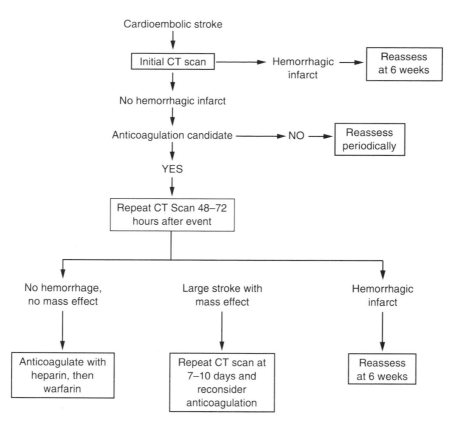

Figure 2 Timing of anticoagulation.

gastrointestinal bleeding. The risk of anticoagulation can be divided into an acute inpatient stage and a chronic outpatient stage. In the acute stage, hemorrhagic conversion occurs in as many as 40 percent of cardioembolic strokes, the majority in the first 48 hours. Although most cases of spontaneous hemorrhagic conversion are not associated with clinical exacerbation, hemorrhagic conversion during anticoagulant therapy can result in neurologic deterioration. Risk factors for symptomatic hemorrhagic transformation have not been well studied, but large infarction size has been noted in some case series. Intensity of anticoagulation and uncontrolled hypertension (blood pressure > 180/100 mm Hg) are also suspected risk factors, although the evidence is scant. A somewhat different set of considerations bears on the risk of long-term anticoagulation. The most consistent association with life-threatening complications has been the intensity of anticoagulation. Persons with a history of falls, a hemorrhagic diathesis or those whose strict compliance with monitoring and dose adjustments is unlikely are also considered to be at higher risk for serious long-term complications. Therefore, the decision to anticoagulate a patient for a probable cardioembolic stroke requires careful patient selection and timing, to minimize the risk of serious anticoagulation-related complications (Fig. 2).

If the computed tomography (CT) study obtained on admission shows a hemorrhagic infarct, anticoagulation is deferred and the patient is reassessed at 6 weeks.

When hemorrhagic conversion has not been associated with worsening and there is a high risk of recurrent cardioembolism, then earlier reassessment may be warranted. If the initial CT scan does not show evidence of hemorrhage and the patient is an anticoagulation candidate, CT is repeated at 48 to 72 hours after the completed stroke. The purpose of this repeat study is to look for delayed hemorrhagic transformation and to assess the size of the stroke. If, on repeat CT, there is no hemorrhage and the stroke is small or moderate-sized without mass effect on midline structures, anticoagulation is begun with heparin.

If the CT at 48 to 72 hours shows the stroke to be large with mass effect on midline structures, the risk of hemorrhagic conversion is increased and consideration of anticoagulation is delayed until 7 to 10 days after the event. If there is no evidence of bleeding on the CT obtained at 7 to 10 days the patient is given anticoagulant medication.

Management of Anticoagulation Therapy

Anticoagulation with heparin is administered by continuous IV infusion delivered by a mechanical infusion pump, the goal being an activated partial thromboplastin time (aPTT) of 1.5 to 2 times the control value. No heparin bolus should be given. In most cases, 1000 units per hour should be administered, the aPTT measured at 6 hours, and the dose adjusted every 4 hours until therapeutic. Once a steady state is achieved, the aPTT should be checked daily. Any neurologic deterioration during anticoagulation should prompt concern about hemorrhagic conversion and an urgent CT scan should be obtained.

Oral anticoagulation with warfarin is initiated after the patient has been therapeutically anticoagulated with IV heparin. Because the prolongation of the prothrombin time (PT) by heparin in therapeutic concentrations is slight, the warfarin dose can be determined without stopping heparin. The goal of oral anticoagulation therapy is a PT value 1.3 to 1.5 times the control value using North American thromboplastin (International Normalized Ratio [INR] = 2-3). This recommendation for the intensity of anticoagulation in secondary prevention of cardioembolic stroke is based on an extrapolation from the results of several large trials of anticoagulation for the primary prevention of stroke in nonvalvular atrial fibrillation.

Initially, warfarin is administered, 10 mg per day unless a dose reduction is indicated. The initial warfarin dose should be reduced for patients older than 80 years, under average weight, or receiving parenteral nutrition; who have an abnormal baseline PT value or significant liver disease or congestive heart failure; or who are taking drugs that potentiate the action of warfarin. The PT should be measured and the dose adjusted daily until the PT is therapeutic and the patient's standard dose has been achieved. However, it should be noted that the anticoagulant effect of warfarin is not fully realized until after 5 days' therapy, including at least 2 days with a therapeutic PT. Once the patient's PT is stabilized with warfarin, the frequency of PT testing can gradually be reduced.

During the first few weeks of warfarin administration, the PT should be measured and the warfarin dose adjusted every few days. Thereafter, the PT is measured every few weeks and simultaneously the hematocrit is measured and the urine and stool are tested for blood. Addition of a drug that alters warfarin's effect should prompt more frequent testing until a steady state is again achieved. Safe, long-term anticoagulation is most easily accomplished by referral to an outpatient anticoagulation clinic.

Coumadin is the proprietary brand of warfarin that is commonly prescribed. Other products, including generic products, are reliable but not interchangeable because of variations in bioavailability.

SPECIAL SITUATIONS

Cerebral Infarction During Anticoagulant Therapy

First or recurrent cerebral infarction while on anticoagulant therapy may represent either failure of anticoagulation or a stroke mechanism other than cardioembolism. If investigations are unrevealing and PTs have been within the range of 1.3 to 1.5 times the control value, then failure of anticoagulation is sus-

pected and higher-intensity anticoagulation should be tried (PT 1.5 to 2 times the control, INR 3 to 4.5), although the attendant risk of bleeding complications is greater. Patients with mechanical heart valves generally receive this higher-intensity anticoagulation. If systemic embolism occurs while the PT is in the range of 1.5 to 2 times the control value (INR 3 to 4.5), then dipyridamole, 400 mg per day, should be added.

Bacterial Endocarditis

Embolic stroke occurs in approximately 20 percent of patients with bacterial endocarditis, the majority before or within the first few days after institution of antibiotic therapy. Optimal treatment consists of appropriate antibiotics and stabilization of cardiac status. Although endocarditis is not an indication for anticoagulation, it is not a contraindication to continued anticoagulation for patients with other indications such as a mechanical valve. The risk of recurrent embolus is small, and it most often occurs in the setting of uncontrolled infection. There is no clear benefit from surgical resection of the valve, unless it is necessary for uncontrolled infection, abscess, or severe valvular incompetence.

Cardiac Surgery

Some probable cardiac sources of emboli, such as atrial septal defect and myxoma, clearly warrant surgical correction. Whether surgical correction of a patent foramen ovale is justified is more problematic, because this is a common abnormality in the asymptomatic general population. Identification of a patent foramen ovale by echocardiography provides only the source of conduit from the venous to the arterial circulation, not the source of embolus. We recommend closure of a patent foramen ovale only if investigation demonstrates a deep venous thrombosis, pulmonary embolism, or other compelling evidence of a potentially recurrent venous source of embolism that antedates the stroke.

DISCUSSION

Embolism from a cardiac source is an important cause of cerebral infarction. We have outlined a cardiac evaluation strategy in which the degree of thoroughness is determined by the index of suspicion for a cardioembolic mechanism. We have discussed measures to prevent stroke recurrence for many common cardiac conditions. During both the evaluation and treatment phases, the care of the patient benefits from close cooperation between neurologist and cardiologist.

SUGGESTED READING

Dalen J, Hirsh J, eds. Third ACCP Conference on antithrombotic therapy. Chest 1992; 102(Suppl).

Hart RG. Cardiogenic embolism to the brain. Lancet 1992; 339: 589–594.

Kittner SJ, Sharkness CM, Sloan MA, et al. Infarcts with a cardiac source of embolism in the NINDS Stroke Data Bank: neurologic examination. Neurology 1992; 42:299–302.

PATIENT RESOURCES

American Academy of Neurology
2221 University Avenue S.E., Suite 335
Minneapolis, Minnesota 55414
Telephone: (612) 623-8115
Patient information guide for neurology.
(E. Wayne Massey, M.D.
Coordinator AAN Practice Committee)

American Heart Association
7320 Greenville Avenue
Dallas, Texas 75231
Telephone: (214) 750-5300

National Stroke Association
1420 Ogden Street
Denver, Colorado 80218
Telephone: (303) 839-1992

INTRACRANIAL HEMATOMA

DANIEL F. HANLEY, M.D.

During the last 15 years, the diagnostic realm of cerebral hematomas has moved from the autopsy room to the computed tomography (CT) scanner. Therapeutic efforts have followed; the benefits of these efforts are not yet clear. The diseases that cause intracranial bleeding are as diverse as their amenability to therapy. Clinically, these hematomas usually present as an acute or hyperacute illness, with headache, coma, and rostral cranial nerve dysfunction (usually oculomotor dysfunction). The neurologic examination and emergency CT are important initial diagnostic efforts that most often reveal a mass lesion, with or without acute hydrocephalus.

Because brain stem dysfunction is an important part of the late natural history of expanding hematoma mass lesions, the lesions present a complex clinical problem and patients exhibit central nervous system, cardiac, and respiratory collapse. Usually, emergency diagnostics and therapeutics are required for each organ system that is dysfunctional. The optimal sequence of diagnostic studies and interventions is not always clear to primary care givers in emergency settings, who are not familiar with diseases of the nervous system. Finally, cerebral hematomas are associated with significant morbidity and mortality.

This chapter is divided into sections describing cranial vault mechanics, methods of localizing and quantitating the mass, a description of clinical presentation for differential diagnosis and emergent therapeutic decision making, and a short review of intracranial pressure (ICP) management with respect to outcome. An appendix describes critical care management of external ventricular cannulas.

LOCALIZATION AND DIFFERENTIAL DIAGNOSIS OF HEMATOMAS

Cerebral hemorrhage presents as a discrete mass lesion or hematoma. The location (and, therefore, signs and symptoms) varies with the precise site of the mass in the neuraxis. For spontaneous cerebral hemorrhages of hypertensive cause, the usual locations include caudate, putamen, and thalamus in the supratentorial compartment, basis pontis and cerebellar white matter of the posterior fossa. Lobar localizations can occur with hypertensive hemorrhage, but they are less common. When hematomas are noted in the anterior or inferior aspects of the frontal and temporal lobes, a traumatic cause should be considered. Subcortical lesions are associated with amyloid vasculopathy. Additionally, ethanol or anticoagulants may have played a role in producing the lesion. Hematomas in the anterior interhemispheric fissure are frequently associated with aneurysmal bleeds from anterior communicating aneurysms. Similarly, sylvian fissure and opercular territory hematomas are frequently associated with middle cerebral artery territory aneurysmal subarachnoid hemorrhage. Because the location of hemorrhage does not accurately define the cause, all hematoma patients should be evaluated for vasculopathy, aneurysm, coagulopathy, and arteriovenous malformation. Once the patient's condition has stabilized, arteriography combined with magnetic resonance imaging (MRI) of the parenchyma provides the best overall screening for these different diagnostic groups.

QUANTITATING THE MASS EFFECT

Two separate variables are currently being investigated as useful adjuncts for describing hematoma and intraventricular hemorrhage. They are lateral shift and hematoma size.

Lateral Shift

For a group of patients who were victims of acute hemispheral masses, lateral shift has been described as a potential mechanism of brain stem injury, and a correlation with level of consciousness was reported. Lateral shift can be described as shift at the level of the pineal gland, the septum pellucidum, or the aqueduct. A correlation with level of consciousness for acute unilateral mass lesions has been confirmed in trauma victims with masses. Unfortunately, to date, no relationship has been identified between degree of lateral shift and outcome. Most examiners do not find a correlation between level of consciousness and vertical displacement of the pineal. However, a study by Feldman does demonstrate this effect. Although lateral shift has been difficult to correlate with outcome, this finding most likely relates to the importance of early surgical reversal of mass effect and the absence of any controlled trials in this area.

Size of the Hematoma

Two different types of volume quantitation are commonly used: (1) a simple measurement of diameter of hematoma or (2) calculation of volume of the entire lesion. The latter calculation must take into account the shape of the hematoma, thickness of CT slices, and number of slices made. Several formulas are available for calculating this variable (Table 1). Simple diameter measurements have been correlated with poor outcome in the case of cerebellar hemorrhage, where poor outcomes with hematomas 3 cm in diameter or larger have been reported. Notably, these patients all had substantial ventricular dilatation as well. Volume measurements have also been correlated with outcome by Andrews and coworkers. These authors demonstrated a significant correlation between hematoma volume and degree of midline shift. They also noted that 41 percent of patients with temporal-parietal lesions had signs of herniation, whereas no patients with frontal or parietal-occipital hematomas of the same size had signs of herniation. Thus, for the temporal-parietal location, lateral shift appears to be most closely linked with herniation and with worse outcome. Within this group of patients who demonstrated temporal-parietal hematomas, hematomas smaller than 30 cc did not show signs of tentorial herniation, whereas seven (64 percent) of 11 patients with larger hematomas did show signs of tentorial herniation.

For spontaneous hemorrhages, the role of mass effect in producing death has been addressed by Tuhrim. His model suggests that factors other than hemorrhage size also figure in the outcome. Empirically, these factors include arterial pulse pressure, Glasgow Coma Scale score, and presence of intraventricular hemorrhage. Precise prediction of death and disability are not yet available for parenchymal hemorrhages, not has a set of clinical factors been identified that can be modified to improve outcome. Caplan probably best summarizes the most rational clinical approach to intracerebral hemor-

Table 1 Cerebral Hematoma Volume Calculations

Author	Formula
Steiner*	$4/3 \pi (ABC)$ [A, B, C are radii of an ellipsoid]
Helweg-Larsen†	Length × Width × Cut thickness
Ropper‡	Hematoma volume in cm^3 = (Greatest diameter × 14) − 14
Broderick§	Σ_1 (Area × Thickness)

*Steiner I, Gomori JM, Melamed E. The prognostic value of the CT scan in conservatively treated patients with intracerebral hematoma. Stroke 1984; 15:279–282.

†Helweg-Larsen S, Sommer W, Strange P, et al. Prognosis for patients treated conservatively for spontaneous intracerebral hematomas. Stroke 1984; 15:1045–1048.

‡Kistler JP, Ropper AH, Martin JB. Cerebrovascular diseases. In Petersdorf RG, et al, eds. Harrison's principles of internal medicine. 13th ed. McGraw-Hill, New York, in press.

§Broderick JP, Brott TG, Tomsick T, et al. Ultra-early evaluation of intracerebral hemorrhage. J Neurosurg 1990; 72:195–199.

rhage prognosis and treatment. He describes three groups of hemorrhages: (1) abruptly developing hematomas that irreversibly damage brain and lead to death; (2) small hematomas that are unlikely to cause mass effect, elevated intracranial pressure, or severe disease (these have an excellent outcome with minimal interventions); and (3) intermediate-sized hematomas that clearly cause mass effect but do not render the patient moribund. It is for this group that aggressive medical and surgical interventions may help improve the outcome. The experience of most neurointensivists supports this contention.

CLINICAL PRESENTATIONS OF TREATABLE CEREBRAL HEMATOMAS

Cerebellar Hematoma With Obstructive Hydrocephalus

Diagnosis of acute obstructive hydrocephalus requires the integration of historical information and the examination findings in such a manner that suspected acute obstruction of the cerebrospinal fluid (CSF) pathways becomes first on the list of differential diagnostic explanations. No one symptom or sign can be relied upon; rather, the complete presentation must be taken into consideration. This is because the presenting symptoms of headache, nausea, and vomiting are non-specific. The history is usually taken from a companion rather than the patient. Complaints of acute onset of headache accompanied by nausea and vomiting are described. These complaints most often occurred for minutes to hours. They are invariably followed by obtundity, and frequently further impairment of the level of consciousness. Many times there is a history of gait difficulties, including axial ataxia and/or frequent falls. Subacute presentations do occur, but they are unusual. Dramatic progression of the ictus is very common; this is usually manifested as abrupt onset of coma, often with associated partial airway obstruction.

Cerebellar hematoma and acute obstructive hydrocephalus in a comatose patient represents a neurologic emergency, as the likelihood of permanent brain stem injury increases rapidly with the duration of coma. These patients usually exhibit no purposeful motor activity, and most frequently extensor posturing of all limbs in response to painful stimulation. Large or middle-sized pupils with little or no reaction to light are the most common eye finding. The vestibulo-ocular response, although it is elicited, may be impaired. The response is often dysconjugate, with bilaterally impaired adduction. Most often, at least one corneal reflex is impaired if the hematoma mass is producing both brain stem compression and obstruction of the CSF pathways. The abrupt onset of these findings suggests a posterior fossa mass rather than the progressive rostrocaudal evolution of signs from supratentorial masses with downward herniation.

CT reveals a uniform cerebellar density, usually in the deep nuclear region. Effacement of the quadrigeminal cistern and rostral migration of the collicular region occurs as part of upward herniation. Patients with a mass at least 3 cm in diameter most frequently require emergent ventricular drainage with concurrent emergent relief of the mass effect via posterior fossa craniotomy.

Hypertensive Hemispheric Hematoma

The presenting symptoms for cerebral hemispheric hemorrhages are quite similar, in that the acute onset of focal neurologic deficits is associated with headache, nausea, vomiting, and frequently stiff neck. For supratentorial masses, the focal neurologic deficit involves some degree of internal capsule level hemiplegia and hemisensory deficit. For anterior lesions, gaze preference ipsilateral to the lesion is noted. For posterior locations such as thalamic bleeds, impaired upward gaze is commonly found. Several excellent detailed descriptions of common localizing neurologic findings are described by Caplan. The single most important clinical finding is the level of consciousness, as this should indicate the need for airway protection and the risks of sedation during imaging studies.

Progression of the patient's deficits occurs more frequently than was previously recognized. Such deterioration is accompanied by an increase in the size of the hematoma over the 24 to 36 hours after presentation. Studies relating the clinical sign to changes in the volume and location of the hematoma mass have not yet been performed. Similarly the relation of these events to blood pressure elevation are not clear. The least disputed sign of progression is the loss of consciousness and the development of a herniation syndrome. New evidence suggests this is related to lateral shift rather than vertical translocation. Regardless of mechanism, the physical signs remain the same: obtundity progressing to coma followed by unilateral or bilateral third nerve paresis. This usually occurs over minutes, though the signs can go unrecognized for a number of hours. An ideal management strategy would allow identification of the hematoma location and initiation of intracranial hypertension management prior to compartment shifts.

As no clear clinical benefit has been demonstrated for aggressive management of hypertensive hematoma subgroups, the clinician must rely on the evaluation of the individual patient, the currently available diagnostic imaging, and physiologic data. Before initiating aggressive medical or surgical interventions, a clinician should be aware that neither cohort nor controlled studies support the hypothesis that patients can be selected for successful intervention. Three locations of mass effect stand out as sites that are potentially amenable to combined surgical and medical treatment: (1) lobar hematomas larger than 30 cc, particularly those in the middle fossa; (2) subependymal hematomas smaller than 30 cc with substantial ventricular extension and hydrocephalus; and (3) 30 to 50 cc putaminal hematomas. With each of these lesions, altered consciousness may be explained by lateral shift or acute hydrocephalus and thus is remediable by ventricular drainage or stereotactic aspiration. Medical management directed at reducing intracranial hypertension before and after such procedures is equally rational. Where available, high-resolution MRI evaluation of the hematoma location may address the possibility that altered consciousness is related to direct extension of the hematoma into the subthalamus and midbrain. In current practice, these anatomic subgroups represent substantially less than half of all "hypertensive hematomas." Independent of the decision to treat, we inform each patient's family that there is no clear beneficial imperative to treat this condition.

Epidural and Subdural Hematomas

A history of acute trauma is usually evident when a patient presents with symptoms. Occasionally, this trauma is minor or more remote. Epidural hematomas are clearly the most rapidly progressing group of hematomas. A patient may be intact after transient loss of consciousness and subsequently develop hemiparesis, hemispheric dysfunction, and obtundity progressing to a second episode of loss of consciousness. A skull fracture may be noted, although not always. Progression is over minutes and often is recognizable as a change from agitation to manageable behavior. Neurosurgical evaluation is best performed in the emergency room setting, as rapid surgical removal or evacuation is necessary. When the surgeon is not immediately available, physician-monitored CT evaluation should not be delayed.

Subdural hematomas also progress rapidly, but they tend to occur more frequently in older persons who have suffered apparently minor trauma or have no history of trauma. The presence of therapeutic anticoagulation or a disorder of coagulation is often a predisposing factor. Additionally, the subdural hematoma can expand slowly over a 2 to 4 week period as clot lysis occurs. Because this late expansion may be the first sign of illness, these patients can present in acute medical coma. Once a patient reaches this stage of presentation, more rapid deterioration is possible, so emergent removal should be facilitated. Surgical treatments are less clearly effective. This is probably not unexpected, as the subdural hematoma is a multifactorial disease that is directly related to aging and alteration of the hemispheric relations to the table of the skull and indirectly related to predisposing disorders, including abnormal coagulation and gait disorders. The majority of patients do benefit from surgery.

Cisternal Hematoma of Aneurysmal Subarachnoid Hemorrhage

Subarachnoid hemorrhage is occasionally associated with hematoma formation in the basilar cisterns, interhemispheric fissure, or sylvian fissure region. Occasionally, high-pressure arterial bleeding produces an extension of the hematoma into the brain parenchyma. The interhemispheric fissure and the circle of Willis region are the two most common sites for this extension. These hematomas are regional accumulations of blood in the subarachnoid space that are also accompanied by more diffuse subarachnoid bleeding. The effects of these masses are not readily separable from those of the subarachnoid hemorrhage. Thus, the patients are indistinguishable clinically from subarachnoid hemorrhage patients without hematoma. Whether postoperative improvement is related to reduction of local mass effect remains a matter of speculation; however, the presence of such a hematoma is a factor that argues in favor of surgical removal and correction of the aneurysmal source. Small parenchymal hematomas with direct extension into the basilar CSF space, interhemispheric fissure, or sylvian fissure should be evaluated angiographically for the presence of, respectively, carotid termination, anterior communicating, and distal middle cerebral aneurysms.

MANAGEMENT OF INCREASED INTRACRANIAL PRESSURE AND OUTCOME

Clinical conditions associated with increased ICP include parenchymal hemorrhage (including lobar, basal ganglia, pontine, and cerebellar), subarachnoid hemorrhage (both aneurysmal and arteriovenous malformation), and head injury with dural hemorrhage. In general, prognosis depends on the location of the mass, the extent of damage to the neuraxis, duration of critical mass effect, and the treatability of the underlying cause of the mass effect. Thus, a parenchymal hemorrhage of the pons can be associated with obstructive hydrocephalus, which can be treated, but the underlying destruction of pontine tissues leads to irreversible neurologic damage and a poor outcome. Conversely, hemorrhage-associated aqueductal obstruction from a surgically remediable aneurysm or arteriovenous malformation can be treated

effectively in the short term with ventricular drainage, and appropriate long-term surgical intervention may lead to complete resolution of all neurologic symptoms without recurrence. Cerebellar hemorrhages and small subependymal basal ganglia hemorrhages may be treated effectively with drainage and/or surgical removal of the mass lesion. However, the patients remain at risk for recurrent hemorrhagic infarction if the predisposing factors (hypertension, coagulopathy, heavy alcohol consumption) are not addressed.

Cerebellar Hematoma

The potential for acute surgical intervention with cerebellar hematoma was first popularized by Fisher. This disease has a rapidly progressive course in the majority of cases. It has been suggested that lesions greater than 3 cm have a potentially fatal course and, therefore, that masses of this size or greater should be treated surgically. Both direct surgical decompression and stereotactic decompression have been performed successfully. Present information appears to suggest that prognosis is related to the patient's condition at the time of surgery, preservation of brain stem cranial nerve functions, and the rapidity with which the hematoma and obstructive hydrocephalus are treated. Overall, the condition appears to be fatal approximately half the time, even with the earliest available treatment.

The monitoring of ICP is not as important as rapid relief of the mass effect. Thus, the absolute level of ICP is not as important as the timing of therapeutic interventions; clearly, the effect of drainage on ICP is a helpful intermediate indicator. But control of supratentorial pressure without relief of brain stem mass effect is of little functional value.

Hypertensive Hemispheric Hematoma

Although location of hematoma is clearly related to deficits and type of long-term disability, it is currently less clear whether location has implications for overall survival. For hematomas of all sizes, a 25 percent mortality rate is expected. In recent randomized studies, cohorts of 21 and 52 patients were treated; the mortality rates were high and there was no difference between patients treated surgically and medically. In both studies, only a small proportion of patients admitted were capable of independent living at home after hospitalization, 19 and 20 percent, respectively. In a Finnish study, the mortality rate for semicomatose and stuporous patients, that is those with Glasgow Coma Scale scores from 7 to 10, was significantly lower in the surgical group than in the medically managed group. This subgroup was quite small. Other data on this issue are retrospective and therefore difficult to evaluate. Several clear trends in case series reviews include the correlation of outcome with presenting clinical status and potential clinical benefits for CT-controlled aspiration of hematomas. Both careful development of new treatment strategies and widespread testing of surgical interventions might lead to either improved prognostication or improved outcomes for this group of patients. Presently, the assessment of each patient for relative effects of acute obstructive hydrocephalus, mass lesions, and parenchymal damage should be made by an experienced surgeon in order to arrive at the optimal care plan. Intracranial pressure has only limited importance as an intermediate variable when drainage of CSF is part of the treatment for hydrocephalus. Attempts to relate ICP control to beneficial outcome have not been successful.

Epidural and Subdural Hematomas

Hematomas in these locations are related to trauma, and their outcome is therefore dependent on traumatic factors that measure the extent of the initial injury to the neuraxsis. Additional important factors are age, duration, and timing of surgical intervention. Older patients have a poorer outcome. When the mass effect presents in a delayed manner, the outcome is usually better; the reason seems to be that the injury is milder and mass effect evolves more slowly. Seelig and Becker have presented strong support for the idea that early surgical intervention is an important treatment variable. In their series of patients, outcome for acute subdural hematoma is substantially better in those who undergo surgery in the first 4 hours after injury. Overall, mortality for both acute subdural and acute epidural hematomas is quite high, usually reported near 50 percent.

ICP per se is not a critical management variable from the point of view of outcome: initiating surgical intervention is more important than the time necessary to acquire another measurement of mass effect often allows for further deterioration. However after surgery, the failure to control or maintain ICP below 35 to 40 mm Hg is a physiologic indicator of poor outcome.

SUGGESTED READING

Andrews BT, Chiles BW III, Olson WL, Pitts LH. The effect of intracerebral hematoma location on risk of brainstem compression and on clinical outcome. Neurosurg 1988; 69:518–522.

Batjer HH, Reisch JS, Allan BC, et al. Failure of surgery to improve outcome in hypertensive putaminal hemorrhage: A prospective randomized trial. Arch Neurol 1990; 47:1103–1106.

Capian LR, Stein RW. A clinical approach. Stroke 1986; :287.

Feldman E, Gandy SE, Becker R, et al. MRI demonstrates descending transtentorial herniation. Neurology 1988; 38:697–701.

Fisher CM, Picard EH, Polak A, et al. Acute hypertensive cerebellar hemorrhage diagnosis and surgical treatment. J Nerv Ment Dis 1965; 140:38–57.

Ott KH, Kase CS, Ojeman RG, Mohr JP. Cerebellar hemorrhage: Diagnosis and treatment. Arch Neurol 1974; 31:160.

Ropper AH. Lateral displacement of the brain and level of consciousness in patients with an acute hemispheral mass. N Engl J Med 1986; 314:953–958.

Ross DA, Olson WL, Ross AM, et al. Brain shift, level of consciousness, and restoration of consciousness in patients with acute intracranial hematoma. Neurosurg 1989; 71:498–502.

Seelig JM, Becker DP, Miller JD, et al. Traumatic acute subdural hematoma. Major mortality reduction in the comatose patients treated within four hours. N Engl J Med 1981; 304:1511–1518.

Seelig JM, Marshall LF, Toutant SM, et al. Traumatic acute epidural hematoma: Unrecognized high lethality in comatose patients. Neurosurgery 1984; 15:617–620.

Tuhrim S, Dambrosia JM, Price T, et al. Prediction of intracerebral hemorrhage survival. Ann Neurol 1988; 24:258–263.

Tuhrim S, Dambrosia JM, Price T, et al. Intracerebral hemorrhage: External validation and extension of a model for prediction of thirty day survival. Ann Neurol 1991; 29(6):658–663.

APPENDIX: PRACTICAL NOTES ON MANAGEMENT OF ACUTE OBSTRUCTIVE HYDROCEPHALUS WITH VENTRICULAR DRAINAGE

Patient Identification

Because the treatment of acute obstructive hydrocephalus is related to the rapidity with which elevated ICP can be relieved, the patient clearly benefits from an organized, team approach to rapidly treating all aspects of the illness. It is best to identify patients at risk of acute hydrocephalus before the definitive neuroimaging diagnosis. Because placement of a ventricular drain requires an operator trained in the neurosurgical skills of ventricular puncture, we identify to the consulting neurosurgeon each patient who is likely to require emergent ventricular drainage before an emergency neuroradiology study is performed. This allows the managing physician to begin the process of defining both the type and location of the procedure to be performed and to consider the proper timing of the procedure. When the managing physician does not have the requisite neurosurgical skills, the neurosurgeon who will be the operator is identified, so that he or she can be immediately available at the completion of the diagnostic testing.

Where to Perform the Procedure

Several locations in the hospital are acceptable for emergency ventricular puncture and drain placement. These include the emergency room, the intensive care unit, and the operating room. The best location for performing the procedure depends on the need for subsequent follow-up procedures such as craniotomy, the availability of a support team to assist the operator in drain placement and other aspects of patient management, and the proximity of the neuroradiologic area to each of the likely sites for performing the procedure. The major prerequisites for hospital environment to perform the procedure include the capability of maintaining a sterile operative field, the presence of a twist drill and drain insertion kit, the availability of appropriate physician and nursing assistance for the operator, and a co-operative patient who is not in acute distress.

Timing Drain Placement and Other Treatments

Ideally, with early diagnosis the patient is obtunded but not comatose and is capable of protecting the airway. Furthermore, at this stage patients are usually maintaining normal cardiac rhythm and blood pressure. Thus, the earliest possible diagnosis and treatment of the obstructive hydrocephalus syndrome involves placement of a drain without airway protection or complex cardiovascular treatments. Frequently this is not the case, because the disease process advances more rapidly than the process of achieving diagnostic certainty. In this situation, the patient is often comatose with major airway compromise and/or cardiovascular instability. If the patient has not been intubated and ventilated prior to the neuroimaging procedure, emergency intubation and ventilatory assistance is required before drain placement. These patients should be immediately hyperventilated with either rapid blood gas assessment or end-tidal capnometry, to determine the level of hyperventilation. As cardiorespiratory management and surgical drainage are both required immediately, two teams of physicians are established, one to prepare and perform the operation and a second to manage the cardiorespiratory status. In such a situation, separate nursing assistance for each physician group is helpful. Many of the patients who present with the acute hydrocephalus syndrome have posterior fossa masses, either in the epidural or in the parenchymal spaces. Relief of brain stem tissue distortion and prevention of upward herniation are best achieved by craniotomy concurrent with or immediately after ventricular drainage. Thus, a significant subgroup of these patients require emergent surgery. For these individuals, the sequence of intubation, drain placement, and craniectomy may be most rapidly and effectively performed in the operating room. Thus, it is often the surgeon's choice to rapidly transport the patient from the diagnostic area to the operating room rather than to an emergency area or to the critical care environment. For patients who have airway protection and mechanical ventilation prior to radiologic diagnosis and who are not responding to hyperventilation, additional medical treatments with loop and osmotic diuretics may be administered as a temporizing measure while awaiting preparation of the operative site. Similarly, when the operative location is not going to be available in a matter of minutes and skilled anesthesiologic supervision is available, we frequently choose to initiate general anesthesia with large doses of barbiturates in the intensive care unit environment. This affords optimal medical treatment of ICP prior to craniotomy and allows the most efficient completion of the craniotomy and ventricular drainage procedures.

Monitoring for the Procedure

For the uninstrumented patient, monitoring during the procedure consists of pulse oximetry, electrocardiography and noninvasive blood pressure assessments every 2 to 3 minutes. This level of monitoring allows safe pursuit of a short surgical procedure in the obtunded patient who is at risk for further airway compromise. For airway compromise or cardiac collapse, more invasive instrumentation is usually necessary. These patients are intubated and undergoing hyperventilation therapy and most often should have arterial pressure monitored directly via an arterial cannula. It is particularly helpful

to follow the end-tidal carbon dioxide tension, as this is a measure of efficacy for hyperventilation treatment. ICP is most rapidly controlled by this maneuver or additional efforts at diuresis. A centrally placed intravenous line is frequently helpful in these patients for administering cardioactive drugs such as dopamine, phenylephrine, atropine, epinephrine, and hyperventilation. For patients who require such a high degree of monitoring and multiple concurrent therapies, several physicians and nurses are used to pursue treatment.

Placing the Drain in the Intensive Care Unit

Practically speaking, we perform this procedure most frequently in the neuro–critical care environment. We choose this environment because it is readily available at almost all times for the immediate pursuit of this procedure. The area is prepared on notification of need for the procedure and is readily available in a matter of minutes (usually the time needed to transport the patient from the neuroimaging area) to the procedure area. A team of a neurosurgeon and a critical care nurse can rapidly and effectively create and maintain a sterile operative field for the appropriate cranial area in most patients. As most patients are obtunded or comatose, they do not need major sedatives or analgesics for this procedure. Furthermore, since rapidly progressive brain stem dysfunction is the predicator for the procedure, it is unwise to prepare the patient with any sedative or analgesic drug that might adversely alter ventilation or cardiac activity. For individual patients who have progressed to the level of complete pontine dysfunction, ventilatory support is required before placement of the ventricular drain. However, for most patients who are obtunded and/or lightly comatose with early midbrain or pontine dysfunction, it is preferable to rapidly place the drain and then reassess airway protection and adequacy of ventilation. This does not represent an excessive risk, as the herniation syndrome usually progresses over a matter of hours and the entire ventricular drainage procedure is usually performed in 10 to 20 minutes.

Intracranial Pressure in the Intensive Care Unit

Once a ventricular drainage system has been established, the single most important physiologic variable is the pressure waveform. The presence of an adequate waveform is necessary to ensure appropriate drain placement, and competence of the drainage system. At low intracranial pressures, the ICP waveform is a low-amplitude version of the normal arterial waveform. This contour is most probably derived from a direct reflection of arterial pulsation from the circle of Willis, and particularly from the choroid plexus. The amplitude of the waveform is 1 to 4 mm Hg when the ICP is less than 10 mm Hg. As ICP rises, the amplitude of this pressure pulse increases. Pressure pulse amplitudes of 10 mm Hg and greater usually are accompanied by mean ICP above 20 mm Hg. So-called "arterialization" of the

ICP trace with large-amplitude pulse pressures (> 20 mm Hg) invariably represents an intracranial hypertensive crisis that if not corrected will threaten brain tissue function. Because ventricular drainage is a main goal of intraventricular catheterization, pressure monitoring is often sacrificed to benefit the goals of CSF drainage and maintenance of a low ICP and adequate cerebral profusion pressure. Hydraulic drainage of the ventricles is best accomplished by gravity feed. Ventricular drainage tubing is taped to the patient's bedside with the uppermost point of CSF transit established 10 to 20 cm above the patient's head. This allows CSF to drain when pressure exceeds that of a 10 to 20 cm column of water. In order to convert this threshold pressure to millimeters of mercury, the height of the column in millimeters should be divided by 13.6. For example, for 20 cm of water that would be (20 cm $H_2O \times 10$ mm/cm) divided by 13.6 mm Hg/mm $H_2O = 14.7$ mm Hg.

This method of drainage is usually adequate to control ICP in acute obstructive hydrocephalus patients and in parenchymal hematoma patients with a large component of intraventricular blood. Ideal goals for ICP control are similar to those for head injury victims: ICP less than or equal to 20 mm Hg and cerebral perfusion pressure greater than or equal to 70 mm Hg. Most prepackaged drainage systems have three stopcocks that allow simultaneous measurement of ICP while drainage is ongoing. Though this is an effective way of following the trend of ICP, it should be noted that this system often underestimates true intraventricular pressure. For that reason, hourly checks of absolute ICP are best performed after temporarily discontinuing drainage for 1 to 5 minutes. This is also an excellent time to record pulse pressure as a measure of cranial compliance.

Frequent assessment of CSF chemistry, cell counts, and microbial culture are recommended with drainage systems. Infections are most frequently related to unplanned breaches of the catheter system with retrograde transit of CSF and air into the ventricular system.

The increased infection risk is also associated with prolonged use of one catheter. For this reason most surgical services recommend re-evaluating, and usually changing, catheters every 5 days. Rising CSF protein and white cell count are particularly helpful clinical indicators to encourage replacement of a drain. The use of prophylactic antibiotics with significant antistaphylococcal activity is strongly recommended. The most commonly used antibiotics include oxacillin, methicillin, and vancocin. For large intracranial masses, additional medical therapies and surgical therapies should be considered as the basis of ICP control.

Management of Intracranial Pressure

The value of ICP control in brain hemorrhage victims with acute obstructive hydrocephalus and/or cerebral hematoma is immediately obvious in most patients. However, a relationship between ICP management and long-term outcome has neither been demonstrated nor seriously evaluated. Clearly, ICP is but one of several intermediate or physiologic variables that must be controlled if a good clinical outcome is to be achieved. Conversely, complete failure to control ICP with medical and surgical treatments is associated with a poor outcome. The clinician should assess the relative contributions of mass effect and of obstructive hydrocephalus and design a treatment strategy that addresses both factors and considers the benefits of intervention and the natural history of the untreated lesion. With the above qualification, aggressive ICP management and other therapeutic modalities can play a major role in avoiding herniation prior to timely surgery and in medically augmenting the decompressive effects of surgery. Ideal therapy may include passive dehydration, intubation with short-term hyperventilation, and the use of osmotic and loop diuretics. A role for high-dose barbiturate coma has yet to be defined, despite several clinical attempts.

RUPTURED INTRACRANIAL ANEURYSM

MICHAEL N. DIRINGER, M.D.

Rupture of an intracranial aneurysm is the most common cause of subarachnoid hemorrhage (SAH) and accounts for approximately 10 percent of strokes. The natural history of the disease is devastating: 1-year mortality is 60 percent. Approximately one-third of patients die of the initial insult, 15 percent die as a result of rebleeding after 1 month, and at 1 year only about 25 percent survive in good neurologic condition. Of those who survive the first year, without surgical obliteration of the aneurysm approximately 3.5 percent rebleed per year.

Of the patients who reach the hospital, about half either die or are left with severe neurologic disability. The major causes of morbidity and mortality are cerebral injury from the hemorrhage, aneurysmal rerupture, hydrocephalus, delayed cerebral ischemia from vasospasm, and complications of medical and surgical therapy. Over the past quarter century, improved surgical techniques and better understanding of the pathophysiology of delayed ischemia have shifted the approach to management of patients following acute aneurysm rupture from noninterventional to one that emphasizes early surgical obliteration of the aneurysm and an aggressive multimodal approach to the treatment of delayed ischemia. This approach requires urgent definitive diagnosis, early surgical and medical intervention, careful monitoring, and medical management until the risk of hydrocephalus and vasospasm has passed. This approach to treatment is best accomplished in special centers that are organized to provide the multidisciplinary expertise required by these patients, and it should improve outcome.

PRESENTATION AND EVALUATION

The classic presentation of aneurysmal rupture is the sudden onset of a violent headache, often associated with syncope, followed by nausea, vomiting, and nuchal rigidity. Often there is confusion, lethargy, and occasionally focal neurologic deficits; however, in a significant number of cases the presentation is less clear, and as many as one-third of cases are misdiagnosed. Therefore, a high index of suspicion is necessary to avoid delay in treatment.

The initial diagnostic test of choice for suspected SAH is a computed tomography (CT) scan. Before being transported to the CT scanner, the patient should be assessed for airway control, level of consciousness, and hemodynamics. Obtunded patients should be intubated, and elevated blood pressure should be controlled. When performed on the day of hemorrhage CT has sensitivity of approximately 90 percent. If CT demonstrates SAH, lumbar puncture is not required, because the diagnosis is established and lumbar puncture may carry a small risk of precipitating rerupture of the aneurysm. When, however, there is strong clinical suspicion of SAH and negative CT findings or if no CT scanner is available, lumbar puncture is indicated. Contrast-enhanced CT may demonstrate an aneurysm, but this does not eliminate the need for angiography.

Angiography should be performed as soon as possible following the diagnosis of SAH. The patient's ability to protect the airway while supine and draped during the long procedure should be assessed. When necessary, intubation should be carried out with premedication (short-acting barbiturates and/or lidocaine), to prevent a hypertensive response to tracheal stimulation. Hypertension should be controlled throughout the procedure (see initial management). Agitated or uncooperative patients should undergo angiography under general anesthesia. While some clinicians delay angiography for fear of inducing rerupture, in a series of more than 5,000 patients this occurred in only seven. Therefore the diagnostic evaluation should not be delayed. Because as many as 20 percent of patients have multiple aneurysms, a selective four-vessel study is necessary for all patients. If angiography does not reveal a cause for the SAH, it should probably be repeated in 1 to 2 weeks. In general, patients with negative angiograms have a relatively benign course.

INITIAL MANAGEMENT

Early surgery (within 3 days of rupture) is becoming the treatment of choice for aneurysmal SAH. This not only eliminates the possibility of rebleeding but also allows aggressive treatment of vasospasm with hypertensive hypervolemic therapy (see below). All patients who present with Hunt and Hess disease grade I through III and many who have grade IV disease (Tables 1 and 2) should be considered for early surgery. Because the incidence of rebleeding is highest in the first 24 hours after hemorrhage, surgery should be performed as soon as it is feasible. If early surgery is performed, antifibrinolytic agents should not be administered, as even a short course is associated with an increased incidence of hydrocephalus and vasospasm. The benefits of early surgery include (1) elimination of rebleeding, (2) obviating antifibrinolytic therapy, which is associated with increased incidence of hydrocephalus and vasospasm, (3) allowing induced hypertension to treat vasospasm (see below), (4) allowing washing out of blood from the subarachnoid space to reduce vasospasm, and (5) potentially shortening hospitalization time.

The initial management of patients after SAH is directed toward prevention of rebleeding, preparation for surgery, and monitoring for and treatment of potential complications. Management strategies are based on the following factors: rebleeding may be associated with hypertension; clinically significant acute hydrocephalus may develop even in the absence of intraventricular blood; SAH patients tend to become volume contracted, and this exacerbates vasospasm; cardiac abnormalities, including arrhythmias, are common; and the incidence of vasospasm is proportional to the amount of subarachnoid blood. Circumstances that could result in hypertension should be avoided.

Table 1 Hunt and Hess Classification

Grade	Signs and Symptoms
I	No symptoms or slight headache
II	Moderate to severe headache and nuchal rigidity but no focal or lateralizing neurologic signs
III	Drowsiness, confusion, and mild focal deficits
IV	Stupor, hemiparesis, early decerebrate rigidity, and vegetative disturbances
V	Deep coma and decerebrate rigidity

Table 2 World Federation of Neurological Surgeons SAH Scale

Grade	Glasgow Coma Scale Score	Motor Deficit
I	15	Absent
II	13–14	Absent
III	13–14	Present
IV	7–12	Present or absent
V	3–6	Present or absent

Therefore, management should include a calm environment, avoidance of excessive stimulation, cardiac and blood pressure monitoring, hydration, and serial neurologic examinations.

The patient is placed in a dark, quiet room, stimulation is minimized, and stool softeners are administered. Agitated patients should be sedated to the point where they tend to fall asleep when not stimulated but can be easily aroused and examined. This should be accomplished with short-acting or reversible agents (morphine, fentanyl, pentothal, midazolam) so that hydrocephalus can be distinguished from drug effect. Analgesics are useful because they treat the headache and can also provide sedation. The traditional use of phenobarbital for sedation and as an anticonvulsant is inappropriate because of its long duration of action and the fact that an anticonvulsant blood level is not achieved for some 1 to 2 weeks. Although the risk of a seizure is small for patients without intracerebral hematomas, anticonvulsants are usually administered for fear that the hyperemia associated with a seizure will precipitate rebleeding. Phenytoin is generally employed, and the loading dose should be administered intravenously because of very slow absorption following oral administration. Corticosteroids are usually administered in the acute period, to reduce meningeal irritation and possibly postoperative swelling. Hydration should be accomplished with isotonic saline administered at a rate slightly above maintenance requirements. Continuous cardiac monitoring is advisable, and blood pressure should be measured frequently. Blood pressure should be maintained at the patient's normal level. If that information is lacking and the patient is normotensive, the blood pressure should be kept below approximately 150 mm Hg systolic and 90 mm Hg diastolic. These limits should be raised for older patients and those with a history of hypertension. Hypertension is often seen in response to a severe headache and can be managed with analgesics. Otherwise, the hypercatecholaminergic state usually responds to beta-blockers (labetalol, propranolol), which are best administered intravenously. Nimodipine may also be helpful in controlling blood pressure and should be administered to all patients (see below).

PERIOPERATIVE MANAGEMENT

In preparation for surgery the patient should be given nothing by mouth and appropriate preoperative studies (electrolytes, blood count, blood type and cross-match, chest film, electrocardiography [ECG]) are performed. Postoperative neurologic evaluation is facilitated by use of an anesthetic regimen that achieves rapid emergence from anesthesia. This allows early assessment of the patient's neurologic status, to help determine if there is postoperative bleeding or if vessels were inadvertently clipped. Many neurosurgeons routinely perform postoperative angiography to check clip placement.

If the aneurysm has been successfully clipped, then the need for sedation and strict blood pressure control is eliminated. Analgesics should be administered as needed, but excessive sedation is avoided lest it interfere with neurologic assessment. Patients tend to be mildly hypertensive, and this should not be treated. Hypotension is unusual and the cause must be sought. It usually results from hypovolemia, as patients often receive mannitol during surgery. If present, hypovolemia should be corrected rapidly, because it increases the risk of symptomatic vasospasm. Some clinicians routinely increase intravenous fluids postoperatively to achieve prophylactic volume expansion in the hope of reducing the likelihood of symptomatic vasospasm.

COMPLICATIONS

Patients who suffer SAH are prone to several complications, including rebleeding, delayed ischemia due to vasospasm, postoperative brain edema, hydrocephalus, infections, and complications of therapy. Careful monitoring facilitates early identification and prompt treatment of complications and improves outcome.

Rebleeding

Prevention of rebleeding is best accomplished by surgically obliterating the aneurysm. Improvements in surgical technique have made early surgery safe, and when it is combined with aggressive treatment of vasospasm outcome is improved. When early surgery is not planned, the utility of antifibrinolytics has not been demonstrated. Although they reduce the risk of rebleeding, the increase in hydrocephalus and vasospasm results in no overall improvement in outcome. Interventional radiologic techniques are becoming available that afford an endovascular approach to obliterate aneurysms. Though these techniques may be useful in unruptured aneurysms, they are associated with rebleeding when applied to recently ruptured aneurysms and should be considered only for carefully selected patients who are not eligible for surgery.

Hydrocephalus

Hydrocephalus is common after SAH and can present either abruptly shortly after SAH or gradually several days to weeks after hemorrhage. Acute hydrocephalus is often associated with intraventricular blood and can develop within hours of SAH. While in some patients it remains static or resolves spontaneously, in about one-third of cases it progresses. If a patient presents with SAH, lethargy, and hydrocephalus, it is probably best to treat the hydrocephalus to determine its contribution to the lethargy. This helps to clarify the prognosis and may prompt a surgeon to proceed with early surgery. Because acute hydrocephalus is frequently obstructive, treatment with ventriculostomy is preferred to lumbar drainage. Care must be employed in placing the intraventricular catheter, to avoid rapidly lowering intracranial pressure (ICP), as this may precipitate rebleeding. It is probably best not to lower the ICP below 20 mm Hg.

Often, acute hydrocephalus may resolve over the course of several days. This can be assessed by periodically stopping cerebrospinal fluid (CSF) drainage and continuously monitoring the ICP response. If after several attempts ICP continues to rise, the patient may require a permanent shunt.

Hydrocephalus may also develop insidiously over days, usually 1 to 3 weeks after SAH. This is almost always a communicating hydrocephalus, and it presents as a gradual decline in the level of consciousness. The diagnosis is easily made by CT and can be confirmed by measurement of ICP and determination of the response to CSF drainage. This form of hydrocephalus can be managed by placement of a ventricular or lumbar drain or by serial lumbar punctures. The need for permanent shunting is determined in the same manner as for acute hydrocephalus.

Vasospasm

Currently, delayed ischemia from vasospasm is the leading cause of morbidity and mortality in hospitalized patients with SAH. At the present time our best understanding of the cause of vasospasm is that hemoglobin slowly released into the CSF from the subarachnoid clot is a major factor in the development of vasospasm. The peak incidence of vasospasm occurs 7 to 10 days after hemorrhage, but it can develop from 3 days to 3 weeks after SAH. The frequency of vasospasm depends on the method used to define it. Angiographic vasospasm develops in 60 to 80 percent of patients following SAH; however, clinical signs occur in 30 to 40 percent. The angiographic pattern may be focal or diffuse and vasospasm is more frequent in vessels distal to the aneurysm. Transcranial Doppler (TCD) ultrasonography is not quite as sensitive as angiography, probably because it samples only a limited portion of the cerebral vasculature.

The clinical syndrome of vasospasm is that of a fluctuating focal deficit or a decline in level of consciousness. The signs are worsened by hypovolemia, hypotension, or severe anemia. When a clinical picture develops that is suggestive of vasospasm, other causes should always be considered. These include hydrocephalus, metabolic derangement, hypoxia, hypercarbia, or infection. Though TCD or angiography is sometimes used to confirm the clinical diagnosis, their value is not absolute. Angiographic or TCD evidence of vasospasm may be present without clinical symptoms, and their absence does not exclude clinical vasospasm. After evaluating other possible causes, many clinicians base treatment on the clinical picture.

Treatment of vasospasm occurs in two stages. Prophylactic therapy is administered to all patients with SAH; aggressive measures are reserved for those who exhibit acute clinical deterioration. Prophylactic mea-

sures include washing out of subarachnoid blood during surgery. This process can be aided with the use of fibrinolytic agents to dissolve the clot. They can be instilled into the subarachnoid space after the aneurysm is clipped, and they are currently being evaluated in clinical trials. Nimodipine, a calcium channel blocker that crosses the blood-brain barrier, has been shown to reduce the number and size of delayed cerebral infarctions after SAH. While it remains unclear whether nimodipine's beneficial effects are a result of action on blood vessels or neuronal membranes, its use is recommended for all patients following SAH. Treatment is started as soon as possible after hemorrhage and continued for 21 days. The recommended dose is 60 mg every 4 hours. The administration of nimodipine can be associated with hypotension, which is best avoided, especially in patients with symptomatic vasospasm. This can usually be avoided by ensuring that the patient is well-hydrated before beginning therapy and starting with a dose of 30 mg and advancing to the full dose, as tolerated. In particularly sensitive patients, administration of smaller, more frequent doses can solve the problem.

Following SAH, complex neuroendocrine disturbances can result in hyponatremia and volume contraction. Though the hyponatremia has been attributed to the syndrome of inappropriate secretion of antidiuretic hormone, treatment with fluid restriction has been shown to dramatically increase the incidence of cerebral infarctions. Several studies have indicated that SAH patients given maintenance volumes of fluids tend to become volume contracted, a particularly dangerous condition when there is vasospasm. A recent study found that prophylactic hypervolemic therapy can prevent volume contraction, and this has become routine therapy following SAH. The hyponatremia is usually mild and asymptomatic. Severe or symptomatic hyponatremia should be treated with hypertonic saline. Diuretics may be helpful, but if they are used fluid administration must be increased to avoid volume contraction.

If, despite all these measures, a patient develops clinical signs of vasospasm, they are treated with hypervolemic hypertensive therapy. This begins with acute volume expansion with 1 to 2 L of either isotonic saline or colloids, in order to optimize cardiac filling pressure and cardiac output. Target pressures are central venous pressure of about 10 to 12 mm Hg or a pulmonary capillary wedge pressure of 15 to 18 mm Hg. Some patients may require as much as 500 ml per hour to achieve and maintain these values. If there is no clinical response in several hours, blood pressure should be elevated. The initial goal is to raise mean arterial blood pressure to 10 to 20 percent above the baseline value. This can be accomplished with a combination of dopamine and phenylephrine. If there is no clinical response, the blood pressure should be raised further. During this therapy the neurologic status must be closely monitored and the therapy titrated to effect so that the minimal therapy that improves the neurologic status is given. If a ventricular or lumbar catheter is in place then the ICP can be lowered to 0 to 5 mm Hg to aid cerebral perfusion pressure. The therapy is maintained for several days and then gradually withdrawn while monitoring the neurologic exam. If symptoms recur, then the therapy must once again be increased. Because vasospasm is a self-limited process, the patient can usually be weaned from hypertensive therapy after several days to 2 weeks. Hypervolemic therapy is usually continued for an additional 1 to 2 weeks.

Hypertensive hypervolemic therapy is not without complications—complications of line placement, cardiovascular compromise, and electrolyte loss, among others. In patients with poor cardiac status it can lead to fluid overload, congestive heart failure, and cardiac ischemia. Use of a Swan-Ganz catheter to monitor cardiac function is essential in these cases, and careful titration of therapy can usually avoid serious difficulties. Serial ECG studies and continuous ST segment analysis are helpful for monitoring for cardiac ischemia. In addition, hypervolemic therapy increases renal loss of potassium, magnesium, and phosphate. Replacement therapy should be guided by frequent (daily) measurement of blood levels of these electrolytes.

Recently, transluminal angioplasty has been applied to cerebral vessels in vasospasm. Initial reports are promising, but the therapy has not been rigorously evaluated. At present, appropriate candidates are probably patients who do not respond to hypervolemic hypertensive therapy or whose cardiac status makes them unable to tolerate it. Angioplasty probably should not be performed if there is an infarct on CT. The clinical response is probably related to the duration of symptoms.

DISCUSSION

Improved surgical techniques, better understanding of vasospasm, and innovative pharmacologic, hemodynamic, and endovascular approaches now provide an aggressive approach to what was previously considered a disease for which therapies had little to offer. The development of specialized centers that command expertise in this wide range of techniques should significantly improve the outcome of patients with SAH.

SUGGESTED READING

Bailes JE, Spetzler RF, Hadley MN, Baldwin HZ. Management morbidity and mortality of poor-grade aneurysm patients. J Neurosurg 1990; 72:559–566.
Hanley DF, Kirsch JR. Cerebral vasospasm: Use of hypervolemic hypertensive therapy. Crit Care Reports 1989; 1:80–87.
Kirsch JR, Diringer MN, Borel C, Hanley DF. Cerebral aneurysms: Mechanisms of injury and critical care interventions. Crit Care Clinics 1989; 5:755–772.
Kistler JP, Heros RC. Subarachnoid hemorrhage due to a ruptured saccular aneurysm. In: Ropper AH, Kennedy SF, eds. Neurological and neurosurgical intensive care. Rockville, Maryland: Aspen, 1988:219.
Solomon CT. Aneurysmal subarachnoid hemorrhage: Detecting and treating complications. Crit Care Reports 1989; 1:75–80.
Solomon RA, Fink ME. Current strategies for the management of aneurysmal subarachnoid hemorrhage. Arch Neurol 1987; 44: 769–774.

ARTERIOVENOUS MALFORMATIONS OF THE BRAIN AND SPINAL CORD

SYDNEY J. PEERLESS, M.D., FRCSC

Vascular malformations of the central nervous system are classified into four subtypes: arteriovenous malformations (AVMs), venous angiomas, cavernous malformations, and telangiectasias. This division is based on (1) the nature of the component vessels, (2) the presence of normal or abnormal intervening neural tissue in and around the malformation, and (3) the clinical features.

Of the four general subtypes, at autopsy venous malformations are the most common. Venous malformations are composed of normal veins separated by normal-looking neural parenchyma, and they usually lie in white matter. The veins have a radial (spoked) configuration, and one or more central ones may be unusually large. No large arterial vessels are obvious in venous malformations, but occasionally there can be a single, dilated vein with a few venous tributaries. These veins are part of the normal drainage system of that area of brain, and the lesions are generally benign with little potential for microscopic or gross hemorrhage. Those found in the cerebellum are thought, without good evidence, to have somewhat greater bleeding propensity. In pathologic studies, small areas of gliosis may be seen in the region of the veins.

Cavernous malformations are composed of a compact mass of sinusoidal vessels with no intervening neural parenchyma. These appear as a discrete, black-brown, multilobulated mass, often with gross and microscopic evidence of recent and remote hemorrhage and hemosiderin-laden macrophages in the adjacent gliotic white matter. Gross hemorrhage from these lesions is rare, but repeated minor hemorrhages are common. They are angiographically occult. Cavernous malformations have become clinically much more important in recent years with the advent of computed tomography (CT) and, in particular, magnetic resonance imaging (MRI); both modalities image the lesions quite dramatically.

Capillary malformations or telangiectasias are composed of small capillary vessels in a spherical mass rarely larger than 1 cm in diameter. The vessels are typically separated by normal neural parenchyma, and there are regions of gliosis and mineralization in the area. Hemorrhage from these lesions is rare.

A fifth form of vascular malformation is the cryptic malformation. This probably represents small AVMs or cavernous malformations which obliterate themselves by moderate to massive hemorrhage in brain or spinal cord, with abnormal vessels, not identified on angiography, but found at autopsy or in the surgical specimen.

True AVMs are congenital lesions that develop between the fourth and eighth week of embryonic life, owing to the persistence of direct communications between the future arterial and venous sides of the primitive vascular plexus and failure to develop of an interposed capillary network. They are not hereditary. AVMs consist of masses of abnormal arteries and veins that on angiography have an easily demonstrable arteriovenous fistula through vessels varying greatly in size and shape. The larger vessels are usually more venous, with little tunica muscularis in the wall and no elastica. Between the vessels is a small amount of abnormal neural tissue, if, indeed, there is any. Histologic examination commonly shows evidence of prior hemorrhage— abnormal stained gliotic tissue and hemosiderin-laden macrophages. The malformation is usually surrounded by a thin layer of gliotic tissue, again with evidence of hemorrhages (variously aged hemosiderin-filled macrophages).

AVMs are uncommon. The incidence, based on small autopsy series, is estimated to be about 3 per 100,000 population, about one-seventh the incidence of cerebral aneurysms. Nevertheless, they are the most common vascular malformation seen in the clinic: about 2,500 new symptomatic cases present each year in the United States. Because the number of asymptomatic persons that harbor AVMs is unknown, critical data necessary for proper natural history predictions are unavailable. Although these are congenital lesions, it is thought that, initially at least, the surrounding vasculature and neural tissue is normal. However, owing to the absence of a capillary-resistant bed, the pressure in adjacent normal arteries is reduced, and the flow increases and may cause subsequent enlargement of surrounding otherwise normal vessels. This gives the appearance of progressive enlargement over time, though the actual congenital vascular anomaly, the nidus of the lesion, remains unchanged in size, and when this nidus is obliterated or removed the surrounding vasculature rapidly returns to normal size and caliber.

CLINICAL FEATURES

AVMs may present with hemorrhage, seizures, headache, or uncommonly, progressive neurologic deficit. In infants, large, fistulous AVMs to large veins (vein of Galen) may present as congestive heart failure or hydrocephalus. The natural history of AVMs is uncertain, because most series are small and selected and the follow-up interval has been relatively short. Perhaps the longest and most complete follow-up came from Troupp in Finland, where 160 cases were followed for an average of 24 years and the rebleeding rate was 4 percent per year with a mortality rate of 1 percent per year, and combined mortality and morbidity were 2.7 percent per year. These rates were similar whether the patient presented with hemorrhage, seizures, or headache without hemorrhage. In a variety of small series in the literature, the hemorrhage rate is estimated to be about 1 to 2 percent per year, with overall 14 percent mortality and 20 percent morbidity rates. The Mayo Clinic series of 164 patients had a 2.2 percent hemorrhage rate with 29 percent mortality and 23 percent morbidity. It needs to be stressed to patients and referring physicians that this hemorrhage rate is quite constant per year and not compounding. It is equally clear that the greater the number of years a patient who harbors an AVM is exposed to the risk of hemorrhage, the cumulative risk of neurologic injury or death for an AVM diagnosed early in life may be quite significant. It has long been thought that small AVMs bleed more frequently than large ones and that hemorrhages from small malformations are often more serious. This appears to be related to the hemodynamics of the malformation: small malformations have a smaller cross-sectional area and, therefore, the pressure drop from the arterial to the venous side of the circulation is more abrupt. Very large AVMs have a proportionately large cross-sectional area. Two-thirds of hemorrhages occur into brain or into an adjacent ventricle, and one-third into the subarachnoid space. Because massive subarachnoid hemorrhage is relatively rare, secondary vasospasm and cerebral ischemia is an uncommon consequence of hemorrhage from an AVM.

Seizures

Depending on the site, some 20 to 70 percent of AVMs are associated with seizures. Approximately half the seizures are focal, 40 percent generalized, and 10 percent partial complex. The cause of seizures is unknown. They may be due to irritation and injury to surrounding cortex by minute or minor hemorrhage or ischemic change from high flow through the AVM.

Headaches

Headaches are a common accompaniment of AVMs, even those that have never ruptured. This is thought to be due to enlargement of feeding arteries and draining veins and involvement of adjacent dura. Many patients with cerebral AVM report typical migraine.

Progressive Neurologic Deficit

Progressive neurologic deficit is an uncommon clinical feature of AVMs, but it has nevertheless been well-documented and may be due to recurrent hemorrhage, progressive occlusion of arterial feeders or draining veins, or high flow through the shunt causing a steal phenomenon or hypoperfusion of the adjacent normal brain.

Associated Lesions

Intercurrent with some 5 to 8 percent of all AVMs is an aneurysm, and 1 percent of all aneurysm patients have an AVM. If both AVM and aneurysm exist in one patient, the risk of hemorrhage is increased. If a patient with both an AVM and an aneurysm presents with subarachnoid hemorrhage (SAH), it is almost always the aneurysm that has ruptured. Usually, aneurysms arise from vessels feeding the AVM, and presumably develop from the high flow through the feeding artery, accelerating the hemodynamic stress to the vessel wall.

IMAGING

The gold standard for radiologic diagnosis of an AVM is four vessel cerebral angiography. Angiography also definitively diagnoses a venous malformation, but cavernous malformations, cryptic malformations, and telangiectasias are invisible to cerebral angiography. CT and MRI will identify most vascular malformations of the brain and spinal cord. Angiographically invisible malformations have a highly distinctive pattern on T1- and T2-weighted images. CT and MR are also valuable in demonstrating recent and remote hemorrhage and ischemic changes in the region of the AVM.

THERAPY

The natural history of untreated AVMs is modestly unfavorable. Deciding whether or not to treat and what form of treatment to use is complex and must weigh several considerations: (1) the presentation and natural history of the lesion; (2) the known results of the available therapeutic alternatives; (3) the patient's age and general medical and neurologic condition; (4) the presenting symptoms (hemorrhage, epilepsy, headache, or none); (5) the physical parameters of the AVM, including its location, size, the number and flow pattern of the feeding vessels, venous drainage; (6) the presence of a recent or remote hematoma; and (7) the site of the lesion (the precise anatomic relationship of the malformation to surrounding brain, cranial nerves, and pituitary gland). For many patients, all that is necessary is symptomatic treatment for headache or seizures and firm reassurance that the risk of living with an AVM is small. Physicians should avoid using such terms as *a time bomb in your head* to predict the future, particularly when an asymptomatic patient's malformation has been detected incidentally while investigating some unrelated complaint. It is also important to remember that the various therapies available for AVMs are directed primarily toward preventing hemorrhage, so that cure of a seizure disorder or reversal of neurologic deficit cannot usually be offered as a therapeutic goal. Furthermore, it is necessary to point out that incomplete treatment of AVMs (i.e., when some abnormal vessels remain) offers no significant protection against rebleeding.

A number of therapeutic options are available for a patient with an AVM. To my mind, the best is complete microsurgical removal. In the hands of an experienced surgeon, microsurgical techniques using effective bipolar cautery, tiny vascular clips, accurate definition and preservation of arterial vessels of passage, precise removal of all of the AVM, and meticulous hemostasis has rendered most small and medium-sized AVMs amenable to direct surgical therapy. The exception is lesions that lie entirely within eloquent areas of the cerebrum or the brain stem. This is the ideal treatment if it can be done safely, but the decision to operate is based on two key variables: the size of the lesion and its anatomic site. The risk of surgical removal increases dramatically with the size of the AVM. In our experience, we have had no morbidity or mortality with small (<2.5 cm diameter) AVMs and just over 15 percent with large (>5 cm diameter) ones (Table 1). The site of the malformation is critical as well. An AVM located in the nondominant frontal pole may be surgically removed with little difficulty and little risk for the patient, but a small, even tiny, malformation within the spinal cord, brain stem, or thalamus may be surgically inaccessible (Table 2). Simple ligation of the feeding vessels of the malformation is completely ineffectual. The fistulous connection between arteries and veins in the nidus of the lesion rapidly recruits surrounding vessels and rapidly makes them as prominent as those that have been ligated.

Embolization

In the hands of an experienced neurosurgeon, the majority of cavernous angiomas can be removed from most locations with microsurgical techniques, even those in the brain stem. This is the preferred treatment, as

Table 1 Risk of Resection of Arteriovenous Malformation with Respect to Size*

Size	Patients (No.)	Risk (%)		
		Good	Poor	Dead
Small (<2.5 cm)	104	100		
Medium (2.5–5 cm)	183	95.6	2.8	1.6
Large (>5 cm)	23	69.7	15	15.2

*Results of resection of supratentorial AVMs in 320 patients in good condition.

Table 2 Risk of Surgery of Arteriovenous Malformation
with Respect to Site

Site/Population	Risk (%)		
	Good	*Poor*	*Dead*
Supratentorial			
320 patients in *good* condition	95	2.5	2.5
51 patients in *poor* condition*	30	50	20
Infratentorial			
86 patients	78	15.1	7

*Underwent operation after hemorrhage and in poor neurologic condition.

embolization and radiotherapy are ineffectual and cavernous malformations exhibit a greater tendency to recurrent hemorrhage or progressive neurologic deficit.

Large AVMs can often be transformed into smaller, low-flow lesions with interventional neuroradiologic techniques by occluding inflow feeders and blocking the nidus of the shunt with particulate material, rapidly setting glue, or metal coils. In my experience, it is rare that a malformation can be completely obliterated by embolization alone, because it is distinctly uncommon for a malformation to have a single feeding vessel. Embolization can, however, be very useful in obliterating deep feeding vessels that are hard to expose and in decreasing the sump effect in the malformation, making surgical obliteration technically more feasible. As a primary treatment, embolization may be all that is necessary in dural AVMs, and in particular for those spinal AVMs that are fed by only one or two dural arteriovenous fistulas.

Radiosurgery

The first systematic use of focused ionizing beams of radiation to AVMs began in Sweden in 1970, using a focused cobalt source in the Leksell gamma knife. Since then, a number of other sources of ionizing radiation have been utilized, including the linear accelerator, the cyclotron-utilizing Bagg-Peak proton beam therapy, and, in a less systematic way, conventional fractionated radiotherapy. The source of the ionizing energy is quite immaterial. The qualitative effects to the vessels that comprise the AVM appear to be the same. The radiation causes endothelial cells and perivascular tissue to swell and degenerate and promotes thrombosis and proliferative fibroplastic repair. With progressive thickening and fibrosis of the abnormal vessel walls, occlusion of the shunt and ultimately obliteration of the AVM occur. The success of these techniques depends on delivery of the ionizing radiation in a precise and focused manner to the malformation using stereotactic principles and avoiding injury to surrounding brain. Using these techniques, Steiner has over the past 20 years treated more than 1300 patients with small AVMs located in deep, eloquent areas of the brain. In about 80 percent of these cases the

malformation was totally obliterated. The success rate increased to 88 percent for lesions less than 1 cc in volume, but for malformations larger than 8 cc, only 60 percent were totally obliterated. The process of obliterating the arteriovenous shunt takes as long as 2 years. In this period, recurrent hemorrhage remains a risk, and at least at the same incidence as the natural history. When an AVM has been irradiated but not completely occluded, some believe abnormal vessels which are still patent are thickened and the risk of hemorrhage reduced, but if this is so, the effect is small and probably not present for several years and, therefore, of limited value. Four percent of the patients suffered permanent neurologic injury from radiation necrosis of surrounding brain tissue.

The radiosurgery of venous angiomas has been less effective, and now it is not considered a treatment alternative for venous malformations. Radiosurgery of cryptic malformations, including cavernous angiomas and telangiectasias, also has been ineffective and the associated complication rate is significantly higher.

Arteriovenous Malformations of the Spinal Cord

AVMs of the cord are rare (4 percent of all spine lesions). They are more common in men than in women and present throughout life, as SAH in 15 percent and as hemorrhage into the cord or progressive neurologic deficit in the remainder. Dysesthetic, radicular pain is a common premonitory symptom. The sudden onset of back pain with SAH is very suggestive of a spinal AVM. Neurologically and radiologically, spinal AVMs are divided into dural and intradural malformations with intra- and extramedullary collections of abnormal vessels. Dural malformations are supplied by the meningeal branches of a radicular artery and drain via a radicular vein into the medullary venous plexus of the cord. These lesions typically present with progressive neurologic decline, which is thought to be due to venous stasis and ischemia in the involved cord segment. Treatment of these lesions by surgical ligation or embolization of the radicular feeder or feeders with closure of the dural AV shunt is very effective and carries little risk. Embolization is simple but less desirable: as many as 75 percent of the occluded vessels recanalize. In contrast, the treatment of true intradural intramedullary spinal AVMs is much more difficult—and potentially hazardous. Microsurgical excision of the malformation is the treatment of choice, but it is difficult to accomplish in true intramedullary AVMs without significant risk of causing neurologic injury. An intradural AVM that is largely extramedullary, particularly if it is located posteriorly in the cord, may be easily resectable. Even so, if the malformation involves a large volume of the cord and is principally fed by anterior spinal artery radicles, it may be quite impossible to remove with any safety. Juvenile AVMs, which involve both extra- and intradural portions of the spinal canal and often extend into surrounding bone, the thoracic cavity, or retroperitoneal space, are generally quite unsuitable for direct excision. Embolization of spinal AVMs may be effective in reducing flow in the intradural and intramedullary forms, though for the latter, the risk of embolic occlusion and infarction of the cord exceeds 30 percent. Radiosurgery generally is not suitable for spinal AVMs because of the increased risk of radiation necrosis to the cord.

MANAGEMENT DECISIONS

The most challenging aspects of caring for a patient who harbors an AVM is to decide rationally on a management strategy. I find it most useful when discussing with patients the treatment possibilities to use four charts (see Tables 1 through 3 and Fig. 1). The algorithm in Figure 1 depicts an annual hemorrhage rate of 4 percent per year and a 1 percent mortality, 1.7 percent morbidity, and recovery without deficit for 1.3 percent of patients who bleed. These figures allow the patient and the referring physician to grasp the risks of living with an AVM for a year or a decade. A more conservative estimate of risk of bleeding—2 percent per year with half the patients returning to normal function and only 1 percent dead or disabled—strengthens the case for leaving the AVM alone and treating only the symptoms (headache, seizures, anxiety). This is particularly true if the patient is older than 50 years and therefore has the prospect of a limited number of years at risk. One should also have available—and be experienced in—the whole range of treatment options (see Table 3): some AVMs are easily and safely treated by one method and are quite unsuitable for others. Finally,

Table 3 Management Options for Arteriovenous Malformation

No intervention
Surgical excision
Embolization and excision
Focused ionizing radiation
    Gamma knife
    Proton Bragg Peak
    Linear accelerator
    Conventional radiotherapy
Combination of the above

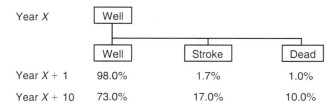

	Well	Stroke	Dead
Year X + 1	98.0%	1.7%	1.0%
Year X + 10	73.0%	17.0%	10.0%

Figure 1 Natural history of AVMs (accruing 4 percent per year hemorrhage rate).

the surgeon's own record of success or failure with these treatment modalities needs to be factored into the decision (see Tables 1 and 2). Armed with these data, it is usually possible to not only modify a patient's fear and anxiety but to arrive at a treatment decision that is logical and ultimately successful.

SUGGESTED READING

Auger RG, Wiebers DO. Management of unruptured intracranial arteriovenous malformations: A decision analysis. Neurosurgery 1992; 30:561–569.

Drake CG, Friedman AH, Peerless SJ. Posterior fossa arteriovenous malformations. J Neurosurg 1986; 64:1–10.

Fults D, Kelly DC. Natural history of arteriovenous malformations of the brain: A clinical study. Neurosurgery 1984; 15:658–662.

Horton JD, Chambers WA, Lyons SZ, et al. Pregnancy and the risk of hemorrhage from cerebral arteriovenous malformations. Neurosurgery 1990; 27:867–872.

Lundquist C, Berthelsen B, Sullivan M, et al. Spinal arteriovenous malformations: Neurological aspects and results of embolization. Acta Neurol Scand 1990; 82:51–58.

Ogilvy CS. Radiation therapy for arteriovenous malformations: A review. Neurosurgery 1990; 26:725–735.

Wilkins RH. Natural history of intracranial vascular malformations: A review. Neurosurgery 1985; 16:421–430.

HYPERTENSIVE ENCEPHALOPATHY

JAMES O. DONALDSON, M.D.

In 1928, Oppenheimer and Fishberg delineated and named the syndrome of hypertensive encephalopathy. Although the diagnosis should be considered in any case of severe hypertension, headache, and altered mental status, the term was bastardized by some in the years thereafter to include any sort of cerebral condition coincident with hypertension. Today we have returned, full circle, to the original clinical description of the syndrome:

> In the course of acute glomerulonephritis, and less commonly in other varieties of chronic interstitial nephritis, there may occur acute episodes of cerebral phenomena, such as epileptiform convulsions, coma, headache, amaurosis, hemiplegia, and aphasia.... Since the beginning of the present century, convincing evidence that these cerebral episodes are not uremic in nature has gradually accumulated. It has become clear that these cerebral symptoms are correlated with hypertension, being a manifestation of circulatory disturbances in the brain consequent on the hypertension. For this reason, we have termed the cerebral syndrome hypertensive encephalopathy.... In most cases, this increase of blood pressure is manifest and, in fact, is usually extreme. We have seen cases in children in which the existence of arterial hypertension was not immediately manifest, only subsequent observation proving such figures as 120/80 to be above the normal for the child.
>
> The onset of the cerebral symptoms is often preceded by an additional rise above the already elevated level of blood pressure. This may occur quickly, particularly in eclampsia gravidarum, or more gradually over a period of several days.... The individual cerebral phenomena come and go, leaving no trace behind them.... The focal cerebral symptoms often change. In the case (of glomerulonephritis) described, the patient had aphasia with the first attack; then his convulsions began on the right side, and later they started on the left side. Sometimes they would affect only the face or an upper extremity, or there would be unilateral convulsions. (Gowers described this in eclampsia in 1888.) ... The occurrence of aphasia in such cases has been described by Osler [in 1911]. Amaurosis is another symptom of hypertensive encephalopathy which is not extremely rare, the nature of the blindness being disclosed by its association with hypertension, its transitory nature, the negative ophthalmoscopic manifestations, apart from possible narrowing of the arteries, and the preservation of the light reflex which shows the cerebral origin.... Headache, which is a frequent—we believe the most frequent—manifestation of the hypertensive encephalopathy ... occurs as the culmination of a rapid rise in blood pressure ... and is relieved by venesection or lumbar puncture.
>
> In the toxemia of pregnancy, the eclamptic seizure invariably occurs in the presence of arterial hypertension (Vaquez and Nobecourt, 1897). The classic form of the eclamptic attack consists in epileptiform seizures in every way analogous to those occurring in glomerulonephritis. The attacks can often be shown to follow an added rise in the blood pressure and to be followed by a drop.

DIAGNOSTIC STUDIES

To this description little can be added except for the findings of neurodiagnostic studies. Lumbar puncture can find cerebrospinal fluid (CSF) pressure to be normal or elevated. The concentration of protein in CSF is typically 50 to 150 mg per deciliter. The electroencephalogram reflects the status of the patient, ranging from mild slowing of the background activity in patients who just have difficulty thinking to delta activity in stuporous patients, often prominently in the posterior regions in patients with cortical blindness. Magnetic resonance imaging (MRI) is an excellent method of showing generalized or focal cerebral edema, which sometimes occurs in arcuate bands through the internal and external capsules. Computed tomography (CT) may not detect some areas of edema in the cortex or visualize petechial hemorrhages; however CT is faster and CT is an excellent method of detecting larger acute hemorrhages like those that can occur in eclampsia. The timing of the appearance of cerebral edema is important. Unlike the delay of several days in the CT appearance of cytotoxic cerebral edema following a common ischemic stroke, vasogenic cerebral edema in hypertensive encephalopathy can be apparent on CT immediately after the crisis, and it often disappears after a few days.

MECHANISMS

Oppenheimer and Fishberg attributed hypertensive encephalopathy to cerebral vasoconstriction and cited as evidence retinal arteriolar narrowing. They noted cerebral edema in some but not all patients with hypertensive encephalopathy. Others attributed cerebral edema in this disorder to ischemic injury to cerebral capillaries, though Oppenheimer and Fishberg sagaciously admitted that the precise mechanism was beyond their ken. The microscopic hallmark of hypertensive encephalopathy is fibrinoid arteriolar necrosis with surrounding ring hemorrhages. These lesions tend to occur in the occipital lobes and in patches that are often watersheds between the territories of major cerebral arteries. Although vasoconstriction can be severe enough to cause microinfarctions, these lesions are always intermixed with ring hemorrhages, which grossly resemble petechial hemorrhages.

The pathogenesis of ring hemorrhages and fibrinoid necrosis can now be attributed to the failure of vasoconstriction at extremely high blood pressures to limit both perfusion through the capillary bed and the pressure exerted on capillary endothelial cells. In pathophysiologic terms, the upper limit of the autoregulation of cerebral blood flow is exceeded in hypertensive encephalopathy. The breakthrough occurs first in the occipital lobes and in the watersheds, which teleologically act as safety valves that protect the rest of the brain. At higher pressures, the process operates throughout the brain and generalized vasogenic cerebral edema results. The upper limit of autoregulation of cerebral perfusion is directly dependent on an individual's customary blood pressure. Thus, those who usually have low blood pressures (e.g., children with acute glomerulonephritis, pregnant teenagers, and pregnant women in unindustrialized regions) develop hypertensive encephalopathy at blood pressures that would be considered acceptable control values for a patient with chronic hypertension. For this reason, obstetricians will never be able to define a universally applicable blood pressure in their criteria for severe pre-eclampsia.

Hypertensive encephalopathy may complicate accelerated hypertension of any cause. Most cases occur in previously normotensive persons — in association with toxemia gravidarum or acute glomerulonephritis, after use of sympathomimetic agents including oral phencyclidine (PCP) often to avoid police apprehension; or phenylpropanolamine, or with tyramine consumption during monoamine oxidase (MAO_a) inhibitor therapy. Quadriplegics and paraplegics who have a complete spinal cord lesion above T5-6 can develop a hypertensive crisis as part of autonomic hyper-reflexia due to a painful visceral stimulus. Lengthening a congenitally short limb can be followed by a hypertensive crisis, which is probably initiated by stretching peripheral nerve. As Oppenheimer and Fishberg noted, hypertensive encephalopathy is infrequent in patients with chronic hypertension, because, as we now know, their upper limit of autoregulation is high, often above 230/150. Nevertheless, exceedingly high pressures can occur in chronic hypertension, often in preterminal stages. Hypertensive encephalopathy has been reported during rebound hypertension during withdrawal of clonidine hydrochloride and a few hours after an infusion of saralasin acetate during investigation for renin-dependent hypertension.

THERAPY

Hypertensive encephalopathy is an emergency. The objectives of treatment are to decrease blood pressure to within the range of autoregulation, to control convulsions, and to manage cerebral edema. The ideal antihypertensive drug for hypertensive encephalopathy would rapidly lower systemic blood pressure within the range of autoregulation, but in a controlled manner in order to prevent overshooting that range. A ganglionic blocking agent such as trimethaphan is effective but too unpredictable for frequent use in an era when other drugs are available. The target zone can be estimated from knowledge of an individual patient's customary blood pressure. If this is not known, mean arterial blood pressure should be lowered 20 to 25 percent. Furthermore, the agent should have minimal effect on cerebral

vessels. To wit, although nitroglycerin decreases systemic resistance, it also dilates cerebral vessels and, so, could worsen hypertensive encephalopathy. It worries me that anesthesiologists often use nitroglycerin during intubation of women with severe pre-eclampsia.

The cause of the hypertensive crisis can define the mode. For a quadriplegic with fecal impaction, enemas may be the ultimate cure, although antihypertensive medication may be needed temporarily. In this case, a drug such as labetalol, which blocks both alpha- and beta-adrenergic receptors, is an excellent choice. Similarly, in the case of renin-dependent hypertension, angiotensin-converting enzyme (ACE) inhibitors, such as captopril and enalaprilat, are effective.

Most often, vasodilators such as sodium nitroprusside, hydralazine, and diazoxide are used to decrease peripheral resistance. Each has advantages and disadvantages. Sodium nitroprusside is the drug of choice for many, but it must be shielded from light and requires constant surveillance that may not be practical. Bolus injections of diazoxide may be effective within 1 to 5 minutes and last 6 hours or more, but blood pressure below the target zone level can occur and cause end-organ ischemia. Hydralazine is the choice of many obstetricians trained in Pritchard's approach to the treatment of toxemia of pregnancy; however, its onset of action is relatively slow, even after intravenous administration — approximately 20 minutes. Nifedipine, a calcium channel blocker, has the advantage of oral administration if intravenous access is a problem. Sublingual or buccal nifedipine takes effect within 5 to 10 minutes, oral doses after 15 to 20 minutes. Usually, doctors use the agent with which they are most familiar.

Many patients with hypertensive encephalopathy, especially eclamptic women, have depleted intravascular volume. Diuretics can worsen the situation. Marked orthostasis and low pulmonary wedge pressures are indications for sodium and fluid replacement.

The best prophylactic anticonvulsant for hypertensive encephalopathy is effective antihypertensive treatment. If convulsions occur, diazepam is a common choice for immediate control. Often, an intravenous dose of 5 or 10 mg stops eclamptic convulsions without having any effect on the fetus. More can interfere with assessment of the level of consciousness and suppress or arrest respiration. Usually the effect of diazepam lasts at least 20 minutes, long enough to load the patient with phenytoin. In the case of eclamptic women, the standard 14 to 18 mg per kilogram loading dose is too much, because in pre-eclamptic women free, protein-unbound, phenytoin is 15 percent of total serum phenytoin instead of the usual 10 percent. Ryan's regimen for pre-eclamptic women is to initially load with 10 mg per kilogram and then repeat with another 5 mg per kilogram in 2 to 6 hours.

Generations of American obstetricians have been wedded to magnesium sulfate as an anticonvulsant for toxemic women. Its use is empiric and without scientific support. Besides being neither an antihypertensive nor an anticonvulsant drug, magnesium sulfate complicates anesthesia, can suppress uterine contractions, and causes neonatal hypermagnesemia. A substantial risk to mother and fetus is the obstetrician's false reliance on magnesium sulfate.

Furthermore, hypermagnesemia restricts ventilation and can cause carbon dioxide retention. This is particularly dangerous for women with severe pre-eclampsia, because a second factor setting the upper limit of autoregulation is partial pressure of carbon dioxide (PCO_2). The upper limit of autoregulation is inversely proportional to PCO_2. Arterial blood gases need to be checked if ventilation is impaired or if respiratory drive is diminished by drugs or central nervous system disease. Women with severe pre-eclampsia can convulse in the recovery room following general anesthesia for cesarean section whose blood pressure before anesthesia was evidently in the zone of autoregulation.

The principles for treatment of the vasogenic cerebral edema of hypertensive encephalopathy rest on the pathophysiologic mechanisms. Hyperventilation seems an obvious first measure, because it both decreases intracranial pressure and increases the upper limit of autoregulation. Second, mannitol can be predicted to be ineffective and sometimes dangerous. The effectiveness of mannitol as an osmotic agent depends on the integrity of the blood-brain barrier formed by the tight junctions between capillary endothelial cells. Vasogenic cerebral edema occurs because those junctions are leaky. Leakage of mannitol, with its sphere of hydration, into brain could worsen patients with widespread vasogenic cerebral edema. Furthermore, mannitol may tip women with severe pre-eclampsia or eclampsia into pulmonary edema and overload patients whose renal function is impaired. Third, corticosteroid therapy could be effective, as it is for vasogenic cerebral edema surrounding tumors metastatic to brain. If no contraindication exists, dexamethasone therapy is reasonable. Usually, the cerebral edema of hypertensive encephalopathy abates soon after blood pressure is controlled. In some cases intracranial pressure may need to be monitored and more aggressive treatment may be needed, including CSF drainage, hypothermia, and barbiturate coma; usually, these patients are eclamptic women with intracerebral hemorrhages. Surgical evacuation is rarely indicated.

SUGGESTED READING

Calhoun DA, Oparil S. Treatment of hypertensive crisis. N Engl J Med 1990; 323:1177–1183.
Dinsdale HB. Hypertensive encephalopathy. Neurol Clin 1983; 1:3–16.
Donaldson JO. Eclamptic hypertensive encephalopathy. Semin Neurol 1988; 8:230–233.
Donaldson JO. The case against magnesium sulfate for eclamptic convulsions. Int J Obstet Anesthesia 1992; 1:159–166.
Oppenheimer BS, Fishberg AM. Hypertensive encephalopathy. Arch Intern Med 1928; 41:264–278.

GIANT CELL (TEMPORAL) ARTERITIS AND CEREBRAL VASCULITIS

RICHARD J. CASELLI, M.D.
GENE G. HUNDER, M.D.

Vasculitic damage to the central nervous system (CNS) may arise from extracranial cervicocephalic arteritis, localized areas of intracranial vasculitis, or widespread intracranial vasculitis (Table 1). Diagnosis and treatment often rest on the clinical findings, arteriographic features (especially cerebral angiography), and histologic confirmation of vasculitis. Biopsy of extracerebral tissue (such as the superficial temporal artery) is sufficient for certain of the vasculitides (such as giant cell arteritis), but others can be diagnosed conclusively only by leptomeningeal and brain biopsy. Some of the inflammatory diseases to be considered are milder processes that produce no reliable radiologic abnormalities and can be conclusively demonstrated only by biopsy of meninges and brain. They may be mistaken for degenerative brain diseases and remain untreated even though some are clearly responsive to treatment. Almost all the conditions listed below produce headache and an elevated erythrocyte sedimentation rate, as do many nonvasculitic diseases. Table 2 summarizes some of the major presenting neurologic features of these diseases.

VASCULITIS PREDOMINANTLY AFFECTING EXTRACRANIAL AND CERVICOCEPHALIC ARTERIES

Giant Cell (Temporal) Arteritis

Giant cell (temporal) arteritis (GCA) most commonly presents as a new type of headache (prevalence 72 percent) in middle-aged or elderly patients and is usually associated with an elevated erythrocyte sedimentation rate (ESR; prevalence 97 percent). Unfortunately, headache is a nonspecific symptom, and an elevated ESR is a nonspecific sign, so that an extensive differential diagnosis must be entertained. Other common clinical manifestations include polymyalgia rheumatica (58 percent), malaise and fatigue (56 percent), jaw claudication (40 percent), and fever (35 percent). Amaurosis fugax occurs in approximately 10 percent of GCA patients.

Table 1 Neurovasculitis and Related Disorders

Disease	Treatment
Extracranial vasculitides	
Giant cell arteritis	Glucocorticoids
Takayasu arteritis	Glucocorticoids
Restricted intracranial vasculitides ("eyes and ears")	
Giant cell arteritis	Glucocorticoids
Cogan's syndrome	Glucocorticoids
Widespread intracranial vasculitis	
Primary CNS vasculitis: granulomatous angiitis of the CNS	
Spontaneous	Glucocorticoids + CTX
Associated with illnesses	
Hodgkin's lymphoma	Glucocorticoids + CTX
Herpes zoster ophthalmicus	Glucocorticoids + CTX
Secondary CNS vasculitis due to systemic inflammatory diseases	
Polyarteritis nodosa (PAN)	Glucocorticoids + CTX
Systemic lupus erythematosus (SLE)	Glucocorticoids + CTX
Rheumatoid arthritis	Glucocorticoids + CTX
Sjögren's syndrome	Glucocorticoids + CTX
Hypersensitivity vasculitides, Henoch-Schönlein purpura	Glucocorticoids
Churg-Strauss vasculitis	Glucocorticoids + CTX
Wegener's granulomatosus	Glucocorticoids + CTX
Relapsing polychondritis	Glucocorticoids
Lymphomatoid granulomatosis	Glucocorticoids + CTX
Infectious diseases complicated by CNS vasculitis	Antibiotics; nimodipine?
Acute inflammatory meningoencephalitis	
Sjögren's syndrome	Glucocorticoids + CTX
Hashimoto's encephalopathy	Glucocorticoids
Behçet's disease	Glucocorticoids + chlorambucil
SLE	Glucocorticoids
Chronic inflammatory meningoencephalitis	
Sjögren's syndrome	Glucocorticoids
Hypereosinophilic syndrome	Glucocorticoids
Sarcoidosis	Glucocorticoids

Key: CTX = cyclophosphamide.

Most patients are anemic and have low-grade thrombocytosis. In the absence of adequate treatment, vasculitis of posterior ciliary and other optic vessels leads to blindness (anterior ischemic optic neuropathy [AION]), which occurs in approximately 8 to 15 percent of patients. Less commonly, involvement of cervicocephalic arteries (carotid and vertebral arteries) leads to stroke. Approximately 7 percent of patients with GCA experience a transient ischemic attack or cerebral infarction, although the relationship of the cerebrovascular event to GCA is not always clear.

The diagnosis is most confidently confirmed by temporal artery biopsy (TAB), and histologic examination of a TAB specimen should not be accepted as negative unless bilateral 5-centimeter segments have been multiply sectioned: GCA is multifocal and characteristically has extensive skip areas. Because most patients require corticosteroid treatment for longer than a year (often 2 years or more) serious complications of steroid therapy occur frequently, including osteoporotic fractures, sepsis, gastrointestinal bleeding, and metabolic disorders, to name only a few. Therefore, despite

the natural reticence of many physicians and patients to pursue an invasive test that often fails to confirm the diagnostic impression (approximately 33 percent of TABs performed at our institution are "positive"), TAB documentation is essential for appropriate long-term management of GCA.

Treatment may be initiated before TAB, but TAB should then be performed within 72 hours, to avoid therapeutic suppression of the diagnostic vasculitic changes being sought in the biopsy specimen. We begin giving prednisone, 60 mg, as a single oral morning dose for most patients, although initial doses may range from 40 to 120 mg per day. In patients with acute ischemic complications, intravenous methylprednisolone, 1,000 mg per day for up to 5 days, may initially be employed; subsequently this is changed to oral prednisone, 60 mg per day. Symptomatic relief, especially of headache and polymyalgia rheumatica, occurs within a day or two, and the erythrocyte sedimentation rate (ESR) falls within days. Ischemic sequelae, however, are often permanent if they have been present for more than a day before treatment is initiated; thus, these should not be taken as

Table 2 Major Presenting Neurologic Features of the Neurovasculitides

Headache alone: GCA
Cranial neuropathy: GCA (II, III/IV/VI, VIII), Cogan's (VIII), sarcoidosis (VII), scleroderma (V, VII), Wegener's granulomatosis (II, V, VII, VIII, IX, XII)
Stroke: GACNS, Takayasu's arteritis, PAN and associated vasculitides, GCA, Henoch-Schönlein purpura (children), Wegener's granulomatosis
Encephalopathy
   Mutli-infarct dementia: GCA, GACNS
   Meningoencephalopathy
      Acute: Behçet's disease, Sjögren's syndrome, hypereosinophilic syndrome, all widespread cerebral vasculitides, Hashimoto's thyroiditis
      Subacute/chronic: Sjögren's (CIME), all widespread cerebral vasculitides, hypereosinophilic syndrome, lymphomatoid granulomatosis
Myelopathy (rare): PAN and related disorders, GCA, GACNS
Peripheral nervous system involvement
   Mononeuritis multiplex and peripheral neuropathy
      Common: PAN and related disorders, Churg-Strauss syndrome, SLE, hypereosinophilic syndromes (with and without L-tryptophan)
      Rare: GCA, sarcoid, Sjögren's syndrome
   Dorsal root ganglionopathy: Sjögren's syndrome
   Myositis: PAN and related disorders, hypereosinophilia-myalgia syndrome, sarcoidosis, SLE, scleroderma/mixed connective tissue disease, Sjögren's syndrome
Hypopituitarism: Wegener's granulomatosis, sarcoidosis

Key: CIME = chronic inflammatory meningoencephalitis; GACNS = granulomatous angiitis of the CNS; GCA = giant cell arteritis; PAN = polyarteritis nodosa; SLE = systemic lupus erythematosus.

Table 3 Model Schedule for Prednisone Taper in Giant Cell Arteritis

Week	Dosage (mg/day)
0	60
3	40
5	30
8	25
12	20
16	15
20	12.5
24	10
28	7.5
32	5
36	4
40	3
44	2
48	1
52	0

reliable guides to treatment response. Prednisone must be tapered carefully, monitoring both symptoms and ESR. The initially effective dose should be maintained for the first 2 weeks and then slowly tapered off. By the end of the first month of therapy, most patients should be taking about 40 mg per day, and gradual (no more than 10 percent every 2 weeks) tapering of prednisone may then proceed. A typical tapering schedule for a hypothetical patient who is to receive 1 year's therapy is outlined in Table 3. *That schedule is merely a guide and should not be adhered to rigidly.* Unlike in many other inflammatory diseases, alternate-day therapy is not effective in GCA patients and generally should not be tried. The patient should be clinically assessed and ESR checked at each of the indicated intervals before the steroid taper is continued. We check fasting plasma glucose and electrolyte values within 2 days of starting prednisone. Severe electrolyte disturbances and extreme hyperglycemia are common, potentially fatal, and readily treated complications that must be vigilantly monitored. We check serum sodium, potassium, and fasting plasma glucose in most instances when the ESR is measured for the first year. Some patients have recurrent GCA symptoms or ESR elevations that require increasing the dose of prednisone at least to the last effective dose. Similarly, treatment complications must be handled on an individual basis, and this may necessitate consideration of a second immunosuppressive agent or more aggressive steroid withdrawal. AION, stroke, and other ischemic complications may occur during periods of too rapid steroid taper, whereas osteoporotic vertebral compression fractures and other complications of chronic steroid treatment attend slow steroid tapering (and can be unavoidable). While the patient is taking more than 15 mg of prednisone daily, concurrent antiulcer therapy may have to be employed. We most often give ranitidine, 150 mg twice daily, but other regimens are acceptable.

Rarely, a patient with TAB-documented GCA does not respond adequately to therapy. The patient may simply have a more resistant form of GCA or another vasculitis that is involving the temporal artery, such as polyarteritis nodosa (PAN). In such cases a second immunosuppressive agent may be required. Several have been tried, but the most effective drug appears to be cyclophosphamide (see the subsequent discussion of Granulomatous Angiitis of the Central Nervous System).

Takayasu Arteritis

Takayasu arteritis is a granulomatous disease of cervicocephalic arteries that principally affects the aortic arch and its proximal branches, including the common carotid arteries. It typically affects children and young women (aged 10 to 30 years), and most reported cases have been from Japan. It is a chronic disease that usually progresses over years while exhibiting occasional spontaneous remissions. Death results from congestive heart failure and cerebral infarction. Prednisone therapy early in the course of the disease may reverse inflammation-mediated arterial stenoses and relieve systemic symptoms of fatigue and low-grade fever. We begin with 60 mg daily and gradually taper the dose, initially following the same schedule suggested for GCA, using symptoms, arterial pulses, and ESR as indicators of disease activity. Patients may need to continue medication indefinitely, taking small maintenance doses of prednisone daily or on alternate days in an effort to delay disease progression to the pulseless phase. Cytotoxic agents such as cyclophosphamide do not appear to confer any additional therapeutic advantage in most patients but occasionally are used in patients whose symptoms appear refractory to prednisone alone.

NECROTIZING VASCULITIDES WITH A LIMITED INTRACRANIAL DISTRIBUTION ("EYES AND EARS")

Giant Cell Arteritis

See the discussion of giant cell arteritis in the preceding section.

Cogan's Syndrome

Cogan's syndrome consists of nonsyphilitic interstitial keratitis (which may present with ocular redness and photophobia) and arteritis affecting the auditory and vestibular divisions of the eighth cranial nerve. Acute onset of unilateral hearing loss should prompt consideration of auditory nerve infarction due to vasculitis; this occurs commonly in Cogan's syndrome. A minority of patients have an associated large artery vasculitis that is histologically similar to PAN and that can affect the aorta. Large-dose prednisone therapy, as described for GCA, is the mainstay of treatment for most patients, but cyclophosphamide or another immunosuppressant should be considered for resistant symptoms or more widespread vasculitis.

NECROTIZING VASCULITIDES WITH WIDESPREAD INTRACRANIAL DISTRIBUTION

The clinical features of any of the entire spectrum of widespread intracranial vasculitides can be very similar. Headache, stroke, encephalopathy, seizures, cranial neuropathies, and meningismus may occur in all of these diseases. The ESR may be normal or elevated. Diseases associated with systemic immune complex deposition may show hypocomplementemia, and some diseases have characteristic serologic abnormalities (for example an elevated rheumatoid factor titer). The angiographic features of cerebral vasculitis include circumferential and beaded arterial stenoses and dilatations, but few features are specific to any particular vasculitic disease. The main distinguishing features are the associated extra-CNS manifestations that may be quite prominent in some, and the histologic features. Treatment of this group of disorders generally consists of prednisone and cyclophosphamide, though some exceptions are noted below.

Primary Central Nervous System Vasculitis

Granulomatous angiitis of the CNS (GACNS) affects meningeal and cortical small arteries and arterioles most severely and carries a 5-year survival rate of approximately 15 percent. Rarely, the superficial temporal artery and spinal cord may be involved. Relapsing and remitting headache, stroke, and encephalopathy are the typical clinical features. Cerebral angiography reveals the vasculitis in 80 percent but is nonconfirmatory in 20 percent. We advocate meningeal and brain biopsy when we suspect this diagnosis, generally directed to the right prefrontal region.

Treatment with corticosteroids alone is usually inadequate, and the preferred regimen is a combination of large doses of prednisone plus cyclophosphamide. We begin prednisone, 80 to 120 mg daily, and gradually taper the dose in a fashion similar to that described for GCA. For fulminant encephalopathy or acute cerebral infarction we begin steroid therapy with intravenous methylprednisolone, 1000 mg daily for the first 3 to 5 days, switching next to oral prednisone, 120 mg for the first few days, and then beginning the slow taper. We often concurrently begin cyclophosphamide, which may be administered intravenously or orally. The oral route is easier to tailor to the patient's symptoms and side effects, and we use approximately 2 mg per kilogram of body weight daily (generally 100 to 150 mg daily each morning). With the combination of prednisone and cyclophosphamide we check complete blood counts twice the first week and thereafter weekly to monthly, because of potentially fatal myelosuppression. We also check electrolytes, fasting plasma glucose, and liver chemistries twice during the first week of treatment, and every 2 to 4 weeks thereafter. The dose of cyclophosphamide must be tapered to maintain the total white blood cell count above 3,000 per microliter, the total lymphocyte count above 750 per microliter, the total neutrophil count above 1,500 per microliter, the hemoglobin level above 11.5 g per deciliter, and the platelet count above 150,000 per microliter. There is generally a 7 to 10 day lag in hematologic effects following dose adjustments, and bone marrow toxicity may become more intense as the prednisone dose is reduced. Patients must be instructed to drink ample amounts of water daily, to lessen the chances of hemorrhagic cystitis. Other side effects and dangers of cyclophosphamide — alopecia, sterility, opportunistic infection, and possible secondary malignancies — underscore the importance of histologic confirmation of the clinical diagnostic impression. Cyclophosphamide should probably be continued for up to a year following the cessation of clinical symptoms.

It is helpful to repeat cerebral angiography if clinical remission is in doubt and before discontinuing cyclophosphamide (approximately 1 year after diagnosis). Following angiographic confirmation of disease inactivity after a full course of immunosuppressive therapy, the cyclophosphamide is rapidly tapered off. Assuming the patient tolerates this without a relapse, the prednisone is then tapered more slowly over 3 to 6 months.

GACNS has been associated with Hodgkin's disease and reportedly may remit with successful treatment of the lymphoma. GACNS has also been associated with herpes zoster ophthalmicus (HZO). Approximately 1 month following HZO, a granulomatous arteritis in the hemisphere ipsilateral to the HZO may produce contralateral hemiparesis due to cerebral infarction. This form of GACNS takes a less severe course than spontaneous GACNS, and 73 percent survive with no therapy. Cerebral angiography may be confirmatory in a larger proportion of patients than in spontaneous GACNS. Immunosuppressive treatment has not resulted in virus reactivation and dissemination in the few patients so treated, and we would treat HZO-associated GACNS in the same way as spontaneous GACNS, depending on the severity of the vasculitis and its course.

Secondary Central Nervous System Vasculitis Resulting from Systemic Inflammatory Diseases

Several systemic inflammatory diseases associated with vasculitis invade the intracranial vasculature with clinical features similar to those of GACNS. These include PAN and vasculitis associated with Sjögren's syndrome, systemic lupus erythematosus (SLE), or rarely, rheumatoid arthritis. We approach treatment in a similar fashion as for GACNS, tempered by the general health of the patient, and particularly the degree of other organ system involvement.

A second group of systemic vasculitides that invade the CNS is systemic vasculitis involving small blood vessels, sometimes categorized as the hypersensitivity vasculitides, which in children includes Henoch-Schönlein purpura. Prednisone therapy alone is generally sufficient for this group.

Churg-Strauss vasculitis is an eosinophilic granulomatous vasculitis that affects small arteries and veins, usually accompanied by asthma due to pulmonary involvement. Its course is variable. Corticosteroids may control the vasculitis, but it is a more aggressive disease than the hypersensitivity vasculitides. In some instances cyclophosphamide needs to be added.

Wegener's granulomatosis is rarely accompanied by a widespread necrotizing cerebral arteritis. Other modes of CNS involvement include direct extension of granulomatous foci from the perinasal sinuses to the base of the brain with cranial nerve involvement, and rarely pituitary gland involvement. Treatment consists of prednisone and cyclophosphamide.

Relapsing polychondritis occasionally is associated with a systemic and cerebral granulomatous vasculitis with giant cell formation that may respond to prednisone, as described for GCA. Neurologic symptoms include a relapsing and remitting encephalopathy.

Lymphomatoid granulomatosis most commonly involves the lungs primarily and usually evolves into an angiocentric T-cell lymphoma, but it may resemble GACNS clinically, owing to involvement of intracerebral vessels. In its early stages treatment with prednisone and cyclophosphamide may ameliorate the encephalopathic symptoms and delay or prevent malignant transformation. The diagnosis must be established histologically.

With most of the diseases discussed above, neurologic involvement is not limited to the CNS, and peripheral neuropathy, mononeuritis multiplex, and inflammatory myopathy may be associated with any or clinically dominate many of these conditions (Table 2).

Secondary Central Nervous System Vasculitis Complicating Central Nervous System Infection

Most purulent meningoencephalitic and parameningitic diseases can induce in some patients a local vasculitic reaction that generally resolves with appropriate antimicrobial treatment. Concurrent administration of calcium channel–blocking agents such as nimodipine may be considered, as for subarachnoid hemorrhage–induced vasospasm, but their efficacy in the former context is currently unknown. Angiographically, vasculitis-like alterations of arteries at the base of the brain are seen in patients with bacterial meningitis, tuberculous meningitis, syphilitic meningoencephalitis, and fungal meningitis.

INFLAMMATORY MENINGOENCEPHALITIDES

The inflammatory meningoencephalitides have a vasculitic component, but vasculitis generally plays a relatively minor pathologic role compared to more extensive perivascular and nonvasculitic leptomeningeal and superficial cortical inflammation. The presenting clinical features are generally those of diffuse encephalopathy: generalized cognitive impairment, hypersomnolence, tremulousness, and unsteady gait. The course can be acute and fulminant, relapsing and remitting, or chronic and progressive with clinical fluctuations. In acute disease, the differential diagnosis includes all other causes of acute delirium. Chronic disease, however, can be misconstrued as degenerative dementia. This is an especially tragic oversight, as chronic inflammatory meningoencephalitis may respond dramatically to glucocorticosteroid treatment, even if it is long delayed.

Acute Disease

Diseases that can cause an acute inflammatory meningoencephalitis (AIME) include Sjögren's syndrome, hypereosinophilic syndrome, Hashimoto's thyroiditis, Behçet's disease, and SLE. Cerebral angiography may show vasculitis in approximately 20 percent of patients with AIME due to Sjögren's syndrome, so that diagnosis generally rests on meningeal and brain biopsy. AIME associated with Sjögren's syndrome does not generally respond to corticosteroids alone, and combined prednisone and cyclophosphamide therapy is recommended.

AIME associated with Hashimoto's thyroiditis and hypereosinophilic syndrome has been reported to respond well to corticosteroid therapy alone, and empiric therapy appears to be warranted in the appropriate clinical setting.

Behçet's disease produces a relapsing-remitting aseptic meningitis that may become complicated by dural venous sinus thrombosis and aneurysm formation, with resultant fatal complications in approximately 10 percent. Treatment consists of prednisone, as described for GCA, and chlorambucil. Chlorambucil therapy may need to be prolonged, and some dangers of treatment include secondary leukemia, sterility, and bone marrow suppression.

SLE is frequently complicated by relapsing and remitting neuropsychiatric complications, including frankly psychotic behavior, seizures, and cerebral ischemia. Pathologic findings include (1) most frequently, multiple small subcortical infarctions due to arteriolar and capillary occlusions not associated with vasculitis, (2) large artery territory infarctions unassociated with vasculitis, (3) rare instances of CNS vasculitis, and (4) cortical lymphocytic perivascular infiltrates. Prednisone has been the recommended therapy: preferred dosage ranges from 30 to 100 mg daily. Immunosuppressive therapy, however, has been relatively ineffective to date. The self-limited nature of most relapses has constrained the use of cytotoxic therapy, but for particularly aggressive neuropsychiatric disease azathioprine or cyclophosphamide might be considered.

Chronic Disease

Chronic inflammatory meningoencephalitis (CIME) is commonly misdiagnosed as Alzheimer's disease or depression. Angiographic findings are generally normal, as are magnetic resonance imaging (MRI) and CT studies. Electroencephalography (EEG) shows severe generalized slowing. Cerebrospinal fluid (CSF) analysis may show modest total protein elevation and increased intrathecal synthesis of immunoglobulins, despite the absence of an elevated leukocyte count. Diseases associated with CIME include Sjögren's syndrome, hypereosinophilic syndrome, and sarcoidosis. In Sjögren's syndrome, antibodies to extractable nuclear antigens are positive for anti-Sjögren's syndrome antigens A and B, and minor salivary gland biopsy shows lymphocytic sialadenitis. In hypereosinophilic syndrome there is hypereosinophilia in peripheral blood smears and in the CSF. CIME responds dramatically to prednisone therapy: clinical improvement is evident within days. We employ a regimen similar to that for GCA, save that alternate-day therapy is effective. We continue daily therapy until we reach a dose of 10 mg and then taper off the alternate-day dose. As the dose of prednisone is tapered, subjective symptoms of mental clouding and dizziness may reappear, with accelerated ESR and an abnormal EEG despite normal findings on cognitive and neurologic examination. In doubtful cases, the EEG has proven to be a reliable indicator of disease activity. It returns to normal within a month of appropriate therapy and becomes abnormal in advance of detectable cognitive impairment. Duration of therapy is currently unknown, and our longest-treated patient has been taking prednisone 3 years and presently takes 5 mg on alternate days. Though this dose is tolerated well, efforts at tapering should continue.

Chronic meningitis due to sarcoidosis is not commonly accompanied by encephalitis symptoms. Cranial neuropathies (especially nerves VII and VIII) and systemic manifestations are more frequent complications and generally alert the clinician to the diagnosis. Contrast-enhanced CT and MRI demonstrate an enhancing meningitis process, which can be confirmed to be sarcoidosis by biopsy of the abnormal area visualized radiologically. Because some patients develop progressive cognitive impairment, baseline neuropsychological testing is advisable for all patients with meningeal sarcoidosis. Treatment with prednisone is sufficient for most patients, and remission of the meningitis process can be visualized with contrast CT and MRI.

SUGGESTED READING

Caselli RJ, Scheithauer BW, Bowles CA, et al. The treatable dementia of Sjogren's syndrome. Ann Neurol 1991; 30:98–101.

Conn DL, Hunder GG. Vasculitis and related disorders. In: Kelley WN, Harris ED Jr, Ruddy S, Sledge CB, eds. Textbook of Rheumatology. 3rd ed. Philadelphia: WB Saunders, 1989: 1167–1199.

Fauci AS, Katz P, Haynes BF, et al. Cyclophosphamide therapy for severe systemic necrotizing vasculitis. N Engl J Med 1979; 301: 235–238.

Hunder GG. Giant cell arteritis and polmyalgia rheumatica. In: Kelley WN, Harris ED Jr, Ruddy S, Sledge CB, eds. Textbook of Rheumatology, 3rd edition. Philadelphia: WB Saunders, 1989: 1200–1208.

Hunder GG, Arend WP, Bloch DA, et al. The American College of Rheumatology 1990 criteria for the classification of vasculitis. Arthritis Rheum 1990; 33:1065–1144.

Moore PM. Diagnosis and management of isolated angiitis of the central nervous system. Neurology 1989; 39:167–173.

TRAUMA

SURVIVORS OF TRAUMATIC BRAIN INJURY

MICHAEL P. ALEXANDER, M.D.

The type of menu of specific treatments that a review of migraine or epilepsy might generate is not a part of this chapter, because few specific treatments exist for survivors of traumatic brain injury (TBI). The mixture of traditional rehabilitation interventions, behavioral managements, and unproven medications that at present characterizes the care of TBI can be understood only if TBI patients are better understood than they commonly are today. The overall goal is that clinical neurologists adopt a systematic model of diagnosis for TBI survivors and learn its relationship to prognosis and management for TBI of all degrees of severity.

DIAGNOSIS

TBI, of course, is a self-evident diagnosis. For severe cases, initial diagnosis and management are neurosurgical problems. The mortality rate is approximately 35 percent, and death usually comes within 3 to 7 days if it is not immediate. Patients with multiple contusions and subdural hematomas, with the lowest Glasgow Coma Scores (GCS) (<7), and those who are oldest are likeliest to die. It is among the survivors that neurologically motivated diagnosis becomes important—and is too infrequently performed. The possible diagnoses each lie in a pathophysiologically distinct event, and the specificity and importance of the diagnoses are clearest if they emerge from analysis of the pathophysiology. The physical mechanisms of closed TBI are inertial forces and contact forces. Rapid deceleration of the head generates inertial forces, most of which are dissipated through widespread microscopic shearing of fragile structures in the long axis of the brain—axons and blood vessels. This phenomenon is diffuse axonal injury (DAI). The vascular injury may be quite variable, ranging from no demonstrable damage, to rupture of capillaries and small veins producing petechial hemorrhages and focal

or diffuse edema, to rupture of small arteries producing deep focal hemorrhages. In summary, although it is labeled diffuse *axonal* injury, the insults are axonal (and, thus, surely transsynaptic) *and* vascular. The critical clinical lesson from experimental models is clear: the clinical deficit is proportional to the severity of the physical injury. DAI always produces at least transient alteration of consciousness; there is no lucid interval. In the mildest cases, so-called *dings,* the patient may only briefly be unresponsive and amnesic. In the severest cases the patient may be unresponsive, with eyes closed, for weeks.

Both inertial and contact forces may produce localized brain damage. The peculiarities of dural attachments and the location of rough bony surfaces are the factors that predispose the inferior frontal and anterior temporal regions to surface abrasions from inertial forces. Contact forces can obviously cause brain abrasions anywhere, depending on the specifics of the head contact. These surface abrasions consist of disruptions of the cortical structure and the surface vessels. The vascular injury can lead to localized intracerebral hemorrhage, infarction, localized edema, and overlying acute subdural hematomas. This injury, again to brain *and* vasculature, is a focal cortical contusion (FCC). It need not be associated with loss of consciousness, and the diagnosis is *strictly* a neuroimaging one.

As noted, both DAI and FCC include vascular injury. If the TBI is accompanied by systemic injury— flail chest, splenic rupture, shock—such that cerebral perfusion is compromised, the risk of hypoxic-ischemic injury (HII) is enormous. HII may be diffuse or focal. Focal HII may be found around regions of local pressure change (e.g., subdural hematoma, FCC) but most often is in the territory of the posterior cerebral arteries (PCA) and is secondary to temporal herniation. The effects of herniation on the midbrain are also due to focal HII. The critical clinical lessons of HII are that there is no certain diagnostic marker for diffuse HII (it is only suggested by the clinical course) and that focal HII is a neuroimaging diagnosis.

In summary, five diagnoses must be considered: DAI, FCC, diffuse HII, focal HII, and herniation HII. Each has its own markers. Each has its own time course of recovery and prognosis. A competent clinical neurologic diagnosis must address each one; otherwise subsequent care will be unmotivated.

NATURAL HISTORY OF THE INJURY

Patients with DAI all have altered consciousness at the outset. From that point, the length of coma (LOC) and the course of recovery are stereotyped, differing, case to case, only in duration of the stages. Patients all open their eyes, but they may seem unaware or have no speech or purposeful attention. If permanent, this condition is referred to as *persistent vegetative state* (PVS). Most gradually become vigilant to environmental stimuli but do not respond to commands or gestures. This is *unresponsive vigilance* and is rarely permanent. At some point, the patient shows directed responsiveness, at first, erratic and detected only by family and therapists who spend much time with the patient. Some patients remain mute long after they are following commands, but generally, as patients become responsive they talk, and it is clear that they are disoriented and confabulatory—in short, in a confusional state. Like all persons in a confusional state, they are distractable and inattentive, at times agitated, at other times lethargic, and frequently fluctuating between the two, depending on stimulation. This period of confusion after TBI is referred to as *post-traumatic amnesia* (PTA). No day-to-day memory is being formed. PTA resolves as the patient becomes aware of daily events, is oriented, and learns the nature of his injury. Although confusion clears (i.e., PTA ends), these patients are in no way cognitively normal. Attention, memory, and executive functions will be deficient for some additional time, but patients now show increasing functional independence, perhaps leading to some degree of social and intellectual independence.

I emphasized that all patients with DAI begin with an interval of altered consciousness then proceed through a series of steps of recovery, which differ only in their duration. At the mild end of DAI are concussions (see below), in which the LOC may be seconds, the unresponsive and vigilant periods compressed into seconds, the PTA 20 to 30 minutes, and evolving independence weeks to months before recovery. At the severe end of DAI, LOC may be many days, unresponsive vegetative state and unresponsive vigilance each days to weeks, and PTA months. These patients may never recover completely, even after years. The differences in duration are proportional to the severity of the brain injury. The evidence for this comes from experimental models and is applicable only to DAI, not to other lesions. Nevertheless, the certainty of this proportional injury is of much value in helping a clinician construct a prognosis or recognize that a case is aberrant in some way, and this fact is often overlooked.

FCC and focal HII show the same natural recovery as vascular lesions of other causes. Local edema decreases after a few days, and then, depending on the extent of ischemic necrosis, the lesion undergoes softening and cavity formation over a few weeks. Recovery is maximal in the first days to weeks after onset but may continue at a very slow rate for a longer time. This is unlike DAI, in which substantial direct improvement may occur for a long time. Prognosis for eventual functional status depends, as it does for other focal injuries, on the number, location, and depth of the lesions. In part because recovery is so poor, the history of diffuse HII will be reviewed below, when residual states are considered.

REHABILITATION MANAGEMENT

Patients in coma or in unresponsive states, vigilant or not, are not candidates for active hospital-level rehabilitation, no matter what the rehabilitation marketers or consumer groups tell you. The primary foci of care are all nursing issues: bed positioning, nutrition, bowel and bladder management, skin care, and passive motion of the limbs. There is *no* utility to individualized programs of coma stimulation. With good nursing care some of these patients improve and become candidates for active rehabilitation.

Patients in vigilant, unresponsive states in particular, need careful reassessments to determine what range of responsiveness and cognitive abilities is present. Reliable methods of demonstrating responsiveness must be identified. The bed and wheelchair positions in which the patient is best able to respond must be established and reinforced. Monoamine agonists, methylphenidate up to 50 to 60 mg daily, or bromcriptine in similar doses, may improve the total interval of responsiveness or shorten the latency of response, although there is scant empirical evidence to support that claim. As patients clearly become responsive, there is often great expectation for their capacities and a burst of enthusiasm for communication boards and the like, but once they are carefully assessed it becomes apparent that the patients are profoundly impaired, even demented. There are a few profoundly injured patients who essentially reach a plateau at this level, thereafter increasing alertness and responsiveness only very slowly over years.

Patients in confusional states (PTA) primarily require protection from themselves because of amnesia, anosognosia, and agitation. It has become customary to deliver this protection in rehabilitation hospital TBI units. Because of the amnesia, no specific learning can take place. Even with PTA, however, there is considerable capacity for procedural learning; that is, patients can learn motor patterns and repeated activities. Thus, they may improve over days in the performance of repeated compensatory motor activities, learn to find their way about the hospital, and even learn to use notebooks or information wallboards when they have no explicit memory of learning these things. Therefore, rehabilitation consists of repetition of concrete, personally relevant activities. There is *no* place for specific cognitive retraining, memory drills, and so on. There is also little role for traditional neuropsychological testing. Although no measure obtained during PTA has any correlation with the eventual functional outcome, an astounding amount of energy is spent proving the obvious (the patient is confused) with high-powered tests. Objective measures of attention and learning may be useful for tracking change.

For agitated patients, behavioral management is usually sufficient: quiet rooms, restricted contacts, a locked or alarmed ward. Maintaining the sleep-wake cycle seems to be helpful. This may require giving a hypnotic drug at bedtime, preferably one without potent effects on learning, such as benadryl, 50 to 100 mg. The dose may be repeated at midnight, but no later for fear of hangover lethargy all through the next day. Then, no matter how difficult, the patient must be kept up the entire next day—by dragging him from appointment to appointment if necessary. When the agitation takes on a paranoid tone or the patient seems very frightened, small doses of antipsychotics are indicated; an attempt should be made to time dosing to prevent daytime sedation. When the patient remains underaroused, monoamine agonists can be continued. Claims for specific effects of other medications for agitation—beta-blockers, anticonvulsants—are even more anecdotal than for the drugs suggested above.

As the PTA clears, patients typically become continent and able to care for themselves (to the extent that physical limitations allow) with only partial supervision. Two new aspects of management become the foci. Specific cognitive impairments related to focal FCC or focal HII can, for the first time, be addressed directly. Only now, as confusion abates, is it possible to ascertain if a patient is aphasic, amnesic, or "frontal" from a known focal lesion. To the extent that the physician believes any of these focal problems to be directly treatable, it is now possible to treat them. The second emerging issue is discharge planning. The patient should be given much responsibility for appointments, schedules, and self-care (with supervision). Families or caretakers-to-be should begin instruction in the nature of required supervision. When it is safe with the supervision available, it is time for discharge from inpatient rehabilitation. Too many patients stay in the rehabilitation hospital far too long.

Over the months or years that it will take to regain independence, outpatient rehabilitation management may generate many practical interventions for the patient. (This is in addition to direct therapy for residual motor or focal deficits.) These interventions are determined by the patient's individual deficit profile and by noninjury factors such as age, family structure, employment or educational status, insurance, and finances. *No single program structure is appropriate for all patients.* Patients with substantial motor deficits but trivial cognitive problems may be best served in programs for independent living with spinal cord injury. Patients with cognitive deficits in planning and organization (so-called executive deficits) may benefit from a structured transitional living program that emphasizes repetition and rehearsal of practical activities of living—schedules, shopping, finances. "Higher-level" patients may require only a vocational program to monitor and to coordinate the rate of their return to work. Patients with behavioral problems might benefit from behavioral management programs, even one with an overtly psychiatric flavor. Planning long-term treatment is greatly aided by collab-

oration with a neuropsychologist. At these later stages of recovery, neuropsychological measures can be very helpful in specifying deficits and guiding appropriate referrals. A case manager familiar with the range of treatment options is also useful for patient referral. There is little evidence that cognitive retraining, whether attention or memory drills, has any generalization or carryover into more practical aspects of long-term management. The last thing in the world that a mildly "frontal" patient needs is to spend 3 or 4 hours each week playing video games to improve attention and eye-hand coordination (Has this helped your son do better in algebra or remember to make his bed?) or completing word puzzles or categorization trials in speech therapy (Does knowing the team history [categorization] of all active baseball players help your son retain American History or remember his bus card? Not mine!) Until *controlled* evidence of efficacy for cognitive retraining of that type is forthcoming, my practice is to move patients directly to pragmatic programs of the type briefly sketched above.

RESIDUAL DEFICIT PROFILES

I am frequently astounded that most neurologists are unfamiliar with the major clinical profiles observed after TBI. I believe that in part it is due to a failure to analyze the contributions of the different types of neurologic injuries independently.

Diffuse Axonal Injury

After PTA clears, cognitive function improves and measurable recovery will be seen for months and years. These patients do not "plateau" until much later than most physicians imagine. By 12 to 18 months postinjury, results of many standard neuropsychological tests will be at premorbid levels or have plateaued, but substantial improvement in learning and executive functions may continue. Many patients recover basic cognitive operations but have reduced information-processing capacity. Thus, their performance deteriorates over time (easy fatigability) and in situations of stress or interference (distractibility). "Treatment" often consists of establishing a "life hygiene" program: regular sleep, regular exercise, no sedatives including alcohol, stress avoidance, and structured work, school, and recreational demands. Patients always respond, "But I never had to do that before," but of course they were never head injured before. Physicians typically cannot, or will not, spend the time to do this life analysis (even for themselves), so referral to a case manager, senior program therapist, or a specialized center may help. In many outpatient "cognitive rehabilitation" programs this sort of application of organization to life is the core of the program.

DAI often produces motor deficits, although I have not emphasized these. Central vestibular problems are particularly common. A mixture of cerebellar outflow and postural (rubral and tectospinal) deficits is the result of predisposition of the dorsolateral midbrain to DAI. The high incidence of DAI lesions in parasagittal and medial frontal white matter underlies the various fragments of bradykinesia, rigidity, postural changes, and paretic ataxia often observed. Vigorous physical therapy, often from a therapist familiar with the odd mix of deficits that may be found, should be started early and maintained while benefit is seen. Again, improvement may go on much longer than is customarily expected by persons familiar only with stroke. Tone abnormalities should be managed aggressively with botulinum or phenol blocks, in addition to traditional therapy modalities.

Focal Cortical Contusion and Focal Hypoxic-Ischemic Injury

FCC and focal HII generally behave like all other focal lesions. Residual deficits are related to lesion number, location, and deep extent. There are, however, four specific lessons about TBI and focal lesions. First, lesions are usually in frontal and temporal limbic regions, notoriously opaque to most neurologists' examination. Any physician unfamiliar with detailed mental state examinations should refer to a specialized center or seek active collaboration from a neuropsychologist. Second, FCCs are often shallow and may be compatible with remarkably good recovery for the extent of the cortical lesion. It is critical to review neuroimaging with an eye to extent and depth. (This often neglected rule is, of course, no different than for lesion relationship to outcome in aphasia or neglect.) Third, FCCs are frequently bilaterally symmetric in limbic cortex, and this likely worsens the prognosis. Finally, the surface effects of frontal FCCs are quite similar to the residual state of severe DAI—blunted awareness, poor executive function, and forgetfulness—but the pathophysiologic differences between cortical ablations and patchy cortical deafferentations are so great that they have *much different long-term prognoses.* This is an essential neurobiologic fact that emerges from understanding the diagnosis of these cases and one that absolutely eludes most insurance companies' claims departments.

Diffuse Hypoxic-Ischemic Injury

There is no specific marker for diffuse HII, only clinical profiles that carry high risk. Here the acute surface manifestations are similar to DAI—confusion, gradually clearing with amnesia and behavioral deficits. But the implications of diffuse HII are much more ominous. Numerous studies have demonstrated that HII that produces coma of 2 days' duration is associated with very low probability of good recovery (or life for that matter) at 1 year. On the other hand, DAI with 2 days' LOC may afford a 70 percent chance of good recovery. Diffuse HII can also cause patterns of impairment that are uncommon with DAI—extrapyramidal movement disorders, visual perceptual deficits, amnesia.

Most patients have mixtures of lesions. The clinical art of caring for TBI survivors involves, in part, devising a mental algebra that can solve for the contributions of the various injuries. Only then can rational plans and expectations be generated. Too many physicians label these patients' problem TBI or specifically identify only the most obvious lesion. This is a simplification of the diagnostic process that would be unconscionable with stroke, for instance.

MILD TRAUMATIC BRAIN INJURY

Although always honored (including here by me), the distinction between mild and worse than mild TBI is essentially without merit. As I emphasized repeatedly in discussing diagnosis, mild TBI (or concussion) is DAI, just less of it than worse than mild TBI. The clinical distinction comes from several sources. First, it is generated by the practical necessities of the emergency room. The patient who is already oriented in the emergency room or who quickly becomes oriented overnight is sent home with a Head Injury Information Sheet and is told to rest for a few days and return as needed. The more severely injured patient is usually referred for rehabilitation services, and management becomes the rehabilitation center's responsibility.

Patients with closed head injury (CHI) often have TBI but not always, and, whether brain injured or not, CHI patients may also have peripheral vestibular injuries, facial injuries, head lacerations, and neck injuries. In addition, milder injuries produce very brief retrograde amnesia, so the patient is very likely to remember all of the terrifying events leading up to the injury. (More severely injured patients will not remember whole days prior to the injury.) Patients with mild TBI will be alert, aware, and at home as the headaches, neck pain, dizziness, and fear settle in. Patients with worse than mild TBI will be intubated in the surgical intensive care unit at the same point in their course. Patients with mild TBI are really recovering from several separate injuries and their interactions, such as those between mood, pain, and sleep. So-called mild cases are better viewed as less than severe cases.

The essential point is that the natural history of recovery from the neurologic injury of TBI is longer than anticipated by patients and physicians alike. Even the mildest "ding" injuries (no coma, very brief PTA) cause neurologic impairments in attention and memory that may take longer than a few days' rest to clear. The modal concussion patient, uncomplicated by any additional injury, with seconds of LOC and 20 to 30 minutes of PTA, may not recover attention to normal levels for *weeks to months.* Demonstration of these deficits is almost certainly not possible on clinical examination. Simple neuropsychological tests of attention (digit span, mental control, simple reaction time) also miss these deficits. More difficult measures of divided attention and sustained attention will, however, be impaired for months, even if the patient has no PCS complaints! This attention deficit is the essential neural injury, and its improvement is the essential natural history of concussion. A "few days' rest" will not do. On the other hand, patients with mild TBI *do* get better, and the rate of improvement is fairly predictable and grossly proportional to severity of injury as measured by LOC and PTA. (Remember, when the patient tells you that he was "out" for 20 minutes, he is telling you his PTA, not his LOC.)

The second essential point is that the natural history of recovery from the mixture of TBI and other injuries, known as the *postconcussive syndrome* (PCS), is more complicated than physicians customarily admit. Overt vestibular symptoms and signs clear in days to weeks, but the positional or movement-induced symptoms can be quite persistent. In the absence of a clear explanation from their physician, other than some vague bowing and scraping toward the "inner ear," patients become quite frightened about activities that intensify symptoms. Patients with vestibular disease have a very high prevalence of agoraphobia and anxiety disorders. If vestibular symptoms persist longer than a few weeks, I refer patients to a vestibular laboratory for more precise diagnosis and then to physical therapy for habituation exercises.

The mechanism of headaches in most TBI is probably related to migraine, even if overt triggers are cervical injury or scalp laceration. Treatment consists of sensible management of local exacerbating factors, the neck primarily, and appropriate specific migraine prophylaxis and/or symptomatic treatment that need not be described here.

Neck soft tissue injury (whiplash) can be quite troublesome to manage. The first principles of management are similar to those for other soft tissue injuries — immobilization, rest, early application of ice, antispasm medications, and anti-inflammatory analgesics, followed by gradual mobilization (physical therapy), antispasm modalities (ultrasound and electrical stimulation), and analgesics. Of course, immobilizing the neck is logistically difficult (without removing the head), and delivery of modality treatments is imprecise. Patients do not stick with treatment regimens and have only fitful improvement. They cannot be referred to physical therapy quickly enough to capture symptomatic and behavioral control of this injury.

Psychological care is often necessary. I refer patients who are not shedding PCS symptoms within 2 to 3 weeks to a clinical psychologist for management of adjustment, anxiety, return to work, and the temporary inactivity. Patients, families, employers, and schools all fail to recognize that the natural history of recovery from the neurologic injury is more than a "few days' rest" and that PCS is a complicated disorder that may be persistent even when properly managed. Patients with mild TBI after CHI have PCS symptoms for weeks (> 50 percent), months (> 20 to 25 percent), or years (10 percent), even when the intrinsic neurologic injury has recovered.

The last essential lesson is that the *neural* injury does recover. Profound persistent PCS is not diagnostic of a *neural* injury. Patients with persistent PCS inevitably have some combination of underlying depression, anxiety, migraine, and whiplash, with or without neural deficits. This cluster of disturbances causes impaired mental function (even to producing pseudodementia), so abnormal neuropsychological test results do not necessarily mean persistent abnormal neurologic function. This is another level at which collaboration between neurology and neuropsychology facilitates management, because there is no acid test, neuropsychological or biologic, that reliably distinguishes between residual TBI and depression, anxiety, or chronic pain. At this time, there are no alternative measures to determine whether, or to what degree, a patient's symptoms are due to neural injury. It is possible that new physiologic measures such as single photon emission computed tomography or brain electrical activity mapping might be more diagnostic, but they have not yet been analyzed against the proper control groups, including patients with depression or chronic refractory headache, to verify that any putative changes of TBI are specific.

DISCUSSION

Future editions of *Current Therapy in Neurologic Disease* should provide more information about specific treatments for head-injured patients. At present there is remarkably little direct medical treatment for mild or severe TBI, in part because diagnosis has been so incomplete. Should different treatments emerge for hypoxia or the axonal transport injury that heralds DAI, at present there is no way, in life, to be certain of the extent of either injury in a given patient. It is simply not known which, if any, rehabilitation interventions actually assist or accelerate recovery. There is no scientific basis for selection of one antiagitation medication over another, except to avoid side effects. There is no basis for identifying which patients are likely to react to monoamine agonists with increased responsiveness. There is no evidence that there is a precise treatment that is specific for post-traumatic headache. Current therapy is an intellectually unsatisfying potpourri of unproven medications, physical treatments, psychological support, behavior management, and pragmatic planning. Until there is precision in diagnosis and characterization of these lesions, mild or severe, therapy may stay that way.

SUGGESTED READING

Gronwall D, Wrightson P, Waddell P. Head injury, the facts: A guide for families and care-givers. Oxford: Oxford University Press, 1990.
Katz DI, Alexander MP, eds. The neurology of head injury. J Head Trauma Rehab 1992; 7:1–116.

PATIENT RESOURCE

National Head Injury Foundation
1140 Connecticut Avenue, N.W., Suite 812
Washington, DC 20036
(202) 296-6443
This is the main organization for patients and families. Most states have local chapters that can provide referrals to specialized centers and state and regional resources.

SPINE INJURY

WISE YOUNG, Ph.D., M.D.

Spinal cord injury essentially disconnects body from brain. Treatment can be divided into four phases based on interval after injury: (1) immediate post-trauma phase (within 1 hour), (2) acute injury phase (first 24 hours), (3) subacute phase (within 1 week), and (4) chronic phase (beyond 1 week). Because each phase has different priorities and treatments (often involving multiple specialists and therapists) I will discuss each phase separately and then describe some promising new pharmacologic treatments for acute spinal cord injury.

IMMEDIATE POST-TRAUMA PHASE (WITHIN 1 HOUR)

The major concerns during the immediate post-injury phase are evaluation, emergency care, immobilization of the spinal column, and rapid transport of the patient to a medical facility for definitive diagnosis and treatment. The evaluation must first rule out life-threatening conditions. For example, if the patient shows evidence of respiratory compromise, ventilatory assistance should be instituted. A neurologic assessment should then be carried out to determine the location and extent of trauma to the brain and spinal cord. The examination should include palpation of the vertebral column for tenderness. If trauma involves the spinal column, even if there are no neurologic signs of spinal cord injury, the patient must be immobilized immediately.

The importance of proper immobilization cannot be overemphasized. A cervical collar alone is not sufficient if cervical spine injury is suspected. The head, body, and hip must be well anchored to an appropriate device that does not allow independent movement of any of these body parts relative to each other. Leg movements, particularly at the hips, should be restricted if lumbosacral instability is suspected. Care must be taken to avoid movement of the spinal column during transport.

If methylprednisolone sodium succinate (MP) is available, the patient should be given an intravenous bolus of 30 mg per kilogram. For a 65 to 70 kg adult, this dose is about 2 g of MP dissolved in 50 ml of vehicle solution delivered over 5 to 10 minutes. For a child, the dose should be reduced according to body weight. This is the initial dose of a protocol found by the National Acute Spinal Cord Injury Study (NASCIS) to improve neurologic recovery after severe and partial spinal cord injuries. Blood pressure should be monitored, because transient hypotension may result from a large bolus dose of MP.

There are three contraindications to MP treatment. The first is a history of allergic responses to corticosteroid drugs (rare). The second is an interval of more than 8 hours after injury: delayed MP therapy may *reduce* neurologic recovery. The third is pregnancy, as a large dose of MP may adversely affect the fetus. Multiple trauma is not a contraindication. MP can be given without complications to spinal cord–injured victims with gunshot wounds. Because MP may salvage more than 20 percent of motor and sensory loss in spine-injured patients, the benefit-risk ratio is high and the risk is justified even in cases where the diagnosis of spinal cord injury has not been established.

ACUTE PHASE (FIRST 24 HOURS)

The patient should be taken to a center with appropriate intensive care, imaging (standard x-ray, computed tomography [CT], and magnetic resonance imaging [MRI] if possible), and neurosurgical facilities. The first priorities on admission are to ensure adequate blood pressure and respiration. If mean arterial pressure (MAP) is below 100 mm Hg, a dopamine drip may be started to restore and maintain MAP above 100 mg Hg. If respiratory compromise is present, intubation should be carried out. A Foley urethral catheter should be inserted. A central venous line should be established. Narcotic analgesics are usually not necessary and may be deleterious to recovery.

A careful history of the traumatic event and detailed neurologic examination must be obtained as soon as the patient is stable. The history should include the time, cause, and specific details of the trauma. The examination should, at minimum, collect the data recommended by the American Spinal Injury Association (ASIA). This includes assessing dermatomes from C2 to S5 for sharp pinprick and light touch sensation at the specified key points (0 = no sensation, 1 = abnormal, 2 = normal) and grading strength of 10 key muscle groups on the standard clinical scale (0 = total paralysis, 1 = palpable or visible movement, 2 = active movement with gravity eliminated, 3 = active movement against gravity, 4 = active movement against moderate resistance, 5 = normal). The neurologic level is defined by the most caudad segment that has normal motor and sensory function (normal is indicated by intact sensation and muscle strength grade of at least 3 for that segment). A rectal examination is essential. Presence of voluntary anal sphincter contraction or sensation at the mucocutaneous junction indicates "incomplete" injury, regardless of other findings.

If the patient has neurologic evidence of spinal cord injury, a continuous MP infusion, 5.4 mg per kilogram per hour), should be started 1 hour after the initial bolus and maintained for 23 hours. Longer duration treatments are not recommended, because increased infection and other complications may result. No clinical evidence supports the use of longer MP therapy. Some data indicate that prolonging MP treatment beyond 24 hours may be deleterious to recovery and lead to complications. If the patient has no evidence of neurologic loss from the injury, the MP infusion need not be started or may be discontinued if it was already started. However, if the patient develops neurologic signs during the first 8 hours after injury, a second bolus dose of 30 mg per kilogram and 5.4 mg per kilogram per hour continuous infusion of MP should be considered.

The radiographic diagnosis and surgical approaches to spine injuries are beyond the scope of this chapter and have been extensively reviewed elsewhere. X-ray studies must include the entire spinal column. Multiple and subtle fractures are common. The studies should include CT, with appropriate immobilization of the patient. Spinal cord damage may occur with minimal radiographic evidence of bony fractures. If traumatic disc herniation is suspected, MRI is preferred to CT or radiography for defining the extent and level of disc herniation(s). If the spinal cord or spinal roots are mechanically compressed, decompression should be accomplished rapidly. This can be done by traction with an appropriate device. If traction does not decompress the spinal column, surgical decompression should be considered and strongly recommended. This is particularly true if the compression is due to a disc herniation, hematoma (rare), or other soft tissue protrusion into the spinal canal.

Some surgeons may choose not to operate immediately if the patients has complete loss of motor and sensory function below the lesion level. However, because MP does restore function in some patients, suggesting that viable spinal axons may be present, definitive surgical decompression should be carried out if traction is unsuccessful. The surgical decision should be made by an experienced neurosurgeon.

SUBACUTE PHASE (WITHIN 1 WEEK)

The spinal column must be stabilized if vertebral fractures or ligamentous injury cause instability of the spinal column. Many approaches are available. At our center, the preferred approach for cervical spine stabilization is posterior or anterior plating. Many fixation devices are available for thoracic and lumbosacral spine injuries. Internal fixation devices effectively stabilize the spinal column. Patients usually do not need bone grafts or postoperative traction. Thoracic and lumbosacral instrumentation often requires abdominal or thoracic surgical approaches. The timing of surgery depends on the patient's condition and the surgical approach.

Intensive and systematic nursing care is critical during this phase. Respiratory therapy should be initiated, especially in patients with cervical spine injuries. The patient must be turned regularly and frequently or placed on an appropriate rotating or moving bed, to prevent formation of decubiti. Limbs must be carefully padded to prevent sores. Histamine H2 receptor blockers should be started to prevent gastrointestinal irritation and hemorrhage. Bladder and bowel care routines should be instituted. For example, intermittent catheterization can be started 1 day after injury. Small doses of heparin may be given to reduce the risk of thrombophlebitis and pulmonary emboli.

If there are no medical contraindications, hyperalimentation may be provided, to retard the progressive negative nitrogen balance that occurs in most spine-injured patients. The therapeutic benefit of hyperalimentation in spinal cord injuries, however, has not yet been demonstrated. Metabolic status should be carefully monitored. One worrisome aspect of hyperalimentation is that it can cause significant hyperglycemia, a condition that has been reported to aggravate ischemic tissue damage in animal models.

The patient, family, and significant friends must be carefully informed of the treatment plan. Spine-injured patients and families should not be told that no recovery will occur. Such statements not only are deeply discouraging but generally are not true. Some recovery is the rule rather than the exception. Even severely spine-injured patients admitted with no neurologic function below the lesion level often recover some function. The recovery may occur over many months, and sometimes years. The recovery may manifest as a descent in lesion level by two or more spinal segments, return of isolated sensory patches and motor function many segments below the lesion level, and improved postural tone. Overly optimistic expectations should be gently and firmly discouraged without eliminating hope. Discussions should emphasize the importance of caring for the body, descriptions of likely complications and what should be done to prevent them, and the need to learn and develop solutions to specific handicaps resulting from the spinal cord injury.

CHRONIC PHASE (BEYOND 1 WEEK)

Rehabilitation specialists should be included in the acute spinal cord injury team to prescribe and coordinate physical therapy. From the first day after injury, they should also begin planning for transfer of the patient to the rehabilitation service. Familiarity with the patient's neurosurgical and medical problems generally facilitates the transfer and minimizes complications.

Unless medical problems (such as infections or respiratory complications) dictate otherwise, the patient should be transferred to a rehabilitation service under the care of an experienced rehabilitation team. Medical diagnosis and care should continue. Intensive physical therapy should be initiated. A urologic evaluation should be initiated with daily urine analyses, cultures when necessary, a urodynamics study, and appropriate radiographs. Orthotic, prosthetic, and other devices should be considered, discussed, prescribed, and fitted.

Physical therapy should focus on progressively bringing the patient to a vertical or sitting position, ensuring that limb joints retain maximum mobility and range of motion, preventing pressure sores, and detecting motor and sensory dysfunctions. A progressive exercise program should be designed and implemented, including swimming. If biofeedback training is available, this can also be started. The patient should focus on strengthening muscles to transfer, carry out intermittent urethral catheterizations if necessary and possible, utilizing muscle stimulators to strengthen selected muscle groups, and training with biofeedback devices to learn better motor control.

Medical diagnosis and care includes a detailed physical examination and blood tests to evaluate hematologic, endocrine, and renal status. Daily vital signs, regular chest radiography, and gastrointestinal assessments should be carried out, including checks of stool for hemorrhage. If the patient has any compromise of respiratory function, systematic respiratory therapy should be initiated and continued. If possible, attempts should be made to wean respirator-bound patients, including by phrenic nerve stimulation. Antispasticity medication (i.e., muscle relaxants and baclofen) should be carefully titrated because of side effects.

Urologic diagnosis and care should include baseline renal function tests, urodynamics, and cystography. These are necessary because urinary tract infections, stones, and spastic bladder are common complications of spinal cord injury. The patient should be trained to do as much intermittent catheterization as possible. To prevent urinary tract infections, appropriate prophylactic antibiotics and a urine acidification regimen should be initiated.

Occupational therapists should begin evaluating the patient, using the Functional Independence Measure. The patient should be trained to perform as much self-care as possible and achieve independence. The training should include transfer techniques, walker, or wheelchair skills, bathing methods, communication methods, self-feeding tools, driving, and other activities of independent living. If necessary, special orthotics and prosthetics should be prescribed, designed, and fitted.

Other important programs includes sex education and therapy, diet counseling, psychological assessments and therapy, and family counseling. In addition, social workers must begin organizing access to community resources, funding, housing, insurance, aides, transportation, and other critical services for the patient. The patient should participate in organized peer group sessions. Finally, follow-up care must be scheduled, with medical, physiatric, urologic, and neurosurgical assessments at regular intervals after discharge.

NEW TRENDS IN SPINAL CORD INJURY THERAPY

The second National Acute Spinal Cord Injury Study (NASCIS 2) found that severely injured patients given large doses of MP within 8 hours after injury

Table 1 Pharmacologic Treatments of Central Nervous System Injury

Type	Drug	SCI	TBI
Glucocorticoids	Dexamethasone	*†	*†
	Methylprednisolone	*‡	*†
Antioxidants	Tirilazad mesylate	*	*
	Vitamin E	*	*
	U-78517F		*
	Chlorpromazine	*	
Opiate receptor blockers	Naloxone	*	*
	Nalmefene	*	*
	Nor-binaltorphimine	*	
Kappa opioid receptor agonist	U-50488H	*	
Thyrotropin-releasing hormone	TRH	*	*
	YM14673	*	*
	CG3703		*
NMDA receptor blockers	MK801	*	*
	Dextromethorphan	*	*
	Dextrorphan	*	*
Other excitotoxic receptor blockers	Kynurenate	*	
	Ketamine	*	*
Calcium channel blockers	Nimodipine	*	*
Monosialic gangliosides	G_{M1}	*‡	
Protease inhibitors	Mixture	*	
Cyclo-oxygenase inhibitors	Indomethacin	*	*
	Ibuprofen	*	*
	BW755C	*	
Serotonin receptor blockers	Mianserin	*	
Free radical enzymes	Superoxide dismutase	*	
Potassium channel blockers	4-Aminopyridine	*	

Key: Drugs have been reported to be beneficial when administered after spinal cord injury (SCI) or traumatic brain injury (TBI).
*Positive animal studies.
†Anecdotal clinical experience.
‡Randomized clinical trial experience.
This is not an exhaustive survey. References are available elsewhere.

recovered 22 percent of lost motor function versus 8 percent for those treated with placebo. MP-treated "incomplete" spine-injured patients recovered 75 versus 59 percent of their lost motor function. Patients given MP longer than 8 hours after injury had worse recovery than placebo controls.

NASCIS 2 has had much impact on clinical care of acute spinal cord injury. Before 1990, spinal cord injury often was not treated as a true medical emergency. Spine-injury victims were often taken to the nearest emergency room, where they might wait hours for radiography and treatment. Now they are rushed to spinal cord injury centers for MP treatment. The observation that MP improved recovery in severe spinal cord inuries has led many clinicians to re-evaluate the long-held clinical dogma that "complete" spinal cord injuries do not benefit from any treatment, including surgery.

One curious and unanticipated development has been the growing practice by neurosurgeons of giving MP to patients before risky spinal cord surgery, to prevent iatrogenic injury. Reasoning that MP should be as effective or more so when given before an injury, they give a 2 g bolus just before surgery. If the patient awakes from surgery with a deficit, they continue the maintenance dose. If not, the drug is discontinued. This practice, although logical, should be put to test in a randomized clinical trial.

Recently, the monosialic ganglioside G_{M1}, 100 mg per day, was reported to improve motor recovery when started 48 to 72 hours and continued for 18 to 32 days after injury after a small-dose course of MP, 250 mg bolus plus 125 mg every 6 hours for 3 days. G_{M1} improved recovery only in the legs (not the arms) of 17 patients, compared to 17 placebo controls. Neither the mechanisms nor the sites of action of G_{M1} are known. A multicenter randomized clinical trial has been started to compare nothing, 100 mg, and 200 mg of G_{M1} per day starting after the standard 24 hour MP course of NASCIS 2.

Dozens of other drugs have been reported in animal studies to be beneficial for acute brain and spinal cord injury. The number of drugs, listed in Table 1, reported to be neuroprotective strongly suggests that secondary injury mechanisms play a role in central nervous system tissue damage. Although the drug mechanisms are not well understood, the observation that drugs as varied as glucocorticoids, antioxidants, receptor and channel blockers, and modulators of intracellular messenger systems have neuroprotective effects suggests that secondary injury involves a complex cascade of endogenous mechanisms initiated by the injury. In the near future, regenerative treatments of chronic spinal cord injury are also likely to become available.

SUGGESTED READING

Bracken MB, Shepard MJ, Collins WF, et al. A randomized controlled trial of methylprednisolone or naloxone in the treatment of acute spinal-cord injury: Results of the Second National Acute Spinal Cord Injury Study. N Engl J Med 1990; 322:1405–1411.

Bracken MB, Shepard MJ, Collins WFJ, et al. Methylprednisolone or naloxone treatment after acute spinal cord injury: 1-year follow-up data. Results of the Second National Acute Spinal Cord Injury Study. J Neurosurgery, 1992; 76:23–31.

Ditunno JFJ, Young W, Donovan WH, et al. Standards for neurological classification of spinal cord injury. Chicago: American Spinal Injury Association, 1992.

Errico TJ, Bauer RD, Waugh T, eds. Spinal trauma. Philadelphia: JB Lippincott, 1991.

Geisler FH, Dorsey FC, Coleman WP. Recovery of motor function after spinal-cord injury—a randomized, placebo-controlled trial with GM-1 ganglioside, N Engl J Med 1991; 324:1829–1838.

Hamilton BB, Laughlin JA, Granger CV, Kayton RM. Interrater agreement of the seven level functional independence measure (FIM). Arch Phys Med Rehab 1991; 72:572.

Young W. Medical treatments of acute spinal cord injury. J Neurol Neurosurg Psychiatry, 1992; 55:635–639.

Young W. Acute, restorative, and regenerative therapy of spinal cord injury. In: Piepmeier JM, ed. The outcome following traumatic spinal cord injury. Mount Kisco, NY: Futura, 1992.

PERIPHERAL NERVE INJURY

ALLAN J. BELZBERG, M.D., FRCSC
JAMES N. CAMPBELL, M.D.

When confronted with a peripheral nerve injury, the physician must first localize and define the lesion. A decision is then made to follow the lesion over time or to refer the patient for surgical intervention. Determining which lesions require surgical intervention and what is the appropriate timing of operation requires an understanding of the pathophysiology of nerve injury and the limitations of spontaneous recovery and surgical repair. Management of a peripheral nerve injury also requires attention to early rehabilitation and pain control.

PATHOPHYSIOLOGY

Regardless of the cause of injury, a nerve responds to an insult in a predictable manner. With mild injuries, local demyelination can produce a conduction block without leading to wallerian degeneration. If the conduction block is complete, the patient may have a dense sensory and motor deficit. The lesion, however, can be fully reversible, with spontaneous recovery over hours to weeks.

More severe injuries can produce axonal interruption. When an axon is divided, wallerian degeneration occurs, so the axon and myelin distal to the injury degenerate and are removed by phagocytic cells, leaving empty endoneurial tubes. The proximal axon begins to regenerate by sending out sprouts. If the sprouts do not reach the distal endoneurial tube or if the tube has been replaced by fibrosis preventing entry, the sprouts form a local tangle or neuroma. Failure of the regenerating axons to gain entry into distal endoneurial tubes precludes a functional outcome and suggests the need for surgical repair.

Axonal breakdown in wallerian degeneration is completed over approximately 2 weeks. The denervated muscle becomes spontaneously active, with electromyography (EMG) findings of fibrillations and denervation potentials. Performing EMG prior to the 2-week point may not show these stigmata of denervation if wallerian degeneration is not yet complete. If after 2 weeks EMG findings are normal, the injury does not involve axonal degeneration, and full recovery is more likely.

When a muscle loses its innervation, it degenerates. By 3 weeks after injury, there are histologic changes in the muscle and the beginnings of muscle fibrosis. The fibrosis gradually replaces the muscle, and by 2 years only scar tissue remains. Typically, the muscle must be reinnervated within approximately 18 months of the injury to provide a functional outcome. Proximal nerve lesions are therefore at greater risk of poor outcome because of the increased time required for axonal regeneration to reach target muscle.

Although there is a 1 to 2 year time limit for muscle reinnervation, no such limit exists for sensory function. While some sensory organs do degenerate over time, reinnervation of skin can still provide a functional outcome in many instances. An example of this is repair of a median nerve injury to provide useful sensory function in the hand several years after injury.

Axons regenerate at a rate of approximately 1 mm per day. The time required for the regenerating axons to cross the lesion and reinnervate the next most proximal muscle can, therefore, be estimated. If there are no signs of reinnervation after an appropriate interval, surgical repair is indicated.

Ectopic mechanosensitivity (Tinel's sign) can be used to assess growth of a nerve. Tapping the regenerating axons of the nerve produces a paresthesia felt in the distribution normally innervated by the nerve. The Tinel's sign should move distally 2 to 3 cm per month, reflecting the advancing axonal growth cone. Failure of Tinel's sign to progress at the expected rate suggests the need for surgical exploration.

When a proximal nerve injury occurs, there may not be sufficient time to await spontaneous recovery of muscle function and still maintain a window of opportunity for surgical repair, if it is required. Intraoperative examination of the nerve injury can be used to determine if there has been axonal regeneration across the lesion without waiting the added time for axonal regeneration to reach the target muscle. Once sufficient time has passed for the axons to regenerate across the lesion, proximal electrical stimulation should result in the recording of a compound nerve action potential distal to the lesion. Failure of conduction across the lesion after an appropriate interval suggests the need for surgical resection.

CLASSIFICATION

Nerve injuries are categorized according to one of two popular schemes. The Seddon classification defines a neuropraxia as a reversible physiologic disruption. Axonotmesis involves interruption of axons and neurotmesis disruption of the nerve trunk, often with loss of anatomic continuity. The Sunderland grading system (Table 1) is useful for purposes of classification, and injuries are usually discussed with reference to this system.

Laceration of nerves produces a grade V lesion. This injury requires surgical repair for a functional outcome. Time can be taken to stabilize associated injuries and assemble a skilled surgical team. Surgery performed within a few days of injury has an equal outcome to that performed in the acute situation.

Stretch, missile, crush, and injection injuries can produce variable injury to the nerve. The lesion may be grade I through grade V, and the damage may extend over a long distance. Acute-phase surgical intervention is contraindicated, except when associated injuries require attention. Surgical repair of the nerve should be delayed, as the full extent of damage to the nerve may take time to manifest itself. Even if it is known that a grade V lesion is present, several weeks should be allowed to pass, to allow the full extent of the lesion to declare itself. If the extent of the injury is unknown, Tinel's sign, sensory function, and muscle function should be followed to determine if recovery is occurring. Failure of Tinel's sign to progress or failure of muscle and sensory function to occur in timely fashion is an indication for surgery. It is important to understand that in the case of brachial plexus injuries, for example, that one part of the plexus

Table 1 Sunderland Classification of Nerve Injury

Grade	Description	Need for Surgery
I	Loss of axonal conduction	No
II	Loss of axonal continuity	No
III	Loss of axonal and endoneurial continuity	Yes for severe injury
IV	Loss of perineural continuity and fascicular disruption	Yes; often requires grafting
V	Loss of continuity of entire nerve trunk	Yes; often requires grafting

may recover spontaneously while another part requires surgical repair (Fig. 1).

CLINICAL EXAMINATION

The clinical history contributes information on timing and cause of the injury. It is essential to know if there has been any change in function after injury. Some traumatic injuries can progress during the first 12 hours, but loss of function after 24 hours requires an explanation. It is also important to know if there are any underlying medical conditions that can produce a neuropathy, such as alcoholism, which may complicate the examination or compromise recovery.

During the physical examination, the physician must identify the location of the lesion in relation to the neural axis. This requires knowledge of the anatomy of peripheral nerves, including their anatomic course and innervation of motor and sensory function. Laboratory testing is often limited to the EMG and nerve conduction study. The production of muscle contraction with stimulation proximal to the injury suggests a partial injury with a good prognosis for spontaneous recovery. Even with dense motor and sensory loss, the presence of motor action potentials or muscle contraction when the nerve is stimulated distal to the injury suggests a grade I lesion and excellent prognosis. It must be remembered that wallerian degeneration takes time and EMG is therefore not of much help if performed within a week of injury.

EMG can also aid in localizing the nerve injury. As each muscle is needled, moving proximodistally along the course of the nerve, the exact level of the injury may become apparent when the most proximal abnormal muscle is identified. Follow-up EMG is a sensitive test for determining if there is evidence of muscle reinnervation.

SPECIFIC NERVE INJURY

Root and Brachial Plexus Injuries

Injury to the brachial plexus is most often seen secondary to stretch injury from motor vehicle accidents and birth trauma. Gunshot and knife wounds to the axilla, tumor involvement, and iatrogenic injury account for most of the remaining injuries of the brachial plexus. In general, lesions of the upper trunk carry a better prognosis than those of the lower trunk, because of the shorter distance for target reinnervation. As after most peripheral nerve injuries, recovery is faster and more complete in children than in adults.

The injury may be localized to a specific component of the plexus, such as a trunk, or more commonly to a combination of elements. Injury to the suprascapular nerve, lateral cord, and axillary nerve is a common combination that may be difficult to distinguish from an upper trunk injury.

Early surgical intervention is rarely indicated for brachial plexus stretch lesions. Our practice is to evaluate the patient immediately and then at monthly intervals, to determine if there is evidence of progressing Tinel's sign and reinnervation of proximal muscle. If, after 3 months there are no signs of recovery, surgical exploration is undertaken. Plexus injuries secondary to birth trauma are generally observed for 4 to 6 months before surgical exploration is considered. An exception is an isolated injury to the lower trunk or medial cord. Because of the great distance required for reinnervation, surgical exploration is considered earlier but prognosis remains poor.

Determining if there has been avulsion of roots from the spinal cord is important because no spontaneous recovery is expected. Physical examination demonstrates decreased or no power in all muscles innervated by the avulsed root. The clue to avulsion injury is the finding that muscles innervated by proximal nerve branches are lost. A flail arm, in combination with serratus anterior palsy, is very suggestive of an avulsion injury. Likewise, Horner's syndrome predicts avulsion of the lower plexus. A myelogram followed by computed tomography or magnetic resonance imaging that demonstrates pseudomeningoceles suggests that root avulsion has occurred.

Electrical stimulation techniques can provide information on root avulsions. The peripheral sensory nerve cell body is located in the dorsal root ganglia (DRG). A lesion proximal to the DRG, such as a brachial plexus avulsion from the spinal cord, does not disconnect the peripheral axon from the cell body. Wallerian degeneration, therefore, does not occur in the sensory portion of the peripheral nerve, and the sensory nerve action potentials remain intact. If, however, the lesion is distal to the DRG, then there is sensory axonal wallerian degeneration and loss of the sensory nerve action potential.

Radial Nerve Injury

Injuries to the radial nerve commonly occur at the mid humeral level secondary to fracture of the humerus. These are most often stretch or contusion injuries and carry a good prognosis for spontaneous recovery. If there is no evidence of recovery at 3 months, surgical exploration is indicated. Because the target muscles are close, surgical repair offers a good prognosis. More distal injuries involving the posterior interosseous nerve are more complex because of branching of the nerve.

Median and Ulnar Nerve Injuries

In general, the median nerve supplies important *sensation* to the hand and the ulnar nerve important *motor function* to the hand. Injury to the median nerve produces sensory loss in the hand, which can be debilitating. Repair of the median nerve, even years after injury, can restore useful sensory function.

A severe ulnar nerve injury that occurs proximal to the elbow is associated with a poor prognosis for functional return of intrinsic hand muscles, because of the distance required for reinnervation of target muscles. An attempt at repair, however, is usually a good idea, if only to obtain innervation to the flexor carpi ulnaris and flexor digitorum profundus III, IV, and ulnar sensory function. With more distal injuries, separation of motor and sensory function into separate fascicles allows more accurate surgical repair and better outcome.

Some patients can suffer severe pain after a median or ulnar nerve injury, often associated with incomplete return of function. These patients may respond to neurolysis. This phenomenon can also occur with other peripheral nerve injuries. Pain, in and of itself, may be an indication for nerve graft repair.

Lower Extremity Nerve Injury

Proximal severe injury is associated with a poor outcome because of the great distances required for reinnervation of target muscle. Civilian femoral nerve injuries are most often iatrogenic. Injury can occur during surgical procedures, such as femoral bypass surgery, and grade V injuries should be repaired acutely

(see Fig. 1). Sciatic nerve injuries are common secondary to hip fracture or hip surgery, injection injury, and laceration injury. External neurolysis may be indicated for pain control if excessive scarring develops around the injury site. Common peroneal nerve injury can occur at the fibular head secondary to fracture. Although anecdotal reports suggests that repair of the peroneal nerve is not associated with a good outcome, this has not been our experience.

TREATMENT

Nonsurgical

During the period of observation waiting for signs of nerve regeneration, pain management can become a problem. Injury to the nervous system can result in pain that is difficult to control pharmacologically. Patients often complain of paresthesia sensations, which may become painful, and of hyperalgesia in the distribution

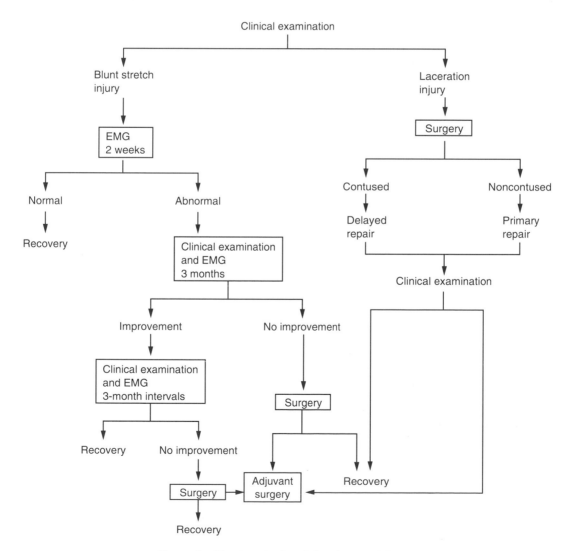

Figure 1 Treatment of peripheral nerve injury.

of the injured nerve. Our initial medication regimen makes use of antiepileptics such as carbamazepine, used just as they would be for epilepsy. If these fail, we add a tricyclic antidepressant such as desipramine. For resistant cases, clonazepan is also sometimes useful. Long-acting opioids are also a very useful adjunct to treatment.

The patient must maintain range of motion in joints, to prevent contractures that would hamper functional recovery. Joint contractures also are often painful. A physical therapist can be most useful in ensuring maintenance of a full passive range of motion.

Daily use of electrical stimulation to maintain muscle while awaiting reinnervation may be of use, but it has not yet been validated. Electrical stimulation to aid nerve regeneration has dubious value.

Surgical

Advances in instrumentation and microscopic technique have improved the outcome of nerve surgery. Certain terms are commonly used in the field of nerve surgery. *Neurotization* refers to the ingrowth of axons into tissue such as a distal nerve stump, or a motor end-plate in a muscle. It can occur spontaneously after an injury to a nerve or after surgical repair of the nerve. *Neurorrhaphy* is the joining together, usually by suture, of the two parts of a divided nerve to enable neurotization. If the nerve ends do not easily come together *interpositional nerve grafts* may be required. *Nerve transfer* refers to the transposition of another freshly cut normal nerve to the distal stump of the injured nerve. It is used when the proximal stump of the injured nerve can no longer provide useful reinnervation (e.g., cases of nerve root avulsion from the spinal cord). The term *anastomosis* should be avoided for nerve repair, as it refers to union of hollow tubes.

Surgical repair is used to restore continuity between proximal axons and distal endoneurial tubes. A complete laceration of the nerve obviously requires repair, which should be done within days of injury. More commonly, a neuroma in continuity is encountered. The Sunderland grade of lesion must then be determined and the need for resection evaluated. A skilled peripheral nerve surgeon can palpate the neuroma and often determine the extent of fibrosis. Additional information can be gained through the use of intraoperative stimulating and recording techniques. If a fibrotic neuroma is divided, no fascicles are seen. The ends are then trimmed back until more normal cross-sectional anatomy is visualized.

A direct suture neurorrhaphy using 2 to 3 epineurial placed sutures is the preferred method of nerve repair. The fewer sutures that are placed, the lesser the chance of fibrosis and the better the prognosis for a functional result. Under certain circumstances, such as a very distal lesion with sensory and motor fibers segregated into separate fascicles, interfascicular repair is indicated, allowing direct alignment of fascicle to fascicle.

A nerve repair resulting in excessive tension on the suture line is unlikely to result in a good outcome. An attempt can be made to gain length in the nerve, thus obviating an interpositional nerve graft. Simple techniques include mobilizing the nerve from its bed and splitting muscle branches from the main trunk. Flexion of the adjacent joint adds to the nerve's length, but the posture must be maintained for 6 weeks to allow the suture line to gain strength before attempting to extend the joint. Nerve transposition, such as anterior transposition of the ulnar nerve at the elbow, may provide enough length to allow end-to-end neurorrhaphy without grafting.

If a large gap occurs it may not be possible to approximate the nerve ends for repair without placing undue tension on the suture site. An interpositional graft using autogenous nerve is used to bridge such a gap. Use of end-to-end repairs when nerve grafting should be done constitutes one of the frequent errors in modern day peripheral nerve surgery. Sensory nerves such as the medial cutaneous nerve of the forearm and the sural nerve serve as examples of useful nerve grafts.

With injuries that result in root avulsion there may not be a proximal end available for repair. A nerve transfer is then required to provide innervation to the distal segment. The intercostal nerves, for example, can be mobilized and provide innervation to the brachial plexus.

After a nerve repair, the appropriate joints are immobilized long enough to allow the neural suture line to heal, generally 4 to 6 weeks. Aggressive mobilization of joints is then employed, to prevent joint contractures.

If reinnervation fails, other measures can be used to provide some function. Tendon transfers are an important adjunct to nerve surgery. In a brachial plexus injury, for example, it may be useful to utilize the wrist extensors to improve the patient's finger flexor function.

SUGGESTED READING

Burchiel KJ, ed. Surgical management of peripheral nerve injury and entrapment. Neurosurg Clin 1991; 2:1.

Gelberman R. Operative nerve repair and reconstruction. Philadelphia: JB Lippincott, 1991.

Mackinnon SE, Dellon AL. Surgery of the peripheral nerves. New York: Thieme, 1988.

Omer GE Jr, Spinner M. Management of peripheral nerve problems. Philadelphia: WB Saunders, 1980.

Sunderland S. Nerve injuries and their repair. New York: Churchill Livingstone, 1991.

NEOPLASMS

CHILDHOOD BRAIN TUMORS

ROGER J. PACKER, M.D.

Primary central nervous system (CNS) tumors of childhood are the second most common form of cancer and the leading type of solid tumor in the first 15 years of life. Unlike adults' brain tumors, those of children are histologically heterogeneous (Table 1). They also vary greatly in site of origin and frequently disseminate through the nervous system early in the course of disease. Approximately half of all childhood brain tumors arise in the posterior fossa, and another 20 percent in the sellar region. Early diagnosis can be difficult in very young children and infants, because primary CNS tumors may produce relatively nonfocal neurologic problems and delayed or arrested development. Magnetic resonance imaging (MRI) has much simplified diagnosis and greatly aided in the staging of disease.

Table 1 Prevalence of Childhood Brain Tumors*

Tumor	Prevalence (%)
Low-grade glioma	20–37
Cerebellar	10–20
Supratentorial	10–17
Medulloblastoma/primitive neuroectodermal tumor	10–25
Brain stem glioma	5–15
High-grade glioma	15–20
Ependymoma	5–10
Craniopharyngioma	5–10
Others	10–15
Choroid plexus carcinoma	
Choroid plexus papillomoma	
Germinoma	
Mixed–germ cell	
Teratoid	
Meningioma	
Pineocytoma	
Teratoma	

*Depends on series

GENERAL PRINCIPLES OF TREATMENT

The management of childhood brain tumors is complicated by their heterogeneity, their tendency to disseminate, and the vulnerability of the developing nervous system to neurotoxic agents required for treatment. Even though some childhood brain tumors are very resistant to treatment and have a poor prognosis, advances in management have been made. More than 50 percent of all children with newly diagnosed brain tumors can be expected to be alive and free of progressive disease 5 years after diagnosis, many cured of their illness. Disease control is possible not only with low-grade, resectable tumors but also for some highly malignant forms of childhood brain tumors, especially primitive neuroectodermal tumors (medulloblastomas) and germinomas. Centralized referral to a multidisciplinary childhood brain tumor center optimizes the chance for long-term survival and may improve the likelihood of an acceptable quality of life for survivors. Multi-institutional randomized treatment trials or pilot therapy programs using newer, possibly more effective, forms of treatment are available at many centers. Two major treatment groups, the Children's Cancer Group and the Pediatric Oncology Group, co-ordinate the performance of the majority of treatment trials in the United States.

The following general principles of treatment have been found useful in the care of children with brain tumors:

Principle 1. Management is individualized to the histologic type of tumor and its location in the nervous system. With the exception of intrinsic brain stem gliomas and infiltrating visual pathway abnormalities in children with neurofibromatosis, adequate material for histologic examination must be obtained before treatment is instituted.

Principle 2. Following histologic diagnosis, patients require staging studies to determine the extent of residual disease at the primary tumor site and at distant sites. Other parameters such as age at diagnosis, biologic properties of the tumor, and specific immunohistochemical findings are often useful for stratifying patients into appropriate risk groups within histologic subtypes. For malignant tumors such as primitive neuroectodermal tumors/medulloblastomas, posterior fossa anaplastic gliomas, and germ cell tumors, the required postoperative assessment includes myelography and cerebrospinal fluid cytologic examination. Magnetic resonance imaging (MRI) of the spine with gadolinium, if done appropriately and in at least two planes (detailed transverse images are recommended), may be as precise as myelography, if not more so.

Principle 3. After staging, most tumors require multimodality management that is designed not only to improve tumor control and survival but also to produce a reasonable quality of life.

Principle 4. The developing nervous system, especially in infants and young children, is vulnerable to standard treatments used for brain tumors, especially radiotherapy. A balance is sought between the likelihood of effective treatment and the probability of significant treatment-related neurologic sequelae.

Principle 5. Because of the poor outcome of many childhood tumors, many patients are candidates for either institutional or multi-institutional treatment trials.

Principle 6. For childhood tumors for which an effective treatment is not known and prognosis is dismal, innovative approaches are warranted.

MANAGEMENT OF SPECIFIC TUMOR TYPES

Primitive Neuroectodermal Tumors/Medulloblastomas

Primitive neuroectodermal tumor or medulloblastoma (PNET/MB) is the most common form of malignant childhood brain tumor. Classification of these neoplasms is controversial. Some believe that tumors that arise in the posterior fossa, commonly named medulloblastomas, have a different prognosis than lesions that arise in the pineal gland (pineoblastomas) or in the cortex (central neuroblastomas). Others contend that because all such lesions are histologically indistinguishable and share similar immunohistochemical features, distinctions based on tumor location are unwarranted. Approximately 20 to 30 percent of all PNETs/MBs have disseminated to the leptomeninges at the time of diagnosis, and another 10 to 20 percent of patients develop leptomeningeal disease in advance of or concurrently with local disease relapse. Postoperative evaluation for postoperative primary site residual disease and leptomeningeal tumor spread is indicated for all patients.

Surgery is an extremely important part of the overall management of PNETs/MBs in children. Extensive resection is indicated for all patients, not only to provide

histologic confirmation but as the basis of effective treatment. Although it has not been proven that total or nearly total resection results in better survival than partial resection, it is clear that patients who undergo only biopsy rarely survive. Postsurgical factors believed to be predictive of outcome include age of the patient at diagnosis, extent of disease at the time of diagnosis, and possibly biologic factors such as ploidy. Based on these parameters, patients with PNETs/MBs can be crudely stratified into two risk groups (Table 2).

Conventional treatment includes craniospinal radiotherapy supplemented with local boosts (local tumor dose 5,400 to 5,580 cGy). The amount of craniospinal radiation required has not been demonstrated by carefully performed dose-response studies. Without craniospinal radiotherapy, disease control is unlikely. Recent randomized trials have demonstrated that craniospinal radiotherapy in a dose of 3,600 cGy produces better control of leptomeningeal disease than 2,400 cGy.

For average-risk disease, treatment with craniospinal irradiation supplemented with local radiotherapy results in 5 year disease-free survival rate of approximately 60 percent or slightly higher. In this group of patients, there is no clear evidence that the addition of adjuvant chemotherapy improves survival. Children with poor-risk PNET/MB treated with standard radiotherapy have a survival rate of approximately 40 percent at 5 years. There is evidence from randomized clinical trials that adjuvant chemotherapy with lomustine (CCNU) and vincristine improves the overall rate of disease-free survival for children with "poor-risk" disease. More recently, the use of vincristine during radiotherapy and postradiotherapy cycles of CCNU, vincristine, and cisplatinum have produced a 5 year disease-free survival rate better than 80 percent for children with poor-risk PNETs/MBs. These survival rates are equal to, if not better than, the survival rates for children with so-called average-risk disease. Based on this type of information, it is my personal bias that all children with PNETs/MBs should receive adjuvant chemotherapy.

The most effective form of adjuvant chemotherapy has not been demonstrated by randomized trials. Results with cisplatinum, CCNU, and vincristine are promising. There is also evidence that cyclophosphamide is active against PNETs/MBs in children. Another significant factor in the planning of treatment for children with PNETs/MBs is the long-term sequelae of treatment. Craniospinal radiotherapy, in the amounts convention-

Table 2 Stratification of Children with Primitive Neuroectodermal Tumors/Medulloblastomas

Variable	Average Risk	Poor Risk
Disease extent	Localized	Disseminated
Extent of resection	Total	Biopsy (?partial): ? brain stem involvement
Age (yr)	Older	<?3, ?5
Location	Posterior fossa	Pineal, ?cortical

ally given, causes significant intellectual and hormonal sequelae. In children younger than 7 years, a sequential drop in intelligence has been seen following 3,600 cGy whole-brain radiotherapy. One approach to minimizing sequelae is to utilize adjuvant chemotherapy in an attempt to reduce the needed amount of craniospinal radiation. In most studies, the amount of local radiotherapy prescribed has remained unchanged, as the local site remains the most likely location for disease relapse and the amount of damage caused by local radiotherapy is unclear. Currently we are participating in a study of reduced-dose craniospinal radiotherapy (2,340 cGy) supplemented with adjuvant chemotherapy, to determine the feasibility of reducing the amount of whole-brain and spinal radiotherapy for children who have localized disease at diagnosis. A multicenter randomized treatment trial through the Children's Cancer Group is soon to begin in which children with localized PNETs/MBs of the posterior fossa who are given reduced radiotherapy will receive adjuvant chemotherapy (cyclophosphamide, cisplatinum, and vincristine) and patients will be randomized to receive either 3,600 cGy or 2,340 cGy of craniospinal radiotherapy. Only a multigroup randomized trial can address these questions.

Treatment for patients with disseminated or "non–posterior fossa" PNET/MB remains problematic. Further intensifications and treatment are planned for these "poor–risk" patients, including large-dose preradiation chemotherapy, and possibly hyperfractionated radiation therapy. Theoretically, this type of radiotherapy allows larger doses of radiotherapy to be given with fewer sequelae.

The neurocognitive sequelae of craniospinal radiation therapy for children with PNET/MB—or for that matter for any child who requires craniospinal radiotherapy—are quite significant, especially for very young children. Various treatment trials have utilized chemotherapy alone for infants and very young children (arbitrarily, those younger than 3 years at diagnosis), in an attempt at least to delay the need for radiotherapy. A variety of different agents have been shown to be effective in 30 to 40 percent of patients. Regimens such as MOPP (mechlorethamine, vincristine, prednisone, and procarbazine) and baby POG (cyclophosphamide, cisplatinum, vincristine and etoposide) have been employed. A controversial question is whether patients who exhibit a complete response subsequently require radiotherapy. It has been our bias to attempt to intensify chemotherapeutic regimens and utilize radiotherapy only when a complete response cannot be obtained.

Brain Stem Gliomas

Brain stem gliomas account for 10 to 15 percent of all childhood brain tumors. Approximately 80 percent of these lesions arise in the pons and cause cranial nerve deficits, long-track signs, ataxia, and sensory abnormalities. There are subsets of patients with brain stem gliomas whose diagnosis is somewhat more favorable—those with low-grade exophytic lesions, focal midbrain (especially tectal) tumors, and possibly those focal lesions or neurofibromatosis—but the vast majority of patients (80 to 90 percent) die of progressive disease within 18 months of diagnosis.

In our opinion, surgery should be reserved for patients with atypical brain stem gliomas. There is some evidence to suggest that cervicomedullary exophytic lesions are amenable to gross surgical resection, and such resection may improve long-term disease control. Similarly, some children with focal, especially midbrain, lesions seem to have a better prognosis. In these types of atypical brain stem gliomas, surgical resection or biopsy is indicated to determine the histologic subtype of the tumor. For the majority of patients who have diffuse intrinsic tumors, surgery has little or no role. Improved surgical techniques such as stereotactic radiosurgery can be utilized to obtain adequate tissue, but it is unclear whether the tissue obtained is representative of the tumor as a whole. Even more important, histologic findings have not been shown to be predictive of outcome with diffuse brain stem tumors. The majority of children with diffuse intrinsic brain stem gliomas, who by biopsy are judged to have low-grade lesions, are frequently found at postmortem examination to have malignant glioma.

As is the case in PNET/MB, stratification into two major risk groups is possible (Table 3). Patients with low-grade cervicomedullary, midbrain, tectal, or focal lesions after conventional radiation (5500 cGy), or in some cases extensive surgical resection without radiotherapy, have a 50 to 60 percent 5 year progression-free survival rate. On the other hand, after similar doses of radiotherapy, children with diffuse intrinsic tumors rarely survive.

Radiotherapy does offer the best chance for transient disease control in children with diffuse, intrinsic tumors and improves symptoms in the majority of patients. Recently attempts have been made to increase the dose of radiotherapy by utilizing different radiotherapy delivery schedules. The greatest volume of experience has been with hyperfractionated radiation therapy, by which multiple doses of radiotherapy are given daily in smaller dose fractions. The rationale is based on theoretical evidence that such a scheduling regimen can increase the amount of radiotherapy tolerated by the normal brain without increasing life-threatening sequelae. More than 170 children have been treated on various hyperfractionated radiotherapy protocols with

Table 3 Risk Factors in Children with Brain Stem Gliomas

Variable	Average Risk	Poor Risk
Location	Midbrain, tectal, cervicomedullary	Pontine
Extent	Focal, dorsally exophytic	Diffuse, pons alone or pons plus
Histology	Low-grade (only if exophytic)	Anaplastic

total doses ranging between 6,400 and 7,200 cGy. Results, to date, have been mixed. There is a bias, which is difficult to confirm, that hyperfractionated radiotherapy is more likely to result in clinical improvement and objective tumor shrinkage. Regardless of response, however, the majority of patients die of their disease within 12 to 18 months of treatment. There is too little evidence to support routine use of hyperfractionated radiotherapy. The toxicity and efficacy of further dose escalations (as high as 7,800 cGy) are currently under study.

Chemotherapy has never been shown to be of benefit for children with brain stem gliomas; however, there is a need to define active agents so that more effective treatment approaches can be undertaken. One method is to use promising agents before giving radiotherapy, in an attempt to determine both response to these agents and whether they improve survival. A form of interferon, beta-interferon, has been shown to be effective in children with recurrent brain stem gliomas. We are presently co-ordinating a study utilizing interferon during and after hyperfractionated radiotherapy, in an attempt to determine the toxicity of this approach and its possible efficacy.

Low-Grade Gliomas

The management of low-grade glioma, the most common histologic subtype of childhood brain tumor, depends on the tumor's location and its degree of resectability. For cerebellar and cortical tumors amenable to gross surgical resection, extensive resection is the treatment of choice. Most centers now favor observation alone for patients who can be treated with total or nearly total resection. Management of subtotally resected low-grade gliomas remains controversial. There is some evidence that radiotherapy increases the duration and frequency of survival, but this has never been proven in a randomized treatment trial. It is my personal bias to recommend repeat resection for patients with subtotally resected tumors. When repeat resection is not feasible, radiotherapy is considered. At the present time there is an open nationwide treatment trial, co-ordinated by the Children's Cancer Group and the Pediatric Oncology Group, to evaluate the need for radiotherapy in children older than 5 years at diagnosis who have subtotally resected lesions; patients are being randomized to treatment with local radiotherapy or observation alone. All patients with totally resected tumors are being observed, and they receive no other form of treatment.

Treatment of children younger than 5 years with residual low-grade gliomas remains unsettled, especially for those with diencephalic masses. Children with neurofibromatosis should be distinguished from other children with low-grade tumors. With the wider utilization of screening studies for all children with neurofibromatosis at the time of diagnosis, a subgroup of patients is being identified who have apparent infiltrating masses in the optic nerve and visual pathway and who

are asymptomatic or have static symptoms. There is evidence to support observation of such patients until they exhibit radiographic or clinical evidence (including visual) of deterioration. Even with progressive disease, there seems to be little reason for surgical intervention. Once the tumor progresses, patients should be treated as any child with a low-grade glioma.

On the other hand, the vast majority of children without neurofibromatosis and infiltrating lesions present early in life with progressive neurologic or visual deterioration, or both. It is my bias that all such patients undergo biopsy and/or resection before treatment is instituted, to confirm the histologic subtype of the lesion, and in some cases to debulk it. Given the potential long-term harm of even local radiotherapy if the radiation portal is large enough, chemotherapy is an important option. In children younger than 5 years of age with progressive lesions there is evidence that chemotherapy can at least delay, if not obviate, radiotherapy. Actinomycin D and vincristine have been used in children with progressive visual pathway gliomas. This combination of drugs achieves objective tumor shrinkage in 20 percent of patients, but more importantly, it halts tumor progression in as many as 80 percent of cases. This allows radiotherapy to be delayed a median interval of 3 years after the date of diagnosis (and for some patients many more years). More recently, carboplatin has been shown to be effective as a single agent against recurrent low-grade glioma. For this reason, a treatment protocol is being performed at our institution and others that utilizes the combination of carboplatin and vincristine for children younger than 5 years who have progressive low-grade gliomas that are not amenable to surgical resection. The objective response rate (tumor shrinkage greater than 25 percent) has been greater than 50 percent for the first 55 children; this seems to be the best short-term result reported to date. It remains to be proven whether this type of approach will result in a greater likelihood of long-term disease control and an even greater delay in the need for radiotherapy than the actinomycin D plus vincristine regimen. Radiotherapy is the gold standard of treatment for children with partially resected or progressive low-grade gliomas, and chemotherapy should not yet be considered standard treatment or utilized unless there is a clear indication or goal.

Malignant Gliomas

Malignant gliomas outside the brain stem account for approximately 10 to 20 percent of all childhood brain tumors. Treatment remains highly problematic. There is evidence that patients with anaplastic gliomas who undergo a more extensive initial resection have a better prognosis. Focal radiotherapy remains the backbone of most treatment approaches; however, a randomized treatment trial has demonstrated that the addition of CCNU and vincristine as adjuncts to local radiotherapy improves the rate of disease-free survival in children with both anaplastic gliomas and glioblastoma multiforme. Overall, the 5 year, disease-free survival rate is as high as 40 percent for children with malignant gliomas after treatment with local radiotherapy (5,500 cGy) and adjuvant chemotherapy, which is considerably better than survival rates reported for adults with tumors of similar histologic type. The reason for these differences in survival are unclear, but it has been suggested that malignant gliomas in adults and children are biologically different.

The overall poor results for this tumor type and their sometimes apparently localized growth pattern has led to the utilization of focused radiation techniques such as implantation and radiosurgery. It is my bias that these types of approaches should be utilized only as part of a clinical trial. Also, given the tendency of these tumors to spread locally and, at least in childhood, to disseminate through the neuroaxis when they lie near the cerebrospinal fluid pathways, the utility of these approaches, when used in isolation, is dubious.

Ependymomas

Ependymomas are a difficult group of pediatric brain tumors to treat. Approximately two-thirds of pediatric ependymomas arise in the posterior fossa. Lesions in both the posterior fossa and the supratentorial space rarely disseminate throughout the neuroaxis early in the course of illness. It is currently our bias to recommend aggressive resection of ependymomas, regardless of their location in the neuroaxis. It is not clear whether histologic features are predictive of outcome.

The 5 year survival rate for children with totally resected ependymomas who then receive local radiotherapy was recently reported to be in the 60 to 70 percent range; however, children with subtotally resected tumors have a poorer prognosis (30 to 40 percent at 5 years). For this reason, even though the benefit of chemotherapy is not proven for this tumor, I recommend that children with totally resected tumors be treated more aggressively. Various different treatments are now being attempted, including hyperfractionated radiotherapy, preradiation chemotherapy, more aggressive postradiation adjuvant chemotherapy, and the combination of hyperfractionated radiation therapy with pre- or postradiation chemotherapy. Given the rarity of this lesion, these treatment approaches should be part of multicenter treatment trials.

Germ Cell Tumors

There is no consensus on how best to treat pediatric germ cell tumors. Although the majority of such lesions occur in the pineal region, approximately 20 to 30 percent arise in the suprasellar area. There are no reliable radiographic parameters that distinguish pineal germ cell tumors from other malignant lesions that can occur in the region. Cerebrospinal fluid markers (alpha-fetoprotein and human chorionic gonadotrophin [HCG]) are useful if elevated, as they are evidence of a mixed germ cell tumor. For tumors with negative marker studies, histologic confirmation is mandatory before therapy is instituted.

All patients with pineal malignancies should have cerebrospinal fluid markers sent for alpha-fetoprotein and HCG. If the markers are positive, treatment for a mixed germ cell tumor can begin. For nongerminomatous (or mixed) germ cell tumors, radiotherapy alone is usually ineffective, and I presently utilize preradiation chemotherapy with cisplatinum and etoposide, followed by craniospinal radiotherapy, supplemental local radiotherapy, and further postradiation chemotherapy.

Treatment for children with pineal germinomas is somewhat controversial. Although there is some evidence that preradiation chemotherapy can shrink tumors in these patients and that relatively focal (? whole ventricular; local) radiotherapy is sometimes effective, it is my bias to treat all such patients with craniospinal and supplemental local boost radiotherapy. Similar approaches are employed for children with suprasellar germinomas.

Craniopharyngiomas

Craniopharyngiomas are the most common sellar tumor of childhood. Management is unsettled, as there are proponents for two approaches, total resections and subtotal resection followed by local radiotherapy. Total resection (no residual lesion on the postoperative scan) results in better than 80 percent 5 year disease-free survival but also may produce significant intellectual and endocrine sequelae. A significant predisposing factor to sequelae is believed to be damage caused by attempts at total resection, as these tumors are often attached to the subfrontal or hypothalamic region. Less aggressive resection may cause less severe surgery-related sequelae, but subtotal resection alone infrequently controls disease. Subtotal resection and local radiotherapy (5,480 cGy) usually controls disease but exposes the developing brain to potentially damaging amounts of radiotherapy. Probably more than for any other childhood brain tumor, treatment of this lesion is left to the expertise and discretion of the neurosurgeon.

PERSPECTIVES FOR THE FUTURE

A great many biases (including my own) color the management of childhood brain tumors. These biases, and the relative rarity of the lesions, have hindered completion of well-designed clinical trials. The only way to truly make progress against the most common childhood brain tumors is to organize such trials. It is also incumbent on treating physicians to refer patients to centers that participate in these trials, both to maximize treatment for any individual patient and to alter the way these lesions will be treated in the future. At the same time, there is room for individualized institutional approaches, especially for the rarer tumors or lesions that carry an extremely poor prognosis. Pilot studies utilizing immunotherapy, new chemotherapy approaches, and alternative radiotherapy schedules and means to deliver radiotherapy are needed for tumors with poor prognosis.

Finally, the long-term cognitive and endocrine sequelae of the tumor and its treatment are significant. Sequential neurocognitive and endocrine follow-up are mandatory components of any brain tumor care program. Formalized educational intervention programs have only sporadically been used for brain tumor survivors and have the potential of improving their overall quality of life. The critical problem in the care of children with brain tumors is reaching a balance between the need to control the tumor's growth and means to improve the overall quality of life of survivors.

SUGGESTED READING

Duffner PK, Cohen ME. Treatment of brain tumors in babies and very young children. Pediatr Neurosci 1986; 12:304–310.

Edwards MSB, Wara WM, Urtasan RC, et al. Hyperfractionated radiotherapy for brainstem gliomas: A phase I-II trial. J Neurosurg 1989; 70:691–700.

Glauser TA, Packer RJ. Cognitive deficits in long term survivors of childhood tumors. Childs Nerv Syst 1991; 7:2–12.

Packer RJ. Chemotherapy for medulloblastoma/primitive neuroectodermal tumor (MB/PNET). Ann Neurol 1990; 28:823–828.

Packer RJ, Nicholson HS, Johnson DL, Vezina LG. Dilemmas in the management of childhood brain tumors: Brain stem gliomas. Pediatr Neurosurg 1992; 17:37–43.

Packer RJ, Sutton LN, Goldwein JW, et al. Outcome of children with medulloblastoma/primitive neuroectodermal tumor (MB/PNET) in the computer tomographic era: Improved survival with the use of adjuvant chemotherapy. J Neurosurg 1991; 74:433–440.

MALIGNANT NEURAL TUMORS

WILLIAM R. SHAPIRO, M.D.

Neoplasms frequently affect the nervous system. Primary tumors of the central nervous system (CNS) are the second most common cancer of children and in adults are more common than systemic Hodgkin's disease. In the United States there are approximately 15,000 new cases of primary CNS cancer each year, representing about 2 percent of the cancer "problem." Of these, more than half are gliomas, the majority astrocytomas. Astrocytomas may be generally classified according to their malignant behavior as low-grade astrocytoma (the slowest growing), anaplastic astrocytoma, and the most malignant, glioblastoma multiforme. Recent epidemiologic data suggest that the incidence of malignant gliomas in elders is increasing. In this chapter I concentrate on the treatment of malignant gliomas and conclude with a comment about low-grade gliomas.

Patients with malignant glioma are usually referred to neurosurgeons and neurologists because of seizures, headache of acute onset, or changes in behavior or personality. The diagnosis of malignant glioma is suggested by computed tomography (CT) or magnetic resonance imaging (MRI) demonstrating a mass lesion that usually, but not always, enhances after administration of a contrast agent. Initial therapy is almost always operative. Traditionally, the radiation therapist has then been responsible for the remaining therapy. In recent years, however, many patients with malignant brain tumors have been offered chemotherapy, and the advent of chemical treatment has added to recent developments in cellular and genetic molecular biology to foster a new scientific interest in brain tumors. Research has been aided by new imaging techniques, including positron emission tomography (PET). To these diagnostic techniques have been added new therapeutic methods such as stereotactic laser surgery and interstitial radiotherapy.

Like the approach to systemic cancer, the treatment of supratentorial malignant astrocytomas is cytoreduction through multimodality therapy, including surgery, radiation therapy, and chemotherapy.

SURGERY

The role of surgical resection in the treatment of malignant gliomas remains controversial, even after 75 years' experience. There is general agreement that only surgery allows a histologic diagnosis to be established during the patient's life. However, some physicians feel that current methods of radiologic diagnosis, including CT and MRI, permit diagnosis of malignant brain tumor without the necessity for operation, thus avoiding the risks of surgery. Such a view denies a role for surgery as "cancer" therapy. There is evidence that surgical reduction of tumor to very small residual amounts can prolong

Table 1 Functional Status in Patients Undergoing Resection for Malignant Glioma*

| | Preoperative Functional Areas Evaluated | Postoperative Status | |
		Improved or Unchanged	Worse
Study 1: 82 patients			
Abnormal	191	151	40
Normal	180	125	55
Study 2: 200 patients			
Abnormal	207	174	33
Normal	661	610	51

*The two studies were performed at Memorial Sloan-Kettering Cancer Center in New York. Functional areas were not identical in both studies, but represented evaluations of speech, personality, and visual, sensory, or motor function. Overall, patients were either better or unchanged by surgery, not made worse.

survival and permit the patient to return to an active life for a year or longer. In one of our Brain Tumor Cooperative Group (BTCG) studies, CT scans from brain tumor patients were studied at several times in their course and compared to the ultimate outcome for respective patients. There was no significant relationship between preoperative tumor size and prognosis, but there was a significant relationship between postoperative tumor size and outcome: a smaller residual tumor was associated with longer survival. This was especially noticeable for patients whose lesion showed minimal or no residual enhancement. When the difference between preoperative and postoperative tumor size was evaluated, there was no significant relationship between percentage of tumor removed and survival, although a trend toward longer survival was seen among patients whose tumor was shrunk by 75 percent or more.

These results support surgical removal of the largest possible volume of tumor that safe operation allows and offer little justification for performing only biopsy or limited resection of accessible tumors. If the surgeon confines his resection to the tumor itself, he rarely induces a major new neurologic defect. In two studies of this subject, patients were examined preoperatively and postoperatively for evidence of abnormalities of speech, personality, or visual, sensory, or motor function (Table 1). Overall, patients were helped rather than hurt by the surgical procedure. Indeed, patients who undergo tumor resection are frequently able to return to a full, active life without needing large doses of corticosteroid hormones to ameliorate incapacitating symptoms.

RADIATION THERAPY

The proper portals and doses of radiation therapy for the treatment of brain tumor have changed with the advent of better imaging techniques. The Brain Tumor Study Group (BTSG) reported in controlled studies that whole-brain radiation therapy increased survival time for patients over that after surgery alone and that patients who received 5,500 to 6,000 cGy lived significantly longer than those who received 5,000 cGy or less. In our BTCG CT study, patients whose tumors did not enhance after radiation therapy had longer survival than those with residual tumor. Patients whose tumor shrank more than 50 percent survived longer than those whose tumors shrank less or increased in size. Other BTCG studies demonstrated that neither increased fractionation of radiotherapy (twice daily) nor addition of the radiosensitizer misonidazole conferred any survival advantage over the conventional postoperative use of whole-brain radiotherapy and bis-choroethylnitrosourea (BCNU, carmustine).

Radiation damages normal brain tissue, and patients who receive whole-brain irradiation often develop cognitive deficits within 2 to 3 years. Such damage may be made worse by associated chemotherapy. Because BTCG studies indicate that partial whole-brain, partial coned-down irradiation was as effective as entirely whole-brain radiation therapy for malignant glioma, most patients now receive their radiation through portals that encompass the tumor mass and spare as much normal brain tissue as possible. This method requires accurate radiation dosimetry based on CT or MRI findings. Even if radiation therapy is only palliative, every effort should be made to spare uninvolved brain tissue from radiation.

Among the newer techniques of radiotherapy is interstitial implantation of radioactive seeds. Prolonged survival has been reported in patients with recurrent malignant gliomas treated with temporarily implanted iodine-125 sources, but patient selection clearly influences such results. The BTCG is currently conducting phase III trial 8701, which randomizes newly diagnosed patients to receive (1) postoperative temporary ^{125}I seed implantation in the residual tumor bed followed by standard external beam radiotherapy plus intravenous carmustine (IV BCNU) or (2) external radiotherapy plus BCNU with seed implantation. The trial tests the value of adding interstitial radiation to the previously best available therapy regimen.

Another technique utilizes radiosensitizers, chemicals that sensitize the tumor cells to radiotherapy. These appear to be especially valuable in hypoxic tumor regions, because radiation therapy is not as effective in the absence of oxygen. One of these, misonidazole, was tested in a number of studies of the treatment of malignant glioma, but in a BTCG study it was not found to enhance the radiation effect. In the same study, hyperfractionation, (i.e., more than one dose per day) was no more effective than once daily fraction, although a number of hyperfractionation regimens are under active investigation.

CHEMOTHERAPY

Chemotherapy completes the technique of multimodality treatment of malignant gliomas. A number of

Table 2 Chemotherapeutic Agents for Malignant Gliomas

Drug	Usual Dose for Single Drug Administration	Route	Toxicity
BCNU	80 mg/m^2 per day for 3 consecutive days; repeat q6–8 wk	IV	Delayed (3 weeks); thrombocytopenia, leukopenia, abnormal liver function tests
CCNU	130 mg/m^2 q6–8wk	PO	As for BCNU
Procarbazine	150 mg/m^2 daily for 28 days; repeat after 28-day rest	PO	Leukopenia beginning in 3 to 4 weeks, rash (rarely)
Combination procarbazine, CCNU, and vincristine (PCV) chemotherapy repeated every 6–8 weeks:			
CCNU	110 mg/m^2 on day 1	PO	See above
Procarbazine	60 mg/m^2 daily on days 8–21	PO	See above
Vincristine	1.4 mg/m^2 on days 8 and 29	IV	Peripheral neuropathy

chemotherapeutic agents have been used, and several are listed in Table 2. In 1983, the BTSG reported that surgery plus radiation therapy and chemotherapy with BCNU (carmustine) significantly extended the survival of patients with malignant glioma as compared to surgery plus radiation therapy without chemotherapy. Patients treated with all three modalities had a median survival time of a year, whereas those with surgery plus radiation survived a median interval of 10 months. The 18 month survivorship was 2.5 times greater among the patients who received carmustine than among those who did not receive chemotherapy. Procarbazine, oral lomustine (CCNU), and streptozotocin are about equally effective as BCNU.

A recently reported BTCG trial indicated that intra-arterial (IA) BCNU was no more effective than IV BCNU and was much more toxic to the brain. Almost 10 percent of patients treated with IA BCNU developed irreversible encephalopathy and CT evidence of cerebral edema, and 26 other patients developed vision loss ipsilateral to the infused carotid artery. Neuropathologically, IA BCNU produced white matter necrosis. Trials of IA cisplatin continue, as this drug produces much less encephalopathy than BCNU when administered IA.

The new BTCG chemotherapy phase III trial 8901 randomizes newly diagnosed patients and those previously diagnosed but not treated with chemotherapy to receive standard IV BCNU, combination IV BCNU plus IA cisplatin, or new chemotherapeutic agents.

PROGNOSTIC VARIABLES

A major consideration in the therapy of this disease is that certain prognostic variables influence survival, often more than therapy does. For example, patients younger than 45 years of age live three times longer than patients older than 65 years, regardless of therapy. Other important prognostic indicators included personality change (which, when present, is associated with earlier death), duration of symptoms (i.e., patients whose symptoms were present longer than 6 months before

operation lived twice as long as those whose symptoms were present under 4 months), and postoperative performance status. The performance status, based on a modification of a scale originally proposed by Karnofsky, semiquantifies the ability of the patient to handle normal living circumstances. The Karnofsky scale is measured in decades, from zero to 100. Generally, patients who are able to work have Karnofsky ratings of 80, 90, or 100; those whose symptoms prevent them from working but who otherwise can take care of themselves have Karnofsky ratings between 50 and 70; and patients who are clinically ill with their disease have Karnofsky ratings of 40 and below. Patients whose postoperative Karnofsky scale is between 70 and 100 live substantially longer than those whose scale is less than 50. The most important prognostic variable is the histopathologic category: patients with glioblastoma multiforme fare much worse than those with anaplastic astrocytoma.

RECOMMENDATIONS

In 1970, the median survival time for patients with malignant glioma who were treated with available surgical techniques and undefined radiation therapy was approximately 6 months. Prospective clinical trials using vigorous multimodality therapy have demonstrated that median survival time can be extended to a year or more, and 25 to 30 percent of patients survive 18 months or longer. In my view, newly diagnosed patients should be referred to a center where clinical trials are performed or should become involved through direct participation of the patient's physician in one of the several outreach programs associated with research centers. For patients who cannot participate in clinical trials the data make it possible to present up to date guidelines for care. Management of malignant glioma should be based on the rationale of cytoreduction through multimodality therapy, including surgery, irradiation, and chemotherapy. Surgical resection of as much tumor as is neurologically safe should be the first step. After surgery, patients should receive radiation therapy to a full tumor dose of

6000 cGy. Chemotherapy should be administered, but its toxicity requires physicians inexperienced in its use to seek the assistance of a medical oncologist. There is no clear-cut choice among a number of agents. Table 2 lists the standard agents, their dosage, and toxicities.

TREATMENT OF LOW-GRADE GLIOMAS

Although at the time of presentation malignant gliomas are often so large as to require immediate therapeutic intervention if the patient is not to deteriorate rapidly, low-grade gliomas (astrocytoma, oligodendroglioma, mixed astro-oligodendroglioma) may present only with a seizure and rarely produce permanent neurologic signs. The advent of CT and MRI has made it far easier to find such lesions, though with earlier diagnosis have come unresolved questions about therapy. Among the most immediate are those related to when and how aggressively patients with low-grade glioma should be treated. The standard dogma of cancer therapy is that early treatment is better treatment. Applying this philosophy to low-grade gliomas would mean that earlier diagnosis should require early and vigorous therapy, although a number of studies question whether early therapy, especially radiation, produces benefit or only brain damage.

The available evidence based on uncontrolled, mostly retrospective, reviews, supports these inferences: Deferring therapy may be associated with a stable clinical course lasting years. Intervention is eventually necessitated by progression of the disease. Deferring intervention does not appear to influence either the incidence or the interval to malignant transformation. The natural history of such tumors may not be significantly affected by the timing of therapeutic intervention.

Since only controlled studies can provide definitive answers, the question remains: Given the initial finding on CT or MRI, are patients with low-grade gliomas better treated immediately, or can they wait until the lesion progresses? I favor immediate biopsy and surgical resection if the tumor is favorably located. For the timing of radiotherapy, I would like to see patients entered into investigative protocols designed to answer questions by testing early versus delayed radiation therapy. The BTCG is currently performing such a study. When radiotherapy is administered, the portal should be confined to the tumor, as delimited by the T2-weighted signal on MRI, and no more than 5,500 cGy should be administered. Chemotherapy should be reserved for recurrence.

SUGGESTED READING

Deutsch M, Green SB, Strike TA, et al. Results of a randomized trial comparing BCNU plus radiotherapy, streptozotocin plus radiotherapy, BCNU plus hyperfractionated radiotherapy, and BCNU following misonidazole plus radiotherapy in the postoperative treatment of malignant glioma. Int J Radiat Oncol Biol Phys 1989; 16:1389–1396.

Recht LD, Lew R, Smith TW: Suspected low-grade glioma: Is deferring treatment safe? Ann Neurol 1992; 31:431–436.

Shapiro WR, Green GB, Burger PC, et al. Randomized trial of three chemotherapy regimens and two radiotherapy regimens in postoperative treatment of malignant glioma: Brain Tumor Cooperative Group Trial 8001. J Neurosurg 1989; 71:1–9.

Shapiro WR, Green SB, Burger PC, et al. A randomized comparison of intraarterial (IA) versus intravenous (IV) BCNU, without or with IV 5-fluorouracil (5-FU) for newly diagnosed patients with malignant glioma. J Neurosurg 1992; 76:772–781.

PATIENT RESOURCES

American Brain Tumor Association
3725 North Talman Ave.
Chicago, Illinois 60618

The Brain Research Fund Foundation of London
111 Waterloo St., Suite 600
London, Ontario N6B 2M4
Canada

Brain Tumor Foundation for Children, Inc.
Suite 9 - 2231 Perimeter Park Dr.
Atlanta, Georgia 30341

The Brain Tumor Society
258 Harvard St., Suite 308
Brookline, Massachusetts 02146

The Children's Brain Tumor Foundation, Inc.
35 Alpine Lane
Chappaqua, New York 10514

The Preuss Foundation
201 Lomas Santa Fe Drive, Suite 340
Solana Beach, California 92075

The Rainbow Foundation for Brain Tumor Research, Inc.
Box 327
Highland Mills, New York 10930

National Brain Tumor Foundation
Suite 510
323 Geary St.San Francisco, California 94102

National Cancer Institute
Building 31, Room 10A18
Bethesda, Maryland 20892

METASTATIC CANCER TO THE BRAIN AND SPINAL CORD

GLENN J. LESSER, M.D.
STUART A. GROSSMAN, M.D.

Metastatic spread of malignancies to the central nervous system (CNS) is common in clinical practice and is an important cause of morbidity and mortality in patients with cancer. Early diagnosis and therapy of these metastases can result in preservation of neurologic function and can dramatically affect the quality and duration of life. Recent advances in neuroimaging and antineoplastic therapy provide new opportunities for clinicians to diagnose and treat brain and spinal cord metastases earlier and with better results.

BRAIN METASTASES

Clinical and autopsy studies suggest that 15 percent of all patients with cancer develop symptomatic intraparenchymal brain metastases and an additional 10 percent harbor asymptomatic brain metastases. More than 100,000 patients in the United States develop brain metastases every year. This far exceeds the incidence of primary malignancies of the CNS, which was expected to be 17,000 in 1992. Approximately 50 percent of all brain metastases arise from primary lung cancers, 20 percent are from breast cancers, 8 percent from gastrointestinal malignancies, and 6 percent from genitourinary tumors or melanomas. These five tumor sites account for nearly 85 percent of all brain metastases. Brain metastases are found at autopsy in approximately 21 percent of patients who die of lung cancer, 10 percent of those who die of breast cancer, and 40 percent of those who succumb to melanoma. About half these patients have single intracranial metastases; the rest have multiple lesions.

Intraparenchymal brain metastases generally arise as arterial microemboli from a primary tumor or metastatic focus in the lungs. These micrometastases travel distally through the cerebral arterial circulation as far as their size permits, frequently lodging at the junction of the gray and white matter in the cerebral cortex. The distribution of brain metastases parallels the relative weight and arterial supply of the various portions of the brain. Eighty percent of all metastases occur in the cerebral hemispheres, 17 percent in the cerebellum, and 3 percent in the basal ganglia and brain stem.

Patients with brain metastases usually present with signs and symptoms that result from increased intracranial pressure or local effects of the tumor and adjacent peritumor edema. Patients characteristically relate a history of days to weeks of headache followed by progressive focal neurologic signs and symptoms. The headache may be mild, nonspecific, and without the classic early morning component characteristic of increased intracranial pressure. The most common focal neurologic findings are hemiparesis and cognitive or behavioral abnormalities. Ten percent of patients present with seizures, and a smaller fraction are first seen for diffuse encephalopathy, ataxia, cranial nerve palsies, sensory loss, acute intratumor hemorrhage, or coma.

The best diagnostic tests for brain metastases are computed tomography (CT) and magnetic resonance imaging (MRI). CT, with or without intravenous contrast medium, is less costly than a comparable MR study and usually provides similar information. The greater sensitivity of MRI may be required in specific situations. Brain metastases are most commonly seen at the gray-white junction as spherical, hypodense lesions that enhance brightly following contrast administration and are surrounded by a region of edema. The tumor plus peritumoral edema may result in considerable mass effect. Although brain metastases have a relatively characteristic appearance on CT or MRI, a recent study of patients with known malignancies who were thought to have solitary brain metastases demonstrated that for 10 to 15 percent an alternate diagnosis was established after stereotactic biopsy.

The systemic evaluation of patients who present with an intraparenchymal brain lesion without a history of malignancy can often be quite abbreviated. A careful history and physical examination coupled with a chest radiograph or CT or MRI of the lungs with a few images of the liver provides most of the required data. More than 60 percent of patients with brain metastases have an abnormal chest radiograph, and the number who have abnormal chest CT or MRI findings is even larger. This occurs because 50 percent of all brain metastases arise from primary lung cancers and because most other systemic malignancies metastasize to the lungs before spreading to the brain. If these studies are not diagnostic, it is unlikely that additional screening procedures will be productive, and biopsy of the intracranial lesion is likely to be necessary to establish a diagnosis.

The development of symptomatic brain metastases is a poor prognostic sign. The median survival time for patients who do not receive specific therapy for these lesions is only 1 month, and death usually results from progressive neurologic deterioration.

Radiation, surgery, and chemotherapy all may play a role in the appropriate treatment of metastatic disease to the brain. Therapeutic decisions must take into account the patient's age and performance status, the extent and histologic type of the systemic tumor, and the potential treatment available for the primary malignancy. In addition, the number, location, and operability of brain metastases also influences treatment plans.

Brain metastases are associated with a proliferation of new blood vessels that lack tight junctions and other physiologic functions characteristic of an intact blood-brain barrier. As a result, intravenous contrast medium extravasates into the tumor and is visible on CT or MRI. These leaky vessels also allow proteins to diffuse into the tumor, which results in accumulation of peritumoral edema. Glucocorticoids partially restore the integrity of the blood-brain barrier within the tumor and reduce peritumoral vasogenic edema beginning 6 to 24 hours after their administration. Maximal steroid effect occurs within 3 to 7 days. The reduction of edema is often accompanied by substantial clinical improvement, and survival for patients treated with glucocorticoids is extended to a median time of 2 months. Although the optimal doses of glucocorticoid are not well-defined, dexamethasone is the preferred drug. A bolus of 20 mg, followed by 16 mg daily, usually suffices for stable patients, whereas doses as large as 100 mg daily may be preferred for those who are critically ill.

Radiation therapy is also beneficial in the treatment of brain metastases. The median survival time for patients treated with cranial radiation is extended to 3 to 6 months, and survival at 1 year is approximately 16 percent. Although most patients experience neurologic improvement with steroids and radiation, local recurrences are common and more than half die of progressive CNS disease. Limited survival is due in part to inadequate local therapy but is even more reflective of the overall status of the patients who develop brain metastases. These patients frequently have extensive systemic tumor that is refractory to therapy, poor performance status, multiple intracranial lesions, and a variety of other serious medical problems.

In the 1970s, several large, randomized, prospective clinical trials were designed to evaluate the optimal treatment schedule and dose of external-beam radiation for brain metastases. A short and intensive course of radiation (30 Gy in 2 weeks) was found to be as effective as the more standard 40 Gy in 4 weeks or the other experimental arms. Seventy-five to eighty percent of those treated improved or had a stable neurologic status for the remainder of their lives. Overall, median survival was 18 weeks, and ambulatory patients survived a median of 21 weeks. Nonambulatory patients survived 12 weeks. Brain metastases were responsible for death in about half the patients in these studies. In a more favorable subset of patients, a subsequent randomized study demonstrated that 30 Gy in 2 weeks was as effective as 50 Gy in 4 weeks. Median survival time in this study was 18 weeks.

These studies have resulted in acceptance of 30 Gy in 10 fractions as standard therapy for metastatic disease. Current data from unselected patients suggest that the median time to neurologic progression after radiation is 14 weeks, survival rate at 1 year is approximately 10 to 20 percent, and 30 to 50 percent of patients succumb to uncontrolled intracranial metastases. Large co-operative group trials and smaller, recent studies have identified a subgroup of patients whose median survival is about 30 weeks. These patients are under age 60 years and have Karnofsky performance scores greater than 70 percent, no other sites of metastatic disease, and a well-controlled primary tumor.

Cranial radiation is potentially toxic to the CNS.

Treatment-induced blood-brain barrier dysfunction may require increased doses of steroids to control peritumoral edema for months following the completion of radiation therapy. Transient somnolence and lethargy can also follow cranial radiation. Of more concern is the development of treatment-related leukoencephalopathy. This occurs months to years after therapy and is most common after large fractional doses and large total doses of radiation to large volumes of brain. Clinically, this disorder presents as a progressive and irreversible demyelinating disorder characterized by dementia, abnormal gait, loss of motor skills, and bowel and bladder incontinence. Striking white matter abnormalities are evident on neuroimaging studies. Patients may live months to years with this slowly progressive and fatal demyelinating disease.

In view of the available information on the efficacy and toxicity of cranial radiation, patients expected to survive only a few months should probably receive the short-duration, large–fractional dose radiation (30 Gy in 2 weeks). Their treatment will be completed rapidly and their limited life expectancy makes it unlikely that they will survive to develop the serious long-term neurotoxicity of radiation therapy. Patients with intracranial metastases who may survive a year or longer should receive smaller daily fractions (180 to 200 cGy), in order to decrease the incidence of disabling or fatal late sequelae of therapy.

Multiple, single-institution studies have suggested that surgical resection of solitary brain metastases can result in clinical improvement and prolonged survival; however, these studies have generally selected patients who have multiple favorable prognostic factors and have compared their results to those of historical controls. The inconsistent use of postoperative radiation therapy confounds the issue further. In a recent prospective trial, patients with a surgically accessible lesion and a Karnofsky performance score of 70 percent or better were randomized to undergo surgery and postoperative radiation or needle biopsy followed by radiation. Both groups received identical radiation therapy, consisting of 36 Gy of whole-brain radiation in 12 fractions. Operative morbidity was 8 percent and operative mortality 4 percent. The median survival time for patients who received the surgery followed by radiation therapy was significantly longer than that for those who received only the radiation (40 versus 15 weeks). The surgically treated patients remained functionally independent longer (38 versus 8 weeks) and had fewer local recurrences (20 versus 52 percent).

Unfortunately, surgery is a reasonable option for only a quarter of patients with brain metastases. Fifty percent of patients have multiple intracranial lesions, and fewer than half of the remaining ones have surgically accessible lesions and controlled systemic disease (or none). Ideally, surgical candidates should also have an excellent presurgical performance status and a long interval between the development of the primary tumor and the intracranial lesion. This further selects patients who are unlikely to develop new intracranial or systemic metastases immediately following resection of their brain metastases.

Patients with non–small cell carcinoma of the lung and single brain metastases represent a common, more favorable subgroup of patients. Median survival time after surgical removal of these metastases and radiation therapy is longer than after radiation alone (19 versus 9 months). In selected series, when solitary intracranial metastases and the primary pulmonary lesions are both completely resected, the survival rate at 5 years is reported to be as high as 21 to 45 percent.

The role of chemotherapy in the treatment of brain metastases has been very limited; however, the blood-brain barrier is disrupted in these lesions, as evidenced by the contrast enhancement seen on CT or MR. This suggests that water-soluble chemotherapeutic agents should be able to enter the tumor much as contrast agents do. There are well-documented reports of intra-cranial metastases from chemotherapy-sensitive tumors (breast cancer, small cell lung cancer, germ cell malig-nancies) that respond to systemic administration of che-motherapy. This therapeutic option should be consid-ered when other therapeutic modalities are exhausted. Chemotherapeutic agents most likely to be effective against the tumor should be chosen in preference to those that can penetrate an intact blood-brain barrier.

Studies documenting improvement in the quality and duration of life following surgical extirpation of solitary brain metastases have led other investigators to study new approaches to the management of these tumors. Radiotherapists now routinely consider larger doses of local radiation for patients with solitary brain metastases who are otherwise excellent candidates for more aggressive therapy. Whole-brain radiotherapy, followed by additional external beam radiation to the smaller tumor-containing region, represents another way to improve local control. Implantation directly into the metastatic lesions of radioactive seeds is an alterna-tive way of providing additional local radiation therapy. Local radionecrosis is a recognized complication of this approach that can be minimized by careful treatment planning. Stereotactic radiosurgery represents another emerging therapeutic technique that is designed to provide very large single doses of ionizing radiation to a small spherical intracranial lesion. This technique min-imizes radiation exposure of normal surrounding brain tissue. Rapid changes in computer and radiation tech-nology are making this technique widely available throughout the United States. Preliminary studies dem-onstrate the feasibility of achieving local control in more than 70 percent of patients with brain metastases of different histologic types. It is also technically possible to administer radiosurgery in multiple dose fractions, and to more than one lesion in the brain. This technique may be used on solitary metastases that are surgically inaccessible.

Future studies are needed to compare the efficacy and toxicity of radiosurgery and surgery in patients with intracranial metastases. Surgery will remain the treat-ment of choice when there is (1) urgent need for decompression or (2) an obstruction to cerebrospinal fluid flow. It is also valuable for acute therapy of intratumoral hemorrhage. In addition, a stereotactic or conventional neurosurgical procedure is required when the cause of CNS lesions is in doubt. Improvements in neurosurgery and anesthesiology have made these pro-cedures quite safe and more available to patients with intracranial malignancies.

INTRASPINAL METASTASES

Intramedullary spinal cord metastases are observed in fewer than 2 percent of cancer patients studied at autopsy. Clinically, they are recognized even less fre-quently. Approximately half of all reported cases are associated with lung cancer. Intramedullary metastases have also been described with breast cancer, lymphoma, colorectal tumors, head and neck cancers, and mela-noma. Despite its rarity, the diagnosis of intramedullary spinal metastases must be considered in the differential diagnosis of most cancer patients who have signs or symptoms of a lower motor neuron lesion or back pain.

In patients with intramedullary spinal metastases the initial neurologic examination almost always dem-onstrates weakness or paralysis. More than 60 percent of patients have a sensory deficit, most commonly a sensory level. Pain, either localized or radicular, is a common early complaint. Most patients progress to flaccid paralysis with a sensory level within 4 weeks of initial presentation. These patients usually have widespread metastases from their systemic malignancy. Liver, lung, and bone metastases are common, as are intraparenchy-mal brain or leptomeningeal metastases. As a result, the prognosis for patients with intramedullary spinal me-tastases is poor. Median survival time is reported to be about 4 weeks, and only 10 percent survive 6 months.

The differential diagnosis of spinal cord disease in cancer patients is extensive. Epidural metastases and neoplastic meningitis are the most common neoplastic disorders that involve the spinal cord, but other real possibilities in some patients include radiation myelop-athy, vascular disorders, paraneoplastic syndromes, and primary intramedullary tumor. A careful history, physi-cal examination, and appropriate imaging studies usually provide the correct diagnosis. It should be noted that severe pain preceding neurologic dysfunction is more typical of epidural cord compression than of intra-medullary metastasis. MRI, with and without con-trast enhancement, is the most sensitive and specific radiographic study for intramedullary metastases. T1-weighted images reveal a hypointense tumor that may enhance with contrast, whereas T2-weighted images demarcate the extent of the tumor and surrounding edema. Myelography demonstrates fusiform expansion of the cord in only 30 percent of patients, plain spine radiographs are uninformative, and lumbar puncture may reveal an elevated cerebrospinal fluid protein value if the flow of spinal fluid is impaired.

Most intramedullary spinal metastases are diagnosed and treated when the spinal cord has suffered irreversible damage. As a result, a minority of patients improve in response to surgery, radiation therapy, or steroids. Early diagnosis and treatment are critical to the preservation of neurologic function. Patients with good performance status and limited systemic disease should be treated aggressively for this debilitating complication of cancer.

SUGGESTED READING

Borgelt B, Gelber R, Kramer S, et al. The palliation of brain metastases: Final results of the first two studies by the radiation therapy oncology group. Int J Radiation Oncol Biol Phys 1980; 6:1–9.

Grem JL, Burgess J, Trump DL. Clinical features and natural history of intramedullary spinal cord metastasis. Cancer 1985; 56: 2305–2314.

Patchell RA, Tibbs PA, Walsh JW, et al. A randomized trial of surgery in the treatment of single metastases to the brain. N Engl J Med 1990; 322:494–500.

Siegers HP. Chemotherapy for brain metastases: Recent developments and clinical considerations. Cancer Treat Rev 1990; 17:63–76.

CARCINOMATOUS MENINGITIS AND ACUTE CORD COMPRESSION BY TUMOR

ALEXANDRA FLOWERS, M.D.
W.K. ALFRED YUNG, M.D.

About 5 to 10 percent of patients with systemic cancers also have disease metastatic to the spine, which often causes severe neurologic deficits. The cancers that most often metastasize to the spine are breast carcinoma, lung carcinoma, prostate carcinoma, and lymphoma. Moreover, as cancer survival rates improve, metastases from melanoma, renal cell carcinoma, and ovarian or colon cancers are increasingly frequent.

The metastatic deposits can form mass lesions that compress the spinal cord or the nerve roots, or they may seed the leptomeninges. The symptoms and signs vary, depending on the site of involvement and the location of the lesion (epidural, intradural, leptomeningeal). Management of metastatic disease to the spine seeks to provide symptomatic relief, decompression, stabilization of the spine, and specific therapy for the tumor. We address all these issues separately for epidural, intradural, and leptomeningeal metastases.

EPIDURAL METASTASES

Epidural metastasis is the most common form of metastatic disease to the spine. In the majority of cases, the clinical presentation is acute spinal cord compression.

Epidural metastases have three major pathogenic mechanisms. The prevalence of hematogenous spread through the paraspinal venous plexus (Batson's) to the vertebral body, and subsequent extension into the epidural space is 85 percent. In another 10 percent of cases, often in patients with non-Hodgkin's lymphoma, the tumor extends through the epidural foramen from a paraspinal mass. The metastatic deposits of leukemias may involve the epidural space directly. The thoracic spine is the most common site of metastasis for epidural spinal cord compression, followed by the cervical and the lumbar spine. The symptoms of spinal cord compression are pain, paraparesis or quadriparesis, sensory loss, and bowel and bladder dysfunction. Progression to paraplegia can be very rapid, occurring over 24 to 48 hours; therefore, in many patients spinal cord compression represents a neurologic emergency. Bilateral radiating back pain, changes in bowel habit (constipation), and paresthesias all suggest possible impending spinal cord compression and warrant immediate neurologic evaluation. The pain is exacerbated by coughing, sneezing, straining, neck flexion, straight leg raising, or Valsalva's maneuver. Motor weakness may vary from monoparesis, to asymmetric paraparesis or quadriparesis, to paraplegia. The pattern is often determined by the site of the tumor mass. Sensory findings help localize the spinal level of involvement. The sensory level may not correspond to the exact site of the tumor but usually falls within two or three vertebral levels. Also, extension of the tumor within the epidural space at several levels may cause asymmetric sensory findings. In cauda equina or conus medullaris syndrome, the sensory loss has a typical "saddle" distribution. When the tumor causes compression of the dorsal columns, the only sensory findings may be loss of vibration and proprioception.

Useful radiodiagnostic studies include radiography of the spine, myelography with computed tomography (CT) follow-up, and, most recently, magnetic resonance imaging (MRI) with gadolinium enhancement. Spine radiographs can demonstrate the presence of lytic or blastic metastatic lesions, vertebral body collapse, or a paraspinal soft tissue mass. Bone scan is more sensitive but less specific for bone metastases. Until high-quality MRI became available, myelography was the gold standard for the diagnosis of epidural masses and spinal cord compression. Myelography also has the advantage of providing cerebrospinal fluid (CSF) for cytologic studies to rule out leptomeningeal metastases. Because it is not invasive, gadolinium-enhanced MRI is rapidly replacing the myelogram.

There are still controversies about the therapy of spinal cord compression by epidural metastases: high-dose versus conventional doses of steroids, the relative merits of surgical decompression and radiation therapy, and the role of chemotherapy. Compression of the spinal cord by the epidural mass obstructs the epidural venous plexuses and causes vasogenic edema. Steroids are the first-line therapy to decrease the edema, reduce the pain, and improve the neurologic deficit. The conventional dose of dexamethasone, a 10 mg intravenous bolus followed by 4 mg every 6 hours, has the same efficacy as the high-dose bolus of 100 mg but fewer side effects. Glycerol was also shown to have a beneficial effect in reducing edema, but its use is still limited. Other substances that have these effects (ketamine, MK-801, indomethacin, Ketanserin) are used only in animal experiments and are not approved for human use.

Decompression of the spinal cord can be achieved through surgical resection, radiation therapy, or a combination of the two. Surgery as the primary modality is indicated when the histologic diagnosis is unknown, the tumor mass is limited, the patient previously underwent radiation therapy to the spine at the same level, or the tumor is "radioresistant." Laminectomy offered no advantage over radiation therapy for treatment of epidural cord compression from radiosensitive tumors. Anterior vertebral body resection with spine stabilization has the advantage of both decompressing the cord and removing the diseased vertebral body. Presurgical embolization can be considered in hypervascular tumors such as renal cell carcinoma.

Radiation therapy is considered the treatment of choice for epidural spinal cord compression. It provides relief of pain and reduces the tumor mass. The dose of radiation depends on the tumor type and ranges from 2,000 to 4,000 cGy. Good results have also been reported with laminectomy followed by radiation therapy. Similar dilemmas arise in the treatment of children with spinal cord compression from metastatic lesions. Surgical decompression followed by radiation therapy or chemotherapy resulted in a better neurologic outcome than either modality alone.

The prognosis in epidural cord compression depends principally on the patient's neurologic status. Ambulatory patients usually have a good functional recovery, whereas paraplegic patients have a poor prognosis.

INTRADURAL METASTASES

Intradural metastasis is less common than epidural metastasis. Metastatic spread in the intradural space occurs by the hematogenous route, by extension along nerve roots from a paravertebral mass, by direct extension from an epidural lesion, or by leptomeningeal seeding. Intradural extramedullary metastasis has clinical manifestations similar to those of epidural spinal cord compression. The main symptoms are localized pain, sphincter dysfunction, and weakness. The diagnosis is based on the clinical findings, especially a definite sensory level; the common association with brain metastases; a positive CSF cytologic examination; and the presence of the metastatic lesion on MRI. Findings of spine radiography are often negative. The progression is more rapid than with epidural disease. Surgical decompression is less successful than for epidural metastases; intradural extramedullary metastasis is, therefore, best treated with radiation therapy and/or chemotherapy.

Intradural intramedullary metastasis is very uncommon: prevalence is about 3 percent for patients with metastatic spinal cord compression. The tumors that cause intramedullary metastases are lung cancer (50 percent), breast cancer (14.5 percent), lymphoma, colon cancer, renal cell carcinoma, head and neck cancers, and melanoma. The presenting symptoms include pain, asymmetric weakness, paresthesia, sphincter dysfunction, and Brown-Sequard syndrome. MRI with gadolinium contrast is the only reliable diagnostic study for intramedullary metastases; myelography can be normal or nonspecific and is diagnostic in only some 35 percent of cases. When positive, the myelogram shows fusiform enlargement of the cord extending over several segments. Differential diagnosis must include epidural spinal cord compression, primary intramedullary tumors, transverse myelitis, radiation myelopathy, and paraneoplastic necrotizing myelopathy.

Radiation therapy and steroids are the best treatment modalities for intradural metastases. Systemic chemotherapy can also be considered. Treatment must be instituted emergently because of the rapid neurologic deterioration associated with this condition. Demyelination and secondary infarction and necrosis of the cord may be present below and above the level of the tumor. Surgery can be an option when the tumor is small, well-demarcated, radioresistant, and the systemic disease is under control. Prognosis is usually poor.

LEPTOMENINGEAL METASTASES (CARCINOMATOUS MENINGITIS)

Leptomeningeal metastasis represents an important neurologic complication of systemic cancer, occurring in 10 to 15 percent of patients with solid tumors and as many as 30 to 50 percent of children with leukemia. Lung carcinoma, breast cancer, non-Hodgkin's lymphoma, and melanoma are the tumors most commonly associated with leptomeningeal metastatic disease (LMD). Prior chemotherapy for systemic disease and prophylactic craniospinal radiation do not prevent LMD from solid tumors, even when the primary tumor is sensitive to treatment. Prophylactic craniospinal radiation has reduced the incidence of leptomeningeal leukemia in children.

Clinically, LMD may be asymptomatic or have a wide variety of clinical manifestations (Table 1); it may be discovered incidentally by MRI. Its most common clinical presentations are cranial neuropathy (cranial nerves III, VI, VII), low back pain, multifocal radiculopathy, and cauda equina syndrome. Mental status changes, meningeal signs, and seizures may also occur. Tumor cells reach the leptomeninges through hematogenous spread or direct rupture of parenchymal metastases into the subarachnoid space or the ventricles. The tumor cells may seed the leptomeninges diffusely or in a nodular pattern. Such nodules can be seen on MRI or myelography as "dropped metastases." They may invade the cranial and spinal nerves and infiltrate the Virchow-Robin spaces with perivascular tumor cuffing, which explains the ischemic events in LMD.

The diagnosis of LMD is based on careful neurologic evaluation and imaging and CSF analysis. Even mild symptoms and signs such as slight ptosis, facial asymmetry, recent hearing loss, asymmetric deep tendon reflexes, or mild change in mental status in a patient with known cancer must raise the suspicion of LMD.

Findings of contrast-enhanced CT of the brain may be normal or show hydrocephalus or contrast enhancement of the leptomeninges. Myelography, besides providing CSF for analysis, may reveal nodules or thickened nerve roots up and down the spinal cord, particularly in the cauda equina region. MRI with gadolinium enhancement is now becoming the preferred imaging modality, because it can detect LMD not seen on CT or myelography.

Although analysis of CSF is the most important test to confirm the diagnosis of LMD, a single negative CSF cytologic examination does not rule it out. Lumbar puncture may need to be repeated three or four times before malignant cells can be detected. Elevated CSF protein and low CSF glucose values are suggestive but not diagnostic of LMD; similar CSF abnormalities can be associated with viral, fungal, or mycobacterial meningitis or granulomatous meningitis. Tumor markers such as beta$_2$-microglobulin, beta-glucuronidase, carcinoembryonic antigen (CEA), and others have been studied as indicators of LMD. Elevated CSF beta$_2$-microglobulin is present in lymphoproliferative disease, and beta-glucuronidase and CEA are seen in LMD from solid tumors. These markers can be useful for monitoring the response to therapy and for early detection of relapse. DNA abnormalities can be detected by flow cytometry in CSF cells of patients with possible LMD, but the use of this approach is still in the experimental stage. Immunocytochemical studies can help identify

Table 1 Symptoms and Signs of Leptomeningeal Metastases

Asymptomatic
Minimal neurologic symptoms and signs
  Diplopia
  Slight ptosis
  Facial asymmetry
  Asymmetric deep tendon reflexes
Headache
Meningeal signs
Encephalopathy
Seizures
Cranial neuropathy
  Ophthalmoplegia (third nerve, sixth nerve)
  Facial nerve paresis (lower motor neuron)
  Hearing loss
  Dysphagia
Back pain
Radiculopathy
Cauda equina syndrome

LMD in leukemia and lymphoma, even when only very few cells are available.

Treating LMD is difficult. Systemic chemotherapy given for control of extracranial metastases fails to prevent LMD, presumably because of the drugs' poor penetration into the CSF through the blood-CSF barrier. Less than 10 percent of the systemic dose penetrates into the CSF, making systemic chemotherapy ineffective for treatment of LMD. Treatment modalities targeted directly at the central nervous system include radiation therapy to the whole brain and/or spine and intrathecal and intraventricular chemotherapy. Craniospinal radiation therapy is especially effective for leukemic or lymphomatous meningitis. More localized radiation therapy can be used for nodular deposits from solid tumors, to relieve pain and prevent or treat cord compression. Chemotherapy for LMD must be administered directly into the CSF. This allows direct exposure of the tumor cells to cytotoxic drugs and the use of much smaller doses than those used for systemic therapy. Chemotherapy can be administered through an intraventricular reservoir (e.g., Ommaya reservoir). This approach provides a higher concentration and better distribution of the drug in the CSF. It is important to confirm the patency of the CSF channels, as blockage may prevent drug penetration into some affected areas and increase local toxicity. Radioisotope CSF scintigraph scan can localize the areas of blockage, and the CSF flow can be re-established with focal radiation therapy.

At present, there is no standard chemotherapy regimen for LMD. Methotrexate is the preferred drug for LMD from solid tumors. In meningeal leukemias or lymphomas, both methotrexate and cytosine arabinoside (cytarabine) have been used, alone and in combination. Combination chemotherapy (methotrexate, cytarabine, and thiotepa) has also been used for meningeal carcinomatosis. The best responses were noted in patients with breast carcinoma and small cell carcinoma of the lung, but remissions were short lived. In one randomized prospective study, a methotrexate/cytarabine combination provided no advantage over methotrexate alone. Furthermore, combination chemotherapy increases the risk of neurotoxicity. The role of radiation therapy given prior to intra-Ommaya chemotherapy is controversial: in some studies it seemed favorably to influence the response to chemotherapy. Other chemotherapeutic agents (ACNU, diaziquinone, AZQ) are also used for intra-Ommaya therapy, but these are still in phase I or II studies.

None of the drugs used so far has significantly improved the overall poor prognosis of patients with LMD. Even with good response to chemotherapy, the time to relapse is short (4 to 24 weeks). Most of these patients have LMD in the setting of widespread systemic metastases. The usual dose for adults is 12 mg methotrexate and 75 to 100 mg cytarabine, initially given twice a week until the CSF is free of tumor cells, then once a week for 2 months, then once a month for 2 months. Pharmacokinetic studies have shown that a *concentration × time* approach, in which smaller doses are administered at more frequent intervals, increases the duration of CSF exposure to the drug, avoids excessively high peak concentrations (thus reducing the neurotoxicity), and delivers a smaller cumulative drug dose. One milligram of methotrexate given every 12 hours for six doses proved as effective as the standard single dose of 12 mg but with a smaller total cumulative dose (6 mg) and fewer toxic effects. Similar results were demonstrated for cytarabine. A dose of 30 mg per day for 3 days maintained a cytotoxic drug concentration in the CSF for more than 72 hours, whereas a single dose of 70 mg did so for only 24 hours.

Neurotoxicity is the most important complication of intraventricular chemotherapy. Encephalopathy, seizures, dementia, and myelopathy are the most dramatic clinical manifestations. Some patients develop extrapyramidal syndrome, headaches, or arachnoiditis. Some of these symptoms are reversible. A rare patient develops a progressive ascending transverse myelitis with subsequent paraplegia or quadriplegia, which is related to high drug concentrations.

Other therapeutic approaches to LMD are intraventricular administration of radioisotopes, monoclonal antibody–linked radioisotopes, and biologic agents. Of the biologic agents, only alpha-interferon and interleukin-2 are used to treat LMD. Encephalopathy and chemical meningitis are the dose-limiting toxic effects of these agents. The results obtained thus far with biologic agents are not very encouraging.

DISCUSSION

Metastatic disease to the spine remains an important neurologic complication of systemic cancer that, overall, has a poor prognosis. The treatment of spinal metastases raises controversial issues and is at the present time mostly palliative. We have addressed some of the problems related to the different therapeutic modalities, as well as the newest approaches to therapy. Research is aimed at developing new cytotoxic drugs that provide good penetration into the central nervous system, good efficacy against tumor cells, and minimal neurologic and systemic toxicity. The addition of hematopoietic growth factors will limit the myelotoxicity induced by systemic chemotherapy.

SUGGESTED READING

Blaney SM, Balis FM, Poplack DG. Pharmacologic approaches to the treatment of meningeal malignancy. Oncology 1991; 5:107–116.

Choucair AK. Myelopathies in the cancer patient: Incidence, presentation, diagnosis and management (part 1). Oncology 1991; 5:71–80.

Choucair AK. Myelopathies in the cancer patient: Incidence, presentation, diagnosis and management (part 2). Oncology 1991; 5:25–38.

Grossman SA, Lossignol D. Diagnosis and treatment of epidural metastases. Oncology 1990; 4:47–55.

Hitchins RN, Bell DR, Woods RL, Levi Y. A prospective trial of single-agent versus combination chemotherapy in meningeal carcinomatosis. J Clin Oncol 1987; 5:1655–1662.

Lipton RB, Portenoy RK, Foley KM. Back pain in cancer patients. Emerg Decisions 1987; 3:33–50.

Nather A, Bose K. The results of decompression of cord or cauda equina compression from metastatic extradural tumors. Clin Orthop 1992; 168:103–108.

Sundaresan N, Choi IS, Hughes YEO. Treatment of spinal metastases from kidney cancer by presurgical embolization and resection. J Neurosurg 1990; 73:548–554.

Vecht CJ, Haaxma-Reiche H, van Putten WLY. Initial bolus of conventional versus high-dose dexamethasone in metastatic spinal cord compression. Neurology 1989; 39:1255–1257.

Wasserstrom WR, Glass JP, Posner JB. Diagnosis and treatment of leptomeningeal metastases from solid tumors: Experience with 90 patients. Cancer 1982; 49:759–772.

PITUITARY ADENOMAS

LEWIS S. BLEVINS, Jr., M.D.
GARY S. WAND, M.D.

Pituitary adenomas account for 10 percent of all intracranial neoplasms. These tumors are almost always benign and are classified by diameter as microadenomas (<1 cm) or macroadenomas (>1 cm). An adenoma may present with symptoms or signs of compression of sellar and parasellar structures, a syndrome of hormonal hypersecretion, or during a neuroradiologic imaging procedure performed for apparently unrelated complaints (Table 1). A sellar mass should be part of the differential diagnosis for all patients when planning therapy (Table 2).

In general, the goals of therapy for pituitary adenoma are to ablate the tumor and reverse mass effects, control hormone hypersecretion and associated medical complications, recognize and treat hormone deficiencies (Table 3), and minimize complications of therapy. The post-treatment evaluation should be designed to determine adequacy of therapy, recognize complications of therapy, and permit early detection and treatment of recurrences. In this chapter we focus on the approach to therapy in patients with a diagnosis of a pituitary adenoma. The reader is referred to standard endocrinology textbooks for discussion of the evaluation and diagnosis of pituitary adenoma.

NONSECRETING ADENOMAS

Twenty-five to thirty percent of patients with pituitary adenoma have no clinical or biochemical evidence of hormonal hypersecretion (Table 4). These patients' diagnosis is generally "nonfunctional" pituitary adenoma; though studies in vitro have demonstrated that the majority of the tumors are, in fact, gonadotropin-producing adenomas.

Patients who harbor a microadenoma or asymptomatic intrasellar macroadenoma do not urgently require therapy and may be followed expectantly. Neuroradiologic and endocrinologic testing should be performed at 6-month intervals for 1 year, and then annually, to allow early detection and treatment of expanding tumors.

Indications for surgical therapy in a patient with a nonsecreting adenoma include extrasellar extension, compression of parasellar structures, pituitary apoplexy, and failure of prior therapy (e.g., radiotherapy, bromocriptine). Trans-sphenoidal resection of a pituitary tumor is the preferred surgical procedure. The transcranial approach may be necessary when the tumor is largely suprasellar, invades the hypothalamus or cerebral cortex, or wraps around the optic chiasm. Visual field abnormalities can be expected to improve in 80 percent of patients following surgery. Anterior pituitary hormone deficits improve in a significant number of patients. Urgent decompression is essential for patients with pituitary apoplexy and may reverse visual field defects, restore anterior pituitary function, and prevent death due to acute adrenal insufficiency or subarachnoid hemorrhage. All patients with a clinical diagnosis of pituitary apoplexy should receive hydrocortisone, 100 mg IV every 8 hours.

Surgical therapy is complicated by diabetes insipidus or partial anterior hypopituitarism in 10 to 18 percent of patients. Optic injury with visual deficits, cerebrospinal fluid rhinorrhea, cranial nerve injury, sinusitis, meningi-

---

Table 1 Clinical Presentation of Pituitary Adenoma

Headache
Visual field disturbances
Ophthalmoplegia (CN III, IV, VI)
Facial pain (CN V_1, V_2)
Hormone hypersecretion syndromes
Anterior hypopituitarism (partial or complete)
Apoplexy
CSF rhinorrhea
Epistaxis
Nasopharyngeal mass
Temporal lobe epilepsy
Hydrocephalus

Table 2 Differential Diagnosis of a Sellar or Parasellar Mass

Pituitary adenoma
Lymphocytic hypophysitis
Metastases (breast, lung, lymphoma)
Craniopharyngioma
Meningioma
Glioma (optic chiasm)
Gangliocytoma
Aneurysm
Granulomatous disease
  Sarcoidosis
  Tuberculosis
  Langerhan's cell histiocytosis
Pituitary cysts
  Dermoid
  Epidermoid
  Rathke's cleft

Table 3 Screening Tests for Hypopituitarism

Hormone	Tests
Adrenocorticotropic hormone (ACTH)	ACTH stimulation test, insulin tolerance test, metyrapone test
Thyroid-stimulating hormone (TSH)	Thyroxine, tri-iodothyronine uptake, TSH
Luteinizing hormone (LH) or follicle-stimulating hormone (FSH)	LH, FSH, testosterone (men) estradiol, menstrual history (women)
Growth hormone (GH)	Insulin tolerance test
Vasopressin	Water deprivation test

Table 4 Screening Tests for Syndromes of Hormonal Hypersecretion

Syndrome	Tests
Prolactinoma	Prolactin
Acromegaly	Insulin-like growth factor I (IFG – I, somato-medin-C), 75 g glucose suppression test
Cushing's disease	24 hour urinary free cortisol, dexamethasone suppression test
Nonsecreting tumor (gonadotropin-producing)	LH, FSH, alpha subunit
Hyperthyroidism (TSH-producing)	Thyroxine, tri-iodothyronine uptake, TSH, alpha subunit

tis, and cerebrovascular insufficiency each occur in fewer than 1.5 percent of cases. The mortality rate is less than 0.5 percent; death may result from hypothalamic injury, hemorrhage from a carotid artery laceration, or a stroke syndrome. The frequency of complications is increased in patients with very large tumors or a history of therapy (surgery, radiotherapy), or when the transcranial approach is employed.

Postoperative endocrinologic and radiologic evaluations should be performed at 1, 6, and 12 months, and thereafter annually. The neuro-ophthalomic status should be reassessed following surgery and then when clinically indicated. All patients should receive cortisone acetate, 25 mg every morning and 12.5 mg daily at 4:00 PM, until normal function of the hypothalamic-pituitary-adrenal (HPA) axis has been demonstrated. Vaso-pressin, thyroid, and sex hormone replacement therapy is withheld until clinical and biochemical evidence of hormone deficiency appears.

Adjunctive conventional radiotherapy is reserved for patients with postoperative residual or invasive tumor. Radiotherapy may be used as a primary treatment modality in an occasional patient when surgical therapy is contraindicated. Radiation is precisely delivered to the pituitary tumor by a 4 or 6 MeV linear accelerator with bilateral moving coronal arc fields and reversing wedge filters. The standard cumulative dose is 45 Gy administered in 1.8 Gy fractions daily. Potential benefits of adjuvant radiotherapy include shrinkage of residual tumor and prevention of tumor regrowth, but prompt reduction in tumor size is rare. Partial or complete hypopituitarism develops insidiously over several years in 40 to 50 percent of patients as a result of radiation-induced hypothalamic injury. Therefore, all irradiated patients must undergo a repeat neuroendocrine evaluation on an annual basis, to permit early diagnosis and treatment of hormonal deficiencies. Additional rare complications include lethargy, optic chiasm or optic nerve injury, cranial nerve palsies, pituitary apoplexy, brain necrosis, vascular ischemia, seizure disorder, and radiation-induced parasellar tumors.

PROLACTINOMA

Prolactinomas account for approximately 40 percent of all pituitary adenomas. Women typically present with a microadenoma and gonadal dysfunction. The spectrum of gonadal dysfunction may include the amenorrhea-galactorrhea syndrome, infertility, decreased libido, or other symptoms or signs of estrogen deficiency, including osteoporosis. Men almost always harbor a macroadenoma and present with symptoms related to the tumor mass, impotence, diminished libido, infertility, and rarely gynecomastia and galactorrhea. Hyperprolactinemia may be associated with a number of conditions that must be excluded before therapy is directed at a presumed prolactinoma (Table 5).

Therapeutic objectives for a patient with a prolactinoma include normalization of the prolactin concentration with restoration of gonadal function, resolution of galactorrhea, and reversal of compressive effects of the tumor. Patients with a microadenoma may be followed expectantly when fertility is not desired and the menstrual cycle is normal. The risk of progressive growth of an untreated microprolactinoma is less than 5 percent.

Pharmacologic therapy with a dopamine agonist should always be the initial treatment for a symptomatic prolactinoma. Attempts at surgical resection of a micro- or macroprolactinoma achieve long-term cure in only 40 to 60 percent and 10 to 40 percent of patients, respectively. Bromocriptine is the only dopamine agonist approved by the U.S. Food and Drug Administration for the treatment of pituitary adenomas. A typical starting dose is 1.25 mg PO at bedtime with a snack. The dose should be increased by 1.25 to 2.5 mg increments every 2 to 3 days, until a dose of 2.5 mg three times daily with meals is achieved. This regimen should minimize side effects and enhance patient compliance. The dose should be increased more rapidly in patients with a macroadenoma and visual compromise. A daily dose as large as 15 mg is often necessary for these patients and is associated with an increased incidence of side effects. Periodic measurement of the prolactin concentration during dose escalation allows identification of the smallest dose required to effectively suppress prolactin hypersecretion. Common side effects of bromocriptine include nausea, headache, orthostatic dizziness, nasal congestion, and fatigue. These usually improve over time and are often diminished by taking bromocriptine with food.

Ovulatory menses are restored in 80 to 85 percent of women within 6 to 8 weeks of achieving normoprolactinemia. Patients with amenorrhea or infertility must

Table 5 Causes of Hyperprolactinemia

Prolactinoma
Acromegaly
Pituitary stalk compression
Empty sella syndrome
Hypothalamic tumor
Hypothalamic infiltrative disorders
   Sarcoidosis
   Langerhan's cell histiocytosis
   Tuberculosis
Drugs
   Antipsychotics
   Antidepressants
   Metoclopramide
   Reserpine
   Alpha-methyldopa
   Verapamil
   Estrogens
Hypothyroidism
Chronic renal failure
Cirrhosis
Neurogenic causes
   Chest wall lesions
   Spinal cord tumors
   Nipple stimulation
Stress
Idiopathic

use barrier contraception during therapy. If pregnancy is desired, measurement of the basal body temperature to predict ovulation should be performed for two or three menstrual cycles following the institution of bromocriptine. Once the cycle length is established, contraception can be discontinued. During subsequent cycles, bromocriptine should be discontinued when the menses are delayed by 48 hours and the serum level of beta-human chorionic gonadotropin should be determined. Pregnancy is usually achieved in 70 to 100 percent of formerly infertile women within 6 months of instituting bromocriptine. Symptomatic tumor expansion during pregnancy occurs in 1.2 percent of patients with microadenomas and 25 percent of those with macroadenomas. Bromocriptine appears to be safe in pregnancy and should be reinstituted when this situation develops.

A decrease in tumor size by 50 percent or more occurs in 64 percent of patients with a macroadenoma. A reduction in tumor size usually occurs within 6 weeks, but it may be delayed up to 12 months. The prolactin concentration normalizes in 50 to 90 percent of patients. Visual field defects improve in approximately 90 percent of patients.

Trans-sphenoidal resection is indicated for patients who cannot tolerate bromocriptine, or who exhibit resistance and persistent hypogonadism or tumor mass effects, or for those who demand surgical therapy. Bromocriptine-resistant or -intolerant patients' disease may be more easily controlled with pharmacologic intervention following partial tumor resection. Conventional radiotherapy may be useful to control tumor mass and hyperprolactinemia.

In general, patients with a prolactinoma require lifelong therapy with bromocriptine, although occasional patients with a microadenoma or a bromocriptine-responsive macroadenoma experience spontaneous resolution. Thus, it is our practice to discontinue bromocriptine every 2 years and measure the prolactin concentration, to determine if continued therapy is warranted.

ACROMEGALY

Some 5 to 10 percent of pituitary adenomas produce growth hormone (GH) and they are the most common cause of acromegaly. Specific goals of therapy include reversal of soft tissue and metabolic complications, decreasing risk of mortality due to colon carcinoma or cardiovascular disease, and control of the tumor mass. Glucose intolerance, hypertension, and cardiovascular disease require appropriate management during the course of therapy.

Trans-sphenoidal surgical resection is the preferred treatment for patients with a GH-producing pituitary adenoma. Biochemical criteria for cure include a basal GH concentration less than 5 μg per liter, suppression of the GH concentration to less than 2 μg per liter following glucose administration, and a normal concentration of insulin-like growth factor (IGF-I, somatomedin-C). An elevated IGF-I concentration is an accurate predictor of persistent tumor, regardless of the GH concentration. A GH concentration less than 5 μg per liter is achieved in 60 percent of patients following surgery; however, a number of these patients relapse and only 30 percent experience a long-term cure. Patients with a large tumor, extrasellar extension, or preoperative GH concentration greater than 50 μg per liter have a less favorable outcome.

Pharmacologic agents are administered to patients with postoperative residual tumor and elevated GH or IGF-I concentrations, and to patients with contraindications to surgery. Bromocriptine relieves the headache and improves the sense of well-being in 70 percent of patients, although tumor shrinkage occurs in only 15 percent, and biochemical evidence of cure is achieved in only 20 percent. Octreotide, a long-acting somatostatin analogue, effectively suppresses GH secretion in patients with acromegaly. The usual starting dose is 100 μg SC every 8 hours. The dose is increased by 50 to 100 μg increments until GH and IGF-I production are adequately suppressed. The maximum daily dose should not exceed 1,500 μg. Occasional patients require continuous subcutaneous infusion or dosing at 6 hour intervals. A majority of patients report immediate relief of headache, and 50 percent experience a decrease in tumor size. The GH concentration decreases in 80 percent and normalizes in 30 percent. Cholelithiasis develops in 40 to 50 percent of patients treated for prolonged periods with octreotide. Other side effects include mild biochemical hypothyroidism, impaired glucose tolerance, malabsorption, nausea, and abdominal discomfort.

Conventional radiotherapy is reserved for cases in which surgery and pharmacologic therapy do not achieve control of GH hypersecretion. Approximately 50 percent of patients can be expected to achieve biochemical cure within 2 to 4 years. Eighty-five to ninety percent achieve a GH concentration less than 10 μg per liter within 10 years when irradiation is used as primary therapy. Adjunctive pharmacologic therapy should be used to minimize the complications of GH excess while awaiting a response to radiotherapy.

CUSHING'S DISEASE

An adrenocorticotropic hormone (ACTH)-secreting pituitary adenoma (Cushing's disease) is present in 80 percent of patients with endogenous Cushing's syndrome. Ninety percent of patients with Cushing's disease have a microadenoma. During the course of therapy, careful attention should be directed to potential complications of hypercortisolism, including hypertension, hypokalemia, glucose intolerance, poor wound healing, and risk of infection.

Initial therapy for Cushing's disease should be directed at the pituitary adenoma. Selective transsphenoidal resection by an experienced neurosurgeon results in a biochemical cure in 70 to 80 percent of cases. Successful outcomes are significantly less frequent with a macroadenoma (less than 50 percent), with dural or bone invasion (25 percent), or when the procedure is performed by an inexperienced surgeon.

ACTH deficiency, or secondary adrenal insufficiency, follows successful resection of an ACTH-producing adenoma and typically lasts 6 to 12 months. Secondary adrenal insufficiency occurs because the normal ACTH-producing anterior pituitary cells have long been suppressed by supraphysiologic levels of cortisol. Therefore, all patients require glucocorticoid therapy in the peri- and postoperative periods. Hydrocortisone, 100 mg IV, should be administered during induction and termination of anesthesia, and at 8 hour intervals during the first postoperative day. The dose should be decreased to 50 mg every 8 hours on day 2, then 25 mg every 8 hours until the patient tolerates oral medication. Glucocorticoid replacement therapy is instituted with cortisone acetate, 25 mg at 8:00 AM and 12.5 mg at 4:00 to 6:00 PM, daily. Occasional patients may require a temporary increase in dose, to alleviate the symptoms of steroid withdrawal. Replacement therapy should be continued until recovery of the hypothalamic-pituitary-adrenal (HPA) axis has been demonstrated by metyrapone or insulin tolerance testing.

The likelihood of surgical cure can be predicted by measuring the early morning cortisol concentration 24 hours after giving the first replacement dose of cortisone acetate. Persistently normal or elevated cortisol concentration indicates surgical failure; levels greater than 4 μg per deciliter identify patients at considerable risk for recurrence of hypercortisolism. Approximately 5 to 25 percent of patients who enjoy initial cure develop a recurrence within 3 to 5 years. Once recovery of the HPA axis has been demonstrated and replacement glucocor-

ticoids have been discontinued, dexamethasone suppression testing and urinary free cortisol determinations are useful tests to evaluate for recurrence of hypercortisolism.

Several therapeutic alternatives are available for patients with persistent or recurrent Cushing's disease. Re-exploration may result in cure of 40 to 90 percent of patients when the adenoma is identified at surgery. Conventional radiotherapy should be administered if re-exploration is not desired, is unsuccessful, or is contraindicated. Approximately 40 percent of patients achieve satisfactory control of hypercortisolism within 12 to 18 months following radiotherapy. When it is employed as initial therapy, 25 percent of adults and 80 percent of children achieve a cure.

Pharmacologic agents that inhibit adrenal steroid biosynthesis are commonly employed while awaiting the effects of radiotherapy or preoperatively to decrease the risks of surgical morbidity and mortality (Table 6). Ketoconazole, an imidazole antifungal agent, inhibits the activity of several adrenal biosynthetic enzymes. A typical starting dose is 200 mg PO twice a day. The dose may be increased to 400 mg twice a day as necessary. The response to therapy is judged by frequent determinations of 24 hour urinary free cortisol excretion. The therapeutic objective is suppression of the 24 hour urinary free cortisol excretion to or below the normal range. Glucocorticoid and mineralocorticoid replacements are administered when necessary. Side effects of ketoconazole include nausea, vomiting, anorexia, headaches, sedation, and symptomatic hypogonadism. Transient mild hepatitis is common; fulminant toxic hepatitis is rare. Liver function tests should be evaluated at 4 weeks, 8 weeks, and then periodically during the course of treatment. Ketoconazole should be discontinued when the serum transaminase values remain persistently elevated.

Bilateral adrenalectomy is reserved for patients whom other therapeutic ventures have failed. Obviously, these patients require lifelong glucocorticoid and mineralocorticoid replacement. All patients should be educated in making necessary adjustments of glucocorticoids during periods of stress. For 2 or 3 days of minor illness, the daily glucocorticoid replacement dose should be increased two- to threefold. An illness that persists longer than 3 days requires careful evaluation, specific treatment, and, possibly, hospitalization. Patients should be supplied with prefilled syringes containing dexamethasone, 4 mg in 1 ml saline. Patient and family should be instructed to administer the injection of dexamethasone and notify the physician immediately in case of severe illness, trauma, or inability to tolerate oral medications. The patient should at all times wear a Medic-Alert tag indicating steroid dependency.

Nelson's syndrome is defined as the development of an aggressive, invasive ACTH-producing pituitary adenoma following bilateral adrenalectomy. Patients typically present with a macroadenoma and hyperpigmentation, which is due to a markedly elevated ACTH concentration. Historically, the syndrome has been

Table 6 Agents to Treat Hypercortisolism

Agent	Daily dosage (mg)	Side Effects
Ketoconazole	200–800	Nausea, vomiting, anorexia, headache, pruritus, hypogonadism, hepatitis
Mitotane	2,000–4,000	Adrenal insufficiency, nausea, vomiting, anorexia, skin rash, ataxia
Metyrapone	500–4,000	Nausea, vomiting, dizziness
Aminoglutethimide	500–2,000	Anorexia, nausea, vomiting, lethargy, sedation, hypothyroidism, skin rash

reported in 10 to 50 percent of patients following bilateral adrenalectomy as primary therapy for Cushing's disease. Nelson's syndrome is less likely to occur when radiotherapy precedes medical or surgical adrenalectomy. Patients with Nelson's syndrome are most effectively treated with trans-sphenoidal surgery and radiotherapy.

THYROTROPIN-PRODUCING ADENOMAS

Thyrotropin-, or TSH-secreting adenomas account for 1 percent of all pituitary tumors. These adenomas generally present with hyperthyroidism, goiter, and inappropriate TSH secretion. Alpha subunit is elevated in 80 percent of patients, and the alpha subunit–TSH molar ratio is usually greater than 1. The general approach to therapy includes trans-sphenoidal resection followed by conventional radiotherapy and medical therapy with octreotide.

SUGGESTED READING

Atkinson AB. The treatment of Cushing's syndrome. Clin Endocrinol 1991; 34:507–513.

Blevins LS, Wand GS. Diabetes insipidus. Crit Care Med 1992; 20:69–79.

Frohman LA. Therapeutic options in acromegaly. J Clin Endocrinol Metab 1991; 72:1175–1181.

Klibanski A, Zervas NT. Diagnosis and management of hormone-secreting pituitary adenomas. N Engl J Med 1991; 324:822–831.

Molitch ME, Russell EJ. The pituitary "incidentaloma." Ann Intern Med 1990; 112:925–931.

Wand GS, Ladenson PW. Management of prolactinomas. Neurology Neurosurgery Update Series 1988; 7(31):2–7.

REMOTE EFFECTS OF CARCINOMA

JOHN E. GREENLEE, M.D.
H. ROBERT BRASHEAR, M.D.

Paraneoplastic neurologic syndromes are remote, nonmetastatic complications of systemic cancer. These disorders are characterized clinically by subacute, progressive neurologic deficits that usually result in profound disability or death. Paraneoplastic syndromes may develop as long as 2 years before diagnosis of the associated neoplasm, after diagnosis, or when the tumor is thought to be in remission. Sera and cerebrospinal fluid (CSF) from many patients with paraneoplastic disorders contain antineuronal antibodies. Recent work indicates that this antibody response also recognizes antigens within patients' tumors. These data suggest that paraneoplastic neurologic syndromes may be autoimmune disorders in which an immune response elicited by the patient's tumor is cross-reactive with specific neuronal proteins.

With a suspected paraneoplastic neurologic disorder the approach to the patient involves three separate diagnostic and therapeutic issues: recognition or suspicion of a paraneoplastic syndrome; use of an associated antibody response as a tumor-specific marker of occult malignancy; and treatment of the paraneoplastic disorder itself.

PARANEOPLASTIC SYNDROMES

Paraneoplastic syndromes may involve the central nervous system (CNS), peripheral ganglia, or the neuromuscular junction. In many patients more than one paraneoplastic syndrome is present initially or develops over time. Paraneoplastic syndromes affecting the CNS include diffuse or regional encephalomyelitis (encephalomyelitis, limbic encephalitis, bulbar encephalitis), cerebellar degeneration, and retinal degeneration. Disorders that affect peripheral ganglia include dorsal sensory neuronopathy and autonomic neuropathy. Syn-

Dr. Greenlee is recipient of a Department of Veterans Affairs Merit Review Award.

dromes affecting the neuromuscular junction include Lambert-Eaton myasthenic syndrome in association with small cell carcinoma and myasthenia gravis associated with thymoma. Several disorders, such as optic neuritis, transverse myelitis, and amyotrophic lateral sclerosis, have been suspected of having a paraneoplastic cause on the basis of a slightly increased prevalence among cancer patients. The diagnosis and treatment of these disorders is little influenced by a possible association with cancer. Major paraneoplastic syndromes are described next.

Paraneoplastic encephalomyelitis is very often associated with small cell carcinoma but occasionally occurs with other neoplasms such as germ cell tumors. Patients may present with evidence of injury involving multiple levels of the neuraxis. Cortical disease shows a predilection for limbic structures. Patients who develop limbic encephalitis exhibit subacute, progressive mental and emotional disturbances, including anxiety and depression, which often progress to dementia. Bulbar encephalitis is characterized by progressive failure of brain stem functions, including control of respiration. Patients with paraneoplastic encephalomyelitis may also show signs of injury to the cerebellum, to anterior horn cells within the spinal cord, and to neurons within dorsal root and autonomic ganglia.

Paraneoplastic cerebellar degeneration occurs in association with ovarian carcinoma (most frequently), and with uterine, adnexal, and breast cancer. Additional cases may occur in the setting of small cell carcinoma of the lung, Hodgkin's disease, or another malignancy. Clinical signs include progressive, often severe ataxia, dysarthria, and nystagmus. Brains of affected patients characteristically show nearly total loss of cerebellar Purkinje cells with variable loss of neurons in the granular layer and deep cerebellar nuclei. Lymphocytic infiltrates are more commonly found in the deep nuclei.

Opsoclonus-ataxia occurs in two clinical settings: in children with neuroblastoma or retinoblastoma, where the condition is often accompanied by myoclonus, and in adult patients with carcinoma of the breast or, less frequently, small cell carcinoma of the lung. Oculomotor abnormalities are disabling and range from ocular flutter and complex nystagmus to frank opsoclonus. The course of paraneoplastic opsoclonus-ataxia differs from that of most other paraneoplastic neurologic syndromes in that it is often remitting and may respond to steroid therapy.

Retinal degeneration has been described in the setting of several different types of malignancy, most commonly small cell carcinoma and breast carcinoma. Patients develop subacute, painless vision loss. Histologically there is loss of photoreceptor cells with variable cell loss in other retinal layers, inflammatory infiltrates, and gliosis.

Dorsal sensory neuronopathy (subacute sensory neuronopathy) occurs predominantly in the setting of small cell carcinoma of the lung and is often accompanied by one or more manifestations of paraneoplastic encephalomyelitis. Patients exhibit progressive sensory loss, often with profound impairment of proprioception. Dorsal root ganglia of affected patients show lymphocytic infiltration and neuronal loss, with secondary degeneration of posterior nerve roots and dorsal columns.

Autonomic neuropathy, like dorsal sensory neuronopathy, is highly associated with small cell lung carcinoma and may be accompanied by other manifestations of paraneoplastic encephalomyelitis or by injury to dorsal root ganglia. Neurons within autonomic ganglia, including the myenteric plexus, are usually involved, and brain stem neurons may be affected. Symptoms include progressive orthostatic hypotension, gastroparesis and other gastrointestinal motility disorders that can mimic acute ileus, and failure of autonomic control of respiration with respiratory failure or arrest.

Lambert-Eaton myasthenic syndrome (LES) occurs in association with cancer in approximately 50 percent of cases (predominantly small cell carcinoma of the lung). The disorder appears to result from an autoimmune response directed against calcium channels in the presynaptic neuromuscular junction, resulting in inhibition of calcium flux and impaired acetylcholine release. Myasthenic symptoms, which usually spare ocular muscles, may be associated with signs of autonomic failure.

AUTOANTIBODY RESPONSE IN PARANEOPLASTIC NEUROLOGIC SYNDROMES

The identification of antineuronal antibodies in serum and CSF of affected patients represented a major advance in our understanding of paraneoplastic syndromes. As mentioned above, this autoimmune response appears to be elicited by tumor antigens which are immunologically cross-reactive with neuronal proteins. Although antineuronal antibodies are found in the majority of patients with classical paraneoplastic neurologic syndromes, their role in the pathogenesis of disease remains undefined.

The pattern of immunofluorescent staining of brain tissue produced by patient serum or CSF and the proteins labeled by patient serum and CSF in Western immunoblots vary according to the specific paraneoplastic syndrome and the histologic nature of the associated neoplasm (Table 1). For instance, sera and CSF from patients with paraneoplastic cerebellar degeneration in the setting of gynecologic or breast adenocarcinoma produce a type I pattern of staining characterized by intense, granular labeling of Purkinje cell cytoplasm with little if any staining of other cell populations. The autoantibodies responsible for this pattern recognize 34 and 62 kd antigens in blots of Purkinje cell concentrates, a response termed *anti-Yo*. In contrast, patients with paraneoplastic disorders and small cell carcinoma of the lung exhibit an antineuronal antibody response (type IIa or *anti-Hu*) that recognizes a group of 34 to 42 kd proteins found in nuclei and cytoplasm of all neurons. Autoantibodies in sera and CSF of patients with

Table 1 Autoantibodies in Neurologic Paraneoplastic Syndromes

Syndrome	Clinical Features	Frequent Neoplasm	Antibody Response by FA	Antibody Response by Blot
Cerebellar degeneration	Ataxia, nystagmus	Ovarian, breast carcinoma	Type I, anti-Purkinje cell antibody	Anti-Yo, 34–38 kd and 62–64 kd proteins
Sensory neuronopathy and encephalomyelitis	Sensory loss; cortical, brain stem, spinal cord deficits	Small cell carcinoma	Type IIa, pan-neuronal antibody	Anti-Hu, 34–42 kd proteins
Opsoclonus-ataxia	Erratic eye movements, ataxia	Breast carcinoma	Type IIb, pan-neuronal antibody	Anti-Ri, 53–61 kd and 79–84 kd proteins
		Small cell carcinoma, neuroblastoma	None detected	None detected
Retinal degeneration	Vision loss	Small cell carcinoma	Antiretinal antibodies	23 kd, other retinal proteins

opsoclonus-ataxia, termed *type IIb* or *anti-Ri,* also recognize nuclear and cytoplasmic antigens found in virtually all neurons. Neuronal labeling is slightly more homogeneous with less nuclear delineation than the pan-neuronal labeling associated with small cell carcinoma, and Western blot analysis of this antibody response reveals that it labels proteins of 53 to 61 and 79 to 84 kd molecular weight. Antiretinal antibodies have been described in patients with paraneoplastic retinal degeneration. Some produce a pan-neuronal pattern of labeling, and reactions with retinal proteins of different molecular weights have been described. When present, antineuronal antibodies are found in high titers in the serum of affected patients. Antibody is also present in CSF, usually with evidence of intrathecal synthesis.

Serum from patients with paraneoplastic LES does not produce a characteristic pattern of immunofluorescence when reacted with neurons. However, the clinical and electrophysiologic features of LES can be duplicated in experimental animals by passive transfer of immunoglobulin G (IgG) from affected patients, and IgG from affected patients has been shown to react with presynaptic calcium channels at the myoneural junction.

Several less common patterns of antibody response have also been detected in individual patients with paraneoplastic neurologic syndromes, but the utility of these variant patterns as specific markers of specific tumor types has not been established. Although antineuronal antibodies have been detected in sera of some patients who develop paraneoplastic neurologic syndromes in the setting of Hodgkin's disease and other lymphomas, other patients have failed to show any identifiable autoantibody response.

APPROACH TO THE PATIENT WITH SUSPECTED PARANEOPLASTIC DISORDER

The major initial concern in patients with suspected paraneoplastic neurologic syndromes is to exclude the presence of metastatic disease or other potentially treatable complications of malignancy (Table 2). While this is being done, sera and (if available) CSF should be

Table 2 Potentially Treatable Nonparaneoplastic Effects of Cancer on the Nervous System

Metastatic lesions
Direct extension of tumor
Metabolic effects
Cerebrovascular disorders
Opportunistic infections
Nutritional deficiencies
Side effects of cancer treatment

sent for analysis for antineuronal antibodies. Screening tests on a commercial or research basis are available through several laboratories, some of which are listed below.

Detection of antineuronal antibodies is followed by extensive search for the associated neoplasm. Evaluation is guided by the clinical syndrome and the pattern of antibody response:

1. Subacute cerebellar degeneration and type I antibody response: female reproductive system or breast cancer.
2. Subacute cerebellar degeneration, encephalomyelitis or sensory neuronopathy, and type IIa antibody response: suspect small cell lung cancer. The rare patient has breast or prostate cancer. Concurrent small cell cancer should be ruled out if any other malignancy is found.
3. Opsoclonus-ataxia and type IIb antibody response: suspect breast cancer. In adult patients without type IIb pattern consider small cell carcinoma.
4. Other patterns of antineuronal antibody response: suspect occult malignancy, but specificity is still unclear.
5. Antibody-negative patients with subacute cerebellar degeneration or other paraneoplastic syndrome: suspect lymphoma.

Appropriate studies usually detect the underlying neoplasm. Occasionally, however, tumor is not found initially in an antibody-positive patient. Follow-up is critical, because a neoplasm may not be detected for up to 2 years after presentation.

SPECIFIC THERAPY

Treatment of paraneoplastic neurologic syndromes is still in its infancy, and it is often frustrating. Because of the infrequent occurrence of paraneoplastic neurologic disorders, information about therapy has been anecdotal. A major need in this area is to determine effective therapy through multicenter co-operative trials.

An aggressive effort should be made to identify and treat underlying malignancy before experimental therapy is considered. This approach is important for several reasons. Detection of occult malignancy is likely to lead to early and more successful treatment of a neoplasm. Most complete recovery from paraneoplastic neurologic syndromes has occurred in cases in which the underlying tumor has been promptly detected and completely removed. In a minority of cases, noncurative therapy of the tumor has also resulted in temporary improvement. Furthermore, clinical and basic research evidence suggest that the autoimmune mechanisms thought to be responsible for paraneoplastic neurologic injury are part of an immune response directed at the patient's tumor. Theoretically, then, immunosuppressive therapy without adequate primary treatment of the responsible neoplasm may increase the chance of tumor growth and metastases.

Immunosuppressive therapy, including plasma exchange, has an accepted role in the treatment of LES, and it is clear that at least some patients with opsoclonus-ataxia respond to prednisone therapy. A minority of patients with other paraneoplastic disorders of the CNS have also exhibited clinical improvement following plasma exchange. In most patients with paraneoplastic encephalomyelitis, cerebellar degeneration, dorsal sensory neuronopathy, or autonomic neuropathy, however, attempts to treat the neurologic disorder by immunosuppressive agents or by plasma exchange have been unsuccessful, even when serum antibody titer has been reduced. In many of these instances, failure of therapy probably reflects the fact that immunosuppressive treatment is often initiated late in the course of disease, after irreversible neurologic injury has already occurred. In addition, chemical immunosuppression may fail because of its limited ability to produce a rapid decrease in antibody titer, and plasma exchange may prove unhelpful because of its inability to remove intrathecally synthesized antibody across an intact blood-brain barrier.

Because of the devastating effects of most paraneoplastic neurologic syndromes, and because occasional patients have benefited from plasma exchange or steroids, our approach has been to initiate careful trials of corticosteroids or plasma exchange, or both, in patients whose disease has been diagnosed early in its course and who continued to get worse despite treatment of the underlying neoplasm. We have also used this approach to treatment in patients with typical type I, type IIa, or type IIb antibody response when no neoplasm can be detected. In both groups of patients, therapy begins with clear clinical end points and the specific goal of reducing antibody titers.

In patients with opsoclonus-ataxia we have used 80 mg of oral prednisone daily until ocular signs improve, at which time the regimen is changed to alternate-day doses of 120 mg, gradually tapered over 2 months as dictated by continued clinical improvement. In patients with other paraneoplastic disorders, we have initiated plasma exchange with the goal of reducing serum antibody titers to less than 1:100. In most patients this has been accomplished with no more than 6 exchanges of about one plasma volume each, replaced with 5 percent albumin and normal saline, carried out three times per week. We have treated patients undergoing plasmapheresis with 60 mg of oral prednisone daily for 2 weeks followed by 100 mg on alternate days, gradually tapered over 1 to 2 months. Serum antibody titers are determined before beginning plasmapheresis and 12 to 24 hours after each plasma exchange. CSF antibody titers are determined before plasmapheresis and 24 to 48 hours following the final exchange. Patients who exhibit no objective evidence of neurologic benefit should have steroids tapered and discontinued more quickly. We have not used other immunosuppressive agents such as azathioprine or cyclophosphamide, but these agents have not been effective in the hands of other workers.

SUPPORTIVE THERAPY

The profound neurologic impairment produced by most paraneoplastic neurologic syndromes is usually a much greater cause of patient disability than either the effects of chemotherapy and radiation therapy or the associated tumor at any point up to its terminal stages. Patients with autonomic failure (usually in the setting of type IIa antibody and small cell lung carcinoma) are at risk for respiratory failure, which may occur without premonitory symptoms. Patients with cerebellar or brain stem syndromes are at risk for aspiration. Profound gastroparesis may develop in patients with either type IIa or type IIb antibody responses. Patients with severe sensory or cerebellar ataxia or with myelitis may remain at bed rest for protracted periods. In such patients, we routinely use small doses of heparin to prevent deep venous thrombosis, and we work closely with the nursing staff to prevent development of decubitus ulcers. Careful passive physical therapy during the subacute phase of the illness, and aggressive, prolonged therapy at a rehabilitation facility, including gait training and appropriate strengthening exercises, are essential to enable patients to achieve optimal use of residual neurologic capabilities. For many patients, however, improvement over time is extremely limited. Issues of disability, concurrent depression, and need for social support are major concerns of patients with paraneoplastic neurologic syndromes who survive their cancer. The obscure nature of the disease and fear of cancer are sources of frustration for patients and family. Compassionate patient and family support from the physician is crucial during the early stages of the illness, when the diagnosis is being made, and during long-term care, to help them deal with the medical, social, and economic ravages of the disease.

SUGGESTED READING

Anderson NE, Cunningham JM, Posner JB. Autoimmune pathogenesis of paraneoplastic neurological syndromes. CRC Crit Rev Clin Neurobiol 1987; 3:245–299.

Greenlee JE, Brashear HR. Antibodies to cerebellar Purkinje cells in patients with paraneoplastic cerebellar degeneration and ovarian carcinoma. Ann Neurol 1983; 14:609–613.

Henson RA, Urich H. Cancer and the nervous system: The neurological manifestations of systemic malignant disease. Boston: Blackwell, 1982.

Luque FA, Furneaux HM, Ferziger AB, et al. Anti-Ri: An antibody associated with paraneoplastic opsoclonus and breast cancer. Ann Neurol 1991; 29:241–251.

PATIENT RESOURCES

The following are laboratories that perform antineuronal antibody assays:

Genica Pharmaceuticals Corporation
Two Biotech Park
373 Plantation St.
Worcester, Massachusetts 01605-9948

Mayo Medical Laboratories
Mayo Clinic
200 First St. SW
Rochester, Minnesota 55905

Specialty Laboratories
2211 Michigan Ave.
Santa Monica, California 90404-3900

University of Virginia Laboratories
Laboratory Special Services
Room 1774 Old Medical School
UVA Hospitals
Charlottesville, Virginia 22908

Neurovirology Research Laboratory (151B)
John E. Greenlee, M.D.
Veterans Affairs Medical Center
500 Foothill Drive
Salt Lake City, Utah 84148

Cancer Neuroimmunology Laboratory
Kurt A. Jaeckle, M.D.
Department of Neurology
University of Utah Medical Center
50 North Medical Drive
Salt Lake City, Utah 84132

PRIMARY CENTRAL NERVOUS SYSTEM LYMPHOMA

MICHAEL L. GRUBER, M.D.
FRED H. HOCHBERG, M.D.

Primary central nervous system lymphoma (PCNSL) is a non-Hodgkin's lymphoma of B-cell origin that arises in the absence of apparent systemic lymphoma. PCNSL accounts for 1 percent of primary intracranial neoplasms. The tumor may involve the brain, the vitreous and retina of the eye, the meninges and ependyma, or, rarely, the spinal cord. In contrast, systemic lymphoma spreads to the epidural space, causing spinal cord compression, invades the meninges, and in 1 to 2 percent of cases directly invades the brain or spinal cord. In the past 15 years, the incidence of PCNSL has increased threefold in apparently immunocompetent patients.

Its association with congenital and acquired (drug- or disease-induced) immunosuppression has also resulted in significantly more cases. PCNSL occurs in 3 percent of the acquired immunodeficiency syndrome (AIDS) population and currently fully one-fifth of all cases of PCNSL are AIDS related. Increased risk of PCNSL accompanies immunosuppression of transplant recipients and chronic granulomatous, inflammatory, and vasculitic diseases. The Epstein-Barr virus genome is identified in biopsy tissue from 80 percent of immunosuppressed patients, suggesting a role for this virus in tumor development.

PCNSL most commonly presents with symptoms related to an intracranial tumor mass and ventricular obstruction. Personality change, a prominent symptom, is seen in 24 percent of patients on admission and in 60 percent whose disease progresses. Tumor deposits in supratentorial locations are three times more common than those in infratentorial sites. There is a predilection for involvement of the periventricular region, corpus callosum, thalamus, and basal ganglia. One-third to half of the patients have multiple lesions, but the margins of these infiltrative deposits are often ill-defined. Infiltration of the vitreous or retina is seen in 15 to 20 percent of patients and may precede brain involvement. As many as 25 percent of newly diagnosed patients have lymphomatous involvement of the meninges. Cytologic techniques may not distinguish between reactive and malignant lymphocytes, and for this reason may provide false-negative results.

The diagnosis is suggested by contrast-enhanced cranial imaging by computed tomography (CT) and magnetic resonance imaging (MRI). Cell surface marker studies of cerebrospinal fluid (CSF) and/or vitreous fluid can identify tumor lymphocytes bearing B-cell monoclonal immunoglobulins in 10 percent of cases. Polymerase chain reaction methods may identify immunoglobulin gene rearrangements. The response to a trial of corticosteroid therapy can be used as a diagnostic test. Dexamethasone, 24 mg per day for 5 days, may result in complete resolution of a radiographic lesion. The benefit often occurs within hours of treatment. Patients treated in this fashion may remain asymptomatic for 6 months or longer, but they generally suffer relapse 1 to 2 weeks after cessation of steroid therapy. In most patients, diagnosis is made following brain biopsy. Staging of patients with PCNSL should include slit-lamp examination of the vitreous, immunocytologic study of the cerebrospinal fluid (CSF), and serologic testing for syphilis and human immunodeficiency virus type 1 (HIV-1) antibody. Routine bone marrow aspiration and CT of the chest and abdomen are not required. In our experience, 10 percent of patients develop evidence of systemic lymphoma.

SURGERY

A CT-guided stereotactic biopsy is the preferred surgical procedure when PCNSL is considered. When it is clinically feasible, corticosteroid therapy should be withheld until after tissue is obtained. Steroids stabilize the blood-brain barrier and have a cytolytic effect on the tumor that may result in disappearance of the parenchymal brain lesions. This creates a problem for the surgeon, who then may no longer have a target from which to take a biopsy specimen; as a result, the pathologist frequently receives tissue that is not diagnostic.

Resection does not improve survival and subjects the patient to the unwarranted risk of mortality and morbidity. On the occasion of communicating or obstructive hydrocephalus or the definition of meningeal or ventricular ependymal tumor, an Ommaya reservoir is emplaced in continuity with a ventriculoperitoneal shunt.

RADIATION THERAPY

Cranial irradiation frequently results in prompt clinical improvement, which can be seen in the first week of treatment following a radiation dose as small as 1,700 cGy. Unfortunately, the tumor recurs in more than 90 percent of cases. In a recent study, the Radiation Therapy Oncology Group (RTOG) evaluated 41 patients who received 4,000 cGy whole-brain irradiation followed by 2,000 cGy to the original tumor volume and to a 2 cm margin defined by a contrast-enhanced CT scan. Median survival time was 11.6 months; 48 percent of patients survived 1 year and 28 percent 2 years. A better prognosis was associated with age younger than 60 years, solitary small masses, and a good level of preirradiation function. Tumor recurrence and treatment failure were local, within radiation fields and in the leptomeninges. The RTOG now recommends that PCNSL patients receive adjuvant chemotherapy prior to undergoing irradiation.

Radiation is the treatment of choice for vitreal or retinal lymphoma. The entire orbit to the inferior orbital ridge is included in the field, to a total dose of 2,000 cGy. This irradiation may be provided concurrently with chemotherapy.

At the Massachusetts General Hospital, cranial irradiation routinely is given after adjuvant chemotherapy is completed, but sooner if there is disease progression. Irradiation to the brain and meninges, including the inferior temporal lobes, the brain stem to the level of C2, and the posterior orbit, is provided as 180 cGy each day for a total dose of 4,140 cGy. In case of parenchymal spinal cord disease or extensive meningeal infiltration, the entire spine can be treated with 3,000 cGy at 150 cGy per day.

CHEMOTHERAPY

The best chance for prolonged survival and cure of PCNSL is initial treatment with chemotherapy. At the Massachusetts General Hospital, we provide patients M-CHOD in 21 day cycles as outlined in Table 1.

Patients are given three cycles of this regimen and then are treated with 4,140 cGy of whole-brain irradiation. In some cases, chemotherapy has been continued for an additional three cycles in lieu of radiotherapy, with good results. Careful monitoring of bone marrow (leukocyte and platelet counts every 7 days) and renal function (creatinine clearance rate before the initial cycle of treatment) is required during therapy. Contrast-enhanced brain-imaging studies (CT or MRI) are performed before the start of each treatment cycle.

Before using this regimen, Gabbai and Hochberg treated 22 patients at the Massachusetts General Hospital with preirradiation (MTX), 3.5 g per square meter every 1 to 3 weeks for three cycles, followed by radiotherapy. Two-thirds of patients exhibited a complete response, and with one exception the remainder had a partial response (decreased tumor size or stable disease). To date the median survival time is 27 months.

Large intravenous (IV) doses of MTX rapidly establish therapeutic concentrations in brain parenchyma and cerebrospinal fluid. Responses were seen in both intracranial and meningeal tumor. Toxicity was minimal and clinical improvement rapid. The development of dementia and myoclonus described in patients given MTX after radiotherapy is rarely seen when MTX is given first. Vitreal and retinal lymphoma did not respond to chemotherapy and required orbital irradiation.

Other groups have reported on their experience

Table 1 Chemotherapy Regimen for Primary Central Nervous System Lymphoma at the Massachusetts General Hospital

Day 1	Cyclophosphamide	750 mg/m² IV
	Adriamycin	50 mg/m² IV
	Vincristine	1.4 mg/m² IV
	Dexamethasone	6 mg/m² days 1–5
Day 15	Methotrexate (MTX)	3.5 g/m² IV
Day 16	Leucovorin calcium rescue begins 24 hr after completion of the MTX infusion. This is a folic acid analogue that replenishes folate levels, competitively inhibits transmembrane transport, and competes with MTX for intracellular protein binding.	

Table 2 BTCG Protocol for Treatment of Primary Central Nervous System Lymphoma

MTX IV	3.5 g/m², weeks 1, 3, 5, 7
Vincristine IV	1.4 mg/m², weeks 1, 3, 5, 7
Procarbazine PO	100 mg/m², daily for 7 days in weeks 1, 5, 9
MTX in Ommaya reservoir	12 mg/dose, weeks 2, 4, 6, 8, 10
Dexamethasone	16 mg/day, weeks 1 & 2
	12 mg/day, weeks 3 & 4
	8 mg/day, weeks 5 & 6
	6 mg/day, weeks 7 thru first 4 weeks of XRT and then fully tapered.

Whole-brain irradiation will be provided approximately 10 weeks from start of chemotherapy. The total dose will be 5,040 cGy, delivered in 28 treatments of 180 cGy.
↓
Cytosine arabinoside (ara-c) 3 g/m² IV, one dose per day for 2 consecutive days
↓
Rest 3 weeks
↓
Cytosine arabinoside 3 g/m² IV, one dose per day for 2 consecutive days

with preirradiation chemotherapy using other regimens, and virtually all identify the same percentage of responders, and survival is simply an effect of the duration of follow-up. The Brain Tumor Cooperative Group proposes the therapy outlined in Table 2.

EVALUATION AND TREATMENT OF PCNSL IN IMMUNOSUPPRESSED PERSONS

PCNSL is seen in AIDS, inherited disorders such as Wiskott-Aldrich syndrome, autoimmune illnesses including systemic lupus erythematosus, granulomatous diseases like sarcoidosis, and during drug-induced immunosuppression for transplant surgery. The clinical picture closely resembles the disease seen in immunocompetent patients, though the lesions seen on cranial imaging studies are not easily differentiated from those of toxoplasmosis or from abscesses of bacterial or fungal origin.

If toxoplasmosis is considered in an AIDS patient, a therapeutic trial of antibiotics is provided and the brain-imaging studies are repeated. If there is no response, CT-guided stereotactic biopsy is performed. Once a diagnosis is made, definitive treatment is provided. Chemotherapy with large doses of MTX, 3.5 g per square meter, has been used safely and with good results in patients with AIDS or AIDS-related complex who have a high CD4 lymphocyte count in the absence of concurrent infection with opportunistic organisms or other neoplasms. At the University of California at San Francisco, unirradiated AIDS patients with PCNSL survived 42 days, compared to 134 days for patients given radiotherapy. A complete or partial response was seen in 70 percent of irradiated patients, and stable disease in 22 percent. For most of these patients, death resulted from opportunistic infection.

Radiation treatment is provided to the whole brain, which includes the posterior orbits, brain, and meninges to the level of C2, as either (1) 150 cGy per day to a total of 4,000 cGy followed by a boost of 2,000 cGy to the tumor bed, or (2) 180 to 200 cGy per day to a total dose of 4,000 cGy. In the transplant population, changes in the use or dosage of the immunosuppressive drugs (e.g., cyclosporine, prednisone, azathioprine) frequently results in disappearance of the lymphomatous deposits.

SUGGESTED READING

DeAngelis LM, Yahalom J, Thaler HT, Kler U. Combined modality therapy for primary CNS lymphoma. J Clin Oncol 1992; 10:635–643.

Gabbai AA, Hochberg FH, Linggood RM, et al. High dose methotrexate for non-AIDS primary central nervous system lymphoma. J Neurosurg 1989; 70:190–194.

Hochberg FH, Loeffler JS, Prados M. The therapy of primary brain lymphoma. J Neurooncol 1991; 10:191–201.

Hochberg FH, Miller DC. Primary central nervous system lymphoma. J Neurosurg 1988; 68:835–853.

Rosenblum ML, Levy RM, Bredesen DE. AIDS and the nervous system. New York: Raven Press, 1988:10.

MOVEMENT DISORDERS

PARKINSON'S DISEASE

MATTHEW B. STERN, M.D.

Parkinson's disease (PD) has remained in the forefront of chronic neurodegenerative disorders since the discovery of levodopa replacement therapy in the late 1960s. Indeed, the steady flow of novel therapeutic strategies for PD and basic research advances have fueled the rapid growth of movement disorders as a neurologic subspecialty. Particularly promising is the recent focus on prophylactic and restorative therapies that are designed to alter the natural history of disease rather than merely treat the symptoms. Moreover, symptomatic treatment of PD has undergone steady refinement in recent years, so that today effective control of disability is achieved while the chances of long-term adverse reactions such as motor fluctuations and dyskinesias are minimized. The clinical approach to PD therefore requires increasing skill in early diagnosis as well as an understanding of the risks and benefits of symptomatic therapies.

LEVODOPA—25 YEARS LATER

The primary biochemical defect in PD is the loss of striatal dopamine, resulting from degeneration of dopamine-producing cells in the substantia nigra. Consequently, the neurotransmitter balance in the brain is altered and clinical symptoms emerge. While inhibiting acetylcholine with anticholinergic compounds was a modestly effective therapy until the late 1960s, the introduction of levodopa as replacement therapy revolutionized treatment and shifted the emphasis toward newer techniques to enhance dopaminergic transmission.

Levodopa combined with carbidopa (a peripheral dopa decarboxylase inhibitor) remains the cornerstone of drug therapy for PD. Its effects can be dramatic, enabling many patients to regain a substantial degree of motor function. While the gastrointestinal side effects of levodopa were largely eliminated by combining levodopa

with carbidopa (Sinemet), the simple and complex motor fluctuations associated with long-term levodopa therapy have proved to be the major therapeutic challenge to clinicians who treat PD patients, and have fostered the ongoing controversy of early versus late introduction of levodopa therapy. While an array of well-described phenomena complicate chronic levodopa therapy, the most common adverse effects include dyskinesias, end-of-dose deterioration (the *wearing-off* effect), and random fluctuations (the *on-off* effect). Numerous studies have attempted to explain the pathophysiology of levodopa-related complications: do they result from chronic, intermittent receptor stimulation and pharmacodynamic alterations, or are they the consequence of disease progression with eventual loss of storage capacity and pharmacokinetic changes? Undoubtedly, disease progression and duration and dose of levodopa therapy—contribute to motor fluctuations. Furthermore, the marked variability in clinical manifestations and rate of progression have hampered our ability to resolve the controversy. Nevertheless, an acceptable "middle ground" is to begin levodopa therapy when a patient's disability affects social or occupational function; this tailors the decision to the individual patient's needs. The dose should be kept low (<500 to 700 mg), and other antiparkinsonian agents should be added early, to combat emerging motor fluctuations (see below). An alternative but acceptable approach, is to begin symptomatic therapy with secondary antiparkinsonian agents (amantadine, anticholinergics) or dopamine agonists (bromocriptine, pergolide) in an attempt to defer the introduction of levodopa, which, in virtually all PD patients, becomes inevitable within 1 to 2 years.

Controlled-Release Levodopa

Controlled-release levodopa preparations were developed in response to observations that continuous dopaminergic stimulation improved motor fluctuations in PD and more closely approximated physiologic conditions. Controlled-release Sinemet (Sinemet CR) and Madopar HBS (hydrodynamically balanced system) have proved to be the most effective of the controlled-release levodopa preparations and have been available for prescription since 1991. Because the bioavailability of

242

levodopa in controlled-release form is about one-third less than that of standard preparations, the total daily dose requirement for levodopa as Sinemet CR is increased, despite the need for fewer daily doses. Advantages of controlled-release preparations include increased total "on" time, improved nocturnal and early morning mobility, and longer dose intervals. However, patients with more advanced PD who already experience dyskinesias and fluctuations are vulnerable to increased involuntary movements and a diminished sense of control over their symptoms. Many patients, therefore, prefer standard preparations or a combination of standard and controlled-release levodopa.

Perhaps more importantly, the maintenance of more continuous levodopa levels with controlled-release levodopa may prove to be a more appropriate strategy for treating PD patients with previously untreated disease. Preliminary observations suggest that this approach avoids some of the eventual response fluctuations and dyskinesias associated with standard preparations. I therefore begin symptomatic therapy with controlled-release Sinemet 50/200, one-half tablet twice daily. The dose can then be titrated to two to four tablets daily. Standard Sinemet, dopamine agonists, or secondary antiparkinsonian drugs can be supplemented when control becomes inadequate (Fig. 1).

DOPAMINE AGONISTS

While levodopa's effectiveness depends on its enzymatic conversion to dopamine in nigrostriatal neurons, dopamine agonists directly stimulate the dopamine receptor. The development of this class of compounds

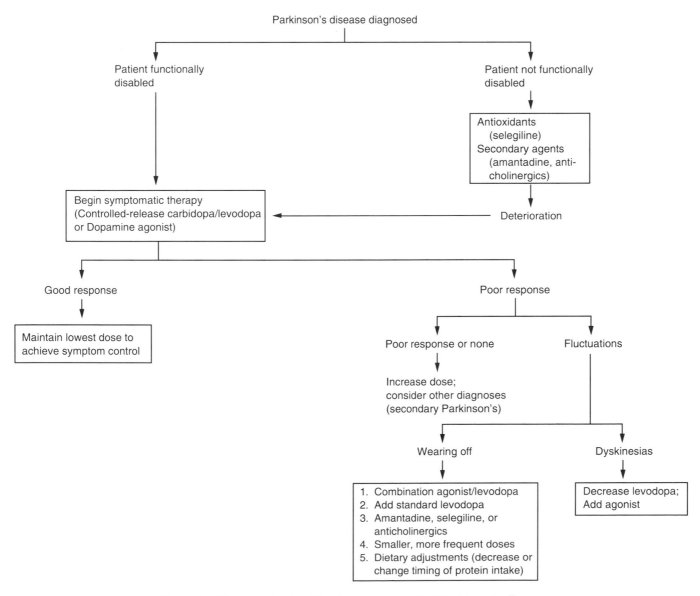

Figure 1 Therapeutic algorithm for management of Parkinson's disease.

has been fueled by levodopa's limitations. Dopamine agonists are not dependent on presynaptic, degenerating dopaminergic neurons; they have long half-lives and are capable of stimulating specific subclasses of dopamine receptors. Dopamine agonists also have the theoretical advantage of sparing the potentially harmful effects of levodopa. By reducing the turnover of dopamine, dopamine agonists might reduce the accumulation of hydrogen peroxide and free radicals, the toxic by-products of dopamine metabolism.

Numerous dopamine agonists have been developed, but only bromocriptine and pergolide are commercially available in the United States. Bromocriptine is an ergot alkaloid with potent D2-receptor agonist properties; pergolide is an ergot preparation that is more potent than bromocriptine and, in addition to stimulating the D2 receptor, pergolide also has partial effects at the D1 receptor. Both drugs appear to be equipotent in clinical studies, and they produce comparable arrays of dopaminergic side effects, including nausea, orthostatic hypotension, confusion, and hallucinations. Although not available in the United States, domperidone is particularly effective in alleviating the gastrointestinal side effects associated with dopamine agonists.

While early clinical studies focused on the utility of dopamine agonists in patients with advanced PD and clinical fluctuations, more recent experience favors their use earlier in the course of disease. An acceptable strategy, for example, is to begin symptomatic therapy with a dopamine agonist, which can, in some instances, delay the need for levodopa for 1 to 2 years. Although few patients can be maintained on dopamine agonists alone for any length of time because of an inadequate clinical response, the combination of levodopa with dopamine agonists has proved to be a useful strategy for taking advantage of levodopa's more potent antiparkinsonian effects while keeping the dose low and avoiding, or at least delaying, the emergence of levodopa-related adverse effects.

In PD patients who are experiencing ineffective symptom control on Sinemet CR (three to four tablets daily) or standard Sinemet (25/100, four to five tablets daily), bromocriptine (Parlodel), 1.25 mg daily, or pergolide (Permax), 0.05 mg daily, may be added and increased slowly (to 15 to 30 mg per day for bromocriptine; 2 to 6 mg for pergolide) until adequate control is achieved.

The future of dopamine agonist therapy in PD is related to our increasing understanding of dopamine receptor subtypes, which can be characterized according to their anatomic location, linkage to specific enzyme systems, and response to pharmacologic agents. Drugs that are specific to a growing number of dopamine receptors will be developed in the quest to maximize antiparkinsonian effectiveness while minimizing adverse reactions. Furthermore, dopamine agonists with prolonged action (i.e., cabergoline) are currently in development, as are transcutaneous preparations. Apomorphine, for example, is a potent D1 and D2 receptor agonist that can be administered subcutaneously. It is particularly useful for patients with advanced PD and severe, unpredictable "off" periods.

MONOAMINE OXIDASE INHIBITORS: THE LATEST CONTROVERSY

Monoamine oxidase (MAO) inhibitors have been used as adjunctive therapy in PD since the mid 1970s. Selegiline (deprenyl) inhibits type B MAO, thus avoiding the dangers of tyramine-induced hypertensive crisis while inhibiting the catabolism of brain dopamine. When selegiline is used as adjunctive therapy, it should be prescribed initially in small doses (2.5 mg daily) and titrated to a maximum of 10 mg. Because of its ability to increase synaptic dopamine, its long half-life, and its metabolism into L-amphetamine and L-metamphetamine, patients can experience untoward effects, including dyskinesias and hallucinations. Therefore, attempts should be made to reduce the dose of levodopa. While selegiline improves motor fluctuations and allows reduction of the levodopa dose, improvement is generally modest and the effects short lived (6 to 12 months).

Interest in selegiline, other MAO inhibitors, and antioxidant therapy blossomed in the late 1980s as a result of a series of observations that implicated oxidative reactions in the causation of PD. Selegiline was found to delay the need for symptomatic therapy with levodopa in patients with early PD (the DATATOP study), suggesting that antioxidant therapies might actually alter the natural history of PD by slowing its natural rate of progression. The mildly symptomatic effects of selegiline cannot be discounted, and they may to some extent explain the observed delay in need for more aggressive treatment. On the other hand, most of the dopamine neuronal system has already degenerated by the time the diagnosis of PD is made. In a sense, the damage has already been done. Whether or not preclinical diagnosis and earlier intervention with "prophylactic therapies" will effectively slow disease progression remains to be seen. Because the scientific rationale for antioxidant therapy in PD remains sound, I begin a patient newly diagnosed with PD on selegiline, 5 mg twice daily, with the caveat that ongoing clinical trials with MAO inhibitors and other antioxidants will undoubtedly refine our approach to early PD.

A WORD ABOUT FLUCTUATIONS AND DYSKINESIAS

The primary goal of symptomatic PD therapy is to improve motor function and avoid levodopa-related adverse effects. Nevertheless, fluctuations and dyskinesias remain the major therapeutic challenge to clinicians treating patients with PD. While our emphasis has appropriately shifted to early management and prevention of diabling fluctuations, it remains common to encounter patients who take frequent, large doses of levodopa for whom each dose produces short-lived action or prominent dyskinesias, or both. Introducing a dopamine agonist is an appropriate first approach to these patients, although titration of the agonist must be accompanied by a concomitant reduction of levodopa if dyskinesias prevail. The addition of controlled-release levodopa, often in combination with standard levodopa preparations, is useful for patients for whom the levodopa effect is short-lived, although the accumulation of levodopa associated with the controlled-release form can often exacerbate dyskinesias. Secondary anti-parkinsonian medications such as amantadine, selegiline, and anticholinergics are also occasionally helpful in the fluctuating patient. Despite the risk of adverse mental effects, anticholinergics can be useful for prominent tremor. Similarly, amantadine has occasionally resulted in marked amelioration of dyskinesias and motor dysfunction in patients with advanced disease and complex fluctuations.

In some patients fluctuations are related to food intake, presumably because of competition with large-chain, neutral amino acids for transport in the gut or across the blood-brain barrier. A reduction in dietary protein, with careful coordination of meals and timing of medication, is often helpful.

Finally, patients' reports of their own fluctuations may vary from those of an objective observer. In some cases, it is appropriate to observe a patient over hours or days to fully understand the pattern of fluctuations and make a rational therapeutic choice.

DEPRESSION, DEMENTIA, AND HALLUCINATIONS

Cognitive problems are universally encountered in PD. Depression affects many patients during the course of their illness and is often overlooked because psychomotor retardation, anorexia, insomnia, and poor concentration are mistaken for PD symptoms. Depression should be treated aggressively with pharmacotherapy, such as tricyclic agents, psychotherapy, and, for severely depressed patients, electroconvulsive therapy (ECT). ECT often produces dramatic improvements in mood and motor function, although its effect on PD symptoms is generally short lived.

Dementia of the Alzheimer's type occurs in approximately 20 percent of PD patients, despite the high frequency of abnormalities detected on formal neuropsychological tests. It is important to consider that confusion, sleep disturbance, frightening nightmares, and hallucinations can also be the consequence of antiparkinsonian medications, particularly anticholinergic compounds. While they frequently require hospitalization and a reduction in medication, in some patients psychotic symptoms induced by dopaminergic compounds can also be treated effectively with the atypical antipsychotic, clozaril. Although somewhat difficult to prescribe because of the necessity for frequent blood monitoring (some cases of agranulocytosis), small doses of clozaril (<50 mg) at bedtime, can ameliorate

insomnia and dopamine-induced hallucinations, and occasionally improve PD symptoms such as tremor.

NONMEDICAL MANAGEMENT

A crucial aspect of managing PD is to employ the wide range of ancillary services available to help the patient cope with the myriad physical, emotional, and psychosocial problems associated with the disease. Physical, speech, and occupational therapy all have key roles in the treatment of PD. The treating physician should be prepared to make appropriate referrals as the disease progresses and assistance in specific areas is required.

The fear, anxiety, denial, and false hope for a cure associated with the initial diagnosis require a comprehensive approach that emphasizes patient education. Well-informed patients undoubtedly fare better in the long run than those who choose the course of physical and emotional isolation. Problems with self-image, changing role in the family, employment and financial concerns, and care-giving decisions are part of PD and should be addressed with appropriate counseling. Patient and care giver support groups, educational material for patients, and the national lay organizations are all valuable resources for PD management (see Patient Resources). The national PD lay societies are particularly helpful in linking patients and their families to local support groups and specialized health care services and providing educational materials on all aspects of PD, including medical treatment, self-help strategies, and research advances.

TOWARD THE FUTURE: SURGICAL AND RESTORATIVE THERAPIES

While advances in pharmacotherapy continue, there is renewed interest in the neurosurgical approach to PD. Although stereotactic thalamotomy was largely abandoned with the development of effective antiparkinsonian medications, refinements in neurosurgical technique—and a clearer understanding of the neurophysiology of the basal ganglia—have ushered in a new era of functional neurosurgery. Early investigations in this area suggest that selected patients may benefit from lesions in the medial globus pallidus or subthalamic nuclei.

Neurosurgery also provides the means for cell implantation in PD, a novel strategy designed to both augment dopamine delivery to the striatum and restore essential nutrients to regenerate or preserve neuronal tissue. A growing number of investigators are pursuing the basic and clinical science of neurotransplantation. Clinical studies have already determined that autologous adrenal medullary transplantation is only modestly effective, but studies using fetal cells are under way, and initial results are promising. Moreover, genetically engineered cell lines designed to deliver both dopamine and specific neurotrophic factors may ultimately prove to be the most effective transplantable tissue.

REMARKS

The remarkable achievements in PD treatment have consistently refined our pharmacologic approach to affected patients. It seems almost contrary to traditional medical teaching that the management of PD from the outset often requires a *combination* of drugs aimed at effective symptom control, prevention of long-term disability, and even slowing of disease progression. New medical and surgical therapies now focus on altering the natural history of PD, and we are using terms such as *neuroprotective, prophylactic,* and *restorative* to describe these novel strategies. Even the most astute among us will be challenged to stay abreast of this rapidly evolving field.

SUGGESTED READING

Koller WC, ed. Handbook of Parkinson's disease. New York: Marcel Dekker, 1992.
Koller WC, Paulson G, eds. Therapy of Parkinson's disease. New York: Marcel Dekker, 1990.
Olanow CW, Lieberman AN, eds. The scientific basis for the treatment of Parkinson's disease. Park Ridge, NJ: Parthenon, 1992.
Stern MB, Hurtig HI, eds. The comprehensive management of Parkinson's disease. New York: PMA, 1988.

PATIENT RESOURCES

National Parkinson Foundation
1501 N.W. 9th Ave.
Bob Hope Road
Miami, Florida 33136-9990
Telephone: (800) 327-4545

The American Parkinson Disease Association
60 Bay St.
Suite 401
Staten Island, New York 10301
Telephone: (800) 223-2732

Parkinson's Disease Foundation
650 W. 168th St.
New York, New York 10032
Telephone: (800) 457-6676

United Parkinson Foundation
360 W. Superior St.
Chicago, Illinois 60610
Telephone: (312) 664-2344

Parkinson's Education Program USA
1800 Park Newport, No. 302
Newport Beach, California 92660
Telephone: (800) 344-7872

SYMPTOMATIC TREATMENTS FOR HUNTINGTON'S DISEASE

SUSAN E. FOLSTEIN, M.D.
CAROL E. PEYSER, M.D.

Huntington's disease (HD) is an inherited neuropsychiatric disorder characterized by abnormalities of movement, cognition, and mood. It is inherited as an autosomal-dominant trait, so each offspring of an affected person, regardless of sex, has a 50 percent chance of inheriting the HD gene and eventually being affected. Symptoms begin most commonly between age 35 and 50 years, but they can begin any time during childhood or adolescence (10 percent) or in old age (10 percent), when they can then be confused with senile chorea. The incidence overall is about 5 or 6 per 100,000 population; the adult population rate is about 12 per 100,000. The average duration of illness is 16 years, although some patients survive for 40 years. The most common cause of death is related to complications of dysphagia. The pathognomonic neuropathology is neuronal loss and atrophy in the neostriatum; however, after many years of illness, atrophy can be widespread. Neuron loss has been documented in cortex, cerebellum, and brain stem. The pathogenesis of HD is unknown.

CLINICAL FEATURES AND COURSE OF ILLNESS

The onset of HD is insidious, often several years in developing, and the presentation may include motor, cognitive, or psychiatric abnormalities or any combination of the three. Diagnosis, though straightforward in a well-developed case with a known family history, can be difficult during the early stages of the illness. The diagnosis is easier if the patient presents with chorea, but many present with clumsiness, bradykinesia, falling, a depressive syndrome, apathy, irritability and aggression, hallucinations (especially in adolescents), or complaining that they cannot think quickly and efficiently. As the disease progresses, however, the characteristic features become more obvious. The motor disorder progresses from mild involuntary movements, usually involving distal muscles, to more frequent and higher-amplitude movements involving more proximal muscles and trunk. Abnormal eye movements and loss of control of voluntary movements progress more predictably than does chorea. Saccadic eye movements become slow and hypometric; eventually patients cannot move their eyes at all. Patients become gradually more clumsy, dysarthric, dysphagic, and ataxic. All body movements, as well as thought, become bradykinetic, until, after many years of illness the patient is bedridden, akinetic, and mute. At this stage chorea may be absent, or present only when the patient is agitated.

The cognitive disorder also progresses gradually. The initial complaints of slow and inefficient thinking can often be documented only on neuropsychologic tests that require speed and changes in strategy. These cognitive changes are disabling for employment. With time, cognition is affected more globally; however, many advanced HD patients can understand simple conversation and recognize their families and surroundings, even though their speech becomes increasingly sparse.

Huntington's disease can present with changes only in emotions, and during the first half of the illness these are often the most distressing features. Patients commonly complain of depressed mood, accompanied by sleep and appetite disturbance, loss of energy, and low self-esteem. Occasionally, patients have depressive delusions (e.g., of cancer or poverty) and the high suicide rate in HD patients is largely attributable to severe depression. About 40 percent of HD patients have such episodes. For approximately 10 percent of patients the mood disorder is bipolar. The hypomanic spells are usually short, but severe mania occasionally is seen.

Some HD patients who are apathetic appear to be depressed because of their slow responses and blank faces, but they deny feeling low and do not have the accompanying sleep disturbance and low self-esteem. Other patients have a "short fuse," becoming angry at slight provocations and remaining so for prolonged periods; a few become dangerously aggressive. Irritability also can be an aspect of a depressive syndrome. Somewhat counterintuitively, patients can be both apathetic and irritable. Quiet and immobile if left alone, they can become angry quickly if their routine is interrupted or if a request is not quickly attended to. Most patients gradually become sexually impotent and uninterested, but a few have strong sexual interest and make constant sexual demands. Others develop abnormal sexual behavior.

EMPIRICAL TREATMENTS

Because the pathogenesis of HD is unknown, treatments are symptomatic and based on clinical experience. Though these treatments cannot forestall the inexorable progression of illness, they are extremely helpful in maintaining the quality of life for HD patients, who must live with the illness for many years. The treatments also ease the burden on family care givers,

who may care for two or even three generations of patients.

It has been common practice for physicians to prescribe only one class of drugs (neuroleptics, traditionally haloperidol) for HD in all of its manifestations. Though neuroleptics can decrease the amplitude of chorea, they are not helpful in treating most other aspects of the illness and can even aggravate several of the signs and symptoms. Each patient must be individually assessed, so that a specific treatment plan can be formulated to address the case-specific symptoms. This plan requires re-evaluation based on the patient's initial response and on changes in symptoms as the illness progresses. Treatment approaches that are appropriate for patients early in the course can be ineffective or even counterproductive later. Also, new symptoms appear that need treatment, and others gradually wane so that treatments for them can be discontinued.

Both pharmacologic treatments and a careful organization of the patient's environment can help alleviate symptoms. For the most part, different treatments are needed for each of the three clinical features—the movement disorder, the dementia, and the abnormalities of mood and perception.

Treatment of the Motor Disorder

Early in the course, the motor disorder does not result in loss of function and generally should not be treated at all. Small doses of neuroleptics usually decrease the amplitude of chorea in mildly affected patients, but these drugs may exacerbate the clumsiness and gait disturbance. Many patients feel dysphoric or drowsy when taking neuroleptics. An occasional patient whose disease is early in its course and who is working (otherwise successfully) worries that the involuntary movements will be noticed. These patients can be treated with very small doses (e.g., 1 mg to start) of fluphenazine. Doses of more than 10 mg do not result in any further improvement of chorea, regardless of its severity; are associated with extrapyramidal side effects such as bradykinesia, rigidity, and akathisia; and carry the risk of tardive dyskinesia. The latter condition can usually be noticed by perioral movements, which are otherwise uncommon in HD.

After a few years with HD, patients' motor response time becomes too slow to allow them safely to drive a car. As the gait disorder worsens (either from chorea or from hypertonia and ataxia), they are at risk for falls and consequent subdural hematomas or broken bones. Most patients stubbornly resist the family's attempts to get them to stop driving, use stair rails, avoid stairs, and use assistive devices such as canes, wheelchairs, and bathroom safety equipment. They are much more likely to respond to a doctor's order. Therefore, rather than suggesting these interventions, physicians should *tell* the patient that these safeguards must be instituted.

Later in the course, some patients develop extremely high-amplitude and continuous choreiform movements. This activity is exhausting and debilitating, and, along with dysphagia, probably contributes to weight loss. Neuroleptic treatment should be instituted, but, again, large doses are unlikely to be more effective than more modest ones and can aggravate existing hypertonia and bradykinesia. As time passes, the chorea becomes relatively unresponsive to neuroleptics, probably because the target receptors are depleted. Such patients occasionally respond to large doses of reserpine, but it should be used with caution in those who have suffered depression. Patients derive the most relief from involuntary movements by being placed in a quiet, highly predictable environment that is free of noise and unexpected stimuli. At this terminal stage of illness, in which the patient may survive several years, it will be very tiring to maintain an upright posture, and the time spent in a chair should be brief. Beds and chairs must be padded. Some patients persist, despite all pleas, in attempting to get out of chairs and beds without assistance. Others fall out of bed because of chorea and can become entangled in the sheets. Falls out of bed can be avoided by placing the bed very close to or actually on the floor, and placing padding around it. This, however, may make it difficult to lift the patient without mechanical assistance.

Treatment of Cognitive Impairment

There is no particular medication that improves patients' slow and inefficient thinking, though these impairments can clearly become worse (as can involuntary movements) in situations where the patient is called upon to perform cognitive tasks. Patients experience significant relief on retiring from a job that has become too taxing. The problem for the physician is to be able to document the cognitive difficulties in a way that is convincing to reviewers of disability applications. Detailed neuropsychological batteries that include tests that require speed and set changes, such as the Wisconsin Card Sort, Trailmaking Test, and the Hopkins Verbal Learning often show marked impairment, even when IQ scores are still well within the normal range. We believe it is most helpful to talk to the patient's employer, who will be able to give many examples of tasks that the patient can no longer perform.

Some patients no longer experience their thinking as a problem after they stop working and their activities become less cognitively demanding. Some get a headache when they attempt exacting cognitive tasks, but usually they become extremely anxious, irritable, and even confused, and may lash out impulsively. This irritability is not limited to the workplace and, in fact, can be more prominent at home. Such outbursts often subside almost entirely as soon as the patient stops working.

A related problem with thinking early in the illness is deciding among several alternatives. Couples are often accustomed to discussing such decisions, but as the HD patient has more trouble thinking this sort of discussion leads to arguments or outbursts of anger because the patient finds it too difficult to think through a problem or because the patient's judgment has become unpredictable. Spouses should be encouraged to limit such discussions and take over the family's domestic planning and decisions. Ideally, this transition is accomplished in a diplomatic way, to minimize its effect on the patient's self-esteem.

As the illness worsens it becomes difficult to understand the patient's speech. Families and other care givers use several strategies. When speech is still relatively intact, comprehensibility can be improved by calming the patient and asking him or her to speak slowly. Later, sentence or letter boards can be devised that include the patient's most common requests. Some patients can spell or write words they cannot speak distinctly.

Treatment of Emotional Disorders

Major Affective Disorder

Many patients have the symptoms of major depression. As in non-HD patients, depression is sometimes psychologically understandable in light of the diagnosis, loss of employment, or limitation of independent living (e.g., cessation of driving). These mood disorders, however, are usually short lived and do not meet the criteria for the syndrome of major depression described above. Depressions often occur in episodes and respond to antidepressant drugs. It would seem logical, given that HD is probably caused by the same gene in all patients, that everyone would respond to the same medication, but this is not the case. In our clinic, we start with nortriptyline, 25 mg at bedtime, and increase the dose as needed to achieve a therapeutic blood level. Should nortriptyline be ineffective or intolerable, we prescribe fluoxetine (Prozac), 20 mg per day, and adjust the dose as needed. Some patients become unable to sleep on that dose and do well on 20 mg every other day; other patients require 40 mg per day. (Weight should be monitored very carefully in patients taking fluoxetine.) Most patients respond to one of these drugs, but we have needed to treat an occasional patient with monoamine oxidase inhibitors. Patients who have depressive delusions or who are so bradykinetic from depression that they are not eating adequately, can be given electroconvulsive treatment (ECT), and they usually respond well. There are no contraindications to ECT in HD patients.

Some patients with bipolar disease do not need pharmacologic treatment for their spells of high mood, which are brief and not associated with dangerous behavior. For those who need treatment, lithium carbonate has rarely been effective in our hands. Carbamazepine is more likely to control the manic episodes. Again, dosing begins cautiously with 100 mg at bedtime and is gradually increased based on symptomatic response and side effects (mainly drowsiness). It is not necessary to achieve the therapeutic range required for seizure control, nor is it necessary to stay within that range. Patients taking carbamazepine need regular monitoring for leukopenia.

Obsessions and Compulsions

An occasional HD patient presents with, or later develops, classic obsessive-compulsive disorder (OCD) with intrusive thoughts and worries that lead to constant checking of lights, locks, or bank papers or to excessive washing and cleaning. Patients so affected usually respond to fluoxetine. To date we have little experience in treating OCD in HD with clomipramine, but we would be glad for information from other clinicians.

Irritability and Aggression

Patients who exhibit irritability and aggression are probably more likely than any other HD patients to be institutionalized long term. Family reports suggest that irritability is somewhat more common in patients who were short-tempered before their HD began. As described in the section on Treatment of Cognitive Impairment, these symptoms can be precipitated when patients are challenged with tasks that are too difficult. Other precipitants include noisy, unpredictable households (common when there are young children), pre-existing marital discord, and unexpected changes in the patient's routine. Some families are able to minimize the occurrence of such precipitants; others cannot.

Some patients for whom environmental manipulations do not suffice do calm down in response to medication. Again, not everyone responds to the same medication. Some patients can be managed with neuroleptics, but these are not the first choice, for reasons mentioned in the discussion of Treatment of the Movement Disorder. Many patients respond to Tegretol, but it makes an occasional patient even more irritable. Some clinicians have reported success with Prozac, but it must be used with particular care in patients with advanced disease, because it can cause weight loss.

Some patients are not particularly irritable in general but become angry when care givers refuse to respond to an unreasonable request, which the patient will make persistently and repetitively, with gradually increasing emotion. One patient became angry every time his wife took him to the supermarket, because the clerk would not "double bag" the groceries. Another patient insisted on keeping two extra cases of soda in the pantry and would become angry when the supply fell below that amount. Other patients become preoccupied with cigarettes. This kind of irritability is much more difficult to treat by environmental manipulation and does not respond particularly well to medication.

If aggressive patients do not respond to a combination of environmental simplification and medication, they may need to live away from home. Some can be better managed in adult foster care by persons who are not family; others require long-term hospitalization. In highly structured setting of an institution, extremely aggressive patients often calm down and require less medicine.

Abnormal Sexual Behavior

Most patients become uninterested in sexual contact, and male patients usually become impotent; some patients, however, desire and pursue very intense sexual activity. The spouse should be asked about this when the patient is not present. Wives, particularly, may be quite distressed and fearful, since male patients can become aggressive if their sexual advances are thwarted. Thus, a wife may be afraid to mention hypersexuality in the presence of her affected husband. Some men also sexually abuse their own or other children. There is no clear treatment for hypersexuality in HD patients. We have treated a few with Provera, with some success. Psychotherapeutic approaches and threats of arrest usually are not effective, probably because the sexual desires are strongly biologically driven by some aspect of the neuropathologic effects of HD. It is nevertheless important to take some action to protect the spouse and children.

MAINTAINING A POSITIVE ATTITUDE TOWARD THE PATIENT

HD patients are generally rewarding to care for, because both they and their families appreciate the ongoing support of an interested and responsive physician. Some patients are very difficult, and in all cases the illness lasts a long time—perhaps half the professional lifetime of the physician. Even the most difficult HD patients respond positively if a few general guidelines are followed. The first is to maintain an attitude of respect toward patients and to approach them in such a way that they know that you expect the same respect from them. It is easier to maintain this approach, sometimes in difficult circumstances, if you keep in mind that patients feel a terrible loss of dignity and bear a seemingly intolerable burden. Most important, patients should be reminded from time to time that you appreciate their tragic plight and admire their fortitude.

SUGGESTED READING

Barr AN, Fischer JH, Koller WC, et al. Serum haloperidol concentration and choreiform movements in Huntington's disease. Neurology 1988; 38:84–88.

Brandt J. Cognitive impairment in Huntington's disease: Insights into the neuropsychology of the striatum. In: Boller F, Grafman J, eds. The Handbook of Neuropsychology. Vol. 5. Amsterdam: Elsevier Science Publishers, 1992.

Burns A, Folstein SE, Brandt J, Folstein MF. Clinical assessment of irritability, agression, and apathy in Huntington's and Alzheimer's disease. J Nerv Ment Dis 1990; 178:20–26.

Dewhurst K, Oliver JE, McKnight AL. Sociopsychiatric consequences of Huntington's disease. Br J Psychiatry 1970; 116:255–258.

Folstein SE. Huntington's disease: A disorder of families. Baltimore: The Johns Hopkins University Press, 1989.

Folstein SE, Chase GA, Wahl WE, et al. Huntington disease in Maryland: Clinical aspects of racial variation. Am J Hum Genet 1987; 41:168–179.

Folstein SE, Jensen B, Leigh RJ, Folstein MF. The measurement of abnormal movement: Methods developed for Huntington's disease. Neurobehav Toxicol Teratol 1983; 5:605–609.

Folstein SE, Leigh RJ, Parhad IM, Folstein MF. The diagnosis of Huntington's disease. Neurology 1986; 36:1279–1283.

Leigh RJ, Newman SA, Folstein SE, et al. Abnormal ocular motor control in Huntington's disease. Neurology 1983; 33:1268–1275.

Peyser CE, Folstein SE. Depression in Huntington's disease. In: Robinson RG, Starkstein SE, eds. Depression in neurologic disease. Baltimore: The Johns Hopkins University Press, in press.

PROGRESSIVE SUPRANUCLEAR PALSY

STEPHEN G. REICH, M.D.

I didn't think that there was any treatment for progressive supranuclear palsy (PSP), is what most will think when they see a chapter on PSP in a text on therapy in neurology. In the strictest sense, PSP is "untreatable," yet that is hardly an excuse to ignore the successful care that can be rendered to patients with PSP and their families. Furthermore, patients easily detect a physician's sense of nihilism and futility. It is therefore paramount, when caring for patients with PSP, that the physician maintain a positive attitude without communicating false hope or unrealistic optimism. We should always seek to improve the state of the patient and the caregiver, if only marginally, and should never underestimate the value of honest communication, compassion, kindness, and close follow-up. In this chapter I set forth the multidisciplinary approach I advocate for patients with PSP.

MAKING THE DIAGNOSIS

The first step toward successful management of PSP is to make the diagnosis. Self-evident as this may seem, most cases are initially either missed or misdiagnosed. Before the correct diagnosis is ultimately made, patients often see several physicians and undergo unnecessary testing, further contributing to the frustration of the disease itself. A full discussion of the clinical features of PSP is beyond the scope of this chapter, but I will "hit the high points" and refer the reader to the references.

PSP is a clinical diagnosis. The *sine qua non* is a parkinsonian syndrome accompanied by slow vertical saccades. As the disease advances, vertical eye movements become limited, particularly downward gaze; the oculocephalic reflex is preserved, hence the designation *supranuclear*. The parkinsonian features include brady-kinesia, rigidity, and impaired postural reflexes. In contrast to Parkinson's disease (PD), the rigidity affects axial muscles more than appendicular ones, especially the neck. There is usually no tremor, and in PSP the impairments of gait and balance appear earlier and are more severe than in PD.

Other features that help distinguish PSP from PD include earlier onset of dysarthria and dysphagia. These symptoms often take patients to an otolaryngologist or gastroenterologist before they consult a neurologist. Patients often complain that they cannot see, leading them to the ophthalmologist, where frequently new glasses (or worse) are prescribed that provide no improvement, before it is discovered that the problem is the inability to move the eyes to the desired target rather than impaired acuity.

The prototypical patient's initial diagnosis is PD, but the condition soon demonstrates a limited response to L-dopa and progresses faster than typical PD, with early onset of falling, dysarthria, and dysphagia. At that point, careful clinical observation usually reveals impaired vertical eye movements and clinches the diagnosis.

TELLING THE PATIENT THE DIAGNOSIS

I explain to patients that PSP is a cousin of Parkinson's disease. I tell them that it is a fairly recently described disease (1964), something about the site of the pathologic changes and a bit about the chemical changes, and I reassure them that it is not familial. The cause is unknown.

Although patients are initially disappointed to learn that treatment for PSP is limited and that it is progressive (though slowly), there is often simultaneous relief in having a name pinned on their condition and receiving appropriate education and counseling. I explain how PSP is different from PD, especially in the sense that the drugs used to treat PD are less effective for PSP. I never tell patients that no treatment is available.

Most patients do not ask how long they have to live. I used to emphasize the positive by saying that the majority of patients live at least 5 years, but that is too often misconstrued: "The doctor said I have 5 years to live." Instead, I emphasize the variable and slow progression and the fact that, in all stages, we can provide some symptomatic relief.

PHARMACOLOGIC TREATMENT

The prevailing attitude among most neurologists is that drugs do not help PSP. That is an overstatement: although dopaminergics never offer as much benefit for PSP as they do for PD, many patients experience some improvement, so a trial is justified. Before starting therapy, I warn patients that the response will be modest at best and that we are looking for any hint of improvement. The most common signs to improve are bradykinesia, rigidity, and occasionally postural instability. Ophthalmoparesis, dysarthria, and dysphagia rarely improve.

My drug of first choice is L-dopa, in the form of Sinemet. Patients begin with one-half of a 25/250 mg tablet with breakfast. I gradually escalate the dose, in increments of one-half tablet every 4 to 7 days, aiming for a maximal dose of four full tablets (1,000 mg), before I decide that the patient is unresponsive to L-dopa. Some specialists advocate increasing the L-dopa dose to as much as 2,000 mg per day.

Although Sinemet is absorbed better on an empty stomach, that also frequently leads to nausea; thus my rationale for beginning treatment with food. Once the drug is tolerated, I gradually have patients take Sinemet one-half hour before meals. Other side effects of Sinemet include confusion, hallucinations, and orthostatic hypotension. Unlike PD patients who take Sinemet, PSP patients rarely develop dyskinesias.

If there is some improvement with Sinemet but the patient remains relatively symptomatic (and they almost always do), I next add a direct-acting dopamine agonist, either bromocriptine (Parlodel) or pergolide (Permax). If there is no subjective or objective response to Sinemet, I instruct the patient to gradually discontinue it. About one-third of the time, patients then notice slight deterioration, proving that Sinemet was helping more than was initially appreciated, and in that circumstance they should continue taking it.

I have not found any major difference between the beneficial and deleterious effects of bromocriptine and of pergolide, but patients occasionally improve with one and not the other or find one more tolerable than the other. Bromocriptine is started at one 2.5 mg tablet per day, and escalated over 10 days to one tablet three times per day, approximately every 8 hours. It usually requires much larger doses of bromocriptine (e.g., 30 mg) to produce a clinically appreciable benefit, but many patients early on develop side effects that limit its use.

From the initial maintenance dose of 2.5 mg three times per day, I attempt to escalate the dose by 2.5 mg every 7 to 10 days, stopping either when the patient experiences intolerable side effects or when improvement seems to have reached a plateau. As the dose is increased, the 5 mg capsule can be employed. Common side effects include confusion, hallucinations, orthostatic hypotension, fluid retention, and nightmares.

If there is no improvement with the maximal tolerated dose of bromocriptine, it should be withdrawn gradually. Again, only then do some patients appreciate that it was providing some benefit, and in that instance, dosing can be continued if a tolerable dose can be determined. If there is no deterioration as bromocriptine is withdrawn, a trial of pergolide should be considered. Pergolide comes in scored tablets of 0.05, 0.25, and 1.0 mg. For patients of advanced age or who have preexisting orthostatic hypotension, I begin with one 0.05 mg tablet per day and escalate slowly by that dose every 3 to 5 days, until improvement or intolerable side effects are observed. Pergolide is given in three divided doses. For younger patients with stable blood pressure, I begin with 0.125 mg per day, increasing slowly using the same criteria. It typically requires at least 1 mg per day of pergolide to demonstrate clinical improvement. The maximal dose is limited only by the patient's tolerance. The side effects of pergolide are similar to those of bromocriptine.

Tricyclic antidepressants (nortriptyline and amitriptyline) are occasionally useful for PSP, particularly if there is intercurrent depression, insomnia, or drooling. Other medications that have been tried but that in my hands have had little or no effect include methysergide, Eldepryl, and anticholinergics. Still, when faced with a relentlessly progressive disease, the threshold for saying, "Let's try this to see what happens" is lower. Medication trials offer patients hope. Still, they should be employed judiciously with tempered optimism, and not infrequently they cause more problems than they alleviate.

For the most part, medications have a limited role in the management of PSP, and most care is supportive. Optimal management is best achieved through a multidisciplinary approach that utilizes physical, occupational, and speech therapists, visiting nurses, and occasionally psychiatrists and other mental health professionals.

GAIT, BALANCE, AND FALLING

Impaired gait and balance are two of the most disabling features of PSP. Most PSP patients eventually become wheelchair- or bed bound. In the early to middle stages, walking can be facilitated with a rolling walker. Standard walkers are usually ineffective. I have two tests that usually predict success with a rolling walker. One is that the patient finds it easier to walk behind a grocery cart. Second, in the clinic, I have the patient walk behind a wheelchair, holding on to the handles, and observe their subjective and objective responses. Rather than sending the patient out with a prescription for a rolling walker, I arrange for a session or two with a physical therapist (one familiar with PSP), who adjusts the height of the walker and instructs the patient in its use. Therapists can provide additional instruction about easier ways of arising from a chair, turning in bed, preventing falls, and executing other movements. An exercise routine should also be prescribed that is directed at preventing contractures and maintaining strength.

Fall precautions include removing throw rugs and other obstacles in the path, providing a well-lit route to the bathroom (or use of a bedside commode), making sure that all stairs have bannisters, and avoiding irregular terrain. Patients who consistently fall on their knees should wear knee pads. Additional safety and assist equipment to consider includes grab bars in the shower, a shower chair, raised toilet seat, and a hospital bed. Occupational therapists and nurses should be consulted to help with the selection of home health aids. I encourage them to carry out a home assessment.

OCULAR SYMPTOMS

"I can't see" is a common complaint. Assuming visual acuity has been optimally corrected, patients need to be educated that their vision problem is the result of inability to move the eyes up or down. The latter is more problematic: patients have difficulty seeing food on their plate, reading, and seeing obstacles in their path. Impaired convergence and square wave jerks also contribute to impaired vision. Moving a plate or reading material to eye level sometimes helps. Vertical prisms may be tried but have not been useful in my experience. Bifocals are impractical, owing to impaired downward gaze, and patients should have separate glasses for near and far vision.

Two additional contributors to impaired vision include blepharospasm and eyelid-opening apraxia. The former is manifested by forceful, bilateral eye closure and can be treated effectively with local injections of botulinum toxin. Eyelid-opening apraxia is manifested by the inability to activate the levator muscle. As the eyes are gently shut, the contracted frontalis muscle attests to the patient's effort to overcome it. This may accompany blepharospasm or appear in isolation.

Eyelid-opening apraxia is difficult to treat, but some patients are able to manually open the eyes for short periods. We have had some success with botulinum toxin, at least enough to warrant a clinical trial. Its mechanism of action in relieving eyelid-opening apraxia is unknown, but it may weaken eye closure. The wife of a recent patient found that the toxin weakened the orbicularis oculi to the point where she was able to keep her husband's eyes open by taping the levator to the forehead, though this runs the risk of exposure keratopathy. This same patient also derived some benefit from bilateral ptosis crutches such as those used for myasthenia. Sustained use was hampered because the crutches made it difficult to change his glasses frequently.

Photophobia is common and can be treated with dark glasses. The diminished blink rate in PSP often causes dry eyes. Patients, or their care giver, should instill methylcellulose eye drops frequently during the day (every 1 to 2 hours) and Lacrilube at night.

SPEECH AND SWALLOWING

Dysarthria and dysphagia are best managed with the help of a speech pathologist experienced in PSP. Most patients eventually become either aphonic or at least so dysarthric that they are unintelligible. This is one of the most frustrating symptoms of PSP.

Patients with adequate manual skills and mentation can use a communication board or electronic communication system. When hyphonia is the dominant symptom, voice amplification should be attempted, although it is ineffective if accompanied by moderately severe dysarthria. Speech therapy alone is rarely beneficial and should not be prescribed routinely.

Dysphagia is the major contributor to morbidity and mortality. Paradoxically, patients may not complain of trouble swallowing, and the physician must be alert to signs, such as coughing or choking during and after meals, frequent "upper respiratory tract infections," and pneumonia. The presence or absence of the gag reflex is not a reliable predictor of dysphagia. In conjunction with a speech therapist, a videofluoroscopy study can help determine the risk of aspiration.

As long as there is little or no aspiration, patients can continue to take food and liquid by mouth. To reduce the risk of aspiration, during meals there should be no distractions (television or reading) and the care giver should supervise. Patients should be advised to eat a soft diet, take small bites, eat slowly, and sit upright. If possible, the head should be in a neutral or slightly flexed position. More specific suggestions, tailored to the individual patient, can be made by the speech therapist. All care givers should be instructed in the Heimlich maneuver.

As PSP advances, most patients either become unable to swallow or are at such risk of aspiration that they cannot swallow sufficient food by mouth. Before they reach this stage, I advocate trying to determine the patient's wishes about a feeding tube. The frankness and timing of this important discussion require careful judgment about just how much the patient wants to know. This determination is not easy and must come from a close and trusting physician-patient relationship.

For a nonambulatory, poorly communicational care-dependent patient, a feeding tube is often viewed only as a device to prolong indignity and delay inevitable death, and they often decide against it. In less advanced cases, especially when dysphagia is more severe than other signs and the patient is relatively independent, most opt for a gastrostomy. Successful management of tube feedings requires a willing and able caretaker.

Discussing the merits of a feeding tube opens the door to discussing the patient's advance directives. If this is not discussed in the middle stages of PSP, patients eventually become either physically or mentally unable to make their wishes known; then the physician must rely on the spouse or children to plan for terminal care. As emphasized above, the extent and timing of this discussion must be individualized, and some patients prefer to remain "in the dark," in which case they should not be force-fed information. When approached tactfully and compassionately, most patients in my experience are ready—and often relieved—to discuss their advance directives as a means of asserting control through all phases of the illness and preserving dignity.

MISCELLANEOUS SYMPTOMS

Autonomic dysfunction, to a mild or at most moderate degree, is common in PSP: impotence, orthostatic hypotension, bladder instability, and constipation. Only the latter two are discussed here.

Constipation is best managed by reducing or eliminating anticholinergic medications. A daily regimen of a stool softener and bulking agent should be prescribed. If that is ineffective, additional measures include mineral oil, suppositories, and enemas. Patients should be counseled that constipation is a part of the disease and that the *regularity* of bowel movements rather than their *frequency* is most important.

Bladder instability can occasionally be controlled pharmacologically, but if not, a condom catheter, diaper, or intermittent catheterization is the preferred alternative to an indwelling catheter.

Drooling can be controlled with a low dose of an anticholinergic such as trihexiphenidyl, 2 to 6 milligrams per day. This may adversely affect the mental state.

Neuropsychiatric complications of PSP include dementia and depression. They may be difficult or impossible to diagnose in advanced cases, when patients cannot communicate either verbally or nonverbally. Although dementia is common in PSP, it should not be viewed as inevitable; therefore, a search for remediable causes is necessary. Furthermore, it is easy to overestimate the degree of cognitive impairment in the setting of aphonia, severe bradykinesia, and bradyphrenia. As such, patients should be approached as if they are mentally competent, and discussion should be directed toward, rather than around, the patient.

THE CAREGIVER

Successful caregiving is the cornerstone of optimal care for patients with PSP, and one of the major determinants of longevity and quality of survival. Caregivers are often ignored during the traditional office visit, when all attention is directed toward the patient. Yet, in chronic degenerative diseases, the caregiver often suffers as much as the patient, if not more. It is the physician's responsibility to recognize the valuable contributions of the caregiver and to be vigilant for symptoms and signs of caregiver distress. "How are you holding up?" are five of the most important words in our armamentarium.

Although there are many positive aspects of care giving, passing—and occasionally persistent—negative feelings include guilt, depression, frustration, anger, and resentment. A full discussion of care giver support is beyond the scope of this chapter, and the reader is referred to the Summer, 1992 newsletter of the *Society for Supranuclear Palsy*.

THE SOCIETY FOR PROGRESSIVE SUPRANUCLEAR PALSY

The Society for Progressive Supranuclear Palsy (SPSP), a patient-run society, was started 3 years ago and is rapidly approaching a membership of 400. All patients with PSP should be encouraged to join, as should physicians who care for them. The SPSP is a useful source for information and gives patients and their families a resource for mutual support and understanding. The society is also a strong advocate and supporter of research.

SUGGESTED READING

Jankovic J. Progressive supranuclear palsy. Neurol Clin 1984; 2:473–486.

Jackson JA, Jankovic J, Ford J. Progressive supranuclear palsy: Clinical features and response to treatment in 16 patients. Ann Neurol 1983; 13:273–278.

Kristensen MO. Progressive supranuclear palsy—20 years later. Acta Neurol Scand 1985; 71:177–189.

Steele JC, Richardson JC, Olszewski J. Progressive supranuclear palsy. Arch Neurol 1964; 10:333–359.

Steele JC. Progressive supranuclear palsy. Brain 1972; 95:693–704.

PATIENT RESOURCE

The Society for Progressive Supranuclear Palsy, Inc.
2904 Marnat Road
Baltimore, Maryland 21209-2420
Telephone: (410) 484-8771

HEREDITARY CEREBELLAR ATAXIA

 OREST HURKO, M.D.

The medical management of cerebellar ataxia is based almost exclusively on specific treatment of the causative disorder, because there is very little to offer in the way of symptomatic treatment. In this sense, the management of cerebellar ataxia is diametrically opposite that of most of the movement disorders, for which there is excellent symptomatic treatment but rarely specific treatment aimed at reversing the underlying neurodegeneration. Whatever the cause in a given patient, the treatment of parkinsonian symptoms is based on dopaminergic stimulation. Unfortunately, no comparable generic cerebellar tonic has yet been discovered.

DIAGNOSIS

In hereditary cerebellar ataxias, the premium is on accurate diagnosis, without which a rational treatment plan cannot be formulated. This is a daunting prospect. McKusick lists 227 mendelian disorders that are associated with ataxia; in his compendium, Baraitser lists 267. Many of these are rare. Only a minority are amenable to treatment with currently available technologies.

The hereditary nature of an ataxic patient's disorder is frequently inapparent. As a general rule, most of the early onset ataxias are recessive conditions and therefore tend to present as sporadic cases: heterozygotes in previous generations are unaffected. Furthermore, since the current average sibship in the United States is smaller than three, the majority of patients do not have an affected sibling. The family history in autosomal-dominant ataxias can also be problematic: many patients do not report the expected history of affected members in previous generations passing on the disorder to half their sons and daughters. Most autosomal-dominant ataxias are disorders of late onset, the symptoms of which are frequently attributed to alcohol, senility, multiple sclerosis, or arthritis. Even when a hereditary disorder is suspected, it is kept from the children as a "family secret," because of misguided efforts to either prevent anxiety or allay guilt. Most cases of mitochondrial DNA deletions and some autosomal-dominant conditions can appear as new mutations, in which the family history truly is negative.

Thus, the first task of the clinician is to distinguish patients with hereditary ataxia from those in whom hereditary considerations are unimportant. In childhood, the foremost differential considerations are tumors, cerebellitis, and infections. In adults, the major considerations are alcohol, direct or remote effects of tumor, vascular insufficiency, cervical spondylosis, multiple sclerosis, thyroid dysfunction, and deficiency of vitamin B_{12}. In all age groups, drug intoxication should also be considered. In most cases, exclusions are straightforward and can be made clinically. It is my practice to supplement clinical evaluation with magnetic resonance imaging (MRI) of the brain as well as determinations of routine chemistry, electrolytes, hemogram with sedimentation rate, vitamin B_{12} and thyroid function tests on all persons who present with ataxia.

Once a hereditary ataxia is suspected, it is no longer sufficient to diagnose "spinocerebellar degeneration." Specific diagnosis of these syndromes, once considered a sterile academic exercise for those with a fondness for Latin names, is of growing practical importance, particularly as pathogenic genes are being located and specific therapies devised. Prognostication for the patient, genetic counseling, identification of comorbidity, and, most important, identification of patients for whom specific medical treatment is possible, requires adequate diagnosis. Standard neurology texts provide old classification systems based on postmortem pathologic studies and thus offer limited guidance for the practitioner who has only clinical information on which to base a diagnosis. Of the published general diagnostic schemes, the best are those of Baraitser, of Harding, and of Bundey; the best source for metabolic information is Scriver; the best general entry into the literature of specific entities is McKusick, whose code numbers, when available, I use to annotate my text (Table 1). Although I attempt an overview, necessity dictates that I focus on the disorders for which there are significant management issues.

INTERMITTENT ATAXIAS

One is most likely to find a treatable disorder if the patient presents with intermittent ataxia. This group of disorders includes those in which ataxia lasts for hours at a time, without progression to other neurologic dysfunction, and a second, larger, category in which cerebellar ataxia is an early phase of a more complex course that can evolve into stupor, coma, and even death if the condition is not recognized and treated. In the former case, the diagnosis can be made clinically and the management can be successfully undertaken in outpatients by generalists. In the second category, more extensive testing is necessary: serum and urine amino acids, electrolyte panel, and serum ammonia. Many of these are complex, life-threatening illnesses, the successful management of which requires considerable biochemical and nutritional expertise as well as the facilities of a tertiary medical center.

In the first category is *periodic vestibulocerebellar ataxia (McKusick No. 108500)*, an autosomal-dominant condition in which attacks of dysarthria, nystagmus, and truncal and appendicular ataxia are precipitated by emotion or exercise. These spells typically last several hours and can be aborted by sleep. Prophylactic treatment with Diamox is very effective. Diamox is started at

Table 1 Selected Ataxic Disorders

Intermittent ataxias
  Periodic vestibulocerebellar ataxia (McKusick No. 108500)
  Pyruvate dehydrogenase deficiency (McKusick No. 208800)
  Late-onset multiple carboxylase deficiency (biotinidase deficiency, McKusick No. 253260)
  Pyruvate carboxylase deficiency (McKusick No. 266150)
  Propionyl-CoA carboxylase deficiency (McKusick No. 232000, 232050)
  Holocarboxylase synthetase deficiency (McKusick No. 253270)
  Ornithine transcarbamylase deficiency (McKusick No. 311250)
  Citrullinemia (McKusick No. 215700)
  Argininosuccinase deficiency (McKusick No. 207900)
  Arginase deficiency (McKusick No. 207800)
  Maple syrup urine disease (branched-chain amino- and keto-aciduria, McKusick No. 248600)
  Isovaleric acidemia (McKusick No. 243500)
  Hartnup's disease (McKusick No. 234500)

Hereditary ataxia associated with structural lesions
  Arnold-Chiari malformations (McKusick No. 207950)
  von Hippel-Lindau syndrome (McKusick No. 193300)
  Turcot's syndrome (McKusick No. 276300)
  Bilateral acoustic neurofibromatosis (NF II, McKusick No. 101000)
  von Recklinghausen's neurofibromatosis (NF I, McKusick No. 162200)
  Hereditary hemorrhagic telangiectasia (McKusick No. 187300)
  Autosomal-dominant cavernous hemangiomas (McKusick Nos. 140800, 116860)

Progressive (more or less) cerebellar degenerations
  Congenital ataxias
    Pelizaeus-Merzbacher disease (McKusick No. 312080)
    Angelman happy puppet syndrome (McKusick No. 234400)
    Galactosemias, secondary to deficiencies of:
      Galactose-1 phosphate uridyltransferase (McKusick No. 230400)
      Galactokinase (McKusick No. 230200)
      Galactose epimerase (McKusick No. 230350)

Table 1 Selected Ataxic Disorders — cont'd

Ataxias presenting in infancy and early childhood
  Ataxia telangiectasia (McKusick No. 208900)
  Xeroderma pigmentosa (McKusick No. 278700, 278710, . . ., 278810)
  Cockayne's syndrome (McKusick No. 216400).
  Deficiency of 5,10-methylene tetrahydrofolate reductase (McKusick No. 236250)
  Transcobalamin II (vitamin B_{12}-binding protein) deficiency (McKusick No. 275350)
  Defective intrinsic factor receptor (McKusick No. 261100)
  Polyglandular autoimmune syndrome (McKusick No. 240300)

Juvenile ataxias
  Friederich's ataxia (McKusick No. 229300)
  Early-onset ataxia with retained ankle jerks
  Hexosaminidase A (McKusick No. 272800)
  Metachromatic leukodystrophy (McKusick No. 250100)
  Sialidosis (McKusick No. 256550)
  Ceroid lipofuscinosis (McKusick No. 204200)
  Multiple sulfatase deficiency (McKusick No. 272200)
  Globoid cell leukodystrophy (McKusick No. 245200)
  Adrenomyeloneuropathy (McKusick No. 300100)
  Kearns-Sayre syndrome (McKusick No. 165100)
  Myoclonic epilepsy, ragged-red fibers (MERRF)
  Refsum's disease (McKusick No. 266500)
  Abetalipoproteinemia (McKusick No. 200100)
  Familial isolated vitamin E deficiency (McKusick No. 277460)
  Cerebrotendinous xanthomatosis (McKusick No. 213700)

Adult-onset ataxias
  Olivopontocerebellar atrophies (McKusick No. 164400, 164500, 164600, 164700)
  Machado-Joseph (McKusick No. 109150)
  Recessive OPCA (McKusick No. 258300)
  Wilson's disease (McKusick No. 277900)

250 mg PO daily and increased, as needed, to 750 mg daily, in divided doses. Perioral paresthesias are frequently an annoying side effect but are usually temporary. More problematic is the increased risk of renal calculi associated with the lifelong treatment that is usually required. Patients are advised to increase their fluid intake. Several authors have proposed addition of valproic acid at anticonvulsant doses to reduce the required dose of Diamox. If there are no other neurologic features, this entity can be diagnosed clinically. Because of reports of an association with *pyruvate dehydrogenase deficiency (McKusick No. 208800)*, however, I determine (1) venous lactate, (2) serum amino acids (to look for elevations of alanine), and (3) electrolyte panel (to check for acidosis). If these tests are negative, I do not determine pyruvate dehydrogenase (PDH) activity in fibroblasts. Some authors further distinguish another category of pure intermittent cerebellar ataxia in which attacks can last for days to weeks but cease with puberty. It is not clear if this group is also responsive to Diamox.

In the second category are a number of disorders in which ataxia and listlessness are the earliest signs of metabolic decompensation, which, if left untreated, evolves over hours or days to stupor, coma, and death. Although complete enzymatic deficiencies are diagnosed in newborn screening programs or after presentation as catastrophic perinatal illnesses, partial deficiencies typically are discovered later in life. In these patients, residual enzymatic activity is sufficient to maintain homeostasis in an anabolic state but not enough to cope with the demands imposed by catabolism. For that reason, metabolic crises are triggered by intercurrent illness or fasting. As the patient becomes catabolic, partially functioning enzymes become overwhelmed by mobilization of endogenous proteins and/or lipids. Therefore, the cornerstone of treatment in almost all these biochemically diverse disorders is rapid induction of insulin, the hormonal master switch that shifts the patient from catabolism to anabolism. If the patient can take oral fluids without vomiting, 1 or 2 ounces of juice taken every hour can frequently avert further decompensation. If vomiting or lethargy ensues, intravenous (IV) infusion of 10 or 15 percent glucose at 1½ times the calculated maintenance dose is required. If the patient has become too depressed to mount an endogenous insulin response, a small priming dose of IV insulin is given along with the glucose infusion. Another frequently encountered feature of many organic acidurias is a secondary deficiency of carnitine, resulting from excessive urinary loss. Whereas free carnitine is readily reabsorbed by the renal tubule, carnitine esterified to an organic acid is not. Therefore, levels of free and esterified carnitine should be determined. If deficiency is documented, carnitine should be replaced. (The current vogue among some practitioners for blind dietary carnitine supplementation of poorly characterized neurologic disorders, however, is properly decried.) In many instances, inappropriate elevation of carnitine level may be harmful, resulting in intramitochondrial trapping of potentially toxic conjugates.

In addition to these general measures, successful management of these intermittent ataxias requires disease-specific treatments, discussed in the following paragraphs.

Late-onset multiple carboxylase deficiency (McKusick No. 253260), deficiency of four biotin-dependent carboxylases (pyruvate carboxylase, methylcrotonyl-CoA carboxylase, propionyl-CoA carboxylase, and acetyl-CoA carboxylase), can present as intermittent or progressive cerebellar ataxia. The combined deficiency state is biochemically heterogeneous, resulting either from deficiency of *biotinidase*, an enzyme responsible for recycling body stores of biotin, or *holocarboxylase synthetase*, the enzyme responsible for attaching biotin to each of the four apoenzymes. In addition, there have been isolated deficiency states of each of these four enzymes, of which *pyruvate carboxylase deficiency (McKusick No. 266150)* and *propionyl-CoA carboxylase deficiency (McKusick Nos. 232000, 232050)* have been associated with intermittent ataxias, usually as part of a "recurrent Reye's-like" syndrome. In severe cases of multiple carboxylase deficiency, onset is in childhood, with seizures, rash, alopecia, hearing loss, and optic atrophy. There are increasing reports of milder, late-onset cases in which cutaneous changes are minimal or absent. The diagnosis is based on demonstration of a characteristic amino aciduria and ketolactic acidosis. For those with *biotinidase deficiency (McKusick No. 253260)*, treatment with biotin, 5 to 20 mg per day PO (obtainable from Hoffman LaRoche), leads to prompt resolution of rash, seizures, and ataxia. Hearing loss and optic atrophy may improve somewhat as well. There have also been reports of improvement with biotin treatment of individuals with *holocarboxylase synthetase deficiency (McKusick No. 253270)*, whereas others are refractory even to larger doses. A trial of biotin is also indicated in *propionyl-CoA carboxylase deficiency (propionic acidemia or ketotic hyperglycinemia) (McKusick Nos. 232000, 232050)*. However, the mainstay of long-term treatment of propionic acidemia is protein restriction (0.5 to 1.5 g per kilogram per day). For acute decompensation, protein is stopped entirely and the patient is given IV glucose, sodium bicarbonate for correction of acidosis, and carnitine replacement as needed. During acute metabolic crises there may be sufficient hyperammonemia to warrant treatment, as detailed in the following paragraph.

Management of the urea cycle disorders *(ornithine transcarbamylase [OTC] deficiency [McKusick No. 311250]; citrullinemia [McKusick No. 215700]; argininosuccinase deficiency [McKusick No. 207900]; arginase*

deficiency [McKusick No. 207800]) depends on reducing the production of waste nitrogen and facilitating its excretion. Long-term management requires a diet that is severely restricted in protein but still provides sufficient amounts of essential amino acids for anabolism and growth. Achievement of such a technically difficult balance requires the skills of a specially trained dietitian and the dedicated support of the family. Protein restriction can be partially relaxed by giving drugs that provide alternatives to urea as pathways for urinary nitrogen excretion. Phenylbutyrate, 0.45 to 0.6 g per kilogram per day, and phenylacetate, 0.4 to 0.5 g per kilogram per day, are the preferred drugs. Sodium benzoate is no longer recommended for long-term treatment but remains useful during metabolic crises. These drugs are currently classified as investigational drugs, available through an IND (Investigational New Drug) to Dr. Saul Brusilow of the Johns Hopkins Hospital. Dosage and diet are adjusted to maintain fasting ammonia, branched amino acids, and serum protein values in the normal range, and the plasma level of glutamine below 1,000 μM. Acute metabolic crises are heralded by listlessness and ataxia and require immediate evaluation. If the plasma ammonia level has approached three times the upper limit of normal, the patient is admitted for emergent IV treatment. Plasma amino acid levels are measured, the hemodialysis team is alerted, and high caloric intake is instituted with intravenous glucose and intralipid, 80 to 100 calories per kilogram per day. In OTC deficiency, the most common of these disorders, a priming infusion of sodium benzoate, 0.25 g per kilogram, sodium phenylacetate, 0.25 g per kilogram, and 10 percent arginine hydrochloride, 2 ml per kilogram, is then given in 25 to 35 ml 10 percent glucose over 90 minutes. Immediately thereafter, a sustaining infusion of the same amounts of these three compounds is given IV over 24 hours. If the ammonia level is not reduced after 8 hours, hemodialysis is begun. If there is increased intracranial pressure, mannitol and hyperventilation are useful temporizing measures; however, the response to specific measures is usually sufficiently prompt that such adjunctive treatment is not necessary. Bicarbonate infusions may be needed to counteract hyperchloremic acidosis resulting from arginine infusion.

Most cases of *maple syrup urine disease (MSUD; branched-chain amino- and keto-aciduria) (McKusick No. 248600)* are recognized in newborn screening programs, permitting early institution of chronic dietary therapy that prevents or ameliorates the development of severe mental and physical retardation. The crux of treatment is restriction of branched-chain amino acids (BCAAs), though these are essential amino acids that must be provided in basal amounts, requirements that vary with the patient's age. Three- to four-hour postprandial amino acid levels provide a useful gauge of the adequacy of treatment. Target values are of 40 to 90 μM for isoleucine, 80 to 200 μM for leucine, and 200 to 425 μM for valine. In addition, all individuals should be given a minimum 3-week trial of thiamine, 5 to 20 mg per kilogram per day, to identify those who respond to pharmacologic doses of this vitamin. Even for thiamine-responsive patients, however, some degree of dietary restriction is still necessary. Metabolic crises are heralded by ataxia, and must be treated with glucose infusion and insulin to reverse the catabolic state. Since the branched-chain amino acids are essential, they must be provided in amounts appropriate for the current metabolic state of the patient. Acute treatment is facilitated through the use of commercially available protein-free powder (Mead Johnson product 80056), BCAA-free formula, and MSUD diet powders. Useful tables of age-specific requirements for acutely ill MSUD individuals are to be found in Scriver.

The chronic intermittent form of *isovaleric acidemia (McKusick No. 243500)* usually presents in the first few years of life as ataxia that rapidly progresses to lethargy and stupor. The two goals of maintenance therapy are (1) reduction of the amount of leucine that is converted to isovaleryl-CoA, accomplished by protein restriction to 1.5 to 2.0 g per kilogram per day; and (2) increasing excretion of isovaleryl-CoA through conjugation to glycine and carnitine. Glycine is given at 250 mg per kilogram per day in three doses, carnitine typically at 20 to 40 mg per kilogram per day. During acute metabolic crises, infusions of glucose and bicarbonate are necessary.

Intermittent ataxia, usually in the presence of additional neurologic signs, has also been observed in some patients with partial deficiencies of *pyruvate dehydrogenase (PDH, McKusick No. 208800), pyruvate carboxylase (McKusick No. 266150)*, or of *mitochondrially encoded enzymes of oxidative phosphorylation*. No consistently effective treatment has been devised for any of these disorders. Because of anecdotal reports of efficacy in some patients, we advocate treatment of PDH-deficient patients with thiamine, 300 to 900 mg per day; patients with pyruvate carboxylase deficiency with biotin, 5 to 20 mg per day PO); and patients with mitochondrial DNA abnormalities with CoQ10, 150 mg per day, the latter available in health food stores. Acute metabolic crises may require treatment with bicarbonate infusions. Dichloroacetate, a potent activator of pyruvate dehydrogenase is available only as an investigational drug, and its use is best restricted to acute decompensations. Although some authors have advocated maintenance administration, we are dissuaded by reports of accumulation in tissues, peripheral neuropathy in humans treated long term; and testicular atrophy, leukoencephalopathy, and cataracts in experimental animals.

In *Hartnup's disease (McKusick No. 234500)*, an autosomal-recessive disorder of neutral amino acid transport, episodes of intermittent ataxia are typically accompanied with psychosis and photosensitive pellagra-like skin rash. Treatment consists of a high-protein diet and supplementation with 50 to 300 mg of nicotinic acid daily. This treatment reliably clears the rash and ameliorates the psychosis and ataxia. The optimal dose of riboflavin has to be determined clinically, because the diagnostic aminoaciduria persists unchanged. A Hartnup's-like illness has been reported with marked ataxia and skin rash, in which the rash but not the ataxia responded to nicotinamide, 100 mg per day PO.

HEREDITARY ATAXIA ASSOCIATED WITH STRUCTURAL LESIONS

Compressive lesions in the posterior fossa frequently have the potential for significant therapeutic intervention. *Arnold-Chiari malformations (McKusick No. 207950)* occur either in isolation or as part of systemic, skeletal, and/or CNS malformation syndromes, only a minority of which appear to be mendelian disorders. We consider surgical decompression to be urgently indicated in all patients who have developed associated hydrocephalus or syringomyelia. In addition, we recommend elective decompression for adult patients who develop disabling symptoms: truncal ataxia, and/or cough-induced headache and light-headedness. Surgical treatment consists of suboccipital decompression with cervical laminectomies at appropriate levels. If present, associated lumbar meningomyelocele or tethered cord requires repair. The need for shunting of associated hydrocephalus and marsupialization or shunting of an associated syrinx should be evaluated individually.

Posterior fossa tumors are frequently encountered in several autosomal-dominant conditions, some of which have been classified as phakomatoses. In our experience, ataxia is most often a presenting complaint in the *von Hippel-Lindau Syndrome (McKusick No. 193300)*, a familial predisposition to cerebellar, spinal, and ocular hemangioblastomas, as well as renal carcinoma, hypernephromas, pheochromocytomas, and abdominal cysts. It is our practice to follow these patients very closely, with a view to detecting early lesions that may be amenable to surgical therapy. Each patient is given a complete neurologic and dilated ophthalmoscopic examination annually. In addition, even asymptomatic patients are examined with annual MRI of the posterior fossa, contrast-enhanced computed tomography (CT) of the abdomen, urinalysis, and determinations of hematocrit, erythropoietin, and metanephrines. Patients with solid tumors are referred for surgical or radiosurgical management, whereas cysts are followed conservatively. We currently take a similarly aggressive approach to patients with the much rarer *Turcot's syndrome (McKusick No. 276300)*; listed as a recessive, but which we have encountered as an autosomal dominant), an association of cerebellar medulloblastoma and/or cerebral astrocytoma, premalignant polyposis coli, and variable thyroid carcinoma. Treatment is mostly surgical. Prophylactic colectomy is advised, as in the more common Gardner's syndrome, of which Turcot's may be a variant. Because of the high frequency of drop metastases associated with medulloblastomas, surgical extirpation of these tumors is followed by craniospinal irradiation.

In contrast, we follow patients with neurofibromatosis more conservatively. If the patient's annual neurologic examination is normal, we do not routinely perform neuroimaging studies, reasoning that there is no therapeutic advantage in presymptomatic intervention for either the benign or malignant tumors associated with these disorders. Ataxia is more likely to be a significant complaint in *bilateral acoustic neurofibromatosis (neurofibromatosis II, McKusick No. 101000)* than in the more common *von Recklinghausen's neurofibromatosis (NF I, McKusick No. 162200)*, which is not associated with acoustic neuromas. Both types of neurofibromatosis as well as the von Hippel-Lindau syndrome have been mapped, allowing presymptomatic diagnosis by linkage.

In passing, we alert the reader to heritable disorders of the cardiovascular system, many of them treatable, that frequently result in secondary cerebellar disease: cerebellar abscesses from disorders associated with cardiac malformations or pulmonary arteriovenous malformations, such as *hereditary hemorrhagic telangiectasia (McKusick No. 187300)*; arteriovenous malformations, chiefly *autosomal-dominant cavernous hemangiomas (McKusick Nos. 140800, 116860)*; and a plethora of disorders associated with coagulopathy, vascular fragility, or premature atherosclerosis.

PROGRESSIVE (MORE OR LESS) CEREBELLAR DEGENERATIONS

To the frustration of the clinician, the most commonly encountered hereditary ataxias fall in this group, and for only a minority is there specific treatment. In virtually all of the static or steadily progressive hereditary ataxias, there are associated neurologic, ocular, and/or systemic features. It is these associated features, as well as consideration of the age of onset and the pattern of inheritance, that are the key to diagnosis. As a general rule, the early-onset disorders tend to be recessive and to be associated with biochemical abnormalities. In contrast, no biochemical correlates have yet been established for virtually any adult-onset, autosomal-dominant ataxias. We can provide only a general overview of diagnosis, with a view to identifying important management issues, and refer the reader to the references for details.

Congenital Ataxias

Although individually rare, heritable disorders account for a significant proportion of congenital ataxias, many of which are static, nonprogressive disorders. In most cases it is not possible to distinguish heritable from sporadic cases. Therefore, it is prudent to counsel a recurrence risk of 1 in 8 for future siblings of infants with "ataxic cerebral palsy." Counseling can sometimes be further refined by clinical or radiographic definition of a recognizable syndrome. The laboratory is usually not much help in this age group, except for *Pelizaeus-Merzbacher disease (McKusick No. 312080)*, an X-linked disorder associated with mutations in the proteolipid

protein gene; the *Angelman happy puppet syndrome (McKusick No. 234400)*, associated with deletions in the q11–13 region of the maternally derived chromosome 15; and *galactosemia*, a biochemically heterogeneous disorder associated with deficiency of one of several enzymes: *galactose-1 phosphate uridyltransferase (McKusick No. 230400), galactokinase (McKusick No. 230200), or epimerase (McKusick No. 230350)*. Of these, treatment is available only for the galactosemias, which are currently detected in newborn screening programs. Galactose restriction ameliorates the development of hepatomegaly, cataracts, and mental retardation that are the hallmarks of the syndrome. Despite optimal dietary management, progressive ataxia and choreoathetosis still occur. Dietary compliance can be monitored by measuring galactose-1-phosphatase activity in erythrocytes.

Ataxias That Present in Infancy and Early Childhood

The most common disorder in this group is *ataxia telangiectasia (AT, McKusick No. 208900)*, an autosomal-recessive disorder that affects both the central nervous system and the immune system. Typically, infants present at 12 to 14 months with truncal ataxia and a distinctive oculomotor apraxia: slowness in initiation of saccades, often requiring head movement. These eye signs can be useful in diagnosis, as the telltale telangiectasias usually do not appear until 3 to 5 years of age. Later in life, these patients develop peripheral neuropathy and then choreoathetosis. The most useful laboratory aids to early diagnosis are elevations in alpha-fetoprotein and carcinoembryonic antigen; low levels of immunoglobulins A, E, and G_2 are frequent but not invariant. The most significant management issues relate to immune-related problems: susceptibility to infection and to neoplasia. About one-fourth of all deaths are related to neoplasia: leukemia and lymphoreticular tumors in childhood; epithelial tumors, including medulloblastoma and glioma in adults. Management of these tumors is especially difficult because of characteristic radiation sensitivity of AT homozygotes: standard doses of radiation can be lethal. Indeed, radiation sensitivity and susceptibility to tumors in otherwise asymptomatic heterozygotes may be a significant public health issue. Although AT homozygotes are rare (1 per 20,000 to 100,000 live births), heterozygotes constitute 1 to 2 percent of the population, and are estimated to account for 8 to 20 percent of breast cancer cases and a significant proportion of radiation-induced injury. Radiation sensitivity is also an important management issue in two other autosomal-recessive disorders associated with cerebellar ataxia, *xeroderma pigmentosa (McKusick Nos. 278700, 278710, . . . , 278810)* and *Cockayne's syndrome (McKusick No. 216400)*.

Also presenting between 1 and 5 years of age are several rarer progressive cerebellar ataxias for which there is effective specific pharmacotherapy. *Deficiency of 5,10-methylene tetrahydrofolate reductase (McKusick No. 236250)* results in a demyelinating disorder somewhat reminiscent of vitamin B_{12} deficiency but with superimposed cerebellar and parkinsonian features, mental retardation, myoclonic epilepsy, and psychosis. Betaine, 8 to 15 g daily, is said to halt the progress of neurologic disease and to reverse ataxia and psychosis. Some authors advocate supplementing betaine with folinic acid, methionine, and vitamins B_6 and B_{12}. Intramuscular injections of pharmacologic doses of hydroxocobalamin have also been reported beneficial in other heritable disorders of vitamin B_{12} metabolism: *transcobalamin II (vitamin B_{12}–binding protein) deficiency (McKusick No. 275350)*, which usually presents as failure to thrive in the first months of life and progresses to a syndrome of spastic ataxia, severe mental retardation, and pernicious anemia; *congenital lack of intrinsic factor (McKusick No. 261000); defective intrinsic factor receptor (McKusick No. 261100)*, in which the clinical picture is further complicated by proteinuria; and *polyglandular autoimmune syndrome (McKusick No. 240300)*, in which there are additional features of hypoparathyroidism, addisonism, and cutaneous moniliasis. Vitamin B_{12} deficiency is encountered most frequently as a cause of pernicious anemia and spinocerebellar ataxia later in life. Although this common disorder of late adulthood does not segregate as a mendelian trait, about half of a proband's siblings and one-fourth of the offspring have demonstrable impairment of vitamin B_{12} absorption.

Juvenile Ataxias

The most common in this group is the autosomal-recessive *Friedreich's ataxia ([FA] McKusick No. 229300)*, with an estimated frequency of 1 in 20,000 to 30,000 live births. Although FA had been used by some neurologists as a wastebasket term to encompass all heritable spinocerebellar degenerations, this is no longer acceptable. FA is a clinically distinct disorder resulting from homozygosity for a mutation on chromosome 9q. It is characterized by onset of progressive truncal and appendicular ataxia before age 21 years; dysarthria developing within 5 years of onset; absent ankle and knee jerks; extensor plantar responses; and normal nerve conduction velocities. In addition to the progressive ataxia, the major management considerations are diabetes mellitus that affects 40 percent of patients, half of whom are insulin dependent, and hypertrophic cardiomyopathy that in late stages may require diuretics and inotropic agents. Less frequently, these patients have deficiencies of parathyroid or thyroid hormone.

FA should be distinguished from *early-onset ataxia with retained ankle jerks* and a host of partial deficiencies of various lysosomal enzymes, complete deficiencies of which constitute the more familiar differential diagnosis of the infantile "amaurotic idiocies": *hexosaminidase A (McKusick No. 272800), metachromatic leukodystrophy (McKusick No. 250100), sialidosis (McKusick No. 256550), ceroid lipofuscinosis (McKusick No. 204200), multiple sulfatase deficiency (McKusick No. 272200), globoid cell leukodystrophy (McKusick No. 245200)*. Although there is no specific treatment for most of these disorders, for a few there are specific disease-related

management issues. Determination of very long–chain fatty acids is necessary for the diagnosis of *adrenomyeloneuropathy (McKusick No. 300100)*, an X-linked paroxysomal disorder in which spinocerebellar degeneration is frequently associated with adrenal insufficiency, requiring replacement therapy. In the so-called *Kearns-Sayre syndrome (McKusick No. 165100)* diagnosed by demonstration of a partial deletion in mitochondrial DNA obtained from muscle (but not blood), cerebellar ataxia and external ophthalmoplegia are not infrequently associated with heart block, diabetes mellitus, and/or parathormone deficiency, which may require treatment. Although there is no proven treatment for this or the other mitochondrial DNA disorder associated with ataxia, *myoclonic epilepsy, ragged red fibers (MERRF)*, diagnosed by demonstration of a point mutation in the tRNA gene for lysine in mitochondrial DNA extracted from blood, urine, or muscle), it is my practice to give CoQ10, 150 mg daily PO, for both disorders.

Although rare, there are several late childhood or juvenile-onset ataxias for which specific prophylactic or curative treatment is available. In *Refsum's disease (McKusick No. 266500, phytanic oxidase deficiency, heredopathia atactica polyneuritiformis)* the cardinal features are cerebellar ataxia, retinitis pigmentosa, and polyneuropathy. Some patients have one or all of several additional signs: ichthyotic skin rash, heart failure, deafness, visual impairment. Treatment is based on dietary restriction of phytanic acid, which is present in the typical American diet in amounts of 60 mg per day. Masters-Thomas et al. (J Hum Nutrition 24:245–256, 1980) provide guidelines for a diet that, using regular food, reduces intake to 10 to 20 mg per day. Exclusive use of a liquid formula can bring intake down to 3 mg per day, but this is a harsh diet. Some clinics advocate plasmapheresis or plasma exchange at the beginning of dietary therapy or once or twice monthly thereafter, to permit liberalization of dietary restrictions. Compliance can be monitored by measuring blood levels of phytanic and pipecolic acid, both of which should decrease. The expectation of therapy should be reversal of ataxia, weakness, rash, and electrocardiographic abnormalities. Auditory and visual changes do not regress, but progression may be halted.

In *abetalipoproteinemia (McKusick No. 200100)*, the spinocerebellar degeneration appears to stem in large part from deficiency of fat-soluble vitamin E. Oral administration of vitamin E, 1,000 to 2,000 mg daily to infants; 5,000 to 10,000 mg daily to adults, halts the progression of the spinocerebellar degeneration and peripheral neuropathy and may ameliorate the myopathy and retinopathy. Other fat-soluble vitamins should also be replaced: vitamin A can be given in a water soluble form; vitamin K should be given if there is a significant abnormality of the prothrombin time, but vitamin D replacement is not necessary because of its independent transport system. Gastrointestinal symptoms are significantly ameliorated by reduction of intake of long-chain fatty acids. This is most practically accomplished by restriction of all fatty foods from the diet. One should not attempt to substitute medium-chain fatty acids because of reports of hepatic fibrosis. Vitamin E replacement, 400 to 1,200 IU of vitamin E PO, daily is also reportedly effective in *familial isolated vitamin E deficiency (McKusick No. 277460)*, an autosomal-recessive disorder in which ataxia, areflexia, and severe proprioceptive loss begin after puberty. Frequently there are xanthomas and elevated cholesterol levels, but the level of beta-lipoprotein is always normal.

Cerebrotendinous xanthomatosis (McKusick No. 213700) is a rare disorder marked by postpubertal ataxia, spinal cord degeneration, and then a final preterminal pseudobulbar phase. Associated signs are xanthomas, premature cataracts, and premature atherosclerosis, all resulting from deposition of noncholesterol sterols in tendons, brain, lung, and blood vessels. The treatment of choice is chenodeoxycholic acid, 250 mg three times a day PO, which has been reported to relieve ataxia and improve BAERS after months of chronic treatment.

Adult-Onset Ataxias

The most frequently encountered adult-onset cerebellar ataxias are the autosomal-dominant *olivopontocerebellar atrophies ([OPCA] McKusick Nos. 164400, 164500, 164600, 164700)*, in which slowly progressive cerebellar degeneration is variably accompanied by extrapyramidal, pyramidal, autonomic, and peripheral nerve dysfunction. Diagnostic classification is difficult because clinical features can vary much among members of a kindred. Some members of the extensively studied *Schut-Haymaker (McKusick No. 164600)* and *Machado-Joseph (McKusick No. 109150)* kindreds had an almost pure cerebellopathy, others a spastic paraparesis, and others had an extrapyramidal disorder with severe polyneuropathy but almost no cerebellar signs. Because of the considerable clinical overlap of some of these phenotypes with those of apparently sporadic Shy-Drager disease or multisystem atrophy, counseling for autosomal-dominant disease can be confidently given only in cases with an appropriate family history. Although *recessive OPCA (McKusick No. 258300)* has been reported, such a diagnosis should always be made with great circumspection, particularly in view of the late onset and variable expression of the established dominant OPCAs. Although the responsible mutation in a minority of OPCA kindreds has been mapped to chromosome 6, such families cannot be distinguished clinically from those that are not linked, which precludes the general use of linkage markers for presymptomatic testing. As there is no specific treatment, management consists in symptomatic treatment of parkinsonian rigidity, spasticity, and autonomic neuropathy, when such problems arise.

An important consideration in the differential diagnosis of adult-onset neurodegenerative disorders associated with ataxia is *Wilson's disease (McKusick No. 277900)*. The movement disorder and psychosis usually far overshadow the cerebellar findings, but given the pleiotropic features of the OPCAs, this disease needs to be considered in the differential diagnosis, particularly when the family history is vague. Wilson's disease is exceptional among the adult disorders, in that it segregates as an autosomal-recessive and is associated with a remediable metabolic error. Although I am listing this as a steadily progressive, adult-onset disorder, Wilson's disease can present as early as late childhood and can be punctuated by acute crises. The mainstay of chronic treatment is D-penicillamine, 1 to 3 g per day in two doses for adults; 500 mg per day for children under 10. Efficacy of treatment initially has to be assessed by documenting copper excretion of 2 mg per day, as it usually takes months to obtain a clinically beneficial response. For the 5 to 10 percent of persons who cannot tolerate penicillamine, I substitute triethylene tetramine at adult doses of 400 to 800 mg three times a day. During an acute crisis, peritoneal dialysis should be performed with added albumin. Liver transplantation has been used in acutely fulminant cases. For long-term maintenance after completion of chelation therapy, 150 mg of zinc as acetate or sulfate is given before meals, three or four times a day.

SYMPTOMATIC TREATMENT

The mainstay of symptomatic treatment for ataxia itself is the provision of occupational therapy. Gait training and instruction in the use of assistive devices to prevent falls and enhance mobility are useful for all ataxic individuals. Some with severe intention tremor benefit from weighted bracelets or similar devices that damp the oscillations. Practical advice and much-needed emotional support are available through a variety of support groups (listed at the end of this chapter).

Symptomatic pharmacotherapy is essentially limited to the treatment of associated symptoms—spasticity, parkinsonian rigidity, autonomic dysfunction, heart failure, and so on—rather than the ataxia itself. Although the literature is replete with anecdotal reports of symptomatic improvement of ataxia in response to any of an extensive variety of drugs—propanolol, physostigmine, choline chloride, lecithin, gamma-vinyl aminobutyric acid, thyrotropin-releasing hormone, gangliosides, L-5-hydroxytryptophan, clonazepam—subsequent control trials have shown no significant benefit. Two possible exceptions currently under investigation are (1) symmetrel, 200 mg per day PO, which was reported to be of modest benefit in FA patients but which I have personally found to have reversibly worsened the ataxia in two adolescent patients with ataxia not of the Friedreich's type, and (2) physostigmine, which has been shown to reduce the ocular dysmetria in individual patients in whom the gain of the vestibuloocular reflex was greater than 1.0. Although I have no moral or intellectual qualms about the use of placebos, it is not currently my practice to use them in the management of ataxia.

In all patients, even when I fail to find a specifically treatable cerebellar disorder or a need for symptomatic treatment of associated symptoms, I recommend annual neurologic follow-up. The clinical phenotype, and the need for adjunctive therapies, can change during that interval. Furthermore, the technology of diagnosis and treatment is finally changing: a condition that today is untreatable may well have a significant treatment developed in future.

SUGGESTED READING

Baraitser M. The genetics of neurological disorders. Oxford: Oxford University Press, 1990.

Bundey S. Genetics and neurology. Edinburgh: Churchill Livingstone, 1992.

Desnick RJ. Treatment of genetic diseases. Edinburgh: Churchill Livingstone, 1991.

Friedman T. Therapy for genetic diseases. Oxford: Oxford University Press, 1991.

Harding AE. The hereditary ataxias and related disorders. Edinburgh: Churchill Livingstone, 1984.

Lechtenberg R, ed. The handbook of cerebellar diseases. New York: Marcel Dekker, 1993.

McKusick VA. Mendelian inheritance in man. Baltimore: Johns Hopkins University Press, 1992.

Milunsky A. Heredity and your family's health. Baltimore: Johns Hopkins University Press, 1992.

Scriver CR, Beaudet AL, Sly WS, Valle D. The metabolic basis of inherited disease. 6th ed. New York: McGraw-Hill, 1989.

PATIENT RESOURCES

National Ataxia Foundation
750 Twelve Oaks Center
15500 Wayzata Boulevard
Wayzata, Minnesota 55391
(612) 473-7666

National Organization for Rare Disorders (NORD)
Box 8923
New Fairfield, Connecticut 06812
(203) 746-6518

Alliance of Genetic Support Groups
35 Wisconsin Circle, Suite 440
Chevy Chase, Maryland 20815
(800) 336-GENE

DYSTONIA

CARLOS SINGER, M.D.
WILLIAM J. WEINER, M.D.

Dystonia is a syndrome characterized by sustained muscle contractions that frequently cause twisting and repetitive movements or abnormal postures. These movements and postures are the end result of excessive muscle activity in which agonists and antagonists co-contract. Dystonia interferes with the smoothness, range, speed, and accuracy of movements in the affected body segment.

Dystonia usually begins in a focal manner involving a foot, hand, or axial muscles. If it remains restricted to a single anatomic area, the dystonia is *focal*. If the abnormal movements involve adjacent body areas, the dystonia is *segmental,* and if the dystonia involves a non-contiguous body area, it is *multifocal. Generalized* dystonia involves three limbs, and usually axial and bulbar structures as well. Age of onset of dystonia is extremely important in determining prognosis. Early childhood–onset dystonia is often progressive, resulting in generalized dystonia, whereas adult-onset dystonia is more likely to remain restricted to focal areas. *Hemidystonia* indicates involvement of half the body and is usually secondary to contralateral hemisphere disease affecting basal ganglia structures (e.g., stroke, trauma, tumor).

Dystonia can be classified three different ways: (1) age at onset (childhood, 0 to 12 years; adolescence, 13 to 20 years; adult, after age 20 years); (2) in terms of cause (Table 1); and (3) in terms of anatomic area of involvement (Table 2). The age at onset and distribution classifications can provide important clues to direct investigation toward a particular cause, and they provide important information on prognosis.

Although rare, some of the paroxysmal dyskinesias may involve dystonic postures and movements. Paroxysmal kinesigenic choreoathetosis (PKC) and paroxysmal dystonic (non-kinesigenic) choreoathetosis (PDC) are the two most important dyskinesias. Their classification into kinesigenic and nonkinesigenic varieties has therapeutic implications.

If neurologic examination suggests involvement of cognition, pyramidal tract, visual pathways, or other neuroanatomic structures outside the basal ganglia, a secondary dystonic disorder is likely. If examination reveals an exclusively extrapyramidal picture, whether generalized or focal, the dystonia is most likely a primary (idiopathic) disorder. There are exceptions to this "pearl," such as Wilson's disease and drug-induced movement disorders.

DIFFERENTIAL DIAGNOSIS

After the clinical diagnosis of a dystonic syndrome is made, the most important clinical decision involves distinguishing between primary and secondary dystonic syndromes. It is extremely rare to discover a symptomatic cause of dystonia in an adult who presents with

Table 1 Differential Diagnosis of Dystonia

1. Primary dystonia (idiopathic torsion dystonia)
   A. Hereditary
      Autosomal-dominant
      Autosomal-recessive
      X-linked recessive
      Autosomal-dominant myoclonic dystonia with dramatic response to alcohol
      Paroxysmal dystonia (kinesigenic, nonkinesigenic)
      Paroxysmal hypnogenic dystonia
   B. Sporadic
      Childhood or adult onset; generalized, segmental, or focal

2. Secondary dystonia
   A. Hereditary neurologic disorders due to identifiable neurometabolic defect
      Wilson's disease
      GM_1 gangliosidosis
      GM_2 gangliosidosis
      Lesch-Nyhan syndrome
      Homocystinuria
      Glutaric acidemia
      Metachromatic leukodystrophy
      Methylmalonic acidemia
      Hartnup's disease
      Triosephosphate isomerase deficiency
   B. Neurologic disorders (often hereditary) with presumed but undefined neurometabolic defect
      Leigh's disease
      Striatal lucencies (with or without vision failure) [? Leigh's disease, ? mitochondrial cytopathy]
      Hallervorden-Spatz disease
      Neuronal ceroid lipofuscinosis
      Dystonic lipidosis
      Calcification of the basal ganglia
      Ataxia telangiectasia
      Chorea acanthocytosis
      Pelizaeus-Merzbacher disease
      Neuronal intranuclear inclusion disease
      Rett's syndrome
   C. "Degenerative" disorders (often hereditary) with no known metabolic defect
      Huntington's disease, usually juvenile Westphal variant type
      Dystonia plus parkinsonism
         Idiopathic Parkinson's disease
         L-Dopa responsive dystonia-parkinsonism, including dystonia with marked diurnal variations
            ("Segawa variant")
      Pallidal degenerations
      Azorean disease
      Other olivopontocerebellar and spinocerebellar degenerations
      Progressive supranuclear palsy
      Corticobasal ganglionic degeneration
      Dystonic amyotrophy
      Familial amyotrophic dystonic paraplegia
      Myoclonic dystonia with nasal malformation
      Dystonia with neural deafness
   D. Acquired dystonia
      Perinatal brain injury, anoxia, kernicterus (athetoid cerebral palsy)
      Anoxia, carbon monoxide poisoning
      Encephalitis
      Heavy metal toxicity, especially manganese
      Drugs
      Focal cerebral disease, usually causing hemidystonia
         Stroke
         Arteriovenous malformation
         Brain tumor
         Head trauma
         Postoperative (thalamotomy)
         Local encephalitis
         Multiple sclerosis
      "Peripheral disorders (e.g., with Sudeck's atrophy)
      Syringomyelia, with cerebellar ectopia: leg dystonia; with spinal cord tumor: neck dystonia
   E. Psychogenic
      Hysterical
      Münchausen's syndrome
      Malingering

From Weiner WJ, Lang AE, eds. Movement disorders: A comprehensive survey, Mt. Kisco, NY: Futura Publishing Co., Inc., 1989; with permission.

Table 2 Classification of Dystonia Based on Distribution

Focal: Involves a single body part (e.g., eyelids, lower face, pharynx, larynx, neck, trunk, limb)
Segmental:
  Cranial: Involves two or more cranial and/or neck muscles
  Axial: Involves neck and trunk
  Brachial: Involves one arm and axial; both arms ± axial
  Crural: Involves one leg and trunk; both legs ± trunk
Multifocal: Involves two or more contiguous parts
Generalized: Crural plus any other segment
Hemidystonia: Involves ipsilateral arm and leg

From Weiner WJ, Lang AE, eds. Movement disorders: A comprehensive survey, Mt. Kisco, NY: Futura Publishing Co., Inc., 1989; with permission.

typical focal or segmental dystonia (e.g., blepharospasm, spasmodic torticollis, oromandibular dystonia, writer's cramp). Younger patients should be screened for Wilson's disease. If onset and progression are typical and there are no additional clues to a symptomatic cause such as additional abnormalities in the examination, additional laboratory testing is not warranted. On the other hand, for patients with progressive or generalized dystonia laboratory investigation is required. In these circumstances slit-lamp examination for Kayser-Fleischer rings, liver function tests, and laboratory values for ceruloplasmin, copper, calcium, electrolytes, uric acid, and organic acids, particularly glutaric acid and methylmalonic acid, should be obtained. Lactate and pyruvate values may also be useful. Urinary amino- and organic acids should be evaluated. A wet smear to examine peripheral blood for acanthocytosis may be useful. Computed tomography (CT) and magnetic resonance imaging (MRI) may provide essential information. Although a cause may be discovered with a thorough investigation, the most important and treatable cause is Wilson's disease. Treatment of Wilson's disease with penicillamine often produces dramatic reversal of the neurologic symptoms.

THERAPY

Levodopa

Once Wilson's disease has been ruled out, the patient with dystonia of undetermined cause, especially with onset in childhood, adolescence, or young adulthood (generalized or more restricted), should undergo a trial of levodopa. Levodopa-responsive dystonia (Segawa's variant) accounts for 5 to 10 percent of patients who present with "idiopathic" dystonia in childhood. Levodopa-responsive dystonia is frequently associated with diurnal variation of symptoms and is exquisitely sensitive to levodopa in modest doses (e.g., one-half to a whole tablet of levodopa/carbidopa 25/100 three times per day). If a patient is unresponsive to 400 mg per day, the chances of therapeutic success decrease, but a full trial should proceed, reaching 800 to 1000 mg per day in more adult persons. Levodopa's effectiveness in this

setting usually does not diminish, and therapy is rarely attended by complications other than mild dyskinesias. It is unlikely that the craniocervical, brachial, focal, or segmental dystonias that present after the third decade will prove responsive to levodopa, but a short trial can rapidly provide the answer before more involved pharmacological treatments are undertaken.

Pharmacologic Treatment

Symptomatic drug treatment is similar for generalized and focal dystonia. Anticholinergics, baclofen, clonazepam, and carbamazepine are first-line drugs. Dopamine agonists, depletors, and blockers have occasionally been used once other measures have failed, but these drugs may exacerbate the movement disorder. An exception to this is tardive dystonia, which has been treated successfully with dopamine depletors. Combinations of two or more of these drugs may be necessary. Slow upward or downward titration is also recommended.

Anticholinergics are often the first drugs to be tried in the treatment of generalized dystonia. They are also frequently used to treat focal dystonias before botulinum toxin is tried. Blepharospasm and hyperadduction laryngeal dystonia (spastic dysphonia) are the two focal dystonias for which botulinum toxin injections have become the treatment of choice. Anticholinergics can also be used as adjunctive treatments to these injections. The best-studied of these drugs is trihexyphenidyl. In children it can be given in very large doses (40 to 80 mg per day). Adults tolerate far less, usually 18 to 30 mg per day. Dryness of the mouth, cognitive dysfunction, focusing difficulty, constipation, urine retention, and aggravation of glaucoma are frequent dose-limiting factors. Treatment should begin with 5 to 6 mg per day, and the dose should be adjusted upward at the rate of 1 mg per week. Dose increments should be added until either the dystonia improves or unacceptable side effects supervene. Once a stable dose has been reached, 5 mg tablets may be easier for the patient to use. Long-acting 5 mg sequels provide the convenience of 12 hour dose intervals.

One of the main side effects of anticholinergics is dry mouth. To counteract this effect, simple measures such as frequent sips of water, sucking on ice chips, and chewing sugarless or xylitol gum or hard candy should be tried. A number of over-the-counter saliva substitutes (e.g., Salivart) can be recommended. Patients may check with their local pharmacist for the available brands (see The Medical Letter 1988; 30:74–76). If peripheral anticholinergic side effects such as cycloplegia or urination hesitancy are intolerable, cautious use of anticholinesterase agents can be considered. Pyridostigmine, in doses of 30 to 60 mg every 4 to 6 hours, may provide some relief with a minimum of side effects.

Carbamazepine, 200 to 400 mg three times daily, has been successful in small numbers of patients with dystonia. We start at a dose of 200 mg per day and gradually increase the dose by 200 mg every 5 to 7 days.

This minimizes side effects such as nausea, vomiting, drowsiness, diplopia, blurred vision, vertigo, and ataxia. Transient mild leukopenia in the initial stages of treatment can be seen. Persistent leukopenia and aplastic anemia are rare, but it is suggested that a complete blood count be obtained at baseline. The timing of subsequent blood monitoring is left to the individual physician. We have not been particularly impressed with favorable responses to carbamazepine.

Baclofen is better tolerated than anticholinergics, although we have seen dryness of the mouth, nausea, urination hesitancy, orthostatic hypotension, generalized "floppiness," confusion, and drowsiness. Although standard recommendations place the maximum dose at 80 mg per day, at times we try as much as 120 mg per day. Doses close to 200 mg per day have been reported to be safe in patients with multiple sclerosis. Baclofen's effectiveness in dystonia is sporadic.

Rarely, clonazepam may offer some relief in dystonia. Its use is attended by drowsiness as the most frequent dose-limiting side effect, and it requires slow upward titration. As much as 20 mg per day may be administered, although patients are unlikely to tolerate more than 4 to 8 mg per day. Periodic monitoring of blood count and liver function tests is advisable.

Occasional reports indicate that amantadine, cyproheptadine, tricyclic antidepressants, and lithium may be useful in the treatment of dystonia. We have not been impressed.

The treatment of drug-induced dystonias and paroxysmal dystonias requires a different therapeutic approach.

Pharmacologic Treatment of Drug-Induced Dystonias

Acute dystonic reactions are manifested clinically as a wide variety of prolonged or short-lived muscle spasms that result in typical dystonic postures and movements. Involvement of the face, tongue, head, or neck is most common. These reactions are the earliest of the neuroleptic-induced movement disorders: 90 percent occur within 5 days after institution of treatment. Acute dystonic reactions have also been reported as a consequence of the use of other dopamine receptor–blocking agents such as metoclopramide.

Acute dystonic reactions can be managed by immediate removal of the offending agent and parenteral administration of 10 to 50 mg of chlopheniramine or 1 to 2 mg of benztropine mesylate. After the resolution of the immediate problem, it may be wise to administer an oral anticholinergic every 4 to 6 hours for the next 24 to 48 hours. This is particularly important if the offending neuroleptic was administered as a depot injection.

Tardive dystonia is a clinical subtype of tardive dyskinesia. When dystonia complicates chronic neuroleptic therapy it may be indistinguishable from that associated with idiopathic torsion dystonia. One clue that it may be tardive dystonia is the occurrence of other drug-induced movements in the same patient.

Tardive dystonia may require treatment that combines a dopamine depletor with one or more of the following drugs: an anticholinergic, baclofen, or a benzodiazepine. If from a psychiatric standpoint it is feasible, the neuroleptic should be discontinued. If further treatment is required, we use reserpine, starting with doses of 0.1 mg per day and we try to increase the *daily* dose by 0.1 mg per week, to a maximum of 1.5 to 2.0 mg per day. Orthostatic hypotension, depression, and parkinsonism are the main side effects. Anticholinergics, baclofen, and benzodiazepines are also employed, in combination or alone. At times it is necessary, from a motor standpoint, to continue the use of a dopamine-blocking agent for a number of weeks or months before slowly tapering the dose.

Tetrabenazine is another drug that both depletes dopamine and blocks dopamine receptors. It can be effective, but it is not available in the United States.

Treatment of Focal Dystonias with Botulinum Toxin

Injection of botulinum toxin A directly into the affected muscles represents an important advance in the therapy of focal dystonias. Botulinum toxin is effective for blepharospasm and in hyperadduction laryngeal dystonia in 90 percent of cases, and for cervical dystonia in more than 80 percent. Jaw closure dystonia and focal dystonias of the upper extremity (e.g., writer's cramp) can also be treated successfully. Its usefulness in hyperabduction laryngeal dystonia, jaw-opening dystonia, and other dystonias requires further study.

Botulinum toxin interferes with the release of acetylcholine at the presynaptic cholinergic terminal, resulting in chemical denervation of the injected muscle. Injections must be repeated every 3 to 6 months to maintain the effect. Side effects are transient and usually mild (Table 3).

The finding of abnormal jitter in single-fiber electromyographic studies in muscles distant to the ones injected has been reported, but to date it appears to have no clinical significance. The eventual emergence of resistance to these injections appears to be linked to the development of antibodies. Studies are under way to evaluate the usefulness of other immunotypes of botulinum toxin.

Treatment of Paroxysmal Dystonias

Paroxysmal kinesigenic dystonia (attacks triggered by sudden movements) are responsive to phenytoin, carbamazepine, phenobarbital, primidone, and diazepam. The nonkinesigenic dystonias do not respond as well to these agents and may warrant a trial of other agents such as acetazolamide, clonazepam, oxazepam, baclofen, or anticholinergics. Neurologic disorders that may mimic these paroxysmal movement disorders include transient ischemic attacks, multiple sclerosis, cerebral palsy, hyperthyroidism, and seizures. Paroxysmal hypnogenic dystonia (attacks occurring during sleep) can be treated with carbamazepine. This condition may represent an overlap with frontal lobe epilepsy.

Table 3 Side Effects of Botulinum Toxin Injections

Condition Treated	Side Effects
Blepharospasm	Ptosis, eye dryness (need for corneal protective measures), ecchymoses, ectropion, entropion.
Cervical dystonia	Neck weakness, dysphagia,* neck soreness, nausea and dizziness, brachial plexus palsy (isolated reports, cause unclear)
Hyperadduction laryngeal dystonia	Hoarseness, voice breathiness, dysphagia, respiratory arrest during procedure†
Jaw closure dystonia	Jaw closure weakness, dysphagia (?)
Hand dystonia	Weakness of injected muscles

*May require close observation, switching to semisolid diet, ingesting liquids through a straw, and caution against aspiration.

†Rare, but the physician performing the procedure should be capable of performing an emergency tracheostomy.

Surgical Treatment and Other Nonpharmacologic Modalities

Surgical interventions include stereotactic neurosurgery, which can be used for severe generalized or hemidystonias, and "peripheral" surgeries designed to address specific types of focal dystonia.

Thalamotomy can be considered in cases of severe generalized dystonia that are unresponsive to intensive pharmacologic trials. These procedures cannot halt the progression of the disease. Severe dysarthria may follow bilateral thalamotomy. Aggravation of motor deficit and actual hemiplegia are unlikely but worrisome outcomes. Unilateral thalamotomy can be considered in hemidystonias, particularly if they are secondary to static lesions.

There are surgical procedures that can be recommended to patients with certain kinds of focal dystonias that have failed to respond to botulinum toxin therapy. Blepharospasm can be treated with orbital myectomy and cervical dystonia with peripheral denervation of cervical musculature (cervical ramisectomy). Both procedures offer a reasonable chance for permanent or longstanding responses. Patients should be referred only to surgeons who have extensive training and exposure to these interventions.

Some patients with spasmodic torticollis derive a sense of better control of their disease if allowed to participate in physical therapy programs, which sometimes include biofeedback. Patients with writer's cramp may learn to use their nondominant hand for writing, although involvement in that hand may develop. Writing-aid devices may also be of help. One of them is the Blackburn writing system device. If unavailable locally, it may be purchased by contacting Cardon Rehabilitation Products, Woodbridge, Ontario.

SUGGESTED READING

Fahn S, Marsden CD, Calne DB, eds. Advances in neurology. Dystonia 2. Vol 50. New York: Raven, 1988.

Fink JK, Ravin PD, Filling-Katz M, et al. Clinical and genetic analysis of progressive dystonia with diurnal variation. Arch Neurol 1991; 48:908–911.

Greene P, Shale H, Fahn S. Analysis of open-label trials in torsion dystonia using high dosages of anticholinergics and other drugs. Mov Disord 1988; 3:46–60.

Jankovic J, Schwartz K, Donovan DT. Botulinum toxin treatment of cranial-cervical dystonia, spasmodic dysphonia, other focal dystonias and hemifacial spasm. J Neurol Neurosurg Psychiatry 1990; 53: 633–639.

Marsden CD, Fahn S, eds. Movement disorders 2. London: Butterworth, 1987.

Weiner WJ, Lang AE, eds. Movement disorders. A comprehensive survey. Mt Kisco, NY: Futura, 1989.

PATIENT RESOURCES

Dystonia Medical Research Foundation
1 East Wacker Drive
Suite 2900
Chicago, Illinois 60601
Telephone: (312) 755-0198

National Spasmodic Torticollis Association
Box 476
Elm Grove, Wisconsin 53122
Telephone: (414) 797-9912

Benign Essential Blepharospasm Research Foundation
2929 Calder Avenue, Suite 304
Box 12468
Beaumont, Texas 77726
Telephone: (409) 832-0788

National Spasmodic Dysphonia Association
Box 1574
Birmingham, Michigan 48009-1574

TORTICOLLIS (CERVICAL DYSTONIA)

MITCHELL F. BRIN, M.D.

Because in most cases torticollis is a form of dystonia involving the neck muscles, it has been called *cervical dystonia* (CD). Torticollis came of age during the 1980s, as better understanding was gained of the diagnostic and therapeutic considerations: We now have markers linked to the gene or genes for dystonia; DYT1 is associated with the gene for childhood-onset Jewish and non-Jewish dystonia; physiologists have begun to unravel the inter-relationships between dystonic tremor and other tremors; and we now have a safe and effective therapeutic intervention, botulinum toxin type A (botox-A). Many questions remain unanswered, and I anticipate that advances during the decade of the brain will further our understanding of the pathophysiology of this focal dystonia and refine our treatment programs.

Dystonia is a syndrome dominated by sustained muscle contractions that frequently cause twisting and repetitive movements or abnormal postures that may be sustained or intermittent. Dystonia can involve any voluntary muscle. Because the movements and resulting postures are often unusual and the condition is rare, it is one of the most frequently misdiagnosed neurologic conditions. The prevalence of the condition is unknown, but we estimate about 50,000 to 200,000 cases of idiopathic dystonia in the United States.

CD is the most common form of focal dystonia presented for treatment. There has been only one epidemiologic study of the prevalence of CD; the incidence of all focal dystonias has been estimated to be 300 per million, nine times the incidence of generalized dystonia. Nutt's estimate of 22,250 cases of CD in the United States (assuming a population of 250 million) is based on a medical record review at the Mayo Clinic. I believe this is likely an underestimate by a factor of four, because this number represents only patients with focal dystonia and we know from our large database that approximately 50 percent of CDs are not focal. In addition, at the time of his study, many affected persons did not come to medical attention; now that we have effective therapy and support groups are better organized, more patients are coming to medical attention. I suspect that there are some 60,000 to 90,000 cases of CD in the United States.

CLASSIFICATION

As a clinical syndrome, we classify dystonia according to clinical symptoms, age at onset, and cause. Classification may be important, as it can provide clues about prognosis and also an approach to management. The classification scheme is outlined in Table 1.

Dystonia may begin at nearly any age. In our experience with more than 1350 idiopathic cases at the Dystonia Clinical Research Center, we have seen presenting signs as early as age 9 months and as late as 85 years (Fig. 1). In general, there is a bimodal distribution of age at onset, with peaks at ages 8 and 42 years. Therefore, we classify disease as "early onset" when the signs appear before age 26 years, and "late onset" at ages 26 years and over. Infantile-onset dystonia is frequently secondary to some insult and is classified separately.

When classified by the distribution, symptoms are categorized as focal, segmental, or generalized. Focal dystonia symptoms involve one group of muscles in one body part, segmental disease involves a contiguous group of muscles, and generalized dystonia is widespread. Common examples of focal dystonia include blepharospasm (forced, involuntary eye closure), oromandibular dystonia (face, jaw, or tongue), CD (neck),

Table 1 Classification of Dystonia

Age at onset
  Infantile (<2 yr)
  Early onset (2–26 yr)
  Late onset (>26 yr)
Cause
  Primary
    With hereditary pattern
      Autosomal-dominant
        Classical (essential) types
        Variant types
          Dopa-responsive dystonia
          Myoclonic dystonia
      X-linked recessive
    Sporadic (without a documented hereditary pattern)*
      Classical (essential) types
      Variant types
  Secondary
    Associated with other hereditary neurologic disorders
      (e.g., Wilson's disease, Huntington's disease, ceroid lipofuscinosis)
    Environmental (e.g., post-traumatic, postinfectious, vascular, tumor, toxic, phenothiazines [tardive])
    Dystonia associated with parkinsonism
    Psychogenic
Distribution
  Focal
    Blepharospasm (forced, involuntary eye closure)
    Oromandibular dystonia (face, jaw, or tongue)
    Cervical dystonia (neck)
    Writer's cramp (action-induced dystonic contraction of hand muscles)
    Spasmodic dysphonia (vocal cords)
  Segmental (cranial, axial, crural)
  Multifocal
  Generalized (ambulatory, nonambulatory)

*The term *sporadic* is in many cases a misnomer (see text).

Dr. Brin conducts clinical trials under the sponsorship of the U.S. Public Health Service (NIH) and Allergan Inc. but does not hold any equity interest in or receive personal remuneration from any commercial sponsor. Preparation of this manuscript was supported by the Dystonia Medical Research Foundation and USPHS grants NS-26656, NS24778, DC-01139 and RR-00645.

writer's cramp (action-induced dystonic contraction of hand muscles), and spasmodic dysphonia (vocal cords). We use the term *cervical dystonia,* because spasmodic *torti*collis implies rotation only, and in addition to rotatocollis we see patients with neck flexion (antero-collis), extension (retrocollis), head tilt (laterocollis), or lateral shift. Patients with CD often present with a combination of these movements. The adjectives *spasmodic* and *spastic* are misleading; there is no evidence that CD is a spastic disorder or due to dysfunction of the pyramidal tracts. Furthermore, the movements are not always spasmodic but may be sustained. From the figure, one observes that generalized dystonia usually has early onset and focal dystonia usually adult onset. The exceptions make patient counseling difficult.

According to the classification by cause, patients with *idiopathic* disease have no evidence by history, examination, or laboratory studies of any identifiable cause for the dystonic symptoms. Therefore, there must be normal perinatal and early developmental history, no history of neurologic illness or exposure to drugs known to cause acquired dystonia (e.g., phenothiazines), normal intellectual, pyramidal, cerebellar, and sensory findings, and normal diagnostic studies. Patients who have abnormalities noted above are classified as having secondary dystonia. The clinical findings are often a clue as to cause.

This classification needs to be revised. Genetic subtypes of dystonia have been identified (see Table 1) in which the only identifiable cause is a gene mutation; the biochemical or pathophysiologic abnormalities are being sought. The subtypes are: (1) autosomal-dominant: classical childhood-onset dystonia, or dystonia musculorum deformans located on chromosome 9q; levodopa-responsive dystonia not linked to 9q; myoclonic dystonia with linkage location unknown; and (2) X-linked recessive: "Lubag." Furthermore, we now have evidence of non-Jewish inherited dystonia that is not due to DYT1. Until the genes for these dystonic conditions are identified and we can differentiate between each genetic subtype and the nongenetic phenocopies, the

term *classical* or *essential* may be preferable for describing the focal, segmental, and generalized cases of *dystonia musculorum deformans* as originally introduced by Oppenheim in 1911 and elaborated by Herz in 1944 and 1945.

Note that the classification distinguishes between inherited and sporadic cases. It has now been demonstrated that most "sporadic" cases of childhood-onset Ashkenazi Jewish dystonia are inherited and are due to the same mutation of DYT1 that is involved in familial cases. This is a classic example of the founder effect.

Inherited dystonia is characterized by incomplete penetrance and clinical heterogeneity: in families with dystonia, various members may have generalized, segmental, or focal dystonia, suggesting that milder manifestations are related to the more generalized cases. It is essential to obtain a complete family history from every patient who presents with any form of dystonia. It is not uncommon to discover that a patient who presents with focal dystonia has a relative who is similarly affected or has symptoms of dystonia affecting another segment of the body.

EVALUATION AND THERAPY

Patients who present with symptoms of CD should have a comprehensive history and neurologic examination. Many patients have signs of dystonia involving other body segments. Sensory tricks often ameliorate dystonic movements and postures, and this maneuver can be effective in different parts of the body. Patients with CD often exhibit a *geste antagonistique* or *Gegendrückphaenomen,* whereby gently touching the chin or back or top of the head relieves symptoms; blepharospastics relieve symptoms by gently touching the lateral canthus. The family history should be carefully reviewed, in addition to careful attention to any factors suggesting secondary dystonia or pseudodystonia.

When evaluating the patient, I introduce the concept of the potential genetic basis of their symptoms. I

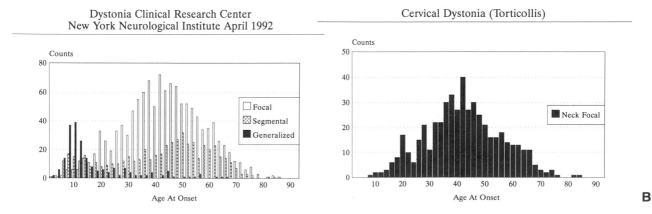

Figure 1 *A,* Age at onset of dystonia in our population of patients. Note that patients with generalized dystonia are younger at onset, and onset of focal dystonia is typically in the adult years. However, there are exceptions: later onset of generalized dystonia and early onset of focal disease. *B,* Patients with focal CD of childhood onset.

obtain a detailed family history, and noting the various clinical presentations of dystonia, search for a history of a movement disorder. The availability of genetic counseling services is discussed. Although by history we may not be able to determine if a particular case of adult-onset dystonia is genetic or a phenocopy, we anticipate being able to make that distinction in the future.

Most patients who present with symptoms of a twisted neck have dystonia, but it is important to evaluate for "pseudodystonic" cases secondary to structural abnormalities (Table 2). Comprehensive lists of diagnostic tests to be performed when secondary or pseudodystonia is suspected are available; findings on neurologic examination that are suspicious for secondary dystonia should be followed-up with appropriate diagnostic studies. All patients should receive screening biochemical studies (SMA-20, complete blood count), in addition to a ceruloplasmin. Although CD would be an uncommon presentation for Wilson's disease, that condition is amenable to treatment. I obtain a magnetic resonance imaging study of the brain or cervical cord if there are any findings on history or examination suggestive of additional neurologic compromise, or secondary dystonia.

The course of CD varies from person to person, *and* any patient's symptoms may vary throughout the course of the illness. Most patients report that their condition stabilizes within the first 5 years after symptom onset.

Reviews of patients referred to movement disorder centers report that about 10 to 20 percent of patients go into remission, and nearly all suffer a recurrence within a few months or years. These studies are biased, however, because patients with mild torticollis who experience remission would have no reason to present for treatment to a physician.

Specific pharmacotherapy directed at the underlying identified biochemical defect is available for only a limited number of symptomatic dystonias; the most notable is Wilson's disease. For tardive CD, the best treatment is avoidance of offending medications when possible, and providing the patient with a list of these medications (Table 3).

Various options are available for treating patients with CD; therapy must be individualized. A treatment strategy must be chosen that keeps the risk to a minimum. Very few systematic drug trials have been conducted on CD; much of what we know about pharmacotherapy has resulted from empiric trials. To avoid causing harm, when evaluating the therapeutic options, surgical therapies and drugs that have the potential to cause irreversible harm (Table 3) should be reserved for patients whom more conservative medical therapies, including botulinum toxin, have failed.

In all situations, *informed consent* must be obtained. This process involves disclosure of the major risks of the treatment or procedure being contemplated, an accurate assessment of the benefits that can be reasonably expected, and a discussion of alternative forms of treatment. Treatment of CD is challenging, and it is wise that the treating physician and associated staff nurture a responsive relationship with the patient. In most situations, I tell the patient that the doctor and the patient "hold hands" as they proceed to explore the treatment options. The dose of medication is carefully monitored and adjusted according to the response benefits versus adverse effects. Patients build a portfolio

Table 2 Classification of Cervical Dystonia

Dystonia associated with abnormal involuntary excessive muscle contraction causing abnormal postures. The causes are diverse (see Table 1)
Dystonia of structural causes
  Orthopaedic
    Atlantoaxial dislocation
    Cervical fracture
    Degenerative disc
    Osteomyelitis
    Klippel-Feil syndrome
  Musculofibrotic
    Congenital torticollis associated with absence or fibrosis of cervical muscles (usually due to local trauma, hemorrhage)
    Postradiation fibrosis
    Acute stiff neck
  Local infectious
    Pharyngitis
    Painful lymphadenopathy, adenitis
  Other neurologic
    Vestibulo-ocular dysfunction (head tilt with fourth nerve paresis, or labyrinthine disease)
    Posterior fossa tumor
    Arnold-Chiari syndrome
    Bobble-head doll syndrome (with third ventricle cyst)
    Nystagmus
    Sandifer's syndrome
    Spinal cord tumor/syrinx
    Extraocular muscle palsies, strabismus
    Head thrusts with oculomotor apraxia
    Hemianopia
    Spasmus nutans
    Focal seizures

Modified from Weiner WJ, Lang AE. Movement disorders: A comprehensive survey. Mt. Kisco, NY: Futura Publishing, 1989; with permission.

Table 3 Drugs That May Cause Dystonia

Acetophenazine (Tindal)
Amoxapine (Asendin)
Chlorpromazine (Thorazine)
Fluphenazine (Permitil, Prolixin)
Haloperidol (Haldol)
Loxapine (Loxitane, Daxolin)
Mesoridazine (Serentil)
Metoclopramide (Reglan)
Molindone (Lindone, Moban)
Perphenazine (Trilafon or Triavil)
Pimozide (Orap)
Piperacetazine (Quide)
Prochlorperazine (Compazine, Combid)
Promazine (Sparine)
Promethazine (Phenergan)
Thiethylperazine (Torecan)
Thioridazine (Mellaril)
Thiothixene (Navane)
Trifluoperazine (Stelazine)
Triflupromazine (Vesprin)
Trimeprazine (Temaril)

of response to therapy; this portfolio is consulted frequently, as each new strategy is considered. An accessible drug treatment list may be kept in each chart.

Mild symptoms may be managed with physical measures or pharmacotherapy. Physical measures include the simple *geste antagonistique* (see above), biofeedback, mechanical braces, and physical therapy. A common problem encountered when treating CD with physical measures is the assumption that the condition results from a spinal or orthopaedic abnormality. In most cases, the brain's disordered central processing commands to displace head position cannot be physically overcome. Therefore, I advise that manipulation-based practitioners (physical therapists, chiropractors) not use such techniques or physical force, as this may result in further discomfort. It is beneficial to help patients to utilize their own resources to improve head control via strengthening and enhanced flexibility.

Pharmacotherapeutic agents in small doses, such as benzodiazepines, baclofen, or anticholinergics, may be useful early in therapy, though, the larger doses we employed before botulinum toxin became available are unacceptable as the disorder progresses, because in most CD patients they are complicated by undesirable side effects. For instance, Greene, in our department, reported that 39 percent of patients with CD improved with anticholinergics (trihexyphenidyl, ethopropazine), but their benefits were often limited by the development of adverse effects (dry mouth, cognitive disturbance, drowsiness, blurred vision, glaucoma, urine retention). Peripheral surgery may be successful in managing patients, but this form of therapy is usually reserved for those who do not respond to more conservative interventions. Thalamotomy and other central nervous system (CNS) procedures have been abandoned by most practitioners because of the significant potential for serious side effects. Most patients with CD have required bilateral operations, which raise the risk of language and swallowing complications. In addition, as our genetic research advances, our concern about ablative CNS surgery has grown. The goal of genetic research is to find out more about the pathophysiology of CD, with the intent to develop specific pharmacotherapeutic interventions. With that goal in mind, we do not want to ablate regions of the brain that may hold important receptors to interventional pharmacotherapy.

Most focal dystonias, including CD, are now effectively treated with local injections of botulism toxin. Safety and efficacy have been established in open-label and double-blind clinical trials in many countries around the world. Improvement in quality of life parameters has also been documented with careful neuropsychiatric testing. Published series report that 70 to 92 percent of the treated patients experience relief of postural abnormality or painful contractions. The average duration of benefit is 12 to 14 months.

In most cases, adverse effects are self-limited and well-tolerated. Immediate side effects include slight pain from the injection, local hematoma, needle irritation of local nerves including the occipital nerve and brachial plexus, and pneumothorax. Subacute side effects are related to an extension of the pharmacologic action of the toxin (i.e., excessive weakness in injected or adjacent muscles). Neck weakness occurs when the patient has a strong response to the toxin; dysphagia is likely due to diffusion into regional pharyngeal muscles. Most patients compensate by temporarily modifying the diet. These complications can usually be avoided by reducing the dose on subsequent treatment. Less frequent side effects include symptoms of generalized weakness without objective signs of weakness and a temporary sense of malaise or headache. A rare patient develops antibodies to the toxin, rendering it inactive. For these patients, other serotypes may be available on research protocol.

Proper selection of muscles for injection is key to a successful result. Usually, the affected muscles can be identified by palpation; the injection is administered through a tuberculin-like syringe and needle. The use of an electromyographic (EMG) examination in conjunction with the clinical evaluation may help identify overactive muscles. The electrode used is a hollow, Teflon-coated monopolar needle that is connected to the EMG machine.

Physical therapy may be a useful adjunct to botulinum toxin treatment when there is less opposition from the dystonic musculature. The goal at this time is to facilitate the patient's increased control over head movement and posture once the antagonists are weakened.

Although therapeutic use of botox in humans has been reported since 1980 without evidence of direct effect of botulinum toxin on uninjected muscles, the long-term consequences of repeated injections are unknown. Weakness or routine EMG changes in muscles distal to the injection site have not been reported; however, there are detectable temporary abnormalities on single-fiber EMG. These findings do not appear to have any clinical significance.

There is a paucity of data on use during pregnancy. In one report, of nine patients treated during pregnancy (dose unspecified), one gave birth prematurely. This was thought not to be related to the drug. Until additional safety data are available, we recommend against injecting patients who are pregnant or lactating.

We have treated some patients with pre-existing disorders affecting neuromuscular junction function and recommend proceeding with caution in treating patients with conditions such as myasthenia gravis, Lambert-Eaton syndrome, and motor neuron disease, particularly when large doses are required, as they are in the treatment of CD. The amount of toxin that enters the systemic circulation after injection is thought to be minute, however, and this theoretical concern should be balanced against the severity of the hyperkinetic symptoms. Patients with Charcot-Marie-Tooth disease and motor neuron disease have been treated with botulinum toxin without experiencing any increase in systemic weakness. Aminoglycosides interfere with neuromuscular transmission and may potentiate the effect of botox therapy. We counsel against injecting a patient who is currently taking aminoglycosides.

Botulinum toxin type A is available in the United States and many other countries around the world from Allergan Pharmaceuticals as Oculinum or BOTOX. It is available in some countries in Europe from Porton Downs (United Kingdom) as Dysport. Although the products show similar efficacy, the side effect profiles are different and the units of measurement are different. Therefore, it is crucial that the physician know which product is being used when comparing treatments. Currently, these products have been approved by the Ministries of Health (Food and Drug Administration) in many countries, including the United States, for the treatment of blepharospasm and associated facial spasms. The toxin is used therapeutically for many more disorders, including CD. The American Academy of Neurology, National Institutes of Health, and American Academy of Otolaryngology–Head and Neck Surgery have issued statements that botox therapy is safe and appropriate for treating CD. We have employed this therapeutic modality since 1984, and in many cases the response has been dramatic. At our institution, CD patients are candidates for treatment with botulinum toxin if conservative pharmacotherapy has failed. In most cases of moderate to severe disease, botulinum toxin is the primary modality of treatment.

Acknowledgments. I am grateful to Deborah de Leon, Susan Bressman, Kathleen Albany, and Judy Blazer for making suggestions.

SUGGESTED READING

American Academy of Otolaryngology–Head and Neck Surgery Policy Statement: Botox for spasmodic dysphonia. AAO-HNS Bull 1990; 9(12):8.

Assessment: The clinical usefulness of botulinum toxin-A in treating neurologic disorders. Report of the Therapeutics and Technology Assessment Subcommittee of the American Academy of Neurology. Neurology 1990; 40:1332–1336.

Brin MF. Interventional neurology: Treatment of neurological conditions with local injections of botulinum toxin. Arch Neurobiol 1991; 54(suppl 3):7–23.

Brin MF, Fahn S, Moskowitz C, et al. Localized injections of botulinum toxin for the treatment of focal dystonia and hemifacial spasm. Adv Neurol 1988; 50:599–608.

Chan J, Brin M, Fahn S. Idiopathic cervical dystonia: Clinical characteristics. Mov Disord 1991; 6:119–126.

Comella CL, Buchman AS, Tanner CM, et al. Botulinum toxin injection for spasmodic torticollis: Increased magnitude of benefit with electromyographic assistance. Neurology 1992; 42:878–882.

Fahn S. The varied clinical expressions of dystonia. Neurol Clin 1984; 2:541–554.

Greene P, Kang U, Fahn S, et al. Double-blind, placebo-controlled trial of botulinum toxin injections for the treatment of spasmodic torticollis. Neurology 1990; 40:1213–1218.

Jahanshahi M, Marion MH, Marsden CD. Natural history of adult-onset idiopathic torticollis. Arch Neurol 1990; 47:548–552.

Jahanshahi M, Marsden CD. Psychological functioning before and after treatment of torticollis with botulinum toxin. J Neurol Neurosurg Psychiatry 1992; 55:229–231.

Jankovic J, Brin M. Therapeutic uses of botulinum toxin. N Engl J Med 1991; 324:1186–1194.

Jankovic J, Fahn S. Dystonic syndromes. In: Jankovic JT, ed. Parkinson's disease and movement disorders. Baltimore: Urban & Schwarzenberg, 1988:283–314.

Jankovic J, Leder S, Warner D, Schwartz K. Cervical dystonia: Clinical findings and associated movement disorders. Neurology 1991; 41:1088–1091.

Jankovic J, Schwartz K. Botulinum toxin injections for cervical dystonia. Neurology 1990; 40:277–280.

Jankovic J, Tolosa E, eds. Parkinson's disease and movement disorders. Baltimore: Urban and Schwarzenberg, 1988.

Kurlan R, ed. The treatment of movement disorders. Philadelphia: JB Lippincott, 1993, in press.

Marsden CD. Investigation of dystonia. Adv Neurol 1988; 50:35–44.

National Institutes of Health Consensus Development Conference. Clinical use of botulinum toxin. 1990; 8(8).

Nutt JG, Muenter MD, Aronson A, et al. Epidemiology of focal and generalized dystonia in Rochester, Minnesota. Mov Disord 1988; 3:188–194.

Ozelius L, Kramer PL, Moskowitz CB, et al. Human gene for torsion dystonia located on chromosome 9q32-q34. Neuron 1989; 2:1427–1434.

Weiner WJ, Lang AE. Movement disorders: A comprehensive survey. Mt. Kisco, NY: Futura, 1989.

PATIENT AND PHYSICIAN RESOURCES

Patient Support Associations
Dystonia Medical Research Foundation
One East Wacker Drive
Suite 2900
Chicago, Illinois 60601-0198
Telephone: (312) 755-0198
Fax: (312) 321-5710

National Spasmodic Torticollis Association
Box 873
Royal Oak, Michigan 48068-0873
Telephone: (800) HURT-FUL
Fax: (313) 362-4552

Resource Handbook
This handbook is a worldwide listing of nonprofit foundations, regional organizations, and local support groups for movement disorders, including dystonia (blepharospasm, torticollis, spasmodic dysphonia), Parkinson's disease and parkinsonian syndromes, tremor, tics, and Tourette's syndrome, Huntington's disease, and myoclonus. Additional resources, including slides, videotapes, and newsletters, are compiled.

WE MOVE Resource Handbook for Movement Disorders
Neurological Institute
Box 22
710 West 178th St.
New York, New York 10032
Telephone: 212-305-1580
Fax: (212) 305-1393
E-Mail: Wemove@movdis.cis.columbia.edu

Resource Journal
Movement Disorders Journal
Raven Press
1185 Avenue of the Americas
New York, New York 10036

TOURETTE'S SYNDROME

ROGER KURLAN, M.D.

Tourette's syndrome (TS) is a hereditary disorder that is defined by the following diagnostic criteria: (1) the presence of multiple motor tics, (2) the presence of one or more vocal tics, (3) onset before age 21 years, and (4) duration longer than 1 year. Despite the formulation of diagnostic criteria, it is now clear that TS is a clinically heterogeneous condition. TS can be considered to represent one extreme of a group of primary tic disorders. Chronic tic disorder (CTD, motor or vocal) differs from TS in that motor or vocal tics, but not both, occur. Transient tic disorder (TTD) differs from TS and CTD by having a duration of less than 1 year. Both CTD and TTD now are generally considered milder variants of TS, and possibly expressions of the same genetic defect. Although the diagnosis of TS is based on the presence of chronic, multiple tics, specific behavior disturbances, including obsessive-compulsive disorder (OCD) and attention deficit hyperactivity disorder (ADHD), commonly accompany tics. Recent family studies indicate that these behavioral disorders may also represent alternative expressions for the TS genetic trait. Other psychiatric diseases, such as conduct disorder and anxiety disorder, have been implicated in the TS clinical spectrum as well. At present, however, the boundaries of the TS behavior disorder have not been accurately delineated. Nevertheless, current information indicates that the clinical manifestations of TS occur along a continuum that includes both motor and behavioral features. Appropriate treatment of patients with TS requires an appreciation of the clinical heterogeneity of the disorder.

TREATMENT APPROACH

Though the diagnosis of a tic disorder can usually be made by simple observation, tics may not be evident at the time of examination, owing to their characteristic waxing and waning quality or to voluntary suppression by the patient. For most individuals affected with TS, tics are mild and severe symptoms are not required for diagnosis. It should be remembered that coprolalia (involuntary obscene vocalizations) may be mild and transient and that it occurs in only a minority of cases.

Given the clinical heterogeneity of TS, it is important to evaluate each patient carefully to determine which aspects of illness are most disabling. For most patients, one or two clinical problems (e.g., tics, ADHD) predominate, and these can serve as specific target symptoms for therapy. We use specific neuropsychological tests of attention, obsessive-compulsive symptoms, and other psychiatric disorders to help sort out the relative contributions of motor and behavioral disturbances for an individual patient.

TREATMENT OF THE TIC DISORDER

Tic-suppressant medication is reserved for patients who are experiencing functionally disabling tics that are not remediable by nondrug interventions. Most patients with mild symptoms who have adjusted well can avoid drug therapy. Psychosocial measures such as educating patients, peers, family members, and school personnel in the nature of TS, restructuring the educational environment, and supportive counseling, may be sufficient to avoid medications. Given the waxing and waning characteristic of tics, periods of tic exacerbation (which often last about 4 months) are usually followed by spontaneous improvement in symptoms. Thus, one can often avoid long-term drug therapy by delaying its institution for some weeks or months.

Drug therapy is indicated for patients whose tics significantly interfere with daily functioning for an extended time. Drugs that block dopamine receptors (neuroleptics) are the most predictably effective (75 to 80 percent response rate) tic-suppressing medications. Neuroleptic dosage is adjusted slowly, in order to determine the smallest satisfactory dose and avoid untoward effects. The maximum dose depends on achieving tolerable suppression of symptoms, which is largely determined by the degree to which they interfere with daily activities.

Haloperidol (Haldol) remains the most commonly prescribed medication for TS, but physicians should avoid prescribing it reflexively upon diagnosis of TS, because many patients do not require tic-suppressing medication. I begin haloperidol therapy with a bedtime dose of 0.25 mg. With this small dose, side effects (e.g., acute dystonia, parkinsonism) that warrant the use of prophylactic anticholinergic medications have not often been encountered. The dosage is increased by 0.25 mg every 4 to 7 days until the lowest satisfactory dose is achieved. A single bedtime dose of haloperidol is generally utilized throughout the course of treatment. Patients and family members are educated in how to judge the effectiveness of medications and to note the appearance of side effects, and during the early course of therapy patients provide frequent telephone calls for progress reports. Most patients respond to 2 mg per day or less, and we generally do not exceed 15 mg. Acute dystonia, parkinsonism, akathisia, and tardive dyskinesia are potential motor side effects of haloperidol and other neuroleptic drugs. Fortunately, although tardive dyskinesia is a real concern, it appears only rarely in treated TS patients. Drowsiness, a common side effect of haloperidol, can often be avoided with a single dose at bedtime, and by having the patient drink coffee, cocoa, or tea in the morning to provide a counteracting stimulant effect. Sedation may be accompanied by an irritable disposition or frank depression, problems that may improve if the dose is reduced. Persistent drowsiness or intellectual dulling may interfere with school and job performance to the extent that the drug must be discontinued. School and social phobias and increased appetite and weight gain are other potential side effects of haloperidol that often are not appreciated by treating physicians.

Pimozide (Orap) is a neuroleptic drug specifically marketed for the treatment of TS. It appears to be about as effective as haloperidol for tic suppression, but it tends to produce less sedation and may, therefore, be better-tolerated. We initiate pimozide therapy at 1 mg at bedtime and slowly increase the dose in order to achieve satisfactory tic control. Although the drug can be administered as a single bedtime dose, two or three daily doses are sometimes necessary. The maximum recommended daily dose is 10 mg for adults and 0.2 mg per kilogram for children. Pimozide may prolong the Q-T interval on the electrocardiogram (ECG), and treatment with large daily doses (60 to 70 mg) has been associated with sudden death. We obtain an ECG before initiating pimozide and avoid giving this medication if the Q-T interval is prolonged. It remains unclear whether monitoring of the ECG is needed for safety reasons during long-term treatment with pimozide in the low doses used to treat TS. Pimozide can cause a spectrum of motor and other side effects similar to those associated with haloperidol and other neuroleptics.

Other neuroleptic drugs such as fluphenazine (Prolixin) and trifluoperazine (Stelazine) appear to have approximately equal tic-suppressing potency when compared to that of haloperidol or pimozide. Switching from one neuroleptic drug to another may be useful for tics that are particularly difficult to control. In addition, patients may vary significantly in their ability to tolerate the adverse effects of different neuroleptic agents.

A variety of other medications can be used to suppress tics in TS, but the response is less predictable than with neuroleptic drugs. Clonidine (Catapres) is an alpha$_2$-receptor agonist that appears to have tic-suppressant effects. It is particularly useful for patients with a combination of mild tics and behavior disturbances such as ADHD (see below). It is a useful drug for initial treatment of tics, so that neuroleptic therapy, with its common attendant adverse effects, may be avoided. We initiate clonidine therapy at 0.05 mg per day, and the dose is gradually increased on a three times a day dosing schedule. The total daily dose usually does not exceed 0.5 mg. The brand name formulation (Catapres) is used because bioavailability of generic products can vary. It appears that prolonged therapy for 3 months or more may be required to achieve optimal clinical benefit. Sedation, dizziness, headache, and insomnia are the most common side effects of clonidine therapy. The appearance of side effects indicates the need for less frequent dose increases or for dose reduction. Reserpine, tetrabenazine (currently available only experimentally), clonazepam (Klonopin), and calcium channel blockers may have tic-suppressing effects for selected patients.

TREATMENT OF OBSESSIVE-COMPULSIVE SYMPTOMS

For some patients with TS, associated obsessive-compulsive symptoms may be more disabling than the tics themselves. Compulsive counting, checking, and perfectionism and obsessive worries or fears are common examples. Antidepressant medications that inhibit serotonin reuptake are effective for treating OCD associated with TS. Fluoxetine (Prozac) is instituted in a single morning dose of 20 mg. Optimal therapeutic effects may not occur for several weeks, and some patients require as much as 60 mg per day in divided doses. The drug is usually tolerated well; anxiety, nervousness, insomnia, reduced appetite, and symptoms resembling mild hypomania are the most commonly reported side effects. Clomipramine (Anafranil) is begun in a dose of 25 mg at bedtime, and the dose can be increased up to about 150 mg per day. With Anafranil therapy, drowsiness and weight gain are more common.

TREATMENT OF ATTENTION DEFICIT HYPERACTIVITY DISORDER

ADHD is characterized by inattention, distractibility, impulsivity, and hyperactivity, and the condition is observed commonly in association with TS. For children with impaired school performance due to associated ADHD we generally initiate therapy with clonidine. Tricyclic antidepressants can also be used. Often, however, these medications are ineffective, and stimulant medications must be used. Although the use of stimulants such as methylphenidate (Ritalin, 5 to 60 mg per day in divided doses) or pemoline (Cylert, 18.75 to 75 mg each morning) can exacerbate or even precipitate tics in some patients, worsening of tics may be tolerable if stimulants prove effective in alleviating hyperactivity and improving attention. A combination of a stimulant and a neuroleptic drug can be used for patients impaired by both ADHD and tics. Modifications of the educational structure, such as one-to-one or small-group teaching, resource room, and special arrangements for testing (separate room, flexible time limits), may facilitate academic progress for children with TS.

GENETIC COUNSELING

It now appears that almost all cases of TS are hereditary. Although the detailed transmission pattern has not been completely determined, current evidence indicates that the disorder is inherited as an autosomal-dominant trait. Penetrance is incomplete and gender specific (affected males are more common than affected females), and expression is variable, including TS, CTD, and OCD. Based on current evidence, an affected parent has a 50 percent chance of passing the TS genetic trait to offspring. Males who inherit the genetic defect have approximately a 95 percent probability of manifesting tics. Among females who inherit the trait, probability of manifesting tics is about 50 percent, probability of showing OCD an additional 20 percent, and the chance of having no clinical evidence of the syndrome (i.e., lack of penetrance) is 30 percent. Such unaffected but TS genetic defect–carrying females can still, however, transmit the trait to their offspring. It is likely that more accurate data for genetic counseling will become available in the future, particularly if current efforts to localize the TS genetic defect prove successful. It is currently impossible to predict the severity of symptoms for persons who express the disorder, although it appears that most cases of TS are mild and not disabling.

SUGGESTED READING

Cohen DJ, Bruun RD, Leckman JF, eds. Tourette's syndrome and tic disorders. New York: Wiley Interscience, 1988.

Kurlan R. Tourette's syndrome: Current concepts. Neurology 1989; 39:1625–1630.

Kurlan R, ed. The handbook of Tourette's syndrome and related tic and behavioral disorders. New York: Marcel Dekker, 1993.

Robertson MM. The Gilles de la Tourette syndrome: The current status. Br J Psychiatry 1989; 154:147–169.

Shapiro AK, Shapiro ES, Young JG, Feinberg TE, eds. Gilles de la Tourette syndrome. 2nd ed. New York: Raven Press, 1988.

Singer HS, Walkup JT. Tourette syndrome and other tic disorders: Diagnosis, pathophysiology, and treatment. Medicine 1991; 70: 15–32.

PATIENT RESOURCE

Tourette Syndrome Association, Inc.
42-40 Bell Boulevard
Bayside, New York 11361
(718) 224-2999

ESSENTIAL TREMOR

JOSEPH H. FRIEDMAN, M.D.

Essential tremor (ET) is a relatively common disorder. Although it is often labeled *benign essential tremor*, it can be so severe as to be physically disabling. It can be socially embarrassing, even when mild. There is frequently a family history suggesting autosomal-dominant inheritance, but the absence of such documentation is also common, owing either to variable penetrance or the common appearance of a genetic mutation.

The tremor may begin at any age, but prevalence and severity clearly increase with time. *Senile tremor* is simply the late-onset form of ET and should not be considered a separate entity. Its onset is insidious, but patients may point to relatively specific dates when the tremor came to attention, when they were embarrassed, perhaps, by poor penmanship or difficulty eating at the dinner table. The tremor is most common in the hands, followed, in order of frequency, by the head and voice; legs, feet, and trunk are involved considerably less often. In the arms the tremor is precipitated by sustained posture and usually increases with movement. It is not usually present at rest. It may affect other body parts, including lips, chin, tongue, eyebrows, and fingers, but not the eyes. When present in the limbs it is almost always bilateral, but the absence of tremor on one side does not exclude the diagnosis. Often, the dominant side is more severely affected. Tremor frequency is very variable but is usually in the upper part of the 4 to 12 Hz range.

DIAGNOSIS

The differential diagnosis of ET is not long, but distinguishing between the possibilities is not always easy. Tremor of the hands in ET can easily be mistaken for Parkinson's disease (PD), especially when tremor is present only at rest or only with sustained posture, or if it is slow. This has generally been the main confounding differential point. Obviously, the lack of the other cardinal features of PD supports the diagnosis of ET, but PD can present with tremor alone. When ET involves more than the hands it typically involves the head or voice, whereas PD rarely involves the head or causes a vocal tremor. PD often causes jaw tremor, which is probably less common in ET.

The second but far less common differential point is dystonia, especially torticollis. This disorder is frequently associated with tremor, and tremor of the head, especially if it is irregular, may evolve into dystonia. Vocal tremor and spasmodic dysphonia can be extremely difficult to distinguish without laryngoscopy.

Hand tremor can be supinator-pronator or extension-flexion, or some combination. Head tremor can be of the yes-no type or complex, with various combinations of the two, or the axis can vary from time to time.

Clearly, a drug history and medical history are important for excluding other diagnoses. Alcohol can ameliorate ET, providing supporting, although not diagnostic, history. Theophylline and hyperthyroidism may produce an enhanced physiologic tremor that can be confused with ET, whereas lithium can induce a tremor that looks like ET or PD. Neuroleptics, on the other hand, induce a parkinsonian syndrome that may suggest a misdiagnosis of PD. The tremor caused by neuroleptics is typically parkinsonian but may have a kinetic component as well.

Tremor studies using surface electromyography electrodes can be helpful in diagnosis by distinguishing whether antagonist muscles contract alternately, as in PD, or simultaneously, as in ET. This is usually not necessary, but it should be considered in difficult cases. Interpretation is clouded by the fact that some ET patients muscles may contract alternately or even change from one pattern to the other over time. Because diagnosis rests on clinical criteria, I do not usually obtain neurodiagnostic studies. Imaging studies are useless, because even autopsy studies of ET patients have been unrevealing. Probably the most important test a physician can do is a quick evaluation of all relatives to assess for subclinical ET.

THERAPY

General Approach

While it is often a happy occasion in the office when I can tell a patient that the tremor is not PD and will not lead to any disability other than what the tremor causes, I find that medications are rarely as effective for ET as PD medications often are for PD tremor. Alcohol may be the most effective medication for ET, but its efficacy is short lived. Concern has been expressed that many ET patients have become alcohol dependent as a result of their empiric observation that drinking improves the tremor. The problem is that the effect of a single drink wears off quickly. In addition, the response diminishes over time, leading to a need to increase the alcohol intake.

Patients whose tremor is only an intermittent problem can be treated on an as needed basis. Some patients have found that a small drink before a cocktail party or social engagement allows them to enjoy the activity more, whereas further intake at the social function prolongs the response. Thus, intermittent small doses of alcohol are a reasonable treatment. Depending on the situation and the individual patient, propranolol might be used in small doses (10 to 20 mg) as it is for "stagefright" in patients who anticipate a stressful situation that will exacerbate the tremor. Whether this effect is placebo or real is unclear. Anxiolytics may also be helpful in this setting.

When treatment is required on a regular basis, the two major drugs that have proven effective in clinical trials are primidone and propranolol. How they work is unclear. Propranalol probably acts on peripheral beta$_2$ receptors, whereas primidone acts centrally. Both drugs act by reducing the amplitude of the tremor and do not alter its frequency. For both drugs the response is variable: some patients respond well and others poorly. No clear distinguishing characteristics have emerged to help predict good or poor response to one drug or the other. Somewhat more than a majority of patients respond to therapy with a measurable reduction in tremor. However, the reduction in the tremor amplitude may produce an uncertain improvement in functional capability, so that a small reduction in tremor amplitude may produce a large improvement in performance and a patient's sense of well-being, just as a large reduction, paradoxically, may not.

At first, propranolol is tolerated well by persons who have no contraindications, but it often causes lethargy and fatigue over time. It is obviously important to exclude patients with asthma, chronic obstructive pulmonary diseases, diabetes, heart failure, or heart block higher than first degree. It should be introduced cautiously in the elderly because the possibility of hypotension and of bradyarrhythmia is important when starting the drug. If a trial is unsuccessful, angina may be induced by withdrawal of the drug. The dose range required for propranolol to be effective ranges up to 320 mg daily. Larger doses are no more effective. No correlation has been found with serum drug levels, so blood monitoring is not useful. The long-acting (LA) form of propranolol is easier to use than the standard preparation. Although the LA form is available as a generic preparation, it is more than twice as expensive as taking the lower-dose form more frequently. Patients who take the standard form do not complain of the drug effect wearing off between doses, so the benefit of the LA form is simply ease of administration.

Primidone, in small doses, is another proven agent that appears to have similar or better efficacy than propranolol. Elble and Koller report, "Aside from ethanol, primidone is the most effective drug for the treatment of ET." Patients who respond to one of these agents may or may not respond to the other. In the usual anticonvulsant dose, however, primidone is poorly tolerated by older patients. To treat ET, much smaller doses are used; some patients respond to 50 mg per day. Even with 50 mg, which is a single children's tablet, some elderly patients at first complain of nausea and dizziness. Attempts to start even lower and build up also are sometimes unsuccessful. No correlation has been found between serum levels of primidone or its metabolite, phenobarbital, and response to tremor. Generally, the maximum effective dose is 250 mg daily, beyond which little extra benefit is derived.

Many other medications have been reported to be helpful in ET, either in case reports or small series. Most popular are the benzodiazepines, particularly clonazepam and alprazolam, which probably work in part by reducing the anxiety that aggravates virtually all tremor disorders and in part by direct anti-tremor effects on the central nervous system. Efficacy has been claimed for phenobarbital in ET, and it may be tried, especially in patients who are intolerant of primidone. Other beta-antagonists, such as metoprolol, more selective for the beta$_1$ receptor than propranolol, are advocated for use in patients with asthma and other pulmonary conditions that contraindicate propranolol. Metoprolol has been found to be helpful for patients who respond to propranolol, whereas atenolol and pindolol have not. It should be noted that metoprolol is relatively but not completely selective for the beta$_1$ receptor, so it must be used cautiously in patients who have contraindications to propranolol. Many other drugs have been reported as being helpful.

Specific Approach

My own approach to treating ET is probably a pretty standard one. The patient is first counseled about the disorder, its probably genetic mechanism, and the implications this has for the family. Information is given about the International Tremor Foundation and its newsletter (see below). Many patients are worried that they have PD, and must be reassured on this score. Because there are some data to suggest that there is a greater than chance association between PD and ET, the physician needs to be a bit cautious about the discussion, but the chances are still very good that PD is not going to emerge.

The discussion about treatment must include the unpredictable nature of the response. Patients must be told that the tremor will probably improve with medication but that the degree of improvement is unpredictable. About two-thirds of patients improve, but only the rare patient's tremor resolves completely. Most important, it must be made clear that treatment is symptomatic only and that no medication cures the tremor. This puts medication in perspective, so that the patient can decide whether the side effects, including cost, justify the treatment.

The central tenet of the symptomatic treatment of a movement disorder is that if a medication is not helpful it should be increased or changed. There is no justification for continuing a medication if the symptoms do not improve. In treating ET, in some sense "the customer is always right." Unlike PD, where a patient may not recognize an improvement that is functionally important, as in safer gait or balance, this is rarely the case in ET. It is, therefore, quite reasonable to adjust medications over the phone. Usually, I have patients call me a week after they begin therapy and then every week or two as medications are being changed.

I usually begin treatment with primidone, 50 mg at bedtime, to reduce the chances of adverse effects. I have the patient increase the medication on a three times daily regimen, as tolerated. Thus, once the patient is tolerating 50 mg at night, the schedule increases to two doses daily and then three. This is then increased to two tablets (100 mg) at the bedtime dose and one at each of the other doses; then two tablets twice daily and a single tablet at the third time; and finally two tablets three times daily. Should a patient either (1) show a satisfactory response to one more dose and no improvement on two further dose increments or (2) fail to tolerate a dose increment, I stop adjusting upward before reaching the maximum of 300 mg per day and if it is not helpful I stop the drug. If the patient were satisfied I would maintain the dose. If not, I would add propranolol, starting with 60 mg of the LA form or 20 mg three times a day, depending on the patient. With the LA form, various adjustment schedules are available, depending on the patient's needs. Usually, I simply increase the dose from once daily to twice daily after a week and then by one tablet daily each week on a twice daily regimen. Thus, a patient takes one a day, then one twice daily, then two and one, then two and two. I generally do not push the dose beyond 240 mg daily, although some patients might benefit from a larger dose. An alternative approach to this dose escalation is to give 1 week's supply of 60 mg and then increase the strength each week, as propranolol LA comes in preparations of 60, 80, 120, and 160 mg.

As with all new prescriptions, a small number of doses should be given initially on a renewable prescription, so that patients don't waste money on a drug that might be discarded after only one or two tablets are taken. If primidone or propranolol or the two together are not helpful, they should be discontinued.

When tremor fails to respond to primidone or propranolol, I usually try clonazepam, starting at 0.5 mg given at night and increased as tolerated. If this is not tolerated I switch to alprazolam and then try phenobarbital, acetazolamide, and clozapine. I obtain informed consent for clozapine because of its potential to cause agranulocytosis. I have never tried using clonidine or theophylline in small doses, but these have been reported to be helpful.

Surgical Therapy

A poor response to large doses of a variety of medications is an indication for thalamotomy. This surgical approach produces good results that are generally persistent. It has the obvious drawbacks of any brain surgery. Though the risk is quite low, the possibility of a disabling stroke must be kept in mind. Since most patients have relatively symmetric tremors, the side to be operated on is generally the dominant hemisphere; this introduces the risk of dominant-side weakness and a language disorder. It is not clear how much lower the risk for bilateral surgery is today than before the era of computed tomography, when bilateral thalamotomy rendered 20 percent of patients mute. One of my patients had a left hemisphere thalamotomy for ET that resulted in severe right arm dystonia, an intractable central pain syndrome, and mild aphasia. Though such effects are rare, they do happen.

Recently, reports have appeared that describe thalamic stimulation as a treatment for tremor. With an implanted electrode and an external stimulator a patient can control the electric current to the thalamus and control tremor. The advantage of this device is that it avoids ablating a region of the thalamus.

A potentially new tool for thalamotomy is the "gamma knife," which is really a radiotherapy tool for delivering highly focused gamma radiation to the brain to ablate a volume of predetermined size that leaves surrounding tissue unscathed. This approach avoids the risks of surgery and even allows better stereotactic localization, but stereotactic surgery allows electrophysiologic monitoring to document localization. With open surgery the response is immediate, so a hole can be enlarged immediately if the response is suboptimal; with the gamma knife the response takes several weeks.

If botulinum toxin is available, a trial should be considered before resorting to thalamotomy, as early data suggest this may be useful. Though there may be some functional weakness after treatment, it wears off in a few months. Clinical trials are currently in progress.

SUGGESTED READING

Elble RJ, Koller WC. Tremor. Baltimore: The Johns Hopkins University Press, 1990.

Guan XM, Peroutka SJ. Basic mechanisms of action of drugs used in the treatment of essential tremor. Clin Neuropharmacol 1990; 13:210–223.

Hubble JP, Busenbark KL, Koller WC. Essential tremor. Clin Neuropharmacol 1989; 12:453–482.

Lou JS, Jankovic J. Essential tremor: Clinical correlates in 350 patients. Neurology 1991; :234–238.

Rajput AH, Rozdilsky B, Aug L, Rajput A. Clinicopathologic observations in essential tremor: A report of six cases. Neurology 1991; 41:1422–1424.

PATIENT RESOURCE

International Tremor Foundation
360 West Superior Street
Chicago, Il 60610

BLEPHAROSPASM AND HEMIFACIAL SPASM

JOHN S. ELSTON, B.Sc., M.D., F.R.C.S.

BLEPHAROSPASM

Idiopathic blepharospasm is a symptom and sign complex characterized by clinical and electrophysiologic evidence of hyperexcitability of the facial nucleus that has no demonstrable underlying cause. It may be isolated or associated with spasms in the face, jaw, or neck (Meige syndrome). Diagnostic difficulty may result from the characteristic variability. For example, the condition often resolves temporarily when emotions are high, during consultation with the doctor, or when the patient is talking. A further source of confusion is the combination in idiopathic blepharospasm of sensory symptoms such as ocular discomfort, photophobia, and dry eyes with relatively minor ocular surface disorders such as blepharitis. The physician should not be misled: treatment of such surface disorders has no effect on the blepharospasm. If the typical history of increasingly frequent and forceful blinking with spasms of eye closure and photophobia is reported, the diagnosis should be made.

Hemifacial spasm (see below) should be clearly differentiated from blepharospasm. The pathogenesis, implications, and to some extent treatment, are different. Rarely, ptosis and defective eye opening due to ocular myasthenia gravis may cause diagnostic confusion, as may myotonia involving the orbicularis oculi. In some patients who complain of difficulty opening the eyes, there is an appearance of passive lid closure with no overt spasm in the orbicularis oculi. These patients often show frontalis overactivity (elevated brows) on attempted eye opening, and the lids go into spasm if the examiner attempts to open them. This has been designated "apraxia of eye opening" but is in fact a variant of idiopathic blepharospasm due to pretarsal and preseptal orbicularis oculi spasm. It may occur as an isolated abnormality or be seen in generalized movement disorders such as Parkinson's disease or progressive supra-nuclear palsy. In the latter condition, stereotyped stroking of the upper lids sometimes results in eye opening. Botulinum toxin injections into the pretarsal orbicularis oculi are worth trying, but the response is less pronounced than in typical blepharospasm.

What To Tell the Patient

Before starting treatment, it is important that the patient have some understanding of the condition and its management. I explain that we believe that it is due to a chemical imbalance in a localized part of the movement control center in the brain. I emphasize that the muscle spasm will not spread to the rest of the body, though cranial dystonia may start with blepharospasm. (Note that some patients use lower facial movements purposefully to achieve eye opening.) Patients may be heartened to know that very rarely idiopathic blepharospasm spontaneously resolves.

We do not know the cause of the problem, and in general, investigation is fruitless. I do not routinely carry out neuroimaging studies or blood tests unless there are unusual features such as early age at onset and other neurologic symptoms or signs. We cannot offer a cure, but we can usually control or reduce the symptoms with botulinum toxin injections. Repeated treatments are necessary, and I reassure patients that although side effects are common they are usually not serious and are always temporary. Patients may be concerned about other family members, and rarely there is a family history of blepharospasm or other adult-onset focal dystonia, and occasionally a patient or family history of eye-winking tic in childhood. In general, however, genetic factors do not appear to play a major role in idiopathic blepharospasm, and reassurance is appropriate. Because of embarrassment about continuous grimacing, patients may become socially isolated, and contact with self-help groups such as The Dystonia Society (in the United Kingdom) is often appreciated.

Treatment

My management schedule is outlined in Figure 1. The treatment of choice is botulinum toxin injections. There are no absolute contraindications. Bruising may

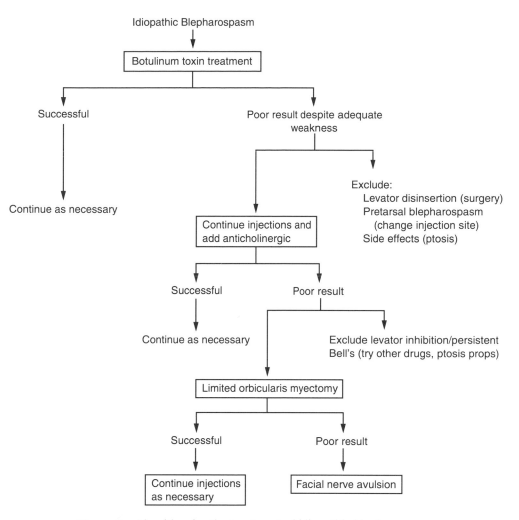

Figure 1 Algorithm for the treatment of idiopathic blepharospasm.

be a problem if the patient has a bleeding diathesis or is taking anticoagulants. Appropriate precautions can be taken, as they can for focal infection in immunosuppressed or immunocompromised patients. Details about the precise dose and location of injections vary but are relatively unimportant, provided overall weakening of the orbicularis oculi without spread to other muscles is achieved. I have used both Oculinum and Dysport (botulinum toxin A). The effect is identical, provided the manufacturer's instructions regarding the unit dose difference are appreciated. Based on clinical experience and assay data, one unit of Oculinum is approximately equivalent to 4 units of Dysport.

I start with three injections of 30 to 40 units of Dysport in 0.15 to 0.2 ml saline (equivalent to 7 to 10 units Oculinum) injected at the junction between the orbital and preseptal orbicularis (Fig. 2). A 27 or 30 gauge needle on a tuberculin syringe is used. It is useful to have a diagram, such as that in Figure 2, in the form of a stamp for the patient's records. Details of the site and dose of injections can then easily be recorded. I tell patients that the treatment will not work at once. Benefit is usually noticeable after 2 to 3 days, but improvement may continue for as long as 2 weeks. Common side

effects are tissue fluid accumulation, bruising, and partial ptosis. Double vision is rare. All side effects are temporary and usually resolve within 1 to 2 weeks.

Monitoring must include an assessment of the sensory symptoms, the visual function, any beneficial effects on middle and lower facial movements, and side effects (Fig. 3). The site and dose of previous treatment, together with information on the response (including side effects) and its duration, are used to plan subsequent treatments. I run monthly clinics, and after the first treatment reschedule the patient to return in 2 months. Thereafter, patients usually return at 2- to 3-month intervals. Some centers may be able to accommodate patients more flexibly, and I am certainly prepared to reinject after 4 to 6 weeks, if necessary.

The response to treatment may be dramatic, and the restoration of normal visual function may prompt a sudden increase in physical activity. Myocardial infarction, (very occasionally fatal), has been described in these circumstances, and a warning to build up exercise tolerance slowly may be appropriate.

Because of persistent weakness in the orbicularis oculi even when symptoms have returned, I use lower

Botulinum Toxin Clinic

Diagnosis: *Blepharospasm*

Date: *17/11/92*

Injections: *40 units at sites marked*

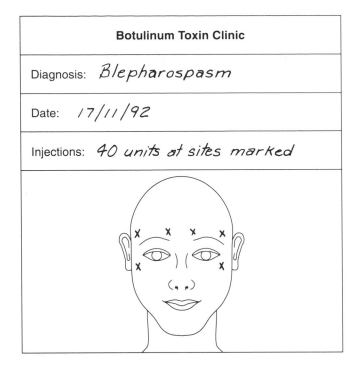

Figure 2 Injection sites for treatment of blepharospasm.

Blepharospasm

Date:

Injection no.

Sensory symptoms

Discomfort	0	1	2	3	4	5
Photophobia	0	1	2	3	4	5
Other						

Visual function

Reading
Watching TV
Out alone
Driving
Working

Side effects

Ptosis
Double vision
Other

Figure 3 Monitoring of patient after botulinum toxin injection must include an assessment of sensory symptoms, visual function, and side effects, as shown on this chart.

doses of toxin for second and subsequent treatments. I usually use 20 to 30 units of Dysport at three locations but am prepared to vary the site of injection considerably if this is indicated clinically. For example, if the pretarsal and preseptal orbicularis oculi muscles are weak but spasm persists, I direct treatment at the orbital portion.

There is a common perception among patients who have been treated for months or years that the injections do not work as well as they did the first time. This is difficult to interpret. There is no evidence for antibody formation at the doses used, and adequate orbicularis oculi weakness is present. In some cases, the underlying dystonia may have worsened and levator inhibition developed. The absence of the marked change in symptoms that follows the first treatment is probably also a factor.

Nonresponders

A group of patients respond minimally or not at all. Others respond for very short periods, say 2 to 4 weeks. Some have a variant, pretarsal blepharospasm (see above), in which case this portion of the orbicularis oculi must be weakened directly. Post-treatment ptosis is usually due to spread to the levator, and it will resolve. However, some patients have a levator disinsertion ptosis caused by or associated with the blepharospasm. The characteristic physical signs of this condition, such as deep upper lid sulci with high lid creases and a good range of levator function, will be present, having been masked previously by the blepharospasm. The ptosis responds well to levator aponeurosis advancement, with or without blepharochalasis surgery under local anesthetic.

If there has been little or no response, I usually repeat the injections two more times. I usually do not increase the dose but vary the site of injection to ensure complete orbicularis oculi paralysis. If there is still no response, the next step is to add an anticholinergic medication (e.g., benzhexol, starting at 2 mg per day), gradually increasing the dose until a response is achieved or side effects supervene. About 20 percent of patients improve to some extent, but unfortunately the response may not be sustained. Other drugs may be helpful in individual patients, but the effect is unpredictable. Tetrabenazine is worth trying, and if anxiety is prominent a benzodiazepine may be helpful. In some cases, secondary depression necessitates psychiatric referral.

Childhood-onset dopa-sensitive dystonia is clinically indistinguishable from idiopathic torsion dystonia. Because of the overlap between generalized and focal dystonia, a trial of levodopa treatment may be worthwhile in cases that have not responded to botulinum and when the diagnostic category is in doubt.

Some patients' visual function remains very poor despite adequate orbicularis oculi weakening, because of levator inhibition or Bell's phenomenon (or a combination of the two). This subgroup of patients must be identified, as surgical treatment is unlikely to help. Rarely, the combination of botulinum toxin injections

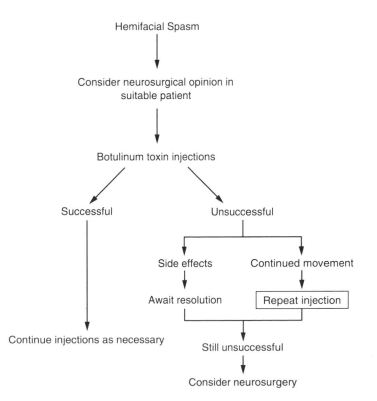

Figure 4 Algorithm for the treatment of hemifacial spasm.

and lid (ptosis) props is useful here. Treatment of blepharitis and dry eyes may have a minor beneficial effect, and systemic medication should be tried.

For visually incapacitated nonresponders, I advise a limited orbicularis oculi myectomy involving the upper lid and lateral orbital and preseptal portions of the muscle plus procerus, combined with brow fixation via

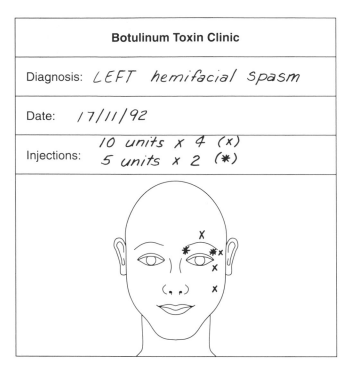

Figure 5 Injection sites for treatment of left hemifacial spasm.

bilateral brow incisions or a bicoronal approach. This modification of the Anderson technique reduces the operative time and difficulty, but botulinum toxin injections to the lower lids may have to be continued. If this fails, the facial nerves have to be avulsed. Side effects, including lid malposition and brow ptosis, are common and require secondary surgeries. Reinnervation may be a problem.

A few patients remain very disabled visually despite these measures. In order to gain access to appropriate social services, the patient may have to be registered ("certified") as being partially sighted or blind.

HEMIFACIAL SPASM

Hemifacial spasm is an intractable embarrassment and a social nuisance, but provided vision is good in the contralateral eye, it has little functional effect. Unlike idiopathic blepharospasm, it can often be cured surgically, and I always refer patients in the younger age group (fourth to sixth decades) for neurosurgical consultation. Healthy older patients can also be referred, provided the risks are understood.

Investigation

In patients in the first two decades, the diagnosis must be regarded with suspicion, as serious intracranial disease (e.g., brain stem glioma) can present with unilateral facial muscle contraction. For this reason, I have a much lower threshold for investigation (neuroimaging) of hemifacial spasm than of blepharospasm. If the condition is long-standing and entirely typical, neuroimaging is not necessarily indicated unless surgical treat-

Hemifacial spasm					
Date:					
Injection no.					
Reduction in movement					
Around eye	0	1	2	3	4	5
Mid-face	0	1	2	3	4	5
Around mouth	0	1	2	3	4	5
Neck	0	1	2	3	4	5
Side effects					
Ptosis Double vision Other Mouth drop					

Figure 6 Chart for monitoring response to botulinum toxin injections. Patients are asked to gauge the percentage reduction in abnormal movements.

ment is being considered. If there are atypical features (e.g., facial sensory change, deafness, sustained chronic contractions) or the patient is outside the normal range of age at onset (sixth to eighth decades) neuroimaging is important. Magnetic resonance imaging is the investigation of choice.

Management

The management plan is outlined in Figure 4. As with blepharospasm, any treatment should be preceded by a discussion of the disease and its management. In my experience, systemic drugs such as carbamazepine have no effect, and the choice of treatment is between surgery and botulinum toxin injections. The latter will not cure the condition, but if carefully "customerized" can reduce the impact to a negligible level.

Because there is often a little pre-existing facial weakness, smaller doses of botulinum toxin than those used for blepharospasm are usually effective. I inject at four to six sites using 20 to 30 units of Dysport. The localization of injections is determined by the symptoms. It is important to avoid or use only very small amounts of toxin medially on the lower lid or mid-face, to avoid spread down toward the mouth. Embarrassing contractions in the platysma can be safely and effectively treated (Fig. 5).

To monitor the response, I ask the patient to gauge the percentage reduction in abnormal movements around the eye, in the mid-face, around the mouth, and in the neck, and to report side effects (Fig. 6). I usually follow patients at 2- to 3-month intervals, but some may go as long as 6 months between treatments. Surgical treatment can be reconsidered at any stage.

Botulinum toxin treatment of blepharospasm and hemifacial spasm is now undertaken by many ophthalmologists and neurologists, usually with highly satisfactory results for both patient and doctor. It is simple, safe, and effective and appears to be repeatable indefinitely. In my view, all major ophthalmologic and neurologic centers should offer this treatment, in order to share the load. This would afford ready access for patients who would not have to travel far and whose treatment could be tailored to individual needs. Also, it is unreasonable to ask individual physicians to treat large numbers of patients, as it can lead to resentment and boredom in the doctor and reduce the quality of patient care.

SUGGESTED READING

Dutton JJ. Treatment of hemifacial spasm and essential blepharospasm with botulinum toxin. In: Wilkins RH, Rengachary SS, eds. Neurosurgery update 1. Diagnosis, operative technique and neuro-oncology. New York: McGraw-Hill, 1990.

Taylor DJN, Kraft ST, Kazdan MS, et al. Treatment of blepharospasm and hemifacial spasm with botulinum A toxin: A Canadian multicentre study. Can J Ophthalmol 1991; 26:133–138.

PATIENT RESOURCE

Benign Essential Blepharospasm Research Foundation, Inc.
755 Howell Street
Beaumont, Texas 77706
Telephone: (409) 892-1339

DEGENERATIVE DISEASES

ALZHEIMER'S DISEASE

LEON J. THAL, M.D.

THE DEMENTIA SYNDROME

The dementia syndrome is clinically defined as deterioration of cognitive functioning that is severe enough to interfere with occupational or social performance, or both. Affected persons suffer memory loss and a variety of other cognitive disturbances, including language and visuospatial difficulties, and frequently problems with calculation, concentration, and abstraction. The level of consciousness remains intact until the late stages of the disorder. This clinical definition describes a state or presentation, but not the cause of the illness.

The dementia syndrome has many causes (Table 1). Patients with Alzheimer's disease (AD) make up the largest proportion: AD accounts for approximately 60 to 70 percent of cases. Another 10 percent have AD plus other disorders known to cause dementia, most commonly coexisting infarcts (mixed dementia). Other causes of the dementia syndrome include vascular dementia, Parkinson's disease, and degenerative and infectious diseases such as Creutzfeld-Jacob disease, encephalitis, and Pick's disease. In some patients, dementia may be arrested, or possibly improved, following treatment; this group includes those who have benign tumors, neurosyphilis, hydrocephalus, or subdural hematomas. Completely reversible dementias must always be sought, though they are found in a minority of patients—those who have, for example, metabolic disturbances such as hepatic disease, hyponatremia, disorders of calcium metabolism, vitamin B_{12} deficiency, thyroid disease, or dementia secondary to drugs or depression.

EVALUATION OF THE PATIENT WITH THE DEMENTIA SYNDROME

Every patient who presents with the dementia syndrome should undergo an evaluation to determine its cause (Table 2). The clinical assessment generally begins with a detailed history, obtained mostly from a collateral source, indicating the onset, duration, and course of the illness. Additional information should be sought by interviewing the patient. Physical examination is performed, with focus on hearing and vision. Mental status testing should include evaluation of recent memory, remote memory, orientation, language, calculation, abstraction, judgment, and visuospatial relations. In addition, I generally supplement my mental status examination with a standardized cognitive test such as the Mini-Mental State Examination (MMSE) or the Blessed Information-Memory-Concentration test, which can then be utilized to monitor the progression of disease.

Table 1 Diseases That Produce the Dementia Syndrome

Disease	Approximate Proportion of Dementia Syndrome (%)
AD	60
AD plus other disorders	10
Vascular dementia	5
Other degenerative disorders	5
Treatable dementia (e.g., tumor, alcohol)	10
Reversible dementia (drugs, depression, metabolic)	5
Miscellaneous disorders	5
Total	100

Table 2 Evaluation of the Patient with the Dementia Syndrome

By the examiner
  History
  Physical examination (especially hearing and vision)
  Mental status testing
  Neurologic examination

Special tests
  Blood for CBC, metabolic screen, thyroid, vitamin B_{12}, syphilis serologic tests, HIV (if indicated)
  Urinalysis
  Chest radiography
  Electrocardiography (ECG)
  Imaging study (CT, MRI)
  Electroencephalography (EEG), if indicated
  Lumbar puncture, if indicated
  Psychometric testing, if indicated

The physical neurologic examination should pay particular attention to the presence or absence of focal motor or sensory findings, gait disturbances, extrapyramidal features, and tremor.

Laboratory evaluation includes blood for complete blood count, metabolic screen, thyroid functions, vitamin B_{12}, syphilis serologic testing, and human immunodeficiency virus (HIV) testing if appropriate risk factors are present. Routine urinalysis should be performed. Chest radiography and electrocardiography (ECG) are helpful to assess cardiovascular status. Brain imaging should be performed at least once on all demented patients to identify structural and potentially treatable causes of dementia such as tumors, hydrocephalus, or subdural hematoma. The role of magnetic resonance imaging (MRI) in evaluation of the patient with dementia is unclear. Simple non–contrast-enhanced computed tomography (CT) is generally sufficient to reveal remediable lesions, but MRI is more useful when vascular disease, acquired immunodeficiency syndrome (AIDS), or multiple sclerosis is suspected. All patients do not need electroencephalography (EEG), but the study may help identify metabolic encephalopathy, seizures, or depression. I no longer perform lumbar puncture routinely but only when I suspect significant systemic illness, cancer, hydrocephalus, or other unusual dementia. Psychometric testing is reserved for difficult or questionable cases. It is particularly helpful for diagnosing early dementia when the in-office mental status testing fails to reveal significant cognitive deficits in spite of a suggestive history. It is useful for separating dementia from depression, as patients with depression often perform inconsistently on different memory tasks during a single test session. It is also useful for establishing baseline performance estimations of an individual patient's ability to work, drive, and live independently.

ALZHEIMER'S DISEASE

AD, the most important cause of the dementia syndrome, afflicts between 5 and 10 percent of the over–age 65 population. In 1990, approximately 3.1 million people in the United States had AD. It usually presents in typical fashion. The most common symptom is memory loss, which affects recent memory relatively more than remote memory. Language disturbances develop early in the course of the disease and include diminished spontaneous output, difficulty naming objects, and, later, comprehension deficits. The majority of patients suffer visuospatial impairment early. Patients often have difficulty drawing a clock and setting the hands to a specified time, such as 3:30 or 11:10. Behavior disturbances are common in AD—depression, delusions, wandering, agitation, insomnia, and disinhibition. Different behavioral disturbances occur during different phases of the disorder. For example, depression, when present, generally occurs early in the course of the illness. In contrast, delusions and hallucinations are more prevalent during the middle stages and diminish in frequency with advancing dementia. Although neurologic findings are generally absent early in the illness, primitive reflexes, disturbances in graphesthesia, and a positive result on the face-hand test may be noted. Extrapyramidal features, principally consisting of rigidity and bradykinesia, occur in about one-third of AD patients, and recent neuropathologic studies have found that many of these subjects have cortical Lewy bodies. Mild gait disturbances, myoclonus, and seizures increase in frequency during the middle and late stages of the disease. The presence of focal finding, ataxia, diminished downward gaze, fasiculations, or resting tremor suggests a diagnosis other than AD.

Patients with AD always decline over time, but there may be prolonged periods of stability. The rate of decline varies, both between patients and within patients during the course of the disease. Many patients with AD reside in nursing homes or related institutions during the later phases of the disease. On average, 20 to 30 percent of mildly affected patients and 30 to 50 percent of moderately to severely affected patients are institutionalized within 2 years. Predictors of institutionalization include early aphasia, incontinence, and loss of basic activities of daily living. The average duration from diagnosis until death is about 6 years.

The cause of the disease is unknown, but a series of risk factors have been identified (Table 3). The most important of these are age and family history. The prevalence of AD roughly doubles for every 5 year epoch beyond age 65. First-degree relatives of AD probands are also at increased risk for AD. A familial AD gene has been located on chromosomes 14 and 21, and possibly one on chromosome 19; however, autosomal-dominant familial AD accounts for far fewer than 1 percent of all cases. Other putative risk factors include female gender, low level of education, history of head injury, and possibly myocardial infarction.

The dementia in AD involves loss of both neurons and synapses. Certain populations of neurons, especially those that contain the neurotransmitters acetylcholine, norepinephrine, and serotonin, are particularly vulnerable. Many investigators currently believe that amyloid, an insoluble protein found in both the senile plaque and the cerebral blood vessels of patients with AD, is neurotoxic and may cause the illness. At this time, however, direct proof of this hypothesis is lacking.

Table 3 Risk Factors for Alzheimer's Disease

Age
Family history
Familial Alzheimer's gene (chromosome 14, 19 or 21)
Female gender
Low level of education
Head injury
Myocardial infarction (?)

THERAPY

Behavioral and Secondary Symptoms

After the evaluation is complete, specific causes of dementia such as thyroid disease, vitamin B_{12} deficiency, and tumors should be treated. While the majority of patients are found to have AD, comorbid conditions such as congestive heart failure, alcohol abuse, or depression should also be addressed. Physicians are commonly challenged to treat behavior disorders associated with AD. There are no absolute rules for treating these symptoms, and pharmacologic intervention, if needed, must be individualized, as it can produce sedation, disinhibition, depression, falls, incontinence, parkinsonism, or tardive dyskinesia. General principles of geriatric psychopharmacology must be emphasized. If a decision is made to use a pharmacologic agent, a specific target symptom should be identified and the smallest possible dose of that agent used. The patient should be monitored frequently. After the symptom has been controlled for some time, the medication dose should be tapered and withdrawal considered. If one medication in reasonable-sized doses does not control the symptom or behavior or produces troublesome side effects, another should be substituted.

Significant depression occurs in about 15 to 20 percent of AD patients (Table 4). The symptom generally occurs early in the course of the illness, when insight is better-preserved. The choice of an antidepressant depends principally on its efficacy and its side effect profile. In general, agents with anticholinergic effects should be avoided in this elderly population. Useful medications include nortriptyline (Pamelor), beginning with 10 to 25 mg daily and increasing as necessary to 75 mg daily. Desipramine in similar doses is also useful. Fluoxetine (Prozac), 10 to 20 mg per day, often both improves depression and decreases anxiety and agitation in AD patients. Trazodone, 75 to 200 mg per day, may help both depression and insomnia. These agents are preferable to others because they induce fewer side effects such as orthostasis, dry mouth, and cardiac problems. Antidepressant agents may be given in a single dose at night, when their mild sedative effect may promote sleep.

Anxiety may occur at any stage, but it frequently occurs early in the course of the disease. It can be treated with a small dose of lorazepam (Ativan), 0.5 to 1 mg daily; alprazolam (Xanax), 0.25 to 0.5 mg two times a day; or oxazepam (Serax), 10 mg once or twice daily as needed.

Agitation is frequently a feature of AD, and it may have verbal and physical components. Precipitating factors for agitation should always be sought, such as physical illness or pain, excessive sensory stimulation, or improper environment. Occasionally, physical agitation can be managed nonpharmacologically by allowing patients to wander outside in an enclosed area; this applies mainly to areas with a favorable climate.

Table 4 Treatment of Behavioral Symptoms of Alzheimer's Disease

Depression
  Nortriptyline (Pamelor), 10–25 mg, maximum 75 mg
  Desipramine, 25 mg, 75 mg maximum
  Fluoxetine (Prozac), 20 mg
  Trazodone, 75–200 mg

Anxiety
  Lorazepam (Ativan), 0.5–1.0 mg
  Alprazolam (Xanax), 0.25–0.5 mg once or twice daily
  Oxazepam (Serax), 10 mg once or twice daily

Agitation
  Thioridazine (Mellaril), 10–20 mg, maximum 80 mg
  Haloperidol (Haldol), 0.5 mg once or twice daily, maximum 3–5 mg
  Consider oxazepam or diphenhydramine

Delusions
  Thioridazine (Mellaril), 10–20 mg, maximum 80 mg
  Haloperidol (Haldol), 0.5 mg once or twice daily, maximum 3–5 mg

Insomnia
  Warm milk
  Trazadone, 50–200 mg at bedtime
  Diphenhydramine, 25–50 mg at bedtime
  Temazepam (Restoril), 7.5–15 mg
  Chloral hydrate, 500 mg at bedtime

Agitation that is sufficiently troublesome and lacks a remediable cause may require treatment. Very few studies have investigated what class of agents is best-suited for treatment of agitation. One recent study demonstrated that benzodiazepines, neuroleptics, and antihistamines were equally effective for agitation: improvement was observed in 20 to 40 percent of patients treated with oxazepam, haloperidol, or diphenhydramine. I generally first try thioridazine (Mellaril), 10 to 20 mg per day. It is a useful drug because in small doses it does not produce extrapyramidal side effects. When the daily dose exceeds 70 to 80 mg, however, it frequently produces increased confusion because of its anticholinergic effects. If thioridazine is ineffective, haloperidol (Haldol), 0.5 mg one or two times daily, may suffice. Unfortunately, doses larger than 2 mg per day frequently cause extrapyramidal side effects, which often become dose limiting. If these two neuroleptics do not control the symptoms, I try oxazepam or diphenhydramine.

Delusions are common in the middle stages of the illness and if mild do not require treatment. If they are significantly disturbing to patients or care givers, thioridazine or haloperidol generally controls or diminishes delusions.

Insomnia is best managed by environmental manipulation. Keeping the patient awake during the day and reducing nighttime fluids frequently help. Taking warm milk at bedtime should be tried before medications are added. Pharmacologic intervention can be attempted with trazodone, 50 to 200 mg at bedtime, or diphenhydramine, 25 to 50 mg at bedtime. These two medications are particularly useful because patients develop relatively little tolerance to their sedative effect. Short-acting benzodiazepines such as temazepam (Restoril), 7.5 or 15 mg at bedtime, may be employed. However, tolerance invariably develops, and intermittent use of these agents is recommended (no more than three doses in 7 days). Chloral hydrate, 500 mg at bedtime, can be utilized, but tolerance develops with continuous administration, and elders may experience morning sedation.

Cognitive Symptoms

At the present time no marketed drug clearly improves memory or cognition in AD. One agent, ergoloid mesylate (Hydergine), a metabolic-enhancing mixture of three ergot alkaloids, has been tested extensively in elders who suffer cognitive impairment. Most studies indicate that patients derive both subjective and mild objective symptomatic improvement in cognitive function, depressed mood, and composite global scores. Studies that use objective tests, however, have failed to document cognitive improvement in AD patients. In my own experience, approximately 5 percent of patients treated with 3 to 6 mg daily seemed to improve in both memory and mood. Side effects of Hydergine are minimal and consist primarily of headache. Because it is the only nonexperimental agent currently available for the treatment of impaired cognition in elderly persons, I treat most mild to moderate dementia with as much as 6 mg per day in three equal doses. If improvement is not seen within 2 or 3 months, I discontinue medication.

Many cholinergic agents have been tried for AD during the past 15 years. The most promising class is cholinesterase inhibitors. At present, none is marketed for treatment of AD; however, tacrine (tetrahydroaminoacridine) has been demonstrated in some studies to produce modest cognitive improvement in AD patients on the MMSE and the Alzheimer Disease Assessment Scale. Global scores improve slightly or not at all, indicating that the effect is small. Tacrine is currently available for the treatment of AD patients under a treatment investigational new drug application; this is a mechanism intended to make drugs available to desperately or seriously ill patients if there is some evidence of efficacy. A pharmaceutical company generally holds the IND, and it may charge for the drug. Treatment INDs have generally been used for drugs to treat AIDS and cancer. Treatment is open, not blind. This treatment IND is a first for AD, and it is designed to expose patients with mild to moderate AD to doses up to 120 mg per day. Treatment begins with 40 mg per day (10 mg four times a day) for 6 weeks; then the dose is increased to 80 mg per day (20 mg four times), and then to 120 mg per day (30 mg four times), if tolerated. Symptomatic side effects include nausea and vomiting. Additionally, tacrine produces elevated liver function test results in 40 to 50 percent of exposed subjects. Therefore, weekly alanine aminotransferase (ALT) monitoring is necessary during dose titration. Dose escalation should be attempted only if the ALT level is normal; if it is three to five times normal the dose should be reduced. At ALT levels greater than five times normal, tacrine should be stopped. Response to therapy can be monitored with the MMSE and a clinical global impression of change. If improvement is not seen, I discontinue treatment after 4 months at 120 per day or the largest dose that is tolerated. Information about this treatment IND can be obtained by calling (800) 829-7575.

SUDDEN CHANGE IN PATIENTS WITH DEMENTIA

In general, AD progresses fairly steadily, although plateaus may occur. On average, patients decline by approximately 3 to 4 points per year on screening instruments such as the Blessed Information-Memory-Concentration test or the MMSE. When sudden deterioration occurs, the physician must suspect a new medical, neurologic or psychiatric event. Evaluation for infections, especially in the urinary tract or respiratory tract, is often revealing. A review of medications and a search for delirium must be undertaken, and possibilities such as cerebral infarct or subdural hematoma should be considered.

OTHER THERAPEUTIC ROLES OF THE PHYSICIAN

The physician who cares for AD patients often serves as the primary family advisor. The nature of the illness, the expected course, and anticipated problems need to be discussed with care givers. Early in the course of the illness, issues related to finances, legal planning, wills, placement, and withholding of treatment need to be addressed. Knowledge about local facilities such as day care centers, Alzheimer's support groups, and sources of information for family members can be as useful in the management of the patient as the writing of prescriptions. Home evaluation for safety and strategies for simplifying the home environment for AD patients should be discussed by the physician, occupational therapist, social worker, or visiting nurse. Discontinuation of driving must be discussed. In some states, reporting to the department of motor vehicles is mandatory, and the physician must be aware of the local law. *The 36-Hour Day,* a book by Mace and Rabins, should be recommended reading for care givers. Contact with the local Alzheimer's Association support group should be encouraged. Knowledge of home health service agencies, skilled nursing facilities capable of handling AD patients, social workers, and legal advisors is a necessary part of the physician's armamentarium.

SUGGESTED READING

Cummings J, Benson DF. Dementia: A clinical approach. 2nd ed. Stoneham, Mass: Butterworth-Heinemann, 1992.

PATIENT RESOURCES

Literature
Mace NL, Rabins PV. The 36-hour day: A family guide to caring for persons with Alzheimer's disease, related dementing illnesses, and memory loss in later life. Baltimore: Johns Hopkins University Press, 1981.

Aronson MK. Understanding Alzheimer's disease. New York: Scribner's, 1988.

Associations
Alzheimer Association
70 East Lake Street, Suite 600
Chicago, Illinois 60601-5997
(312) 853-3060.

AMYOTROPHIC LATERAL SCLEROSIS

LORA L. CLAWSON, R.N., B.S.N.
JEFFREY D. ROTHSTEIN, M.D., Ph.D.
RALPH W. KUNCL, M.D., Ph.D.

The work of the neurologist who *cares* for the amyotrophic lateral sclerosis (ALS) patient is to dissuade both the patient and himself that the condition is untreatable. In a recent article in the *New England Journal of Medicine,* Bulkin and Lukashok make the following observation on physicians' approach to incurably ill patients.

> Physicians are trained to investigate, diagnose, prolong life, and cure. When these goals are no longer relevant, physicians often feel they have no skills to offer and distance themselves from the patient. Some turn the patient over to other care givers. Many, like the physician in Tolstoy's *Death of Ivan Ilyich,* continue to prescribe cures in an effort to hide the reality that the patient is dying. The family is then placed in the position of Ilyich's wife, insisting that the patient adhere to the doctor's protocol and refusing to acknowledge the truth. Thus, the patient's final act of living is denied validity, and the patient and family are deprived of the opportunity to come to terms with it and with each other. All are left with the perception that there is some sort of shame attached to being incurably ill, and the patient is left with a sense of having been abandoned at the time of greatest crisis. Yet in truth, there remains much that the physician can offer the patient when curing skills are no longer required.

Few patients are as needy as those with ALS. Paradoxically, there are few patients for whom neurologists provide worse continuing care. Many patients with ALS—perhaps most—leave the doctor's office with the idea that they ("the average patient") will die in 3 years and that ALS is untreatable. Thus, this chapter might be subtitled "What to do when there is nothing to do," or "Treating the untreatable."

WHAT PATIENTS SAY THEIR DOCTORS NEED TO KNOW

Because of the sense of having been abandoned that ALS patients experience, and because of the psychological problems that arise, we began an ALS support group in the early 1980s in Baltimore, with the collaboration of the Muscular Dystrophy Association (MDA). What the pressing needs of ALS patients are, which solutions work best, what unspoken questions patients harbor—these things we have learned best by simply listening to members of the support group in a setting removed from the formality of the medical office. When asked, What is the worst part about having ALS? patients' answers have included these: "I was in the dark for 6 months without a diagnosis." "Not being told about the MDA." "Nothing ever truly helps; things only become temporarily more tolerable." "The fear of the respirator: not being *on* it, but the machine itself, sort of like the fear some people have of using a computer. But it was much easier than I'd ever anticipated."

When asked, What are the most important things you learned and who did you learn them from? patients answered as follows: "No physician can help." "We improvise. It's a matter of living with it . . . self discovery." "I found out I was too afraid of the gastrostomy; it was no big deal." "I handled each symptom as it came up, through the support group and my doctor and my therapist." "Doctors need to learn how to talk to patients with ALS."

Talking to Patients with ALS

There seem to be two extremes in how doctors talk to patients with ALS. The first extreme is avoidance, whether deliberate or unconscious. It naturally evolves from the doctor's feeling of helplessness about the disease. It leads to withdrawal from the patient, a curt manner, obfuscation concerning the diagnosis, concentration on documenting the inevitable neuromuscular decline without discussing solutions to the problems of everyday living, and even to formal discharge of the patient to the care of other previously unengaged specialists such as pulmonary physicians or internists. Of course, it often works in reverse. The patient may withdraw from the doctor because of embarrassment or of anger about the diagnosis or about the way it was given or received. This combination of avoidance behaviors no doubt explains the common switching of doctors that occurs with this disease early in its course.

The opposite extreme is the physician who actively engages the patient, transmitting his or her great experience with the natural history of the disease or its multiple symptoms and treatments by launching into a nonstop treatise on every conceivable outcome. Such speeches are seldom heard during the clinician's first encounter with the patient, and what is heard is probably very frightening. The advice of experienced ALS clinicians is always to schedule a second visit after a short time for reflection, in order to discuss the prognosis and its implications for activities of daily living. It is then important to take the occupational therapists' approach: to attempt to "fix" only what the patient perceives is "broken." To do otherwise leads to overload and a feeling of hopelessness. Thus, for example, extensive conversations or demonstrations about communication problems and the many devices available to aid communication are rarely of value to patients who have no trouble speaking. Despite our best intentions to prepare people well in advance for any contingency, human nature is such that most of us do not prepare for future risks. Inundating patients with information about their illness is to be avoided in favor of focusing on one or a few distinct current problems.

A final point on talking to patients with ALS is that it pays to kneel or sit when talking to any patient in a wheelchair. This brings doctor and patient eye to eye, removing the patient's need to strain weak cervical paraspinal muscles to crane the neck during conversation, and it avoids the position-of-authority body language.

DIAGNOSIS

The diagnosis of ALS is usually straightforward. *Progressive* weakness accompanied by other lower motor neuron signs such as atrophy or fasciculation must be present. It is important to note that fasciculation is a lower motor neuron sign that is associated with many disorders, and it is *not,* in and of itself, pathognomonic of ALS. Further, although the tongue is always examined, at the time of diagnosis it is denervated in only one-fourth of patients. The definite diagnosis of ALS requires the presence of *widespread denervation* (Lambert's criteria) that is not explainable by neuropathy or radiculopathy and that occurs in the presence of upper motor neuron signs but in the absence of significant

Table 1 Suggested Studies for the Diagnosis of ALS

Electrophysiologic tests
  Electromyography with evidence of denervation (fibrillation potentials or positive sharp waves, in the context of large-amplitude, long-duration motor potentials) in at least three major muscle groups supplied by motor neurons arising from different brain stem and/or spinal cord levels.
  Nerve conduction studies to rule out significant neuropathy not explained by other disease (e.g., diabetes) or evidence of conduction block seen in multifocal motor neuronopathy

Radiologic studies
  If indicated, MRI of cervical, thoracic, and lumbar spine; or CT-myelography
  If indicated, MRI of brain (especially for bulbar presentations)

Laboratory tests
  Creatine kinase
  Ca^{2+}
  Heavy metal screen
  Thyroid functions (thyroid-stimulating hormone, thyroxine)
  Vitamin B_{12}
  Cerebrospinal fluid tested for cells, glucose, protein*
  Hexosaminidase A
  Serum and urine protein immunofixation electrophoresis*
  Antiganglioside antibodies (IgM anti-GM_1)
  In addition, vital capacity and negative inspiratory force are tested on initial evaluation of all patients.

*Note: If paraproteins are found, or a high CSF protein (>70 mg/dl) is observed (in the absence of spinal structural lesions), a bone marrow aspiration and biopsy are suggested to rule out lymphoma and plasmacytoma.

sensory, bowel, or bladder abnormalities. Although easy to recognize in approximately 80 percent of cases, ALS remains a diagnosis of exclusion. This requires ruling out disorders that mimic it, such as cervical and lumbar spondylotic myeloradiculopathy, multifocal motor neuropathy with conduction block and antiganglioside antibodies, plasma cell dyscrasias, polymyositis, lead intoxication, adult hexosaminidase deficiency, hyperthyroidism, hyperparathyroidism, chronic inflammatory demyelinating polyneuropathy, and other primarily motor neuromuscular diseases. A few patients with ALS present with breathing difficulty from diaphragmatic paralysis as their first symptom. This is an important differential diagnostic point, because few neuromuscular diseases present with predominant respiratory weakness. The few that do include myasthenia gravis, polymyositis, adult acid maltase deficiency, amyloid myopathy, and ALS. Rarely is an unusual presentation of multiple sclerosis or Parkinson's disease misdiagnosed as ALS.

In addition to a thorough neurologic examination looking for upper and lower motor neuron signs, there are a number of electrophysiologic and radiologic studies and laboratory tests that help establish the diagnosis of ALS, primarily by excluding other diagnoses (Table 1).

THERAPEUTIC APPROACHES

Weakness

The rule for treating weakness associated with ALS is that autonomy equals therapy. Weakness is functionally important only insofar as it prevents a particular activity. This is the premise of the occupational therapist who inquires about activities of daily living. One will never know that the patient needs a prescription for a raised toilet seat until the patient is asked whether he or she can rise from it and about his or her feelings of helplessness. One will never know that the patient needs a card-holding device until he or she is asked about hobbies and it is discovered that the patient's whole social life circles around the game of bridge. One will never know that the patient needs a wrist splint until it is learned that he can no longer shave himself and that this depresses him. These basic but essential problems are not likely to be addressed in the course of a half-hour return visit to the hurried but compulsive neurologist who is busy documenting semiologically how the patient's muscles have worsened since the last visit. The number of devices that can help patients suffering from symptomatic weakness are as legion as the number of activities that can be limited by this disease. The breadth of the problem and what we and our patients have found to be the most helpful solutions are shown in Tables 2 and 3, but a picture is worth a thousand words. It is a good idea to lend your patient a catalogue of self-help aids (such as that by Sammons) to thumb through at home, and to keep a copy as an office reference. The

Table 3   Durable Medical Equipment

Four-pronged cane
Forearm crutches
Upright rolling walker (adapt with forearm supports, vertical grip handles, and basket)
Manual wheelchair, measured and fitted by physical therapist (best is lightweight, portable, with removable armrests and swing-away removable leg supports [e.g., Quikie II, Compax]; add high-density foam cushion, sheepskin, wheelchair tray, and carryall bag/pouch)
High-backed recliner electric wheelchair, measured and fitted by physical therapist (should be adapted with changeable control switch) [i.e., joystick, suck/blow controls] and with space under seat for respirator or computer as weakness progresses; should have removable armrests, swing-away removable leg supports, cushion and sheepskin, wheelchair tray and carryall bag/pouch)
Portable suction machine, with Yankar oral/tonsil adaptor
Fracture bedpan/urinal
Hand rails/safety bars for tub/shower and toilet
Hospital bed (electric preferred; with high-density egg crate mattress and sheepskin)
Overbed table with tilting top
Mechanical patient lift (portable preferred) with full body sling (e.g., Hoyer)
Drop-arm bedside commode
Accessible shower stall with rolling shower/commode chair (or tub chair, bench with back and side support)
Electric reclining seat-lift chair
Outdoor ramps
Stairway glide
Van adapted with electric hydraulic lift for wheelchair passenger

Table 2   Most Useful Adaptive Aids for Weakness in ALS

Personal hygiene
  Long-handled sponge
  Wash mitt with soap pocket
  Soap on a rope
  Lightweight built-up handles for toothbrush, comb, razor, nail file
  Electric toothbrush with suction brush device
  Electric razor
  Hand-held shower head
  Raised toilet seat
  Nail brush/clipper with suction cups

Dressing
  Button hook
  Zipper ring, hook, loop
  Dressing stick
  Long-handled shoehorn
  Velcro clothing closures
  Suspenders
  Sock and shoe aid

Positioning
  Ankle-foot orthosis (AFO)
  Cock-up wrist splint
  Transfer board
  Foam wedge cushion (bed)
  Cervical collars: open Kydex frame collar with Plastozote padding; Philadelphia collar; soft collar (e.g., Freeman, Newport)
  Head strap
  Lightweight resting hand splint
  Cervical pillow

Feeding
  Mobile arm support, ball-bearing feeder
  Nonskid foam (DYCEM)
  Plate guard
  Rocker knife
  Lightweight built-up silverware (tubular foam)
  Lightweight mugs with easy-grip handles
  Utensil hand clip/ADL universal cuff

Meal preparation
  Long-lever jar opener with adaptive turning knob
  Lap tray (beanbag; bed tray/table)
  Lightweight built-up handles for cooking utensils, pots
  Adapted paring board
  Twist-off bottle opener
  Milk carton holder

Other
  Lamp extension switch
  Triangular pencil grip
  Book holder
  Card holder
  Page turner (hand-held, mouth-held)
  Rubber thimble
  Speaker phone with automatic dialing
  Telephone holder; hand clip
  Operator headset
  Lightweight reachers
  Adapted built-up key holder
  Doorknob extension lever
  Self-opening scissors
  Antiembolism (TED) stockings
  Wanchik's Writer

issue of exercise is discussed separately later in this chapter.

Swallowing

Conservative measures and helpful eating strategies (Table 4) go a long way toward improving swallowing and preventing aspiration. When swallowing is first jeopardized and aspiration is a risk, patients and their families should be trained in the Heimlich maneuver and cardiopulmonary resuscitation. They should obtain a portable suction machine to help clear secretions and retrieve from the posterior larynx boluses that cannot be expectorated and that jeopardize the airway. With the conservative measures outlined, many patients are, surprisingly, able to eat (though with great caution) despite severe corticobulbar dysfunction and severe impairment as measured by cine-esophagography.

When the patient's intake of food provides inadequate nutrition, some form of tube feeding must be considered in consultation with a trained nutritionist. Patients may mistakenly place a feeding tube in the same category as all tubes, including an endotracheal tube, as if it were a "heroic" measure. This can be demystified by demonstrating the devices or referring the patient to another patient who uses the device. There are many options. Simple nasogastric tubes are often the easiest solution. Keough tubes have the advantage of smaller size and greater flexibility and comfort, but with long use they frequently become occluded. The most easily tolerated surgical procedure, and currently the best option, is endoscopically guided gastrostomy performed while the patient is under local anesthesia. We do not find cervical esophagostomy or feeding pharyngotomy with cricopharyngeal myotomy useful.

Sialorrhea is a difficult and humiliating problem. The problem with all treatments for drooling is that an excessively dry mouth may in fact make swallowing more difficult. We have only occasionally found permanent procedures, such as parotid gland irradiation or tympanic neurectomy, helpful. Unfortunately, such procedures may make residual saliva tenacious, difficult to expectorate, or even inspissated—a cure worse than the original symptom. Most patients end up using a suction apparatus or a cloth in the mouth as the most practical solution. Over-the-counter antihistamines may be tried. Amitriptyline has the advantage of being a very potent anticholinergic agent for sialorrhea as well as an antidepressant and hypnotic agent (although the drug is not indicated for sole use as a hypnotic over the long term). There are, of course, many anticholinergic agents, but the most convenient is the scopolamine patch. Its convenience is its relatively constant therapeutic effect without the patient's needing to swallow anything, but its chief disadvantage, as with all anticholinergic agents, is potentiation of glaucoma, urinary retention, or adverse central nervous system effects. The chief advantage of glycopyrrolate, a quaternary anticholinergic agent, is that it does not cross the blood-brain barrier.

Communication

Because the low volume of the voice is rarely the only problem, amplification devices are rarely or briefly usable. For some patients who have limited use of certain fingers, portable hand-held printout devices, such as the Light Writer, are a quick way to produce a written message. For those who can produce few recognizable spoken words and whose hands are weak there are still numerous strategies for communication (Table 5). Speed is the most frustrating aspect. ETRAN display boards are an old standard. Letters, phrases, or words can be indicated by eye movements or pointing. The pointer can be as simple as a soda straw held in the mouth if lip muscles or neck muscles are strong enough. A clear Lucite communication board is an ideal way to improve eye contact between "speaker" and interpreter. Simple eye blink (yes/no) strategies cost nothing and rely on the inventiveness of the patient and family in developing the quickest strategies for scanning the alphabet or developing codes. The disadvantages of such systems are that they become idiosyncratic and do not transfer to friends or multiple therapists. Personal computers have the potential for speed and permanent printout. Input can be linked to any residual movement (eyebrow, finger flicker, eye movement) via microswitch. Many kinds of software exist, and a popular one in our

---

Table 4 Helpful Strategies for Swallowing

Position: Sit upright 45–90° angle (high Fowler's), head bent slightly forward
Attention: Concentrate on swallowing: avoid communication and other distractions at mealtime and eat in a comfortable, unhurried setting
Adjustment of taste, texture, and temperature: Avoid excessively sweet or sour foods, as they increase saliva production: avoid bitter and salty foods, as they increase thirst
Use soft, cooked, moist foods and gelled, pureed, strained foods; add sauces
Avoid extremes of temperature
Common sense: Take frequent small meals (6 per day)
Cut food into small, bite-sized pieces
If adjustment of food texture limits nutrition, use high-calorie, high-protein supplements
Instruct patient and family in Heimlich maneuver.

Table 5 Communication Aids

Note pad
Magic slate
Call device: dinner bell, clicker, intercom system, Speak & Spell toy
Letterboards: ETRAN, letter cuff (alphabet list worn on forearm); word or picture communication books, (e.g. Daily Communicator, Picture Communicator)
Electric typewriter
Hand-held computers with printout device (Lightwriter)
Personal computer (desktop)
Computer augmentation devices:
    Specific software capabilities adapted to patient needs such as Words Plus
    Voice synthesizer
    Switches adaptable to head movement, eye blink, or suck/blow.

clinic is Aurora. The more complex the algorithm of the software, such as the ability to predict the next letter or word from known common spelling patterns or rules of grammar and rhetoric, the speedier the output. Inefficiency and slowness of certain scanning programs make patients put their computers back in boxes and revert to simpler eye blink and alphabet board strategies. An advantage of computers is that the output can be linked to a speech synthesizer to add a human speech quality to communication, to printers to allow for correspondence, and to modems to allow telephone interaction. An important new national volunteer agency, Volunteers for Medical Engineering, helps provide and train handicapped patients with such devices. One should not forget that the old-fashioned pencil and note pad and the 29 cent magic slate are communication tools far superior to "high-tech" devices if the patient can use his or her hands.

Some speaking habits that care givers develop are particularly irritating to ALS patients. These include speaking to family members rather than directly to the patient, speaking without eye-to-eye contact with the patient, standing far above the patient when addressing him or her, speaking loudly as if the patient were deaf, pretending to understand speech that is not understandable, completing patient's sentences and thoughts, or speaking in a manner or tone of voice one might use with a child.

Breathing

Respiratory impairment is the most serious sign in ALS. To the physician, the patient, and the family members it may appear to represent the beginning of the end. Pneumonia or aspiration, as secondary complications of severely weakened respiratory and bulbar muscles, is the usual cause of death.

Assessment

The two most important measurements for assessing neuromuscular respiratory impairment are vital capacity (VC) and negative inspiratory force (NIF). VC is the single most important measurement, as it can be easily measured by spirometry. As a global indicator of lung function, VC should direct the physician's care in dealing with impending respiratory insufficiency. NIF begins to decline into a useful measurable range when the VC falls below 1.5 L or half the patient's predicted baseline value. It is a useful indicator of respiratory *muscle* status (with contributions from intercostals, diaphragm, and accessory muscles of respiration), exclusive of parenchymal lung disease. Arterial blood gas evaluations are rarely useful, because serious changes are only late indicators of respiratory muscle failure in ALS. PaO_2 levels remain well preserved until late in the course of the disease. Carbon dioxide retention to levels greater than 45 mm Hg is a poor prognostic sign, common in patients who present with severe respiratory failure (Fig. 1).

Symptomatic Care

Treatment should be directed toward maintaining and improving the patient's ventilation by instructing family members in chest physiotherapy, nasopharyngeal suctioning, assistive cough techniques (Heimlich maneuver used synchronously with the patient's cough attempt), and use of intermittent positive pressure breathing (IPPB). Episodes of acute respiratory difficulty should not be automatically attributed to the progression of ALS but should be properly diagnosed by examination of sputum, body temperature, respiratory rate and effort, and by chest x-ray examination. Acute upper respiratory tract infection, aspiration, or dehydration should be treated early with intravenous fluids and/or antibiotics, as they further compromise an already poor respiratory status. Bronchodilators, such as metaproterenol sulfate or albuterol (preferably administered by a nebulizer), may be given if indicated by bronchospasm associated with mucus plugging. Long-acting theophylline compounds are used as well (because of their putative direct effects on muscle) to relieve respiratory muscle fatigue. Adequate hydration to liquefy secretions and nutrition to maintain strength should be emphasized.

Mechanical Ventilation

The issue of mechanical ventilation should be openly and supportively discussed with the patient and the patient's family as soon as involvement of respiratory muscle is observed. Whereas symptomatic treatments may alleviate the initial symptoms, the underlying problem of respiratory muscle fatigue and eventual paralysis will not be solved until a decision is made on the use or refusal of mechanical ventilation. Although this decision is difficult, most patients and family members have difficulty grasping the consequences of their choices and are grateful to the physician for the opportunity to discuss them. There is no simple way to direct such a discussion other than to adopt an unhurried, honest approach. Discussion of a living will may be a catalyst in this conversation. The living will outlines in writing one's desire to use or not to use mechanical ventilation to sustain life. Many states have adopted the living will as a legal right; federal law mandates patients be informed and allowed to give advance directives on admission to hospital. These documents can be obtained easily through a lawyer. The patient should understand that the decision does not have to be made immediately and that it is revocable.

The optimal family situation for home ventilator use requires many resources. Proximity to an acute care hospital, supportive care by a dedicated nurse and physician, a home health agency, insurance coverage, financial support for that family member who will become the primary caretaker, respite care, emotional support for patient and family members, and equipment and necessary electrical adaptations for the home are a few of the tangible and intangible resources necessary to improve the transition to total ventilator support. Most

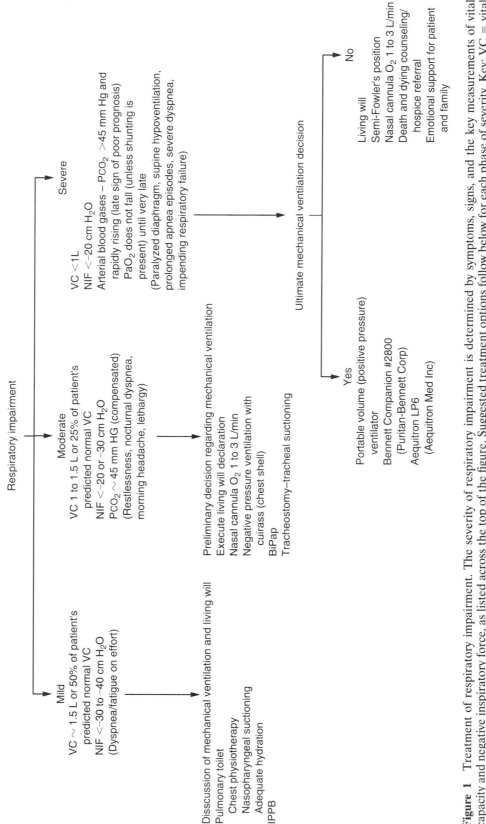

Figure 1 Treatment of respiratory impairment. The severity of respiratory impairment is determined by symptoms, signs, and the key measurements of vital capacity and negative inspiratory force, as listed across the top of the figure. Suggested treatment options follow below for each phase of severity. Key: VC = vital capacity; NIF = negative inspiratory force; IPPB = intermittent positive pressure breathing; BiPap = bilevel positive airway pressure.

insurance companies assist financially with the cost of nursing care and respiratory therapy to allow the patient to remain in the home. Some agencies, such as the MDA, assist in the purchase of electric wheelchairs that, when modified, can include space for a portable ventilator, to afford the patient mobility. After some initial adjustment, many patients can be weaned from the ventilator for several hours during the day. Outings are made possible by a wheelchair-accessible van equipped with a hydraulic lift. While the picture is not entirely rosy, it is not the same picture that one may envision of the patient attached to a large, noisy respirator in a socially isolated hospital ward. If appropriate support is available, the patient can live a life with quality, although necessarily experiences become increasingly more vicarious.

Tracheostomy by itself is an option for the patient whose problem with aspiration of food or secretions predominates over respiratory impairment. This procedure can be performed relatively easily and can increase comfort when the airway is jeopardized by aspiration. After some time, the patient can have a talking tracheostomy tube inserted, or in some cases may be able to speak simply by deflating the tracheostomy cuff.

For the patient with moderate to severe respiratory difficulty who decides against using mechanical ventilation, other supportive measures can still be used (see Fig. 1). Negative pressure ventilation, though only a short-term solution, is possible with a cuirass device that uses a shell through which a vacuum motor provides intermittent negative pressure to the chest wall, thus enabling the patient's chest to rise and fall. The newest-generation cuirass machine (Life Care NEV-100) is pressure/flow sensitive, and thus compensates for air leaks in the shell; it can be cycled by the patient's breathing. BiPap (Bilevel Positive Airway Pressure) is the newest generation of continuous positive airway pressure ventilatory support systems. Use of sophisticated electronics provides variable pressure and flow co-ordinated with inspiration and expiration. In patients whose respiration is otherwise marginal, ventilation can be maintained for long periods using cuirass or BiPap at night and a continuous IPPB apparatus during the day to force open atelectatic airways. Low-flow oxygen (1 to 3 L per minute via nasal cannula) can be used, particularly at night, to combat the typical supine hypoventilation that causes eventual hypoxia. Patients should sleep in semi-Fowler's position (30 to 45 degrees) to aid ventilation.

Sleeplessness and Breathing

In the context of respiratory insufficiency, sleeplessness may become a more significant problem. It can easily be treated with small doses of triazolam or flurazepam hydrochloride, but these should be used intermittently for short periods. Anxiety symptoms may be helped by these or other benzodiazepine derivatives administered in small doses. If cough is the problem, short-term codeine also promotes rest. Alcohol or over-the-counter antihistamines should not be used as hypnotics: they are less effective, are prone to suppress rapid eye movement (REM) sleep, and cause adverse side effects when taken in overdose. For moribund patients, administration of morphine—with the full knowledge of the potential for further respiratory suppression associated with the use of all anxiolytics and hypnotics—allows patients partial mental detachment from their situation. At this stage of the disease, however, the majority of patients may be already naturally sedated or lethargic from carbon dioxide narcosis and usually die quietly in their sleep. Long before this point, referral to a local hospice agency may provide much-needed support for the patient and family members. The professional counseling and physical and emotional support that this multidisciplinary team can provide are invaluable for patients at this stage of ALS.

Any ALS patient has the right to change his or her mind about mechanical ventilation at any time. Whatever decision the patient makes, the physician should seek to understand it from the patient's perspective. In fact, the physician needs to become the student of the patient. Openness, flexibility, and most of all *caring*, are essential in treating all aspects of this disease but especially when treating the respiratory insufficiency that eventually progresses to respiratory failure.

QUESTIONS ALS PATIENTS ASK

"What Do I Have?"

The answer to this question should be simply "ALS." It is now the name that the lay public know and use in North America. A more generic and unfamiliar (e.g., British) term like "motor neuron disease" is often used as a form of medical obfuscation. Such a term should be reserved for truly atypical cases that fail to meet the criteria for the diagnosis of ALS. If a more specific form of motor neuron disease can be diagnosed, the specific correct term (e.g., progressive bulbar palsy, spinal muscular atrophy, primary lateral sclerosis, multifocal motor neuropathy) should be used and explained to the patient. To prevent common confusion, physicians should explicitly distinguish ALS from Alzheimer's disease (the other "A" disease), multiple sclerosis (the other "sclerosis"), and muscular dystrophy.

One should be honest when discussing the diagnosis and then during the first two visits let the patient limit the discussion. One should allot an unhurried hour for this discussion. In explaining the meaning of ALS, avoid the impulse to say, "That's what Lou Gehrig had." Everyone is familiar with the picture of a stooped, tearful Lou Gehrig in his uniform. It evokes a sense of hopelessness, early retirement, and early death. Nowadays, it is much more helpful to say something like, "It's what Senator Jacob Javits had," because this evokes hopefulness, visibility, acceptance, and continued productivity.

"How Long Do I Have to Live?"

The wrong answer is, "God only knows when *any* of us will die. We could be hit on the highway tomorrow by a truck. The average patient dies in 3 years." To someone who is already assured of death, it is not comforting to be told that he may be hit by a truck as well, and such a comment immediately conveys to the patient that the doctor does not really understand the dilemma. Further, quoting a specific survival time is always wrong, since the patient can only assume that he is like the "average patient." A much better answer evokes hope: "Half of the patients who come to us are alive 3 years after onset of the disease, and many live a much longer time, even as long as 10 years or more." One may convincingly add at that point, "All along the way, there will be many treatments we can offer you for every problem that might arise." Such hopefulness is quite a different message to receive than the more typical 3 year "death sentence" that many patients end up hearing.

"Should I Exercise?"

One should resist the urge to answer in a scholarly way, "There is really no research on it, but if you do exercise, don't do too much. Don't exert yourself to the point of fatigue." We see a surprising number of patients with ALS who have been forbidden by their physician to exercise or even warned to quit active exercise programs to which they were previously accustomed, out of some unspoken fear of the harmfulness of fatigue or an unfounded idea about motor units "wearing out." Telling a patient to exercise but not to exert himself to the point of fatigue is like telling a child to have fun swimming but not to go near the water. ALS is in fact marked by reinnervation of muscle, as evidenced by electromyography and muscle biopsy. One should capitalize on this. Motor units *need* use to prevent atrophy of innervated muscle fibers. Movement of joints is essential to prevent both disuse and contracture. The simplest of all reasons to prescribe exercise is that exercise feels good. It can produce a sense of euphoria and encourages hopefulness. Of course, there are no new converts to exercise; a sedentary person unaccustomed to exercising is unlikely to take up the challenge as a new way of coping with the diagnosis of ALS. Passive stretching exercises should certainly be encouraged. This is particularly important for families to learn in order to prevent contracture of shoulder joints, which, aside from being painful, can make such simple activities as dressing difficult.

When an active exercise program is undertaken, it should be designed and supervised by a physiotherapist or physiatrist who specializes in exercise evaluation and prescription. One common formula for a resistance exercise program begins by determining for the target muscle the maximum resistance for ten repetitions of an exercise. Prescribed exercise then consists of a series of graded efforts as follows: five to ten repetitions each at 50 percent maximum resistance, at 75 percent, and then 100 percent, each cycle interspersed with 2 minutes rest. Such programs, targeted at particular muscles that are functionally important for the individual patient, can be combined with cardiac fitness exercise programs using swimming, stationary bicycling, or other sustained activity, depending on the abilities of the patient at that stage of the illness. Overexertion can be prevented by using some fairly liberal rules of thumb, so that the level of exercise is reduced if any of the following signs occur: (1) tachycardia greater than two times the baseline heart rate, (2) persistent tachycardia more than 10 beats per minute over baseline heart rate 10 minutes after exercise has ceased, (3) dyspnea for more than "a few" minutes, (4) angina, (5) excessive pain and fatigue on the *day after* exercise.

"What Do I Do Now?"

Resources

In response to this question, the first advice one should give is to contact the Muscular Dystrophy Association, which is the single largest provider of money for both research and patient services for this disease in the world. It is surprising how few patients are referred early to the MDA or to the ALS Association (a research- and educational-oriented association). Given the gravity of the diagnosis, the second piece of advice should be to obtain a responsible second opinion. The physician should then suggest that the entire family join a support group for ALS patients and families. Such support groups are now offered by every major clinic supported by the MDA or the ALS Association. Support groups offer a place to vent anger and frustration, share common solutions to vexing problems (such as coping with insurance companies or determining which of the many available orthopaedic and occupational aids are truly useful), deal with the sense of abandonment by physicians or friends of family, discuss the problem of respite care, and provide a forum where psychological needs can be expressed and heeded to carry patients and their families through phases of depression. In addition, probably the most important function such groups serve is that of creating a network that provides the most practical education about the disease and that gives friends some understanding of what it feels like to have ALS.

Clinical Trials

The final prescription may be to encourage patients to participate in valid clinical research. The physician should firmly resist the urge to provide placebo therapy in the hope that it "might help keep the disease from progressing." The extensive menu of such placebos (from bee pollen to pancreatic enzymes) changes with time, but they are always used with the misguided rationale that "at least they won't do any harm." Expensive quack treatments like snake venom and transfer factor injections can be truly harmful by virtue of their expense alone. Placebo responses last weeks to months. Their eventual failure leads to withdrawal of patients from health professionals and to hopelessness; they do not encourage attendance at clinic, nor do they provide the psychological support often intended. Rather, regular visits to a specialized multidisciplinary clinic that offers the services of social worker, patient service coordinator, nurse clinician, physician, occupational therapist, orthopaedist, physiotherapist, speech therapist, and dietician offer infinitely better therapy and psychological support than all the prescribed cures of Ivan Ilyich's doctor.

A valid, controlled clinical trial is a real expression of hope. More than half of patients with ALS will want to participate in a clinical trial at least once. The physician's work is to be an advocate and to help the patient evaluate the validity of a particular trial. Quackery abounds with this disease as much as it does with cancer. Besides advocating participation in valid research, the physician needs to be a resource to help patients screen out quackery. The following obvious "red flags" can be offered to ALS families that should alert great caution: (1) treatments that are good for many seemingly unrelated diseases, (2) treatments for which no formal protocol can be produced, (3) a rationale or an experimental trial that is neither written nor explainable to the referring physician, (4) the absence of control subjects, (5) supporting literature that relies on testimonials, (6) nonsponsored research that has not undergone some form of peer review, (7) high costs that are *all* borne by the patient. Any one of these should prompt caution, but several should be indicative of quackery.

Current clinical research available to participants with ALS in the United States includes trials of neurotrophic factors, agents that disrupt neurotransmitter glutamate actions, and immunomodulators (Table 6). The best sources for current information on controlled clinical trials are the MDA and the ALS Association.

FINAL SUGGESTIONS

1. When you make the diagnosis of ALS, plan two sessions: the first to give conclusions and the second to lay out your plans.
2. Know and connect the patient with essential public resources such as the MDA.
3. Do not discuss all possible outcomes and available devices at an early stage. This only leads to information overload and feelings of hopelessness.
4. Prescribe exercise. It is invigorating and encourages hopefulness. It prevents the development of frozen joints and subsequent pain, capitalizes on the potential for reinnervation of muscle, and is

---

Table 6 Current Clinical Trials for ALS

A. Trophic factors
  1. Ciliary neurotrophic factor (CNTF)
      Organizers: Regeneron Pharmaceuticals, Inc. (Tarrytown, NY) and Synergen, Inc. (Boulder, CO)
      Actions and principles for use: CNTF is a naturally occurring peptide that promotes survival of embryonic motor neurons and injured motor neurons.
  2. Myotrophin
      Organizer: Cephalon, Inc. (West Chester, PA)
      Actions and principles for use: Cephalon's Myotrophin is an insulin-like growth factor (IGF) that also permits motor neuron survival in cultured motor neurons. Fewer data are available on its effects on injured motor neurons in vivo or in animal models of motor neuron degeneration.

B. Glutamate antagonists or metabolic inhibitors
  1. Branched-chain amino acids (L-leucine, L-valine, L-isoleucine)
      Organizer: Available for individual use or in a clinical trial organized by A. Plaitakis, MD, Mount Sinai Hospital, NY, NY.
      Actions: At high concentrations these amino acids may alter glutamate oxidation. Some clinical trials, though not all, have suggested that chronic oral administration slows the rate of deterioration.
  2. Dextromethorphan
      Organizer: Available for individual use; also clinical trial organized by T. Munsat, MD, New England Medical Center, Boston, MA.
      Actions: Active ingredient in cough syrup, can act as a weak glutamate receptor (NMDA subtype) antagonist. Limited data on its clinical efficacy, small clinical trials have not shown any clinical benefit.

C. Immunotherapy
  1. Cyclophosphamide
      Organizer: Available for individual use; also clinical trial organized by D.B. Drachman, M.D., Johns Hopkins University, Baltimore, MD; *not appropriate for use outside of peer-reviewed, IRB-approved protocols*
      Actions: Potent immunosuppressant that is effective in immune based multifocal motor neuropathy.
  2. Intravenous human immunoglobulin
      Organizer: Available for individual use; also clinical trial organized by M. Dalakis, MD, NINDS, NIH, Bethesda, MD.
      Actions: Immunomodulator thought to be effective in patients with multifocal motor neuropathy.

D. Genetic studies
  1. Patients with familial ALS can be referred to T. Siddique, MD, Northwestern University, Chicago, IL, or R.H. Brown, MD, Massachusetts General Hospital, Boston, MA.
  2. Twins with ALS can be referred to International Twin Study, University of Southern California, School of Medicine, Parkview Medical Building B-105, 1420 San Pablo, Los Angeles, CA 90033-1042 (800) 421-9631.

not harmful if certain rules of thumb regarding limits are followed.

5. Be knowledgeable about aids for activities of daily living; buy a Sammans catalogue or its equivalent. Read it and discuss it with a knowledgeable occupational therapist. Question patients on their needs and abilities, and when particular needs arise, have them try occupational aids. Use occupational therapists, nurse clinicians, or other professionals *experienced* and *interested* in ALS.

6. Start a support group for ALS patients and their families. Use other patients with ALS as a resource. You will learn everything that will be useful to you in treating these patients from the patients and families themselves.

7. Encourage the patient to participate in valid research at least once. This fulfills altruistic motives and is morally rewarding for the patient. It is an activity that inspires hopefulness. Become an active advocate to help patients screen various research opportunities.

Acknowledgements. We gratefully acknowledge the dedicated assistance of Blair Ertel. Our ALS research and patient care have been generously supported by the Jay Slotkin Fund for Neuromuscular Research, the Baltimore Relief Foundation, and the Muscular Dystrophy Association. We are indebted to our colleagues in the Neuromuscular Division, and most of all to the many members of the Baltimore ALS Support Group and our ALS patients whose courage, patience, and guidance contributed much to the content of this chapter.

SUGGESTED READING

Caroscio JT, ed. ALS: A guide to patient care. New York: Thieme, 1986.

Kuncl RW, Crawford T, Rothstein JD, Drachman DB. Motor neuron disease. In: Asbury AK, McKhann GM, McDonald WI, eds. Diseases of the nervous system. Philadelphia: WB Saunders, 1992:1179.

Rowland LP. Advances in neurology. Vol 56. Amyotrophic lateral sclerosis. New York: Raven, 1991.

PATIENT RESOURCES

Associations
The Muscular Dystrophy Association is a nonprofit national organization (information and referral agency) whose main focus is to provide funds for medical care, equipment, education, support groups, research, co-ordination, and financing of clinics for many neuromuscular diseases, including ALS.

Muscular Dystrophy Association
3561 East Sunrise Drive
Tucson, Arizona 85718
Telephone: (602) 529-2000

The Amyotrophic Lateral Sclerosis Association is a nonprofit national organization (information and referral agency) whose main focus is to provide funds for education and research and to sponsor chapter groups for patients with ALS.

Amyotrophic Lateral Sclerosis
21021 Ventura Boulevard, Suite 321
Woodland Hills, California 91364
Telephone: (800) 782-4747

The Volunteers for Medical Engineering is a nonprofit national organization of engineers who donate equipment, time, and ingenuity to solving specific problems of disabled persons.

Volunteers for Medical Engineering
UMBC-TEC
5206 Westland Boulevard
Baltimore, Maryland 21227
Telephone: (410) 455-6395

Literature
Appel V, Callender M, Sunter S. ALS: Maintaining mobility—a guide to physical therapy and occupational therapy. Houston: Muscular Dystrophy Association, 1988.

Appel V, Calvin S, Otte I. ALS: Maintaining nutrition. Houston: Muscular Dystrophy Association, 1990.

Appel V, Calvin S, Smith O, Woehr D. Meals. Houston: Muscular Dystrophy Association, 1987.

ALS Association: Five Manual Series. Manual I: Finding help; Manual II: Muscular weakness; Manual III: Swallowing difficulty; Manual IV: Breathing difficulty; Manual V: Communication difficulty. Woodland Hills, California: ALS Association, 1986.

Fred Sammons Catalogue
145 Tower Drive, Dept. #423
Burr Ridge, Illinois 60521-9842
(708) 325-1700.

Enrichments Catalogue
Box 579
145 Tower Drive
Hinsdale, Illinois 60521
(800) 323-5547

THE OTHER DEMENTIAS

RICHARD MAYEUX, M.D.
THOMAS K. TATEMICHI, M.D.
NED SACKTOR, M.D.

Although Alzheimer's disease (AD) is the most frequent cause of dementia, it accounts for only 40 to 60 percent of dementia cases in most published series. In fact, before age 60 years, a number of other diseases account for the nearly half the causes of dementia. Among those forms of dementia, stroke and other types of vascular disease, Parkinson's disease (PD) and Huntington's disease, and acquired immunodeficiency syndrome (AIDS), as well as a variety of metabolic disorders, are most frequently encountered.

Little has been written about the management or treatment of these forms of dementia. As we hope to indicate, some of these frequently encountered disorders have viable treatment options, which should be noted and employed when possible.

DEMENTIA ASSOCIATED WITH CEREBROVASCULAR DISEASE

Cerebrovascular disease (CVD) is considered the second most common cause of dementia after AD. Approximately 50 to 60 percent of cases are due to AD, 20 to 25 percent are attributable to stroke alone, and another 10 to 15 percent may be explained by a combination of the two disorders. Thus, CVD plays a significant role in a large proportion of elderly persons with dementia. In some populations, especially those at high risk for stroke (e.g., Japanese, Chinese, and nonwhite samples in the United States) the prevalence of vascular dementia exceeds that due to AD. On this basis, it has been suggested that, worldwide, vascular disease may be the most common cause of mental deterioration in elders.

The contribution of CVD to dementia may have been underestimated, in part because of diagnostic difficulties, the populations examined, and the source of information used (clinical series, population-based sample, or pathologic material). The counterargument has been that vascular dementia is overestimated because of the tendency to attribute significance to trivial CVD, even when the primary cause is likely to be degenerative. Nonetheless, even if the dementia is a result of multiple or mixed causes, including AD, it is the vascular component for which preventive or treatment options are available. The management of dementia associated with CVD thus begins with its recognition and discrimination from other forms of dementia, followed by identifying risk factors and the underlying vascular cause, and finally taking specific steps to treat the vascular component.

Three essential elements are required for diagnosis (Table 1). In evaluating the dementia syndrome from stroke, a common problem is distinguishing focal neurobehavioral syndromes from multifocal or global effects consistent with dementia. We rely on neuropsychological testing to assist in this discrimination, although when aphasia is present the results may be difficult to interpret. As in other dementias, memory impairment combined with other cognitive deficits should be present, in keeping with the *Diagnostic and Statistical Manual of Mental Disorders* (DSM-III-R) criteria. Although the neuropsychological profile in vascular dementia overall is not clearly distinguishable from AD, distinctive vascular subtypes may be recognizable, especially forms due to subcortical infarction. These patients typically display frontal lobe features, including psychomotor slowing, abulia, inattention, and mild memory impairment.

Evidence for CVD may be clinically obvious, as in major territorial brain infarction with disabling physical and cognitive consequences. These patients are readily codified by ischemia scores, which emphasize clinically evident strokes. More problematic are minor attacks or subtle strokes (whether they are classified as transient ischemic attack [TIA], reversible ischemic neurologic deficit [RIND], or minor completed stroke is unhelpful, and probably irrelevant). Some of these occur in areas strategic for higher cerebral function and may not be associated with symptoms or signs (e.g., hemiplegia) typically expected with stroke; others result in cumulative damage to the cerebral white matter resulting in progressive but not apoplectic cognitive impairment. In both of these circumstances, brain imaging is critical.

After recognizing the presence of both dementia and CVD, the central diagnostic problem is to determine what constitutes significant (and therefore causally related) vascular disease of the brain (see Table 1). Perhaps the most important feature that distinguishes vascular dementia from AD is the occurrence of mental deterioration following a clinically obvious stroke. Similarly, a course with stepwise declines or fluctuation

Table 1 Diagnostic Criteria for Dementia Related to Cerebrovascular Disease

1. Dementia (and not circumscribed neurobehavioral deficit)
2. Cerebrovascular disease (history, examination, or brain imaging)
3. Evidence that (1) and (2) are causally related. Features that support causality include:
   Temporal relationship between stroke and dementia
   Stepwise deterioration or fluctuation in mental function
   Supportive brain imaging findings

Adapted from Roman CG, Tatemichi TK, Erkinsuntti T, et al. Vascular dementia: Diagnostic criteria for research studies. Reports of the NINDS-AIREN International Work Group. Neurology (in press), with permission.

Support for this work was provided by the following federal grants to the authors, AG07232, AG08702, and NS26179, and from the Parkinson's Disease Foundation.

should support the diagnosis, regardless of whether clinical stroke events are associated. It is often not possible to obtain reliable information on temporal sequence or course retrospectively. Lacking these data, we are often forced to turn to brain-imaging evidence and are faced with a different diagnostic challenge: interpreting the clinical significance of ischemic lesions on computed tomography (CT) or magnetic resonance imaging (MRI). In any given patient, the effect of localized brain injury may be highly variable, depending on age, co-existing disease, and functional reserve.

The role of diffuse white matter disease (leukoaraiosis [LA]) deserves further comment. As a brain-imaging abnormality, LA has been identified in normal healthy elders, those who have suffered or are at risk for stroke, and in AD, with a variable relationship to cognitive impairment. We have all encountered patients with strikingly abnormal brain images who are clinically normal. Thus, it is not difficult to see why the specificity and clinical relevance of LA have been questioned. Hypoattenuation on CT or hyperintensity on T2-weighted MRI mainly in the periventricular zones corresponds pathologically to areas of gliosis and demyelination, consistent with "incomplete infarction" of uncertain pathogenesis but most likely related to disease (including arteriosclerosis or amyloid deposition) involving the deep medullary vessels that branch from larger surface arteries. As a form of chronic white matter ischemia rather than infarction, the mechanism involved in producing mental changes has also been uncertain, although cortical disconnection is a favored thesis. As with gray matter damage, whether due to infarction or plaques and tangles, we believe that both a threshold quantity of white matter damage and location-specific effects are most likely responsible for cognitive impairment or dementia.

It has been commonly assumed that the risk factors for dementia associated with stroke are the same factors that increase the risk of CVD in general. Thus, factors such as hypertension, atrial fibrillation, congestive heart failure, coronary heart disease, carotid bruit, diabetes, cigarette smoking, hyperlipidemia, peripheral vascular disease, TIA, and stroke have all been cited as potential precursors of vascular dementia. Risk factors for CVD that are precursors of vascular dementia are important to identify in the individual patient, as preventive measures for stroke in general should also apply to vascular dementia in particular. Specific attention should be directed to factors that may result in small vessel disease (e.g., diabetes mellitus), as the result could be clinically occult, or "silent," stroke delaying recognition of a potentially treatable condition.

The underlying vascular causes of dementia are as varied as the causes of ischemic CVD in general. When dementia occurs in the setting of CVD, evaluation for underlying vascular causes should be initiated. At the minimum, this should include brain and vascular imaging studies (CT or MRI and Doppler ultrasonography or magnetic resonance angiography [MRA]) and assessment of vascular risks (e.g., recording blood pressure;

performing cardiac examination and electrocardiography (ECG); obtaining a family history, and measuring glucose, lipids, and sedimentation rate as a screen for occult inflammatory disorders). In patients who lack risk factors for thromboembolic disease, additional studies might include a search for prothrombotic conditions (e.g., lupus anticoagulant or anticardiolipin antibodies) or consideration of unusual disorders (e.g., granulomatous angiitis or moyamoya disease). The need for more detailed or invasive studies would be guided by the initial results (e.g., uncovering occult cardioembolic sources with transesophageal echocardiography, defining surgically relevant hemodynamic carotid artery disease with cerebral angiography, and identifying perfusion failure from carotid disease or coexisting AD by functional brain imaging with single photon emission computed tomography or positron emission tomography).

Although we have focused on ischemic vascular disease, brain hemorrhage may also result in dementia. The clinical syndrome is usually obvious in the setting of either subarachnoid or parenchymatous bleeding. A single lobar hemorrhage in an elderly person without hypertension, or multiple lobar hemorrhages (in rare instances, simultaneous) should suggest amyloid angiopathy as the diagnosis; dementia may become evident early or late in the course.

Treatment

Therapies for prevention of stroke recurrence are established and should be applied to all patients with vascular dementia. Depending on the underlying vascular cause, antiplatelets, anticoagulants, or carotid endarterectomy would be appropriate. For most patients, aspirin, 325 mg daily, is effective and the safest option. Some evidence suggests that ticlopidine may be more effective than aspirin for intracranial vascular disease, although there has been no antithrombotic trial that has examined dementia as an endpoint. Hypertension and other vascular risks must be monitored and controlled; however, overaggressive antihypertensive treatment may be deleterious, possibly aggravating white matter ischemia. Currently, there is no recognized effective therapy specific for the vascular dementias, although several approaches are under investigation (Table 2).

Finally, we have a comment on symptomatic treatment. Although the concept of "depressive pseudodementia" has been widely discussed in the literature, we suggest the alternate possibility that apparent "depression" may be an indication or early sign of dementia. Thus, elderly depressed patients, especially those with frontal lobe features, may have an underlying dementia due to focal or multifocal vascular disease (i.e., have "pseudodepression of dementia"). There is increasing evidence that depression in elderly persons should prompt a search for CVD. Even if CVD is found, antidepressant medications should be considered as well. Nortriptyline is effective and tolerated well by stroke patients.

Table 2 Treatment Options for Vascular Dementia

Prevention of stroke recurrence
  Antithrombotics
    Aspirin, ticlopidine, warfarin
  Surgical
    Carotid endarterectomy
    Extracranial-intracranial bypass surgery†

Specific treatments for vascular dementia
  Calcium antagonists*
  Hemorrheologic (trental)*
  Dopaminergic enhancement (bromocriptine)†
  Cholinergic enhancement*
  Vasodilators†

*Under investigation
†Efficacy doubtful or uncertain

DEMENTIA ASSOCIATED WITH MOVEMENT DISORDERS

Parkinson's Disease

The idiopathic form of PD is one of the most common neurologic disorders, estimated to affect between 80 and 200 people per 100,000 in the general population. The number of affected persons rises steeply with increasing age. Epidemiologic studies have implied that environmental factors play a major role in the cause, although no specific factor has been identified. Dementia frequently accompanies Parkinson's disease, particularly when the motor manifestations begin after age 70. Overall, parkinsonian dementia is the third most common form of dementia in adults. Identification of dementia is critical, because it is the single most important factor that limits the standard therapy for PD.

Clinically, demented patients with PD have both a recent and retrograde memory disorder similar to that observed with Alzheimer's disease. This is accompanied by a loss of complex skills such as visuospatial perception, and it may often be associated with periods of confusion and delirium precipitated by levodopa, other dopamine agonists, or anticholinergics. Major depression can be an antecedent to dementia and is occasionally a coincident feature.

There are at least three distinct pathologic features associated with dementia in PD (Table 3). These features can appear alone or concurrently, but no single pathologic substrate has been identified. In addition to decreased concentrations of brain dopamine, reductions in serotonin and acetylcholine have been implicated in the pathogenesis of dementia in PD.

Treatment

There is no specific treatment for dementia associated with PD. When therapy is instituted with levodopa or another dopamine agonist, we have noticed that many patients report feeling more alert, but this effect is seldom sustained and is not apparent at all with severe dementia. Selegiline, a type B monoamine oxidase inhibitor, also has this awakening effect initially in new

Table 3 Pathology With Dementia in Parkinson's Disease

Coincident AD: neurofibrillary tangles, senile (with and without neurities) plaques and neuronal loss
Lewy body formation in cortical and subcortical areas
Primary medial nigral degeneration

patients; however, dementia is seldom present early, when such therapy is first given. We have used daily doses ranging from 5 to 10 mg in patients with dementia. Although clear improvement in cognitive function has been observed in early previously untreated patients, we have seen a general increase in alertness and improved self-care in some demented patients. We strongly recommend that anticholinergics not be given to demented patients and that dopamine agonists be used in very small doses, to maintain motor function.

To date, there have been only two controlled clinical trials specifically intended for the dementia of PD. Sano and co-workers at Columbia University in New York found no improvement with piracetam, a drug purported to enhance metabolic activity. Phosphatidylserine has been found to increase the speed of the background activity in computerized electroencephalography (EEG) and reduce anxiety, but it has little direct effect on cognitive function in demented patients. Several research groups are exploring the use of cholinergic agonists such as physostigmine and the monoamine oxidase B inhibitor, selegiline.

Lewy Body Disease

A number of researchers have called attention to an unusual disorder defined at postmortem examination as "diffuse Lewy body" disease. At this time, it is not clear whether diffuse Lewy body disease represents a unique disorder or a variant of either AD or PD. Moreover, the frequency of the disorder is unknown. The clinical syndromes associated with Lewy bodies fall into at least three categories, depending on the location of the Lewy inclusion body. The predominant manifestations include dementia with psychosis and extrapyramidal signs of varying degrees of severity. Until better criteria are developed, we recommend the diagnostic criteria proposed by the Nottingham Group for the study of neurodegenerative diseases, be used for the diagnosis of dementia associated with cortical Lewy bodies. These include provisions for the occurrence of both dementia and parkinsonism at some point during the course of the illness, with the exclusion of other causes of dementia or parkinsonism. These criteria await verification but seem a reasonable approach to the problem in diagnosis.

The pathologic hallmark is a small intracytoplasmic eosinophilic inclusion. Most often, Lewy bodies are restricted to the brain stem, as in typical PD, but in two other forms of this disease the distribution can include the brain stem, diencephalon, and cerebral cortex. Reduced brain acetylcholine has been found in the cortical form of this disorder, so-called diffuse cortical Lewy body disease.

Treatment

We have found that dopamine agonists may be useful in some forms of this disorder but are not helpful when psychotic features are present. Traditional antipsychotics may provoke extrapyramidal signs and intensify the psychosis. Therefore, we recommend clozapine, because it has been effective in limiting the psychosis without increasing parkinsonism in our experience. Except for experimental therapies, no treatment for the dementia of Lewy body disease has been established.

Progressive Supranuclear Palsy

Characterized by supranuclear gaze palsies, pseudobulbar palsy, rigidity, dystonic postural changes (particularly of the neck), and a disturbance in gait, this disorder is rare (age-adjusted prevalence in the population over 55 years of age is 7 per 100,000). The usual age at onset ranges from 60 to 70 years. Dementia is a constant feature, although it differs from that associated with PD. Classified as "subcortical" or "subfrontal" dementia, the major manifestations include slowing of thought processes, memory loss, personality change, and defective processing of visual information. Dysarthria leading to mutism is very common. The personality changes include indifference, apathy, and depression.

Pathologic changes in brain include neuron loss, gliosis, and neurofibrillary tangle formation in substantia nigra, the basal forebrain, and other subthalamic areas. Variable reductions in dopamine, acetylcholine, and gamma-aminobutyric acid (GABA) occur in these same regions.

Treatment

Although treatment for progressive supranuclear palsy has been generally disappointing, we believe that most aspects of the disorder can benefit from symptomatic treatment. We have relied on levodopa and other dopamine agonists (including bromocriptine and pergolide) for treatment of the motor manifestations and we give such a drug in doses smaller than those typically used for PD. Tricyclic antidepressants are useful for treating the emotional aspects of the disease and improving swallowing. Again, we recommend small initial doses and gradual increments. Physostigmine may improve visual attention and long-term memory, but a research protocol is needed to establish its efficacy. Idazoxan, a selective alpha$_2$ presynaptic inhibitor that increases noradrenergic transmission, also is being investigated.

Normal-Pressure Hydrocephalus

The characteristic triad of slowly progressive gait disorder, urinary incontinence, and dementia in association with evidence of hydrocephalus by brain imaging and normal intracranial pressure by cerebrospinal fluid examination is suggestive of the diagnosis of *normal-pressure hydrocephalus*. This rare form of dementia accounts for fewer than 5 percent of all cases, but it is potentially treatable. Antecedent factors associated with this disorder include subarachnoid hemorrhage, trauma, meningitis, invasive neurosurgery, and diencephalic or posterior fossa tumors, but a third of cases are idiopathic.

The clinical syndrome is characterized by a mild degree of intellectual decline, with disorientation, impaired abstraction, apathy with and without depressive features, and urinary incontinence. The gait disturbance has been described as "magnetic," with short, shuffling steps. Evidence of spasticity in the legs may be present. CT or MRI should indicate dilatation of the ventricular system and rounding of the frontal horns. Periventricular lucencies may be apparent with normal or obliterated cortical sulci. Lumbar puncture findings should be entirely normal, especially the opening pressure.

A number of diagnostic tests have been used to predict the best response to surgical intervention, but we have found that no one test is better than another. We recommend at least three separate lumbar punctures with removal of 30 to 50 ml of cerebrospinal fluid or continuous drainage by placement of a catheter into the lumbar subarachnoid space to observe clinical improvement. Videotaping of gait, neuropsychological assessment, and other objective bedside measures are useful for predicting surgical response. We also recommend having a colleague review the results of these brief assessments who does not know whether they were done before or after removal of spinal fluid. Should a clear beneficial response be noted, the probability of a good surgical outcome is increased.

Treatment

Ventriculoperitoneal shunt is the primary treatment, although the rate of recovery is highly variable (range 25 to 80 percent). We recommend careful consideration of the patient's response to the spinal fluid studies described above, because complications occur frequently. Shunt malfunction, subdural hematoma, seizures, and infection are the major problems.

Huntington's Disease

Huntington's disease is an autosomal-dominant disorder genetically linked to the short arm of chromosome 4. The disorder is rare, affecting about three to seven individuals per 100,000. Unlike PD, Huntington's disease begins during early middle age, the peak age at onset being between 35 and 50 years. The typical clinical features include various dyskinesias in addition to chorea, ocular motor dysfunction, and impaired performance of fine movements of the arms and legs. As incapacitating as these features may seem, cognitive impairment (characterized by memory loss and difficulty in performing complex or sequential mental activities) probably accounts for most of the early disability attributed to Huntington's disease. With disease progression, however, chorea, postural instability, and dementia all impair function significantly. A number of psychiatric problems occur with and without dementia. Apathy (with or without depression), irritability, and poor impulse control are among the most common emotional disorders. Psychosis with delusions and hallucination is rare.

The most striking pathologic change in Huntington's disease is atrophy or flattening of the caudate nucleus and putamen where it serves as the ventrolateral wall of the lateral ventricle. Cerebral white matter is decreased in volume, and there is extensive nerve cell loss and astrocytosis. Neurons containing GABA, enkephalin, substance P, and dynorphin are reduced in number, and brain concentrations of GABA and of glutamic acid decarboxylase are decreased.

Treatment

Symptomatic therapy for chorea and psychiatric disturbances is generally successful but its value is limited. Various dopamine antagonists, such as tetrabenazine, are effective in reducing chorea but eventually lead to rigidity or other features of parkinsonism. Antipsychotics such as haloperidol produce similar results. Depression responds to standard doses of tricyclic antidepressants, and monoamine oxidase inhibitors have also been shown to be useful. Propranolol can be used in moderate to high doses to reduce impulsive behavior. A test dose for safety, followed by gradual increments, produces the best results. No specific treatment for dementia or other cognitive loss has been found. Strong social support and avoidance of neuroleptics, when possible, limit the extent of disability from dementia.

OTHER DEMENTIAS

Acquired Immunodeficiency Syndrome Dementia Complex

Dementia associated with AIDS, or the AIDS dementia complex (ADC), is a syndrome of cognitive impairment, behavioral change, and motor dysfunction in patients with antibodies to human immunodeficiency virus type 1. The annual incidence of dementia among AIDS patients is estimated to be 14 percent.

Cognitive impairment begins in the early stages of infection and seems to parallel the systemic disease. Dementia usually occurs in the latest stages of AIDS, and on occasion is a presenting symptom. Forgetfulness, loss of concentration, confusion, and diminished verbal recall all are features of ADC. Apathy and social withdrawal are less constant features. Motor signs associated with dementia include gait and posture disturbance, diminished finger and hand movements, spasticity, and weakness. As the disease progresses, akinesis, mutism, incontinence, paraplegia, myoclonus, and seizures appear.

Diagnostic studies help to distinguish secondary infection and malignancy from primary dementia. CT, MRI, and functional brain imaging such as photon emission tomography are very useful and can reveal patterns related specifically to AIDS. Cerebrospinal fluid studies allow identification of dementia from infections such as cryptococcal meningitis.

The brain disease associated with ADC consists mostly of frontotemporal atrophy with pallor in the myelinated areas of the centrum semiovale. Multiple small nodules containing macrophages, lymphocytes, and microglia can be scattered throughout the brain and brain stem. Multinucleate giant cells are also present and their presence correlates with the severity of dementia during life.

Treatment

Zidovudine (AZT), 250 mg every 4 hours, was found to improve cognitive function more than placebo in demented patients with AIDS. Increased metabolic rates noted by functional brain imaging support the improvement seen with this drug. Zidovudine may also reduce the likelihood of developing dementia, but this needs to be substantiated. We recommend 500 to 600 mg for patients with dementia and AIDS; doses of 1000 to 1200 mg daily would be recommended for patients who show no improvement and can tolerate larger doses. Careful attention must be paid to identify toxic effects such as bone marrow suppression, headache, nausea, and myalgia. Patients with depression respond well to tricyclic antidepressants and psychostimulants such as methylphenidate in small doses. Dextroamphetamine may also be of use, but the side effects include arrhythmias, hypertension, and psychosis. Newer agents such as dideoxyinosine, peptide T, L-acetyl carnitine, naltrexone, and nimodipine are all under investigation.

Miscellaneous Causes

A number of other degenerative diseases are associated with dementia, but the treatment for dementias related to cerebellar atrophy and some biochemical disorders is very limited. Recognition is the first step in management.

Some partially or completely treatable disorders are important to recognize. Drug intoxication, particularly benzodiazepines or other tranquilizers, may induce in elderly patients a "chronic" confusional state that looks like degenerative dementia. Depression can also mimic dementia and can be reversed by treatment, but depression can also be an important antecedent feature of various degenerative dementias such as AD and PD. Neoplasms, subdural hematomas, and common metabolic disturbances such as congestive heart failure, renal or hepatic failure, hyper- or hypothyroidism, and calcium disorders can be identified easily by a series of routine laboratory studies used to evaluate dementia. Treatment usually, but not always, restores function.

SUGGESTED READING

Stroke

Chui HC, Victoroff JI, Margolin DT, et al. Criteria for the diagnosis of ischemic vascular dementia proposed by the State of California Alzheimer's Disease Diagnostic and Treatment Centers. Neurology 1992;42:473–480.

Roman CG, Tatemichi TK, Erkinjuntti, et al. Vascular dementia: Diagnostic criteria for research studies. Report of the NINDS-AIREN International Work Group. Neurology (in press).

Tatemichi TK. How acute brain failure becomes chronic. A view of the mechanisms of dementia related to stroke. Neurology 1990;40:1652–1659.

Parkinson's Disease

Gibb WRG. Dementia and Parkinson's disease. Br J Psychiatry 1989;154:596–614.

Mayeux R. The mental state in Parkinson's disease. In: Koller WA, ed. Handbook of Parkinson's Disease. 2nd ed. New York: Marcel Dekker, 1992:159.

Mayeux R, Denaro J, Hemenegildo N, et al. A population-based investigation of Parkinson's disease with and without dementia: Relationship to age and gender. Arch Neurol 1992;49:492–497.

Diffuse Lewy Body Disease

Hansen L, Salmon D, Galasko D, et al. The Lewy body variant of Alzheimer's disease. Neurology 1990;40:1–8.

Kosaka K, Tsuchiya K, Yoshimura M. Lewy body disease with and without dementia: A clinicopathological study of 35 cases. Clin Neuropathol 1988;7:299–305.

Progressive Supranuclear Palsy

Barr AN. Progressive supranuclear palsy. In: Vinken PJ, Bruyn GW, Klawans HL, eds. Handbook of clinical neurology. Extrapyramidal disorders. Amsterdam: Elsevier, 1986;49:239–254.

Ghika J, Tennis M, Hoffman E, et al. Idazoxan treatment in progressive supranuclear palsy. Neurology 1991;41:986–991.

Grafman J, Litvan I, Gomez C, et al. Frontal lobe function in progressive supranuclear palsy. Arch Neurol 1990;47:553–558.

Jankovic J, Friedman DI, Pirozzolo FJ, et al. Progressive supranuclear palsy: Motor, neurobehavioral, and neuro-ophthalmic findings. In: Streifler MB, Korczyn AD, Melamed E, et al, eds. Advances in neurology. Parkinson's disease: Anatomy, pathology, and therapy. New York: Raven, 1990;293.

Steele JC. Progressive supranuclear palsy. Brain 1972;95:693–704.

Normal-Pressure Hydrocephalus

Black PMcL, Ojemann RG. Hydrocephalus in adults. In: Youmans JR, ed. Neurosurgical Surgery. 3rd ed. Philadelphia: WB Saunders, 1990:1277.

Cummings J, Benson F. Hydrocephalic dementia. In: Cummings J, ed. Dementia: A clinical approach. 2nd ed. Boston: Butterworth-Heinemann, 1992:267.

Huntington's Disease

Burn A, Folstein S, Brandt J, Folstein M. Clinical assessment of irritability, aggression and apathy in Huntington's disease and Alzheimer's disease. J Nerv Mental Dis 1990; 178:20–26.

Shoulson I, Odoroff C, Oakes D, et al. A controlled trial of baclofen as protective therapy in early Huntington's disease. Ann Neurol 1989;31:293–298.

AIDS Dementia Complex

American Academy of Neurology AIDS Task Force. Nomenclature and research case definitions for neurologic manifestations of human immunodeficiency virus-type 1 (HIV-1) infection. Neurology 1991;41:778–785.

Fernandez F, Adams F, Levy JK, et al. Cognitive impairment due to AIDS-related complex and its response to psychostimulants. Psychosomatics 1988;29:38–46.

Navia BA, Jordan BD, Price RW. The AIDS dementia complex: 1. clinical features. Ann Neurol 1986;19:517–524.

Price RW, Sidtis JJ. The AIDS dementia complex. In: Wormser GP, ed. AIDS and other manifestations of HIV infection. New York: Raven, 1992:373.

Schmitt FA, Bigley JW, Mckinnis R, et al. Neuropsychological outcome of zidovudine (AZT) treatment of patients with AIDS and AIDS-related complex. N Engl J Med 1988;319:1573–1578.

TOXIC DISEASES

OPIATE OVERDOSE AND DEPENDENCE

GEORGE A. RICAURTE, M.D., Ph.D.
UNA D. McCANN, M.D.

Treatment of opiate abuse and dependence has been a persistent and challenging medical problem. Although accurate figures on the prevalence of opiate addiction are difficult to ascertain, it has been estimated that in the United States alone there are more than 500,000 opiate narcotic addicts. Of these, approximately 50,000 require emergency medical services each year, the vast majority for heroin overdose. Although many of these patients will be seen in emergency rooms, others may come to a physician's attention in a hospital ward, and still others may present for routine office visits. Thus physicians of all specialties need to be prepared to recognize and manage patients addicted to opiate narcotics. In this chapter we outline strategies for treating acute opiate intoxication and managing opiate dependence, but because optimal therapy requires a basic understanding of opiate pharmacology and toxicology, we begin with a discussion of these topics.

PHARMACOLOGY

The term *opiate* refers to morphine-like compounds that interact with opiate receptors in the peripheral and the central nervous systems (PNS and CNS). Originally, opiates were thought to be exclusively exogenous; however, with the discovery of enkephalins, endorphins, and dynorphins (endogenous peptides with morphine-like pharmacologic activity), this view has changed, and there is now evidence that morphine itself may occur naturally in the mammalian brain. Whether exogenous or endogenous, opiates exert their effects largely by interacting with tissue recognition sites (opiate receptors), of which there are several types. According to the nomenclature proposed by Martin and colleagues, mu (morphine) and kappa (ketocyclazocine) receptors are probably involved in opioid-induced supraspinal anal-

gesia, respiratory depression, and pupillary constriction, whereas delta (enkephalin) receptors play a role in spinal analgesia. Sigma (norallylnormetazocine or SKF 10,047) receptors, though originally thought to belong to the opiate receptor class, are now regarded as probable phencyclidine (PCP) recognition sites. The widespread distribution of opiate receptors in the nervous system is in keeping with their multitudinous pharmacologic effects, which, in addition to analgesia, miosis, and respiratory depression, include hypothermia, bradycardia, sedation, suppression of the cough reflex, and gastrointestinal paresis. For the first-time user, the psychoactive effects of opiates are often unpleasant and accompanied by nausea and vomiting; however, in accustomed users, these untoward effects become less prominent, and a tranquil sense of well-being (euphoria) predominates. It is this aspect of the opiate experience that no doubt accounts for the abuse liability of opiates, though the threat of withdrawal (see below) also plays a role.

The range of pharmacologic effects described above is thought to result from the interaction of opiate *agonists* with opiate receptors. Interestingly, when narcotic *antagonists* interact with opiate receptors, the effects are few, at least in persons who are not physically dependent on opiates. In an opiate addict, however, narcotic antagonists can precipitate an acute withdrawal syndrome. In its mild form, opiate withdrawal resembles a "flulike" illness, whose prominent signs and symptoms are rhinorrhea, lacrimation, gooseflesh, and diffuse myalgias and arthralgias. In its severe form, opiate withdrawal is characterized by tremulousness, tachycardia, mydriasis, vomiting, diarrhea, extreme anxiety, and sometimes myoclonic jerks and convulsions. The effects of opiates depend not only on the state of the person but on the particular narcotic drug in question: its potency, duration of action, onset of action, and its ratio of agonist-antagonist activity.

In addition to direct actions at opiate receptors, opiate drugs exert a number of pharmacologic effects by interacting with nonopioid neurotransmitter systems in the CNS and the PNS. These include the cholinergic, dopaminergic, serotonergic, and histaminergic systems. Although the contribution of these other transmitter systems to the pharmacologic actions of opiates is variable and incompletely defined, cholinergic systems appear to be involved in the gastrointestinal, cardiovascular, and respiratory depressant effects of opiates; dopamine systems appear to play a role in the reinforcing actions of opiates; serotonin systems appear modulate, and in some instances may mediate, analgesic effects of opiates; and histaminergic systems have been implicated in the hypotensive effects of opiates.

TOXICOLOGY

To a large extent, the toxic effects of opiates represent an exaggeration of their pharmacologic effects. As such, opiate overdose generally results in slow, shallow respirations, coma, and miotic pupils. Other common effects of opiate overdose include hypothermia, bradycardia, muscular flaccidity, hyporeflexia, and, with certain opiates such as meperidine and propoxyphene, myoclonic jerks and seizures. Of these toxic effects, respiratory depression is by far the most serious, as it can be life threatening. Although miosis is a helpful clue to opiate intoxication, its absence should not exclude the diagnosis, because extreme hypoxia secondary to respiratory depression can induce dilatation of the pupil, as can some of the opiate drugs themselves (e.g., meperidine [Demerol]).

CLINICAL MANAGEMENT

Acute Opiate Overdose

As mentioned above, acute opioid overdose is a medical emergency. Generally, the most pressing concern is severe respiratory depression. If the patient is apneic, an airway should be established immediately and manual or mechanical ventilation should be supplied. In addition, reversal of the respiratory depression should be attempted with the pure narcotic antagonist naloxone (Narcan). Naloxone should be given intravenously (IV) at an initial dose of 0.4 mg. When IV access is a problem (not uncommon in drug addicts), naloxone can be given intramuscularly (IM) using the same dose, recognizing that naloxone given IM will take longer to act and act longer than naloxone given IV. The effects of IV naloxone are generally evident within 2 to 3 minutes, and they include deeper, more rapid respirations, increased pupil size, and any sign of arousal. When the effects of naloxone are negligible or in doubt, another 0.4 mg dose should be given. (Recall that addicts may require larger naloxone doses, particularly if they have recently ingested an unusually large dose of an opiate agonist or if they have taken an opiate of inordinate potency [such as 3-methylfentanyl]). In sufficient doses, naloxone reverses the respiratory depressant effects of virtually all opiates, including heroin, morphine, fentanyl, propoxyphene, codeine, meperidine, and methadone. As much as 10 to 20 mg of naloxone can be given without causing significant side effects. It is critical to bear in mind, however, that naloxone is relatively short acting (in normal adults, its plasma half-life is approximately 1 hour after IV administration) and that repeated dosing is necessary within 45 to 70 minutes of the initial dose. Depending on the opiate involved in the overdose, repeated naloxone administration may be needed for longer than 24 hours. For example, in the case of overdose with methadone, continued use of naloxone for 48 to 72 hours is needed while the patient is closely monitored for signs of respiratory insufficiency. When prolonged opiate antagonism is needed, continuous IV infusion of naloxone should be considered, at a recommended starting infusion rate of 0.2 to 0.4 mg per hour. The dose can be increased as needed, as side effects of naloxone are rare. The only significant complication of naloxone therapy is precipitation of acute withdrawal, but this occurs only in opiate-dependent persons and generally subsides within 1 to 2 hours of naloxone administration. Given the apparent involvement of cholinergic systems in the respiratory depressant effects of opiates, the use of physostigmine in the treatment of heroin overdose has also been proposed.

A second, less common, complication of acute opiate overdose is pulmonary edema. Because opiate-induced pulmonary edema is generally not of cardiac origin, it has been designated noncardiogenic pulmonary edema (NCPE). NCPE should be suspected when there is a picture of respiratory insufficiency and evidence of interstitial edema without cardiomegaly on the chest radiograph. Although the underlying pathophysiology of NCPE is unclear, it carries a significant mortality rate and should be treated aggressively while central venous and left ventricular end-diastolic pressures are monitored. Fluid restriction, along with ventilatory support using positive end-expiratory pressure and oxygen, should also be implemented. Notably, NCPE does not respond to diuretics and is not reversed by naloxone. Most often, NCPE is a complication of heroin or codeine overdose. Thus, a urine or blood drug screen may be helpful.

The third serious complication of acute opiate overdose is profound *hypotension.* It is thought to result from release of histamine in the periphery, as well as from a centrally mediated cardiodepressant effect. Opiate-induced vascular collapse is best treated with pressor agents, IV fluids, and plasma expanders while central venous pressure is monitored. Again, naloxone is of little proven benefit.

In addition to immediate life-threatening complications of opiate overdose, several other complications may require medical attention. Convulsions may occur as the result of extreme hypoxia or may be drug-induced (propoxyphene [Darvon] is a common offender). Other complications of acute opiate overdose include hypothermia (due mainly to vasodilatation with consequent heat loss), rhabdomyolysis (usually due to pressure necrosis), and infection (often secondary to phlebitis or unsterile drug solutions). Two infectious complications of intravenous opiate narcotic abuse that merit special attention are hepatitis and human immunodeficiency virus (HIV) infection. Detection and management of these infections are of utmost importance. In general, treatment of the foregoing complications should first be directed at the primary cause (e.g., in the case of convulsions the hypoxia should be corrected) and then at the complication itself (e.g., hydration to prevent myoglobinuric renal failure in the setting of rhabdomyolysis).

Dependence

As noted by Ling and Wesson, the diagnosis of opioid dependence calls for the presence of a combination of cognitive, behavioral, and physiologic symptoms reflecting impaired control over drug use and continued use despite adverse consequences. Neither the presence of tolerance (reduced sensitivity to a given dose of drug) nor a withdrawal syndrome suffices. Currently, there are three approaches to dealing with opiate addiction: (1) agonist maintenance, (2) maintenance with antagonist drugs, and (3) detoxification. The principal form of agonist therapy used today is methadone maintenance. Agonist therapy with methadone can be regarded as a form of substitution therapy, as the pharmacologic effects of methadone are qualitatively similar to those of heroin or morphine. However, methadone has the advantages of longer action and medical sanction. As such, methadone maintenance offers the addict the opportunity to alter his or her lifestyle, particularly when methadone is dispensed in the context of a therapeutic support group under medical supervision. To ensure adequate dosing, methadone should be given at a dose of 50 to 100 mg per day; doses smaller than 40 mg per day are insufficient for most addicts. The major goal of agonist therapy is to eliminate IV narcotic abuse and drug-seeking behavior. When successful, methadone maintenance programs reduce needle sharing among opiate addicts and decrease the risk of HIV infection and hepatitis. Ideally, methadone maintenance leads subsequently to detoxification, though persons who are dependent on methadone are not incapable of leading productive lives.

Two other agents that have been tried in agonist therapy are levo-alpha-acetyl-methadol (LAAM) and buprenorphine hydrochloride. Though both agents have shown promise, neither has come into wide use. LAAM offers the advantages of slower onset of action and longer action than methadone. Buprenorphine is attractive from the standpoint that, in addition to its agonist effects, it has antagonist properties, which become more prominent as the dose of buprenorphine is increased. This makes abuse of buprenorphine less likely. Symptoms of withdrawal from buprenorphine are also said to be less severe, leading some to suggest that buprenorphine may be useful for facilitating opiate detoxification.

In addition to agonist drugs, opiate antagonists have been tried for treatment of opiate dependence. Because in opiate-dependent persons opiate antagonists can precipitate acute withdrawal (and possibly induce craving), use of narcotic antagonists should be limited to opiate-free subjects who seek to prevent relapse. The principal agent tested for this purpose has been naltrexone (Trexan), another pure narcotic antagonist chemically related to naloxone but much longer acting. A single 150 mg dose of naltrexone can block the euphorigenic effects of a 25 mg dose of heroin as long as 3 days. Naltrexone is well-absorbed after oral administration, is not addictive, and is extremely effective in blocking the reinforcing effects of a wide range of opiate agonists. Its long duration of action obviates frequent clinic visits. Not surprisingly, naltrexone has been most effective for highly motivated persons. When compliance is a problem, naltrexone is unlikely to be of benefit.

Detoxification calls for gradual reduction of opiate dose, with the ultimate goal of complete abstinence. Various strategies have been employed to facilitate complete cessation of opiate use. One has employed gradually decreasing doses of agonist drugs such as methadone and LAAM, whose advantages over heroin and morphine already have been mentioned. Another has involved the use of clonidine (Catapres), an alpha$_2$-agonist that suppresses many of the symptoms of opiate withdrawal and makes abstinence more tolerable. The usual starting dose of clonidine is 0.2 mg given every 4 to 6 hours while monitoring for signs of postural hypotension. For treatment of opiate withdrawal, the dose of clonidine can be increased to 1.2 mg per day in divided doses. Yet another approach has called for the use of an antagonist drug such as naltrexone (an orally active opioid antagonist that has greater affinity for opioid receptors than heroin or morphine), alone or in combination with clonidine. It is fair to say that all these approaches remain experimental and that each should be undertaken under close medical supervision in a structured therapeutic environment.

The search for an opiate analgesic that is devoid of abuse liability should (and no doubt will) continue; however, even when available, it is unlikely that such a nonaddicting opiate will eradicate nonmedical use of opiates. Accordingly, successful medical management of opiate intoxication and dependence will continue to challenge the clinical skills of specialists and generalists alike.

SUGGESTED READING

Annual emergency room data, 1990 data from the Drug Abuse Warning Network. National Institute on Drug Abuse Statistical Series. Rockville, MD: U.S. Department of Health and Human Services, Public Health Service, Alcohol, Drug Abuse and Mental Health Administration, 1990.

Bradberry JC, Raebel MA. Continuous infusion of naloxone in the treatment of narcotic overdose. Drug Intell Clin Pharmacy 1981; 15:945–950.

Handal KA, Schauben JL, Salamone FR. Naloxone. Ann Emerg Med 1983; 12:438–445.

Heel RC, Brogden RN, Speight TM, Avery GS. Buprenorphine: A review of its pharmacological properties and therapeutic efficacy. Drugs 1992; 17:81–110.

Henry J, Volans G. Analgesics: Opioids. Br Med J 1984; 289:990–993.

Jaffe JH, Martin WR. Opioid analgesics and antagonists. In: The Pharmacological Basis of Therapeutics. New York: Macmillan, 1991:485.

Kulberg A. Substance abuse: Clinical identification and management. Pediatr Toxicol 1986; 33:325–361.

Ling W, Wesson DR. Drugs of abuse—opiates. West J Med 1990; 152:565–572.

Martin WR, Eades CG, Thompson JA, et al. The effects of morphine- and nalorphine-like drugs in the nondependent and morphine-dependent chronic spinal dog. J Pharmacol Exp Ther 1976; 197:517–532.

Pasternak GW. Opioid receptors. In: Melzer HY, ed. Psychopharmacology: The third generation of progress. New York: Raven, 1987.

Person PH Jr, Retka RL, Woodward JA. Technical paper: A method for estimating heroin use prevalence. Rockville, MD: U.S. Dept. of Health, Education, and Welfare, Public Health Service, Alcohol, Drug Abuse, and Mental Health Administration. (ADM) 77–439.

Ruprecht J, Dworacek B, Oosthoek H, et al. Physostigmine versus naloxone in heroin overdose. Clin Toxicol 1983; 21:387–397.

Weddington WW. Use of pharmacologic agents in the treatment of addiction. Psychiatr Ann 1992; 22:425–429.

Weitz CJ, Lowney LI, Faull KF, Goldstein A. Morphine and codeine from mammalian brain. Proc Natl Acad Sci USA 1986; 83:9784–9788.

Yaksh TL, Wilson PR. Spinal serotonin terminal system mediates antinociception. J Pharmacol Exp Ther 1979; 208:446–453.

BIOLOGIC TOXINS

EDWIN B. GEORGE, M.D., Ph.D.

Biologic toxins produce a wide spectrum of neurologic syndromes, and intoxication may occur via a number of routes. Although many of these intoxications are rare, early diagnosis is the key to effective management, and often the neurologist is the first physician to suspect the diagnosis. A brief review of the pharmacology of each toxin is provided, and the symptoms, diagnostic considerations, and currently available therapy are described.

BACTERIAL TOXINS

Botulism

Botulinum toxin is a potent protein neurotoxin produced by *Clostridium botulinum* bacteria. There are eight antigenically distinct types that differ in potency. Types A, B, and E are most frequently implicated in human intoxication. Spores of types A and B are found in soils throughout the world, whereas spores of types E and F are found in fresh water and marine sediments, respectively. Types E and F are usually associated with contaminated fish products, though the latter is a rare cause of human intoxication. Types C and D are almost exclusively associated with animal intoxications. Although the toxin types differ in size and peptide sequence, all inhibit presynaptic release of acetylcholine.

Botulinum toxin usually enters the body through the gastrointestinal tract after consumption of contaminated food, although *C. botulinum* may proliferate and produce toxin in wounds or in the gastrointestinal tract of infants. *C. botulinum* is a strict anaerobe, and spores can survive temperatures of 100°C for several hours, resulting in a substantial risk of toxin contamination in improperly canned food. Spores are destroyed by exposure to temperatures of 120°C for 30 minutes, and the toxin is more heat labile. Wound botulism usually results from a penetrating injury, and the wound may appear unimpressive. Wound botulism has occurred in parenteral drug abusers in association with abscess formation at injection sites. Soft-tissue radiographs occasionally reveal evidence of gas production in the wound. Colonization of the intestine with *C. botulinum* occurs in infants who ingest spores. The peak incidence is at 2 to 7 months of age, and infant botulism is one cause of sudden infant death syndrome.

After ingestion of botulinum toxin, there is an asymptomatic interval of 8 to 36 hours, which may be followed by gastrointestinal symptoms such as nausea and diarrhea. Subsequently, the characteristic neurologic progression is external ophthalmoparesis followed by loss of pupillary reactions, bulbar involvement with dysphagia, and then generalized weakness, often in a descending pattern, leading to respiratory insufficiency. Paralytic ileus frequently occurs. Tendon reflexes are lost only as the weakness becomes profound, and sensation remains unaffected. In infants the disease presents as a previously well baby who develops ophthalmoparesis and bulbar weakness with generalized hypotonia, usually preceded by 24 to 48 hours' constipation.

The differential diagnosis in adults includes the Miller-Fisher variant of Guillain-Barré syndrome or another form of cranial polyneuritis, diphtheria in unimmunized persons, and tick paralysis; in infants sepsis and poliomyelitis must also be considered. The initial phase of brain stem cerebrovascular events may also mimic the syndrome. The pupillary involvement and loss of reflexes serve to differentiate botulism from myasthenia gravis and Lambert-Eaton syndrome. Identification of an outbreak from a common food source helps suggest the diagnosis. Laboratory studies include testing of blood and stool for toxin, stool culture for *C. botulinum*, and nerve conduction studies. Botulism results in normal conductions with reduced-amplitude evoked muscle potentials and an incremental response to repetitive stimulation. Diagnosis of food-borne botulism mandates prompt notification of public health authorities and a search for both the source and other potential victims.

Critical aspects of treatment are early diagnosis and ventilatory monitoring and support, as death is due to respiratory failure. Frequent monitoring of vital capacity in an intensive care setting is imperative, and the decision to intubate should be based on decline in vital capacity. Respiratory failure may be precipitous, and the arterial blood gas values are abnormal only after hypoventilation begins. Infants cannot be effectively monitored for impending respiratory failure. They require early intubation and prolonged respiratory support, with continued observation in an intensive care setting after extubation. In adults, nasogastric suction and enemas may help to remove unabsorbed toxin from the gastrointestinal tract after paralytic ileus occurs. Penicillin therapy is indicated to eradicate the organism in cases of infant botulism and wound botulism, but it is of doubtful value for adults with food-borne botulism. Surgical debridement is essential for wound botulism. Trivalent (ABE) equine* antitoxin can be obtained at any hour from the Centers for Disease Control (see Resources at the end of this chapter). The recommended dosage for adults is one vial intravenously and one vial intramuscularly every 2 to 4 hours. The antitoxin is not recommended for treatment of infant botulism.

Tetanus

Tetanus toxin is a protein neurotoxin produced by another ubiquitous species of *Clostridium, Clostridium tetani*. Tetanus and botulinum toxins are similar in molecular weight and have about 33 percent sequence homology. Tetanus toxin cannot be absorbed through the gastrointestinal tract, and intoxication occurs only by toxin production at an infected site. Tetanus toxin is capable of preventing presynaptic release of acetylcholine at the neuromuscular junction, but the clinical manifestations of infection arise from retrograde transport of the toxin in motor axons to the spinal cord and brain stem, where it blocks presynaptic release of inhibitory neurotransmitters, including gamma-aminobutyric acid and glycine. This disinhibition results in repetitive sustained muscle contractions, which may be triggered by reflexes and a variety of other stimuli. The spasms may begin locally in the wound-bearing limb, but only 1 percent of cases remain localized. Generalized

tetanus typically begins with bulbar muscles, including masseter spasm (trismus) and facial spasms (risus sardonicus), and spreads to paraspinous and axial muscles, causing opisthotonos and apnea. Cognitive and sensory function are spared.

Susceptible persons include neonates of unvaccinated mothers (particularly those born in potentially contaminated environments) and unvaccinated adults. A primary series of three tetanus toxoid doses, followed every 10 years by booster doses, is recommended for previously unvaccinated adults. In the United States, more than half the cases of tetanus occur in persons aged 50 years or older whose immunization is not current. Intravenous drug abusers are also at risk because they suffer recurrent skin infections and frequently lack adequate immunizations.

For clean minor wounds tetanus prophylaxis consists of a tetanus-diphtheria booster for persons whose immunization status is unknown or not current. All other wounds should be cleaned and debrided, and a tetanus-diphtheria booster should be administered unless the patient's immunization is current and the most recent booster was given in the last 5 years. If the patient is not known previously to have had at least three doses of tetanus toxoid, passive immunization with at least 250 units of human tetanus immune globulin by intramuscular injection is also recommended. Antibiotic therapy should be based on the condition of the wound, and is of secondary importance in tetanus prophylaxis.

Treatment of clinical tetanus requires surgical debridement of the wound and supportive care in a critical care setting. Penicillin is part of general wound care. Antitoxin is recommended, but it serves only to clear circulating toxin. Once the toxin is taken up by peripheral nerves for retrograde transport to the central nervous system, it is inaccessible to antibodies. The recommended dose is 3,000 to 6,000 units of human tetanus immune globulin given by intramuscular injection.

Prevention of severe recurrent spasms is important to avoid fractures, renal failure consequent to myoglobinuria, and apnea. A quiet, dark environment helps to minimize the stimulus-sensitive spasms. This can be achieved even in a modern intensive care setting, but should not prevent appropriate monitoring. In more severe cases, benzodiazepines (diazepam) can be used prophylactically on a regular basis with additional doses to treat spasms. The total daily dose may exceed 5 mg per kilogram, and ventilatory support must be available. Intubation or tracheostomy followed by curarization should be instituted promptly if the spasms cannot be controlled with diazepam without causing respiratory depression.

Severe generalized tetanus is a prolonged illness with a mortality rate of 42 percent among patients over 50 years of age. Patients often develop ileus, requiring nasogastric suction and parenteral nutrition. Severe constipation should be prevented, and enemas should be avoided when possible because of their potential to induce spasms. Careful attention must be paid to fluid

---

*Many of the antisera mentioned in this chapter are currently available only as equine preparations. Patients should be tested for sensitivity to horse serum before they receive these antisera. Horse serum or antivenin should be diluted 1:10 in normal saline and no more than 0.02 ml injected intradermally. If there is a history of reaction to horse serum, an initial test using a 1:100 dilution should be performed. A wheal and flare reaction after 10 minutes indicates a positive reaction, and a decision to proceed with desensitization must be based on the clinical status of the patient. A negative test result does not preclude horse serum allergy, and patients must be watched for signs of serum sickness for 8 to 10 days after receiving the equine antiserum. Pretreatment with intravenous antihistamine may be useful, and intravenous corticosteroids are recommended for children or for adults who require large doses of antisera.

and electrolyte balance, and subcutaneous minidose heparin is recommended as prophylaxis against pulmonary emboli.

All patients who recover from tetanus must receive active immunization with three consecutive doses of tetanus toxoid. The amount of neurotoxin released into the circulation during clinical tetanus is insufficient to produce immunization, and recurrent cases of tetanus are well-documented in patients who did not receive active immunization.

Diphtheria

Diphtheria toxin is a protein neurotoxin elaborated by *Corynebacterium diphtheriae*. Most often, clinical infection occurs in the oropharynx or nasopharynx, but cutaneous infections also occur. The toxin spreads to areas of the peripheral nervous system with greater permeability of the blood-nerve barrier and causes demyelination by inhibiting protein synthesis in Schwann cells. The toxin is also myotoxic, and the myocardium is particularly susceptible.

Palatal paralysis, often unilateral, is usually the first neurologic manifestation, and it occurs during the first 2 weeks of disease. Subsequently, paralysis of accommodation develops, followed by generalized polyneuropathy, which peaks in the sixth or seventh week. At this stage, electrocardiographic changes reflecting early myocarditis appear. Examination of the cerebrospinal fluid shows elevated protein without pleocytosis. The manifestations may closely resemble those of Guillain-Barré syndrome, with cranial and somatic nerve palsies. The diagnosis is made by finding the site of infection. The bacterium can be demonstrated on methylene blue–stained smears or by culture.

The neurologic manifestations of diphtheria are late sequelae that can be prevented by early therapy with antibiotics (erythromycin or penicillin) and antitoxin. Ideally, equine antitoxin should be given within 48 hours of the earliest signs of infection. A single dose of 20,000 to 120,000 units, depending on the location and severity of the infection, is recommended. It is useful to obtain blood for culture and immune titer before giving the antitoxin. Respiratory compromise is unusual, but the pharyngitis and palatal weakness may prevent normal feeding, and intubation may be required to protect the airway.

Diphtheria is a preventable disease, and immunization at 2, 4, and 6 months of age with boosters at 18 months, 4 to 6 years, and every 10 years thereafter is recommended.

ENVENOMATION

Black Widow Spider Bite and Other Arachnidisms

Spiders of the genus *Latrodectus* are found in many parts of the world. *Latrodectus mactans* is the true black widow, though other *Latrodectus* species are also called black widows. The female spiders produce alpha-latrotoxin, a protein that causes presynaptic release and depletion of cholinergic vesicles at the neuromuscular junction. Often, the victim does not notice the bite, but within a half hour severe local pain develops and generalized symptoms of diaphoresis, salivation, sinus arrhythmias, muscle rigidity, and fasciculations. The symptoms peak 1 to 6 hours after onset and usually resolve after 24 to 48 hours. The differential diagnosis includes other forms of cholinergic toxicity. Identification of the spider or its remains is useful.

Atropine relieves the autonomic manifestations, and muscle spasm may be treated with diazepam (or curarization in severe cases) as described for tetanus. Calcium gluconate relieves many of the symptoms via an unknown mechanism. The usual dose is 10 ml of 10 percent calcium gluconate given intravenously over 10 to 20 minutes with cardiac monitoring, and it may be repeated as necessary. An equine antivenin is available but should be reserved for high-risk cases. Death from latrodectism occurs in fewer than 5 percent of cases, usually from respiratory distress or cardiac failure. One vial of equine antivenin is mixed in 50 ml of saline and given intravenously over 15 minutes.

Other arachnids that produce neurotoxins include ticks (discussed in the following section), funnel-web spiders, tarantulas, and scorpions. Funnel-web spider toxin contains calcium channel inhibitors, which can produce neuromuscular blockade. Treatment is primarily supportive, and an antitoxin is available. The neurotoxin produced by tarantulas is thought to be similar to that of *Latrodectus* species. Scorpion stings may contain a variety of neurotoxic peptides as well as a coagulant. The most pronounced neurotoxic effect of scorpion venoms is presynaptic depolarization leading to neurotransmitter release. The treatment outlined above is useful for both tarantula bites and scorpion stings. An antivenin is available for scorpion stings. Patients may also require treatment with anticonvulsants.

Tick Paralysis

Tick paralysis is caused only by the bite of a pregnant female tick. Several species of tick can produce the toxin: *Ixodes holocyclus* and *Ixodes cornatus* in Australia, where human cases are most frequent; *Rhipicephalus evertsi evertsi* in South Africa, and *Dermacentor andersoni* in North America. *D. andersoni* is found mostly in the western and southeastern United States and in British Columbia in Canada. The toxin is found in the salivary glands of the pregnant tick and most likely is not a protein, as toxin isolated from *I. holocyclus* is resistant to several proteases. Studies in animals suggest the toxin interferes with presynaptic acetylcholine release at the neuromuscular junction but also can affect conduction in small-diameter motor and sensory axons.

Weakness begins several days after the tick attaches, often spreading in an ascending pattern, although proximal or focal weakness may occur. Children are most frequently affected. The weakness progresses over days, leading to diffuse areflexia and dysphagia. The pupils, cognition, and sensation are spared, although some patients report paresthesias. Apparent ataxia is usually due to weakness. Blood and cerebrospinal fluid examinations remain normal, while electrophysiologic studies usually show normal sensory and motor conduction with reduced evoked muscle action potentials.

Tick paralysis is rare even in areas where the offending ticks are found. Differential diagnosis includes the Guillain-Barré syndrome and botulism. The former is distinguished by examination of the electrophysiologic findings and cerebrospinal fluid and the latter by the pupillary involvement. The diagnosis is made by finding one or more ticks. The treatment is to remove the tick by grasping the sides of the mouth parts with forceps and lifting it with a levering motion. The patient generally begins to improve by 24 hours, and full recovery usually takes a few days to 2 weeks.

Snakebite

Accurate statistics on the incidence of snake bite are scarce, but it is estimated that each year in the United States, approximately 8,000 people are bitten by venomous snakes and that in Australia, where venomous snakes are more common, there are 2 to 3½ pediatric cases of venomous snake bite per 100,000 children annually. Venomous snakes are found in three families of Serpentes: Viperidae, Elapidae, and Colubridae. The Viperidae group encompasses both the true vipers and the pit vipers (Crotalidae). The Crotalidae include rattlesnakes, copperheads, cottonmouths, and massaugas, which comprise the bulk of the venomous species in North America. The Elapidae are absent from Europe but constitute the majority of species in Australia and include the coral snake in the United States, the *Bungarus* species of Asia, and many of the clinically significant species found throughout the world, notably cobras, mambas, and kraits. Sea snakes (Hydrophiinae) are relegated by modern taxonomy to a subfamily of Elapidae. The Colubridae include approximately 60 percent of snake species, but only about 30 percent of colubrids are technically venomous, and only a few species are considered dangerous to humans.

Snake venoms are composed of enzymatic components and low–molecular weight peptides. In general, neurotoxicity is a major component of elapid bites and plays a minor role in viper envenomation, which produces primarily coagulopathy and (cardio)myotoxicity. Neurologic symptoms in the latter case are often secondary to compartment syndromes or diffuse intravascular coagulation and should be managed accordingly. Most elapid venoms contain a combination of pre- and postsynaptic toxins. Both notexin, a peptide of 119 amino acids, and taipoxin, a sialoglycoprotein, cause presynaptic inhibition of acetylcholine release as well as myotoxicity, whereas a variety of toxins, including the well-known alpha-bungarotoxin, block nicotinic acetylcholine receptors at the neuromuscular junction.

First aid for all snakebites consists of a thick gauze pad placed directly over the bite and held firmly in place by a wide circumferential bandage, which should be tight enough to occlude lymphatic, but not arterial, circulation. The bite wound should be held at or below the level of the heart. This technique has proved effective in Australia. Tourniquets applied in the field often do more harm than good, and the controversial incision and drainage procedure should be performed only in a clinical setting and within the first 10 minutes after a bite, which is rarely practical. If possible, the snake should be killed and brought in for identification, with the caveat that assistance with first aid and a good description of the snake are much more useful than a second victim. Freshly killed snakes must be handled with care, as the reflexes which produce striking and envenomation, may remain active for a half hour or so.

In contrast to viper bites, elapid bites often do not cause localized pain. Neurologic symptoms usually begin within 1 hour but may be delayed up to 8 hours; these consist of extremity paralysis, trismus, ptosis, and external ophthalmoplegia followed by bulbar paralysis and respiratory embarrassment. Coagulopathy and myoglobinuria often accompany the neurologic manifestations. The treatment is the appropriate equine antivenin and supportive therapy. In Australia, the Commonwealth Serum Laboratories in Melbourne produces a venom detection kit that may help to identify the involved snake, as well as a variety of antivenins. In the United States, the Arizona Poison Information Center maintains an index of antiserum availability (see Resources at the end of this chapter).

Marine Envenomations

Venomous marine vertebrates include stingrays and some sharks, catfish, weeverfish, scorpionfish including the stonefish, and sea snakes. Sea snake envenomation and treatment is described above. Stingray venom contains a protein toxin as well as serotonin, phosphodiesterase, and 5′-nucleotidase. Stonefish venom contains a high–molecular weight protein that has direct toxic action on muscle.

Neurologic manifestations of catfish envenomation consist of muscle spasms and fasciculations. Stingray envenomation also produces muscle spasms and fasciculations, as well as central nervous system effects such as headache, vertigo, and seizures. Weeverfish and scorpionfish venoms are reported to cause headache, delirium, and seizures.

Treatment begins with immersion of the wound in hot water (40.5°C) for 30 to 90 minutes or until pain subsides (the toxins are heat labile). The wound should be irrigated with normal saline, explored, and débrided. Intravenous calcium gluconate, as for black widow spider bite, may be helpful for weeverfish sting, and an equine antivenin is available for stonefish sting. Other treatment is supportive. If the wound becomes infected, the laboratory must be informed that a marine-acquired organism may be present, as special culture media are required.

Marine invertebrates with neurotoxic venoms include the Portuguese man-of-war *(Physalia physalis)*, box jellyfish *(Chironex fleckeri)*, the Australian spotted or blue-ringed octopus *(Hapalochlena lunulata* and *H. maculosa)*, and cone shells. There are more than 400 species in the genus *Conus,* most of which are venomous, and at least 18 species have been implicated in human envenomations. *P. physalis* is found in tropical and semitropical areas of the Atlantic and Pacific oceans, and the venom is poorly characterized. Neurologic manifestations are headache, delirium, vertigo, ataxia, paralysis, and obtundation. *C. fleckeri* is found in the Indo-Pacific oceans, and the toxin produces muscle spasm followed by muscular and respiratory paralysis and hypotension. Stings from either should be washed with 5 percent acetic acid to detoxify the clinging nematocysts. Exposure to fresh water prior to detoxification stimulates toxin release. The patient and physician should be aware that acetic acid does not relieve the pain from toxin that has already been discharged. An ovine antivenin is used to treat *C. fleckeri* stings (risks are similar to those from equine antivenins), and other therapy is supportive.

Hapalochlena and cone shells are found in Indo-Pacific waters. The octopus venom, maculotoxin, acts as a sodium channel antagonist in peripheral nerve. Conotoxins include several proteins that act as sodium and calcium channel antagonists. Both venoms produce neuromuscular blockade similar to curarization as well as sensory disturbances. Soaking with hot water may help inactivate conotoxins. Pressure immobilization therapy, as for snakebite, is recommended first aid for both. No antivenin is available, and treatment consists of ventilatory support. The effects of maculotoxin usually last 4 to 10 hours. Disseminated intravascular coagulation is a rare sequela of cone shell envenomation.

INGESTIONS

Marine Toxins

Marine toxins that may be ingested include ciguatera toxin (ciguatoxin), brevetoxins, saxitoxin, tetrodotoxin, and domoic acid. All can be produced by marine micro-organisms, although puffer fish appear to synthesize their own tetrodotoxin. Blooms of these micro-organisms are publicized by public health authorities and should alert physicians to the possibility of seafood intoxications.

Ciguatera toxin is produced by the dinoflagellate *Gambierdiscus toxicus,* which attaches to microalgae along coral reefs. The toxin is concentrated as it passes up the food chain to a variety of reef-dwelling fishes that may be consumed by humans. Ciguatera toxin is a lipid-soluble polyether with a molecular weight of 1,112 that opens voltage-gated sodium channels. Symptoms may appear immediately after consumption but typically are delayed 2 to 12 hours. Severe gastrointestinal distress with vomiting and diarrhea are followed by paresthesias

and altered temperature sensation, paresis, and myalgias. Severe cases may proceed to coma and cardiac conduction abnormalities, but fatalities are rare. The symptoms resolve over several weeks. Intravenous 20 percent mannitol, 500 mg per hour to a dose of 1 g per kilogram, produced rapid improvement by an unknown mechanism in a small series of patients.

Brevetoxins are produced by another dinoflagellate, *Ptychodiscus brevis* (formerly classified as *Gymnodinium breve)*, found off the southeast coast of the United States and in the Gulf of Mexico. The toxins are lipid soluble polycyclic methylated polyether compounds with a "ladder" structure that bind to sodium channels at the same site as ciguatoxin. There is some evidence that at least one of the brevitoxins may affect potassium and calcium channels as well. Ingestion produces paresthesias, gastrointestinal distress, and ataxia. An antiserum has been investigated in laboratory animals, but is not currently available for clinical use.

Saxitoxin is produced by the dinoflagellate *Gonyaulax catenella* and by some bacteria. It is concentrated in plankton-eating shellfish, which may in turn be consumed by humans. Saxitoxin is a tetrahydropurine base with a molecular weight of 299 that blocks sodium channels. It produces prompt oral and distal numbness, followed by paralysis that progresses over 2 to 24 hours. Treatment is as for tetrodotoxin, described below.

Tetrodotoxin is concentrated in the ovaries of puffer fish species, genus *Tetraodontidae,* also known as blowfish or globefish. The toxin has been detected in other fish species, as well as in California newts, octopuses, frogs, and marine bacteria. It has been suggested that puffer fish acquire the toxin through the food chain, but there is also evidence that toxic puffer fish may synthesize and excrete the toxin. Puffer fish dishes, known in Japan as *fugu,* are considered a delicacy, partly because of the tingling oral sensation they produce. Fugu is prepared by specially trained chefs who select fish on the basis of species, season, and sex to minimize the toxin content, and carefully remove organs in which the toxin is concentrated. Puffer fish may occasionally be consumed inadvertently.

Tetrodotoxin is a heterocyclic guanidine, aminoperhydroquanizoline, and has a molecular weight of 319. It is not inactivated by cooking or freezing. It inhibits sodium channels and binds to the same site as saxitoxin. Eating fish that contain an excessive amount of residual toxin produces circumoral paresthesias, typically within 30 minutes of ingestion. Numbness of the tongue and limbs is followed by a rapidly progressive paralysis, and in severe cases, myocardial depression. The symptoms may progress as long as 24 hours. The toxin often induces emesis, but if necessary toxin can be removed from the stomach by lavage with 2 percent sodium bicarbonate. Activated charcoal should be instilled following emesis or lavage. Other treatment is strictly supportive, and the mortality rate is high.

Domoic acid was identified as the toxin in a major outbreak of food poisoning in Canada in late 1987. An algae, *Nitzschia pungens,* was found to be the source of the toxin, which contaminated blue mussels. Domoic acid is a glutamate analogue with excitotoxic activity at the kainic acid receptor, resulting in lesions in the hippocampus and amygdala. Severe gastrointestinal distress with vomiting and diarrhea occurred within 24 hours of ingestion, followed by headache, confusion, seizures, hemiparesis, ophthalmoplegia, and decreased level of consciousness. Three cases were fatal, and severely affected patients who survived had residual anterograde memory deficits and a predominantly motor polyneuropathy. Electromyography and nerve conduction studies showed denervation and reduced evoked motor potentials with relatively preserved conduction velocities. There is no specific therapy, but studies in mice suggest a combination of kynurenic acid and probenecid might be of potential benefit.

Botanic Toxins

Botanic intoxications are most frequent in young children, and in adults commonly occur when plants are consumed for "drug effect" or toxic mushrooms are inadvertently consumed. A wide variety of plants contain neurotoxins, and many neurologic agents used clinically or as drugs of abuse are derived from plants (atropine, scopolamine, curare, colchicine, taxol, opiates, marijuana, to name only a few). Table 1 summarizes the neuropharmacology of several important plants found in North America. A complete discussion is impossible, but a few toxins merit special mention, as well as some general principles.

The diagnosis of botanical ingestion is usually made from the history. Treatment of all noncaustic ingestions begins with induction of vomiting, if it has not already occurred and if the patient is able to protect the airway. If the patient is obtunded or has bulbar paralysis, gastric lavage should be performed. Observation of the gastric contents obtained may also provide clues to the nature of the ingested material. If the plant species ingested can be identified, regional poison control centers can usually provide information on the toxins involved and any available specific therapy. Otherwise, activated charcoal, symptomatic therapy, and supportive therapy are the mainstays of treatment.

Mushrooms can be divided into two groups: those that produce early symptoms of toxicity (within 6 hours after ingestion) and those that produce delayed symptoms (6 to 40 hours). In the former group are *Amanita muscaria* and *A. pantherina,* which look like mushrooms from a fairy tale, with red hoods and white dots. They contain biotinic acid, muscazon, and muscimol. These toxins are antagonists at muscarinic cholinergic and gamma-aminobutyric acid synapses, and produce agitation, confusion, muscle spasms, ataxia, and mydriasis. When the anticholinergic symptoms are severe, physostigmine may be beneficial. *A. muscaria* contains clinically insignificant amounts of the cholinergic agonist muscarine, but small brown and white mushrooms of the genera *Inocybe* and *Clitocybe* also contain muscarine and are usually responsible if cholinergic symptoms such as sweating, salivation, lacrimation, myosis, and hypertension dominate. Atropine is useful to counteract these

Table 1 Pharmacology of Toxic Plants

Plant	Symptoms of Toxicity	Treatment
Anticholinergic:		
Bittersweet	Fever	Physostigmine
Black henbane	Headache	
Nightshades	Confusion	
Black nightshade	Hallucinations	
Deadly nightshade	Dry mouth and skin	
Jimson weed	Mydriasis	
Potato leaves, sprouts, and tubers		
Jerusalem cherry		
Lantana, red sage, wild sage		
Wild tomato		
Depressant:		
Calico bush	Obtundation and coma; many	Respiratory and cardiac support
Death camass	plants also cause cardiac	
Lambkill	and gastrointestinal irritation	
Mountain laurel		
Sheep laurel		
Convulsant:		
Carolina allspice	Seizures	Respiratory and cardiac support
Chinaberry	Carolina allspice contains the	
Moonseed	strychnine-like toxin caly-	
Pinkroot	canthine	
Water hemlock		

Modified from Goetz CG. Neurotoxins in clinical practice. New York: Spectrum Publications, 1985; with permission.

symptoms. The hallucinogenic mushrooms of the *Psilocybe* genus also produce early symptoms, which include altered mood, hyperkinesis, vertigo, ataxia, mydriasis, weakness, and paresthesias in addition to the desired effects of hallucinations and synesthesias. The sensorium remains clear, in contrast to intoxication with *A. muscaria* or *A. pantherina*. The toxins are psilocybin and psilocin, thermostable indoles structurally related to serotonin. Symptoms usually resolve after approximately 12 hours, but accidental ingestion in children has resulted in high fever, seizures, and death.

Mushrooms that produce delayed symptoms include *Amanita phalloides* (death cap, which is the agent of the majority of fatal mushroom ingestions), several other *Amanita* species, and several species of the genera *Galerina* and *Gyromitra*. The *Amanita* and *Galerina* mushrooms contain amanitins, cyclopeptide RNA polymerase inhibitors that produce hepatic and renal cytotoxicity. Neurologic symptoms are secondary to the ensuing metabolic derangements. Therapy for amanitin ingestion remains controversial, but aggressive removal of toxin from the gastrointestinal tract, forced diuresis, early charcoal hemoperfusion or plasma exchange, and intensive metabolic support are the mainstays. Large doses of penicillin (300,000 IU per kilogram per day), silybin (20 to 50 mg per kilogram per day in four doses), and thioctic acid (5 to 10 mg per kilogram per day in four doses with monitoring for hypoglycemia) are likely to be beneficial. *Gyromitra* species contain monomethylhydrazine, an inhibitor of pyridoxine-dependent enzymes. Hepatotoxicity ensues, but direct central nervous system toxicity also produces seizures. Circulating methemoglobin can be detected early in the course, and may be used to diagnose monomethylhydrazine exposure. Intravenous pyridoxine is used to combat the toxicity.

Consumption of several varieties of the chickpea, genus *Lathyrus*, may result in a spastic paraplegia. These plants contain the neurotoxins alpha-amino-beta-oxalyaminoproprionic acid and alpha-amino-gamma-oxalyaminobutyric acid, as well as much manganese, which also appears to play a role in the toxicity.

Chickpeas produce neurologic symptoms when they account for more than one-third of the caloric intake. Typically, the syndrome begins with lumbar pain and mild fever, followed by several days of progressive spastic paraplegia and sensory disturbance. The sensory disturbance usually resolves over a few weeks. Sphincter control is spared. Severe cases may involve the upper extremities, and peripheral neuropathy may occur. The most common neuropathology is anterolateral sclerosis in the thoracolumbar cord. There is no specific therapy.

SUGGESTED READING

Baden DG. Brevetoxins: Unique polyether dinoflagellate toxins. FASEB J 1989; 3:1807–1817.

Goetz CG. Neurotoxins in clinical practice. New York: Spectrum, 1985.

Kincaid JC. Tick bite paralysis. Semin Neurol 1990; 10:32–34.

McGoldrick J, Marx JA. Marine envenomations; part 1: Vertebrates. J Emerg Med 1991; 9:497–502.

McGoldrick J, Marx JA. Marine envenomations; part 2: Invertebrates. J Emerg Med 1992; 10:71–77.

Piqueras J. Hepatotoxic mushroom poisoning: Diagnosis and management. Mycopathologia 1989; 105:99–110.

Schantz EJ, Johnson EA. Properties and use of botulinum toxin and other microbial neurotoxins in medicine. Microbial Rev 1992; 56:80–99.

Symposium on domoic acid toxicity. Can Dis Weekly Rep 1990; 16 (suppl 1).

RESOURCES

Botulism Antitoxin and Diphtheria Antitoxin
 Centers for Disease Control
 Drug and Immunobiologics Service
 1600 Clifton Rd., Bldg. 1, Rm. 1259
 Atlanta, Georgia 30333
 8:00 AM to 4:30 PM EST: (404) 639-3670
 Nights/weekends/holidays: (404) 639-2888 (emergency requests only)

Index of Antivenin Availability (Snake and Other Animal Venoms)
 Arizona Poison Control Center
 Telephone: (602) 626-6016

NEUROTOXICITY OF CYTOTOXIC AGENTS

MARK R. GILBERT, M.D.
MIRIAM L. FREIMER, M.D.

The importance of the neurotoxic effects of cytotoxic drugs in patient care is increasing. Oncologic treatments, and some recent therapeutic approaches to neurologic disorders, use cytotoxic agents in large doses. The incidence of neurotoxicity from the use of these agents is increasing for several reasons:

1. For most chemotherapeutic agents, there is definitely a dose-response relationship, which dictates use of larger doses. Consequently, there have been tremendous improvements in supportive measures and treatments for the systemic toxicity of chemotherapy. For example, the recent advent of colony-stimulating factors allows the use of drug doses that previously would have produced severe bone marrow toxicity. Unfortunately, no methods are known to reduce nervous system exposure and toxicity, and the increasing drug dosing has increased the incidence and severity of neurotoxicity.
2. Duration of survival is increasing for many malignancies. As a consequence, treatment-related neurotoxicity with a long-latency is more likely to manifest neurologic signs, as evidenced in the early 1970s in children with acute lymphocytic leukemia. When prophylactic cranial radiation and intrathecal methotrexate (MTX) were introduced, the incidence of leukemic meningitis declined markedly and the cure rate increased dramatically. Several years later, however, some of these children developed severe dementia and many others lost cognitive ability.
3. The development of new agents or novel routes of administration that specifically target disease in the nervous system, such as brain metastases or primary brain tumors, is likely to amplify the development of neurotoxicity. Treatments that increase exposure of tumors in the brain generally also expose normal brain cells. The use of blood-brain–barrier (BBB) disruption before intra-arterial or intravenous infusion of chemotherapy markedly increases the exposure of normal brain tissue to the drug, to a degree that exceeds the relative improvement in delivery of drug to the tumor. Preliminary results also indicate an increased incidence of neurotoxicity in these patients.

Continued improvements in the treatment of cancer and immune-mediated neurologic disorders will prolong survival and increase the rate of cure. Therefore, long-term morbidity—particularly irreversible neurotoxicity—should be a critical concern.

Chemotherapy-related neurotoxicity is often difficult to diagnose. Table 1 lists the chemotherapy agents that are most commonly associated with neurotoxicity. All other potential causes of neurologic dysfunction, those related to the patient's malignancy and those that are not, need to be considered. For example, patients who develop loss of dorsal column function after treatment with cisplatin should undergo evaluation for vitamin B_{12} deficiency and syphilis. Patients with radicular or cranial nerve findings should be evaluated for neoplastic or infectious meningitis. In addition, treatment- or cancer-related immunosuppression can make the patient more susceptible to infection. Specifically, encephalopathy from viral infection may mimic treatment-associated leukoencephalopathy, delaying diagnosis and institution of antiviral therapy.

GENERAL CONCEPTS

Blood-Brain and Blood-Nerve Barriers

Most chemotherapeutic drugs do not readily cross the BBB. The ability of a chemical to cross the BBB depends on the molecular weight of the agent and its lipid solubility. Agents such as the nitrosoureas are lipid soluble and small and, therefore, easily cross the BBB. On the other hand, vincristine, though lipid soluble, is large and therefore crosses the BBB poorly. Vincristine, however, is able to cross the blood-nerve barrier and causes peripheral neuropathy, a dose-limiting toxicity.

When given in large doses, drugs that cross the BBB poorly can cause significant neurotoxicity. For example, only a small percentage of MTX crosses the BBB when given IV, but when massive doses (>3 g per square meter) are administered, a sufficient amount enters the brain and can cause significant neurotoxicity, particularly when cranial irradiation has been given.

Sensitivity of the Nervous System to Chemotherapy

In high enough concentrations all chemotherapeutic agents are neurotoxic to exposed brain or spinal cord. The concentration that is sufficient to cause damage varies, so some drugs (i.e., MTX, cytosine arabinoside [Ara-C] and thioTEPA) can be administered directly into the cerebrospinal fluid (CSF). Other drugs cause severe toxicity even in very low concentrations. For example, several reports indicate that accidental intrathecal administration of small doses of vincristine causes rapid and fatal destruction of the brain and spinal cord.

Toxic Synergy with Other Treatment

Injury to the nervous system from exposure to cytotoxic agents is often most severe in patients who had previously existing neurologic disease. Prior disease is

Table 1 Neurotoxic Effects of Chemotherapeutic Agents

Agent	Class	Neurotoxicity	Notes
Methotrexate (MTX)	Antimetabolite	Acute somnolence, chronic leukoencephalopathy, mineralizing microangiopathy, myelopathy from intrathecal injection	Acute syndrome may be helped with folinic acid. CSF elevated during early stages of myelopathy.
Cytosine-arabinoside (Ara-c)	Antimetabolite	Irreversible cerebellar syndrome, chronic leukoencephalopathy, myelopathy with intrathecal injection	Purkinje cell destruction seen with cerebellar dysfunction. Synergy with MTX in myelopathy.
Cisplatin	Non-classic alkylating agent	Predominantly large fiber sensory polyneuropathy; hearing loss, tinnitus; possible optic neuropathy, retinal cone dysfunction	New agents (Org 2766, WR2721) may help prevent neuropathy. Hearing loss is generally irreversible.
Vincristine	Vinca alkaloid, microtubule depolymerizer	Sensorimotor polyneuropathy, autonomic neuropathy, cranial neuropathy, syndrome of inappropriate antidiuretic hormone secretion (SIADH), possible encephalopathy, myositis	Toxicity worse with underlying neuropathy. Gastrointestinal dysmotility after treatment indicates severe toxicity; no more vincristine should be given.
5-Fluorouracil (5-FU)	Antimetabolite	Cerebellar dysfunction, transient confusion and disorientation, Wernicke-Korsakoff-like syndrome, optic neuropathy, parkinsonism (rarely)	Cerebellar signs are partially reversible. Confusion and other toxicity may be related to effect on normal thiamine metabolism.
Cyclophosphamide	Alkylating agent	SIADH	SIADH seen with large-dose treatment.
Ifosfamide	Alkylating agent	Reversible encephalopathy; extrapyramidal signs: athetosis, myoclonus, opisthotonic posturing	Frequent (20% of patients). Low serum albumin, elevated creatinine, pelvic tumor, and prior cisplatin treatment are risk factors.
L-Asparaginase	Antimetabolite	Organic brain syndrome with psychosis, depression, intracranial hemorrhage and thrombosis, seizures, hyperglycemia	Organic brain syndrome may result from reduced L-asparagine and L-glutamine. Alters clotting mechanisms. Controversial treatment: fresh-frozen plasma (FFP) vs. FFP + heparin vs. FFP + antithrombin III
BCNU, CCNU	Nitrosoureas, alkylating agents	Necrotizing encephalopathy with intra-arterial injection, retinal toxicity with common carotid injection	Focal brain necrosis probably secondary to streaming phenomenon. Minimal neurotoxicity with IV injection.
Procarbazine	Alkylating agent	Peripheral neuropathy, encephalopathy with large dose	Penetrates blood-brain barrier. Has monoamine oxidase properties.
Interferon	Biologic response modifier	Encephalopathy, progressive vegetative state with intraventricular injection, parkinsonism with intraventricular injection, hearing loss	May cause diffuse cerebral edema. Some patients have persistent cognitive deficits after systemic treatment.
Taxol	Tubulin polymerizer	Peripheral neuropathy, autonomic neuropathy, seizures (rare)	Neuropathy is predominantly sensory. Onset of neuropathy may be rapid.
Misonidazole, metronidazole	Radiosensitizers	Peripheral neuropathy	Neuropathy is the dose-limiting toxicity.

thought either to make the neuronal elements more susceptible or to cause further loss of functional neuronal elements, resulting in a more dramatic loss of function because of reduced capacity for compensation. Patients with diabetic neuropathy develop severe neuropathy from smaller doses of vincristine than patients without underlying peripheral neuropathy, and the effects appear more rapidly. In fact, the overwhelming majority of deaths from neurotoxicity secondary to

systemic vincristine administration have occurred in patients who had an underlying neuropathy.

NEUROLOGIC SYNDROMES ASSOCIATED WITH CHEMOTHERAPY

Dementia

The use of intrathecal chemotherapy, intracarotid chemotherapy, and direct instillation of chemotherapy into the brain are all associated with the development of cognitive impairment. The dementia associated with intrathecal chemotherapy has been studied extensively. Cognitive changes usually occur 6 months to 2 years after therapy. The dysfunction may be progressive and can result in coma or even death. The syndrome is not, generally, reversible. Prior cranial radiation treatment markedly increases the risk and severity of the neurologic dysfunction. Pathologically, the process appears to affect principally white matter. On histologic examination, regions of axonal swelling or loss with accompanying demyelination are seen. Other histologic changes include calcification of blood vessels and coagulative necrosis of white matter regions.

Acute encephalopathy is associated with several cytotoxic treatments. High doses of intravenous MTX or Ara-c cause a reversible encephalopathy that is generally accompanied by lethargy. The pathogenesis of this acute, reversible confusional state is not known, but animal studies and positron emission tomographic studies in patients have shown a temporary global reduction in brain metabolic activity — both glucose utilization and protein synthesis. In the case of MTX, the administration of folinic acid (leucovorin) has been associated with improved metabolic activity in laboratory studies and in clinical studies. The immunostimulant levamisole causes reversible encephalopathy that occasionally is accompanied by seizures. Other agents that can cause encephalopathy include vincristine, ifosphamide, procarbazine and L-asparaginase. Biologic response modifiers such as the interferons and interleukins routinely cause reversible encephalopathy, but recent evidence suggests that some permanent neurologic sequelae may develop with prolonged interferon use.

Findings of early clinical trials with the experimental agent spiromustine underscore the axiom that cytotoxic agents are neurotoxic if they are accessible to the nervous system. Spiromustine, an alkylating agent (nitrogen mustard) bound to a hydantoin, is specifically synthesized to improve drug delivery to the brain in an attempt to provide a new therapy for metastatic and primary brain tumors. Initial phase I studies were stopped early because profound psychosis resulted, even with the smallest doses. Physostigmine blocks the neurotoxicity, but it may also inhibit the antitumor effect of this drug.

The administration of many chemotherapy agents results in altered mental status by creating a secondary metabolic derangement. Cyclophosphamide and vincristine can stimulate inappropriate ADH secretion. The resulting hyponatremia can lead to encephalopathy and seizures. Likewise, cisplatin can cause a salt-wasting nephropathy, resulting in hyponatremia and encephalopathy. Other agents can cause hepatic or renal dysfunction with secondary neurologic findings. Corticosteroids, L-asparaginase, or streptozocin may lead to glucose intolerance, which, if not controlled, can result in nonketotic hyperosmolar coma.

Seizures

Many chemotherapeutic agents have been associated with seizures, most commonly generalized tonic-clonic seizures. In most cases, seizures resulting from chemotherapy toxicity are accompanied by encephalopathy, suggesting a more global effect of the agent on higher cortical function. Usually, however, focal seizures are seen when cerebral hemispheres suffer structural damage. For example, MTX-induced leukoencephalopathy causes areas of focal necrosis, which can then cause a focal seizure. Likewise, cerebrovascular events, both hemorrhagic and bland, resulting from L-asparaginase–induced coagulopathies, can also lead to focal seizures. Cisplatin can cause seizures, perhaps by inducing vasospasm of a cerebral vessel and causing transient ischemia, thus providing a seizure focus.

Cerebellar Dysfunction

Several chemotherapeutic agents, most commonly cytosine arabinoside (Ara-c) and 5-FU, are known to cause dose-related cerebellar toxicity. Ara-c and 5-FU are specifically toxic to the Purkinje cells, making this toxicity irreversible. Clinically, patients exhibit midline cerebellar dysfunction with truncal ataxia, unsteady gait, dysarthria, and nystagmus. Appendicular ataxia is less common. Rarely, MTX-induced leukoencephalopathy affects the cerebellum. Dorsal column dysfunction with loss of proprioceptive sense may mimic cerebellar toxicity, but the absence of eye movement abnormalities, truncal ataxia, and dysarthria with dorsal column injury should distinguish it from cerebellar dysfunction.

Cranial Neuropathy

Cranial nerve palsies are a rare complication of chemotherapy. Vinca alkaloids, particularly vincristine, are known to cause cranial nerve palsies, the most common involving the facial nerve. In addition, intraventricular administration of chemotherapy or biologic agents such as interferon-alpha can cause cranial nerve palsies, which are generally transient. The pathogenesis of this temporary dysfunction is not known, but in some cases abnormalities in cerebrospinal fluid (CSF) circulation delay clearance of anticancer drugs from the ventricles and basal cisterns after intraventricular administration.

Optic Neuropathy and Ocular Toxicity

Optic nerve and retinal toxicity are most commonly seen with intracarotid injection of chemotherapeutics, particularly when the infusion occurs at or below the level of the common carotid artery. Both nitrosoureas and cisplatin are associated with this toxicity. In addition, systemic administration of cisplatin has been shown to cause optic disc swelling, and optic neuropathy has been reported with 5-FU.

Spinal Cord Toxicity

Myelopathy, a rare complication of cancer treatment, occurs almost exclusively with lumbar intrathecal administration. Both intrathecal MTX and Ara-c are associated with focal spinal cord dysfunction. Initial symptoms usually appear hours to days after treatment. Patients can experience sensory changes, a combination of upper and lower motor neuron dysfunction, and radiating pain similar to Lhermitte's phenomenon. Often, there is a prodrome: the patient experiences transient pain after a previous intrathecal treatment. Some studies have shown that CSF myelin basic protein levels are elevated during the early phases of myelopathy and that further treatment is associated with progressive neurologic dysfunction. Prognosis is variable. Some patients show gradual, and occasionally complete, recovery, whereas others have a progressive myelopathy that is often ascending and fatal. Systemic administration of cisplatin can cause damage that is limited to the posterior columns, and patients may complain of Lhermitte's phenomenon. Pathologic findings in the spinal cord from cisplatin toxicity are similar in appearance to subacute combined degeneration; however, a recent study failed to show a connection between vitamin B_{12} level and cisplatin toxicity.

Peripheral Neuropathy

Peripheral neuropathy is a frequent complication of cancer. It is estimated that 10 to 20 percent of patients with cancer develop a sensorimotor polyneuropathy during their illness, generally in the later stages. Distinguishing this apparent paraneoplastic neuropathy from the changes associated with cachexia or from treatment-induced neuropathy is often difficult. There are, however, several agents that cause a dose-related stereotypical neuropathy. The manifestations of the neuropathy are directly related to the probable underlying neurotoxic mechanism. Vincristine causes disruption of microtubules and so affects both small and large peripheral nerves, although small fibers are affected earlier and more severely. Conversely, cisplatin causes aggregates of neurofilaments; therefore, large sensory fibers are involved most profoundly. Taxol, a novel antimicrotubule agent that promotes tubulin polymerization and aggregation, causes a mixed sensorimotor neuropathy similar to that seen with vincristine toxicity. Other agents, such as procarbazine, can cause a stocking-glove sensorimotor polyneuropathy. The radiation sensitizers misonidazole and metronidazole produce dose-limiting peripheral neuropathy.

Autonomic neuropathy, presenting with orthostatic hypotension or intestinal dysmotility, is most commonly seen with vincristine, particularly when an underlying neuropathy (e.g., diabetic) is present. Cisplatin and procarbazine have occasionally been associated with mild autonomic dysfunction. Early reports indicate that taxol has autonomic toxicity similar to that of vincristine.

Myopathy

Cancer chemotherapeutic agents that have toxic effects on muscle are uncommon. Reports of myositis from vincristine and taxol indicate that it is a rare complication. Interferon administration can result in myalgias plus other influenza-like symptoms. Cisplatin can cause muscle cramping as a result of hypomagnesemia that is a direct consequence of nephrotoxicity. Many agents, particularly biologics, cause myalgias but apparently without muscle damage or dysfunction.

TREATMENT

No specific treatment exists to reverse the neurotoxic effects of chemotherapy. There are some preliminary reports of protective agents, such as Org 2766 and WR 2721, that may have a role in limiting cisplatin neuropathy without adversely altering its antineoplastic activity. The use of leucovorin for MTX-induced somnolence has also been suggested. For the majority of the agents, therefore, careful observation for early signs of toxicity and dose modification or cessation are the only available treatment strategies. Several clearly defined situations mandate cessation of treatment:

1. *Patients, particularly those with underlying neuropathy, who are treated with vincristine should be carefully monitored for intestinal dysmotility.* Treatment should be stopped if obstipation is detected, as subsequent treatment will likely lead to increasing dysfunction. Fatal vincristine neuropathy is most often secondary to bowel motility problems and perforation.
2. *Patients receiving intraventricular chemotherapy should undergo an Indium-111-DTPA CSF flow study by injecting the tracer into the reservoir system and observing tracer clearance.* Failure of the tracer to flow over the cortical convexities indicates a degree of communicating hydrocephalus and abnormal retention of fluid in the lateral ventricles. Injected drugs remain within the ventricles in very high concentrations, markedly accelerating the development of leukoencephalopathy. If abnormal flow exists, cranial radiotherapy may be used to destroy tumor cells that are blocking the arachnoid granulations and obstructing CSF absorption.
3. Localized back pain or the development of Lhermitte's phenomenon in patients receiving lumbar chemotherapy may indicate early chemotherapy myelopathy. The myelin basic protein level in CSF has been shown to be elevated before signs of myelopathy develop. Therefore, if a patient develops symptoms, intralumbar administration should be stopped, the CSF myelin basic protein (MBP) level measured, and, if the MBP level is elevated, lumbar intrathecal administration of chemotherapy should be avoided. Alter-

nate locations, such as intraventricular administration, can be used, as the myelopathy is probably due to diminished local CSF flow because of arachnoiditis associated with frequent chemotherapy treatments.

DISCUSSION

Drug neurotoxicity is an important problem in cancer treatment. The incidence of neurotoxicity is increasing as improvements in supportive care permit escalation of treatment doses and prolonged survival uncovers toxicities with long latencies. Most toxic effects are diagnosed by their characteristic presentation, though a thorough evaluation is required to exclude other treatable causes. Although some potentially useful new protective agents are being developed, treatment is now limited to recognizing early signs of toxicity to allow treatment modification, identifying pre-existing conditions that increase the risk of developing toxicity, and avoiding treatments that have known neurotoxic synergy.

SUGGESTED READING

Chamberlain MC, Corey-Bloom J. Leptomeningeal metastases: [111]Indium-DTPA CSF flow studies. Neurology 1991; 41:1765–1769.

Mollman JE, Glover DJ, Hogan WM. Cisplatin neuropathy: Risk factors, prognosis and protection by WR-2721. Cancer 1988; 61:2192–2195.

van der Hoop RG, et al. Prevention of cisplatin neurotoxicity with an ACTH(4-9) analogue in patients with ovarian cancer. N Engl J Med 1990; 322:89–94.

METABOLIC DISEASES

ACUTE HEPATIC PORPHYRIA

HENRY A. PETERS, M.D.

In the plant kingdom, porphyrins, in the form of chlorophyll, are "complexed" with magnesium. In animals, porphyrins complexed with iron make up hemoglobin, but in the nervous system the porphyrins coproporphyrin III and protoporphyrin are combined with zinc and are deposited along with the myelin in the white matter of the central nervous system and in the peripheral nerves. Klüver and other pioneer researchers have suggested a major role in nerve conduction for these zinc-complexed macromolecules. When attacks of acute intermittent porphyria (AIP) involved the nervous system, early reports described mortality rates as high as 90 percent. Much of the descriptive literature about AIP was derived from fatal cases.

For years, investigators have been looking for a porphyrin precursor or an altered toxic porphyrin molecule to account for the precipitation of often life-threatening attacks of AIP. But all of the normal porphyrins and porphyrin precursors have been injected into man and beast without reproducing signs or symptoms of an attack. Only hematoporphyrin, which is created unnaturally by treating hemoglobin with sulfuric acid, was found, on intravenous administration, to produce intense photosensitivity, an observation later used to induce sensitivity in tumors for localization and to enhance sensitivity to laser and x-ray therapy.

All animals excrete porphyrins and porphyrin precursors in their urine, so the presence of these compounds does not in itself establish the diagnosis of AIP. During attacks of AIP larger than normal volumes of the porphyrin precursors porphobilinogen (PBG) and delta-aminolevulinic acid (D-ALA) are excreted in urine, as well as coproporphyrin (COPRO) and uroporphyrin (URO). This increased excretion may be constant, intermittent or short lived. Some AIP patients may excrete very abnormal volumes in urine and be asymptomatic or in remission, and others may occasionally "normalize" in the middle of life-threatening attacks. Although AIP attacks have been seen as early as 2 to 5 years of age, this is exceptional; onset at puberty or later is more likely.

In recent years, there seem to be increasing numbers of patients who have been erroneously diagnosed as having AIP. Once it is misdiagnosed, it is difficult to remove the label of porphyria. Because the basis for diagnosis of AIP is not clear and some of the treatments are hazardous, it seems appropriate to discuss diagnostic criteria before treatment options are considered.

When AIP is suspected the physician looks for an excess of porphyrin precursors in the urine. The simplest, and perhaps best, method is to collect a fresh urine sample and have it quantitatively analyzed for PBG and D-ALA. The same specimen can be used for quantitative determination of COPRO and URO. The great number of spectroscopic peaks now often reported is confusing and may lead to misinterpretation and erroneous diagnoses. Twenty-four hour urine samples may not give accurate information, because the precursors change to mature porphyrins with time, even in the urinary bladder. Done correctly, a Watson Schwartz test for PBG is helpful, but the diagnosis of AIP cannot be ruled out on the basis of a negative result (around 20 mg of PBG may be required to give a positive result). Quantitative estimates on fresh urine samples will be much more reliable. Values above 2 mg per liter for PBG and 4 mg per liter for D-ALA mean that the patient should be watched and the tests repeated. Values for COPRO over 150 µg per liter and URO above 40 mg per liter may be significant. Part of the porphyrin levels may represent porphyrins derived from the precursors in the bladder or in vitro while the urine was aging.

Medications such as the sulfones, sedormid, estrogens, barbiturates, phenytoin, primidone, and sulfa drugs and their derivatives may increase the levels of COPRO and URO, even in some nonporphyric patients. This is due to induction of the enzyme D-ALA dehydrase (D-ALA-D) also noted in attacks of AIP, an observation that gave rise to the idea that AIP was the first inborn error of metabolism discovered to be caused by overactivity of an enzyme.

Observations that the chelating agents intravenous ethylenediaminetetra-acetic acid (EDTA) and intramuscular dimercaptopropanol (BAL) seemed successful in reversing severe AIP attacks (with ultimate recovery) resulted in our postulating since 1954 that an enzymatic block caused by an excess of zinc, or other cations, at the stage between PBG and URO could lead to a porphyrin deficit in the nervous system and might be the cause of attacks. Metal-complexing agents, by removing these excess cations, might unblock the enzyme and improve availability of mature porphyrins that had been withdrawn or not replaced in the white matter. The presence of a great excess of PBG and D-ALA in the liver of patients who died during AIP attacks seemed to give weight to the theory that a block at the PBG level was causing this porphyrin deficit.

That enzyme was found and was named uroporphyrinogen synthetase (URO-S, also known as porphobilinogen deaminase). In AIP patients, activity of URO-S, measured in red blood cells, was found to be reduced by 50 percent or more. When present, this blockage of enzyme activity is strong evidence for AIP, but the presence of the block does not mean that the patient is having an attack or needs treatment. Moreover, some of our AIP patients with blocked URO-S function who had unmistakable attacks with severe polyneuropathy, psychosis, seizures, and heightened levels of porphyrins and precursors and who were treated with intravenous EDTA, were shown during and after successful treatment to have normalized their URO-S activity. Although we found reduced URO-S activity in a group of retarded epileptic patients who were treated with carbamazepine and valproate, they did not exhibit AIP symptoms. The question is, What other medicines or chemicals might inhibit URO-S activity.

Experience with Turkish porphyria (TP), in which inadvertently ingested hexachlorobenzene (HCB, a fungicide)-treated seed grain induced a mixed type of porphyria in 3,000 to 4,000 patients, after 30 years or more has revealed that some of the TP patients are showing depressed function of URO-S. Also, DALA urinary excretion is elevated above control values in almost half the patients tested. Elevation of COPRO and URO as well in a few others indicates that long-lasting (for years), nongenetic porphyria may be chemically induced.

Once thought rare (1.5 per 100,000 population), the incidence of AIP is now estimated to approach 1 in 1,000 in northern Scandinavia and in Ireland. In South Africa, a mixed porphyria (variegate) affects 1 to 4 percent of the Boer white population; this determination is relatively easy to make because of a persistence of abnormal fecal porphyrins and the presence of an X porphyrin in the feces. AIP, cutanea tarda (CT), and varigate forms of hepatic porphyria are thought to be autosomal-dominant traits.

CLINICAL SIGNS AND SYMPTOMS OF AIP ATTACKS

Based on more than 130 hepatic porphyria patients identified and followed as long as 39 years, it is possible to describe the signs and symptoms of AIP attacks. Because high levels of urine porphyrins, porphyrin precursors, and depressed URO-S can even be present in asymptomatic AIP patients, how does one determine if the clinical picture represents an attack? We have seen AIP patients with pain and colic caused by a retained surgical sponge, back pain related to a fall and dorsal fracture of the spine, and abdominal problems from a ruptured appendix, for example. The diagnosis relies heavily on the clinical and laboratory findings.

In severe AIP attacks there is often tachycardia and tachypnea. Hyperventilation (as in phobic neurosis) may be difficult to separate at first from incipient respiratory failure. AIP patients who in the past have experienced severe attacks with neuropsychiatric signs and symptoms may become so fearful that they demand intervention when none is indicated. Much of the information written about porphyria is frightening; opiate addiction, drug habituation, and dependence on inappropriate medical therapy are common.

Pyramidal tract signs are seldom seen unless there is an additional cause, such as a stroke. Extrapyramidal symptoms may be secondary to medications such as the phenothiazines, which can induce parkinsonian symptoms and akathisia, especially with prochlorperazine. Parkinsonian symptoms due to AIP are rarely seen, but after 30 years TP patients are beginning to show early extrapyramidal involvement (about 30 percent of 275 cases followed). This may result from long exposure to the toxic effects of HCB (which is fat soluble and measurable in milk and fat) rather than to induced porphyria.

Abdominal or visceral symptoms may be entirely absent in some AIP patients. Attacks may be associated with colic, constipation (alternating at times with diarrhea), and sometimes flank pain suggesting renal colic. The abdomen may be tender to slight pressure, the pain not localized by muscle wall splinting. A plain x-ray study of the abdomen may show areas of spasm and dilatation, and the patient may adopt the knee-chest position as the most comfortable one.

When adhesions (often from multiple operations) result in partial obstruction, localized pain may be present. Obstipation can give rise to severe impaction. One patient had not defecated for a month, and the impactions were dissolved with rectal infusions of papase (Adolph's Tenderizer).

Recurrent dysesthesias of the fingers and toes and sensory loss, generalized or local and including at times the saddle area, may be present. Backache may mimic sciatica, disc disease, or even kidney stone. Polyneuritis may ascend as in Landry's, may suggest Guillain-Barré syndrome, and may be asymmetric or symmetric, proximal or distal. Urinary incontinence or retention may be seen. When paralysis is fulminating, gross fasciculatory shivering of weakened or paralyzed muscles occur.

We have seen brachial plexitis, mononeuritis multiplex, and drop foot after crossing the legs or squatting. Three patients developed unilateral recurrent laryngeal nerve palsy along with generalized polyneuropathy.

Pinkish urine may stain the sheets although the patient may not mention or be aware of discolored urine.

Placed in the window, especially if acidified, sunlight may change the urine's color from normal to red, brown, or black. (This may be due to other chromagens and not the porphyrins themselves.)

During an attack the level of consciousness may be lowered and responses to questions or commands delayed. One patient, after treatment with EDTA/BAL was instituted, for the first time complained of pain in the shoulder, and radiography showed a fracture dislocation.

Hysteroid behavior, and also neurologic signs of hysteria, may be labeled functional. Waldenström was said to have remarked, "If a patient from northern Sweden is hysterical and dies of respiratory failure, the correct diagnosis is acute porphyria."

Other psychiatric symptoms may be present—a delerioid state resembling the delirium tremens (an AIP patient may also be an alcoholic), catatonic excitement, paranoid psychosis, and, less often, depressive symptoms. Both visual and auditory hallucinosis have been seen, as well as micropsia and macropsia or Brobdingnagian phenomenon. These so preoccupy patients that they may be uncooperative or uninterested in being examined. Patients may not volunteer that their mind is playing tricks on them, and some have a degree of insight into their experience, especially after they recover from the attack. Even today, the patient may be taking bromides, and the blood level should be checked, especially if visual hallucinosis, rash, ataxia, folliculitis, nausea, or tracheitis is present.

Increased melanosis or a metallic appearance of the facial skin may be present and, during an attack, a "malar gloss" of the face is sometimes seen. The patients with variegate, CT, TP patients due to HCB and the congenital porphyrics (which will not be discussed here) may all react to sun exposure: bulla formation, Nikolsky's sign (epidermis is rubbed off with slight trauma) and rashes predominating. Solar reactions should alert one to the possibility of these conditions, which may include neurologic and psychiatric signs and symptoms as in TP and variegate forms.

Grand mal or temporal lobe seizures and status epilepticus may occur, possibly the result of withdrawal of medication or electrolyte imbalance, which should be appropriately studied including magnesium levels. Both hyper- and hyponatremia are frequently present and need prompt attention.

ATTACK-PRECIPITATING FACTORS

AIP attacks are most often caused by barbiturates (especially pentothal) and sulfa drugs and their derivatives. Some medicines have added barbiturates, such as Donnatal. Thiazide-derived hypoglycemic, diuretic, and antihypertensive preparations should be identified, stopped, and replaced if necessary. The sulfones were the first sedatives implicated in AIP and other agents such as glutethimide may be at fault. We have seen an AIP patient who began regular use of seconal in her late teens but did not have major attacks until she discontinued the drug as an adult and then resumed taking it after several months.

Some patients became symptomatic after ingesting sucaryl, a sulfa drug used for some time as an artificial sweetener; saccharine also may cause trouble. Starvation will induce AIP attacks, and reliance or bingeing on diet drinks might obscure the fact that the AIP patient is really fasting and may even be hypoglycemic.

A Hmong mother of three developed seizures, which were made worse by phenytoin therapy. She was hospitalized and overnight became ventilator dependent from progressing severe polyneuropathy associated with unilateral laryngeal palsy, psychosis, incontinence, and recurrent seizures. After 5 days on respiratory support, lorezepam, fluid and electrolyte correction, her condition was worse. She was then treated for 1 day with intravenous (IV) EDTA and improved for 2 days but then began to lapse. After 4 more days, IV EDTA was resumed for 5 days, resulting in progressive improvement. The cause of the recurrent fever and the 30,000 white cell count was obscure until she was found to have a severe hookworm infestation (which may have killed her 5 year old son a month before her attack). Deworming ended her pleocytosis and recurring fever. The starvation secondary to the parasite infestation very probably caused her AIP attack. Ventilator dependency lasted 2 months, and complete motor recovery took about 2 years. This case called attention to a warning that unexplained sudden death was common in the Hmong population in their native land. If our patient (who had been in Asia a month before onset of her attack) had stayed at home in her village, she might have suffered unexplained sudden death.

Exposure to oil-based paints and solvents precipitated symptoms in half of our AIP patients and for seven was a chief precipitant of major attacks. For example, a woman had two attacks, the first erroneously diagnosed as Guillain-Barré, which coincided with painting and redecorating her restaurant. Steroid administration and supportive measures improved her enough for discharge. A second more severe episode followed a similar indoor paint exposure and resulted in more severe polyneuropathy which, after diagnosis of AIP, responded to EDTA/BAL. She has had no further recurrences. Her 47 year old daughter had AIP attacks on two occasions when she was exposed at work to indoor painting and redecorating. After cessation of exposure, recovery took several months. A URO-S block and increased urine porphyrin precursors and porphyrins persisted in mother, daughter, and a number of other members of this family, but only those exposed to paints became symptomatic.

Screening of family members is indicated, because AIP is an autosomal-dominant trait and protection of AIP patients by avoidance of precipitating factors is very important. A URO-S determination, looking for a block of around 50 percent, may be done at any age and positive tests would be reliable evidence. A fresh urine test for quantitative D-ALA, PBG, COPRO, and URO would provide adequate screening. In the event of suggestive symptoms, if the patient is going to need anesthesia for surgery, or if the patient is very young (attacks are infrequent before puberty), these tests should be repeated, even if results are at first normal.

A family history of multiple operations, reactions to drugs of the barbiturate or sulfa group, reactions to paints or solvents, long recovery from anesthetic agents, seizures, delerium-like reactions, or other neuropsychiatric illness should increase the suspicion of AIP. In addition, the feces should be screened for above average levels of COPRO, URO, and PROTO (as might be seen in the variegate type of porphyria so common in the white population of South Africa). Here, there may also be an X porphyrin in the feces, and fecal porphyrins will be increased even during disease remission. Hereditary coproporphyria (HC) also may be marked by persistent elevation of fecal porphyrins, though the urine may be normal between attacks. In HC the phenothiazine medications may aggravate symptoms!

TREATMENT OF ACUTE EXACERBATIONS

When a patient does not have confirmatory laboratory evidence of AIP but has a history of reacting to barbiturates or sulfa drugs or to paints and solvents and has signs and symptoms suggestive of porphyria or relatives with known AIP, we have used the label *paraporphyric*. The patient is then advised to avoid all factors that seem to have provoked symptoms in the past as well as known precipitants of AIP. For colic, chlorpromazine or related drugs of this type may be given in small doses; opiate-type medications are avoided or, if indicated, withdrawn. Occasionally, some of these patients later show laboratory evidence of AIP, and in the meantime, the patient has not lost anything by avoiding possible precipitating factors. This regimen may be continued indefinitely without hardship.

In recent years it seems that we are seeing fewer florid examples of AIP, probably because barbiturates are being used less and the phenothiazines are being used more.

When a patient is having a true attack of AIP, the avoidance of or removal of all drugs of the sulfa or barbiturate series and their derivatives (including oral antidiabetes agents such as glyburide, thiazide diuretics, and antihypertensive agents) should have high priority. If a thiazide diuretic is still essential for cardiac purposes, we would cautiously introduce minimal doses of furosemide.

The anticonvulsants diphenylhydantoin (Dilantin), primidone, phenobarbital, ethosuximide, phensuximide, and valproate should be gradually phased out, especially if chelation therapy is used (provided no structural lesion is causing the seizures). If an anticonvulsant still needs to be used, carbamazepine, though it may induce D-ALA-D, is in our experience tolerated in AIP if introduced slowly. Lorazepam has also been used as a anticonvulsant and as a relaxant and sedative for respirator-dependent patients. Paraldehyde may be used for seizures if the patient is not asthmatic. Clonezepam (Klonopin) has also been reported to be tolerated. On rare occasions bromides have been used, but they require careful laboratory control to prevent ataxia, undue sedation, and hallucinosis. Ethanol is contraindicated for CT, variegate, and possibly HC patients, but some AIP patients seem able to tolerate moderate drinking. Patients with all types of porphyria may suffer from chronic alcoholism.

We emphasize again careful regulation of electrolytes, including magnesium, because inappropriate antidiuretic hormone (ADH) is a problem and hyponatremia is often seen. Thiamine might be given and vitamin B_6, the latter because chelating agents may lead to a pyridoxine deficiency.

Although a high carbohydrate intake has been thought to be helpful in AIP attacks, we have seen patients who have been taking oral and parenteral carbohydrates for months without experiencing reversal of the neurologic and psychiatric symptoms (which then responded to IV EDTA). Other patients become morbidly obese and even diabetic when carbohydrate regimens are used, and this approach does not prevent recurrences.

Pain (including colic, with nausea and sometimes emesis) may be handled with phenothiazines, preferably in small doses, meperidine only if necessary, and avoidance of habituating medications. If the patient is addicted to opiates we substitute chlorpromazine and withdraw the offending substance. Methadone replacement may be useful, after which withdrawal may be easier. The great majority of patients can stop taking pain medication (especially with chelating regimens). Sedative drugs like meprobamate, chlordiazepoxide, and diazepam may exacerbate porphyria and have great potential for abuse. Lithium is tolerated but usually is not necessary, and it needs careful laboratory control.

Because of the severity of the neuropathy, which is a combination of demyelinating and axonal, physical therapy should be employed early to prevent contractures, scoliosis, and often severe muscle atrophy. Complete recovery occurs in even the most severe cases of sensorimotor neuropathy, though several years may pass before full return of strength and muscle volume. Orthoses may be useful only for a time (until drop foot recovers, for example). Personnel working with porphyria patients should have an understanding and optimistic manner, because patients are often devastated by their illness.

CHELATING REGIMENS

If the measures described are unsuccessful in reversing an attack, we resort to EDTA and/or BAL. At times the patient may be so sick that we choose to begin this therapy right away. Since 1953, we have collected more than 130 patients with hepatic porphyria and have resorted to chelating in 52 cases; the others recovered with time after causative factors were removed.

Out of the selected group (13 of whose disease was grade 4) who in total had more than 100 AIP attacks, response to EDTA/BAL was very good in more than two-thirds. Recurrent attacks were few, and they responded to the same treatment. Only one death related to AIP occurred, this from sepsis. Treatment response was often immediate with disappearance of psychosis, evidence of increasing strength, and cessation of seizures. Once improvement starts, it will usually continue with recovery from severe polyneuropathy being complete in 1 to 2 years, depending on the degree of axonal involvement. Excellent nursing and other supportive measures are invaluable. Since our initial report in 1954, a dozen or more reports in the literature have described similar responses to complexing agents in AIP and CT attacks.

Our protocol for EDTA is to administer disodium calcium EDTA (versenate), 1.5 to 2.00 g per day IV in 1,000 cc 5 percent glucose in water over a 3 to 4 hour period for 5 to 7 days. Total daily fluid intake should be about 3,000 cc. The side effects are minimal, and only at 2 to 3 times this dose (4 to 7 g) have (reversible) lower nephron changes been reported. Tetany does not occur, because the patient is taking the calcium salt. The 5 to 7 day course can be repeated as necessary, although response to treatment is seen as early as the first day and, once improvement is evident there is usually continued progress and ultimate recovery.

On some occasions we have added intramuscular (IM) injections of BAL, 25 to 50 mg several times a day. It is helpful to have blood and urine lead determinations, as in an adult with a high lead burden BAL alone may not form a stable complex. Under these circumstances EDTA is used for several days before BAL is added. Theoretically, a pyridoxal phosphate (vitamin B_6) deficiency secondary to chelating agents may arise, so we have added vitamin B_6, 50 mg, after treatment is instituted. A pattern of increased kynurenine and xanthurenic acid in the urine after tryptophan load of AIP patients suggests vitamin B_6 deficiency, but this corrects with EDTA administration, even without B_6 replacement.

Kynurenic and xanthurenic acid, the sulfhydryl pool, histidine, and the porphyrins themselves are all natural chelating mechanisms subject to exhaustion from a variety of causes, including heavy metal poisoning, barbiturate and sulfa drugs, AIP itself, and HCB poisoning as in TP. In TP, some of the patients who were least symptomatic showed the most excessive volumes of porphyrin excretion, suggesting that the induced porphyria may have played a protective role.

We have already described the normalization of URO-S blockage during and after treatment with EDTA/BAL. In some cases the normalization has continued for years, even in patients who had the worst attacks. In time, urine porphyrin and precursor levels also move toward a more normal pattern or become completely normal. The patient's treatment should not,

however, use either the enzyme activity or porphyrin excretion as the only guide; rather, the clinical status of the patient is most important.

The explanation as to why a metal-complexing agent should seem to alter an attack of porphyria must be related to the way the metals are handled by a normal, healthy body, as opposed to AIP patients with a block in porphyrin synthesis. Excess cations such as zinc can block a number of enzyme activities. When a patient with AIP is in an attack associated with development of neuropsychiatric signs and symptoms, determinations of urine zinc excretion demonstrates a level of zincuria (before any chelating agents are administered) that ranges from 2 to 36 times the normal value. The increased amount of excreted zinc was more proportionate to the clinical symptoms than the amounts of porphyrin precursors and porphyrins.

Normally zinc is excreted into the gut, not the urine, and zincuria implies an overabundance of available zinc with spillover into the urine. We have also seen zincuria in patients with arteritis, heavy metal intoxication, delirium tremens, and Wernicke's encephalopathy. With the introduction of IV EDTA or BAL, there follows enhanced zinc excretion that may reach normal levels, even with continued administration of the complexing agents. In remission there is no zincuria. We have also noted that, during and following the EDTA administration normalization of URO-S enzyme activity may occur, which persists in recovery. We believe such normalization is due to the removal by the complexing agents of excess zinc (or another cation) that is responsible for the block. When normal persons are stressed by barbiturates or sulfa drugs, paints and solvents, or starvation, the pathway for maintaining normal porphyrin supply does not shut down enough to cause trouble. In AIP patients, whose porphyrin supply is marginal owing to the enzymatic (URO-S) block, the same stress may bring on an attack.

Penicillamine has been used for chronic porphyria (CT), but it is a good chelator of copper, not zinc, and is associated with side effects that include vasculitis, neuropathy, and polymyositis.

Histidine, a powerful naturally occurring zinc chelator, has been described as helpful in AIP, but it may induce vitamin B_6 deficiency, which must be anticipated and treated. ACTH and steroids reduce colic but exacerbate AIP if given when the nervous system is involved. For a severe case of AIP with quadriparesis during the recovery phase of treatment with EDTA, we used small doses of steroids and found that they relieved edema for which it was given and was tolerated at that stage. Did the EDTA/BAL therapy that preceded the steroids protect?

Desferrioxamine, an iron and aluminum chelator, cholestyramine resin, EDTA and BAL, as well as phlebotomy have all been used to treat CT. Others have made therapeutic attempts with ovulocyclic agents, which can create attacks as well as help some AIP patients, so this approach must be explored with caution and individualized.

Hypertension may occur during attacks, but it responds to EDTA/BAL therapy and goes away in recovery. Propranolol has been recommended for high blood pressure, and some claim that it may help AIP patients if they are not asthmatic. Calcium channel blockers such as nifedipine may be used, as well as other nonthiazide agents, including reserpine.

In recent years, hematin therapy has been recommended as a means of reducing the formation of porphyrins at the D-ALA stage via negative feedback on porphyrin synthesis. This approach presupposes that porphyrin precursors, porphyrins themselves, or some aberrant porphyrin molecules are toxic and are the cause of the AIP attacks, which should cease if the production of these substances is curtailed or stopped by hematin.

We have commented on the failed attempts to demonstrate symptoms analogous to AIP attacks by injecting natural porphyrins and porphyrin precursors into humans and animals and the lack of correlation of extremely high precursor and porphyrin excretion with clinical symptoms in latent or AIP patients in remission.

Results of a symposium on hematin and heme-arginase in 1986 indicated that hematin preparations, especially the earlier forms, produced intravascular coagulation and bleeding in more than 30 percent of the patients. Very fresh hematin (produced when it was to be used) was recommended, but vascular problems persist, even with the newer forms of hematin (heme-arginase). Silberberg and Schutta in 1967 demonstrated that when added to cultures of cerebellar tissue hematin is even more toxic to the tissue than bilirubin.

According to the hematin group's consensus, though hematin seemed to stop colic in AIP and "normalized" porphyrin and precursor excretion, it did not prevent recurrences of the attack, even if given prophylactically. Moreover, once the patient began to show neurologic and psychiatric symptoms, hematin had little or no effect. They recommended that hematin be given as early as possible. One could postulate that this advice could result in inappropriate hematin therapy and that the drug might even be given before the diagnosis of AIP had been established.

Moore and coworkers described an AIP patient who survived many recurrent attacks when treated with glucose, phenothiazines, and propranolol but who, after hematin was introduced, experienced flurries of attacks and a fatal outcome despite six courses of hematin. A recent report by King and Bragdon described hematin therapy that produced clearing of psychosis and colic as well as reversal of white matter demyelinized lesions on magnetic resonance imaging that they felt might be vascular in origin. Although the white matter lesions vanished, perhaps the needed porphyrin replacement was not possible since the quadriparesis remained. Follow-up in this case and others will be very important, as the role of hematin in the nervous system is unclear.

Many authors have called attention to the similarities between AIP attacks and lead poisoning. Both disorders induce D-ALA-D and produce marked porphyrinuria. In lead poisoning there is no URO-S block as in AIP. Lead poisoning, after the sulfhydryl groups are exhausted, causes the porphyrins to assume a chelation role in which zinc is replaced by lead in the porphyrin molecule and then the toxic lead complex is excreted from the body.

D-ALA-D activity increases in response to the porphyrin deficit in the nervous system, which deficit accounts for the neurologic symptoms in plumbism. In AIP attacks there is also induction of D-ALA-S, which produces more precursors to make up for the block in URO-S activity and to replace porphyrins removed from or not replaced in the nervous system.

Attempts to use hematin for lead poisoning have demonstrated that it does not work, and this may be because its action is to shut down D-ALA-D, and thereby the production of precursors needed to restore porphyrins to the nervous system. The advisability of using hematin to treat lead poisoning—or severe AIP attacks—seems very debatable.

By contrast, IV EDTA, with or without BAL, is effective for lead poisoning, and, in our experience, for the treatment of AIP attacks when the nervous system is involved. The outlook for AIP patients should be good: if precipitating causes of attacks are eliminated most can expect to lead a normal existence without relapses or early death. Those with severe neurologic symptoms that require additional measures should be treated as if they had a severe case of lead poisoning, using a complexing agent, and they should respond positively, as we have seen in more than two-thirds of the patients treated in this manner.

SUGGESTED READING

King PH, Bragdon AC. MRI reveals multiple reversible cerebral lesions in an attack of AIP. Neurology 1992; 41:1300–1302.

Moore MR, McColl KEL, Rimington C, Goldberg A. Disorders of porphyrin metabolism. New York: Plenum, 1987:110–114.

Mustajoki P: New therapeutic approach to hepatic porphyrias. Presented in a workshop held in Basel, Switzerland, October 12, 1986.

Peters HA, Cripps DJ, Gocmen A, et al. Turkish epidemic hexachlorobenzene porphyria. A 30-year study. Ann NY Acad Sci 1987; 514:183–190.

Silberberg DH, Schutta HS. The effects of unconjugated bilirubin and related pigments on cultures of rat cerebellum. J Neuropathol Exp Neurol 1967; 26:272.

REYE'S SYNDROME

DAVID A. STUMPF, M.D., Ph.D.

DIAGNOSIS

Reye's syndrome (RS) is a metabolic encephalopathy. Typically a catabolic process triggers RS; viral infections and fasting (often together) are common antecedents. Anorexia and vomiting are followed by progressive deterioration in the level of consciousness. Decorticate posturing will, with continued progression, deteriorate to decerebrate posturing and then flaccidity. With posturing, respiratory compromise develops, necessitating intubation and ventilation. Characteristic laboratory changes include hyperammonemia, elevated liver enzymes, prolonged coagulation parameters, lactic and fatty acidemia, and, particularly in young persons, hypoglycemia. Bilirubin is normal. This picture is easily discernible, making the diagnosis relatively straightforward. Liver biopsy is the "gold standard" and is helpful in doubtful cases or research protocols. Staging (Table 1) is helpful in determining the intensity of therapy required.

ETIOLOGY

RS has many potential causes. Most commonly it follows a viral illness. Host and viral factors contribute. The antecedent catabolic state exhausts glycogen stores and requires the host to switch metabolism to fatty acids and protein. Some hosts may have underlying metabolic disorders of fatty, amino, or organic acid catabolism that are "unmasked" by the catabolic illness. Influenza and varicella are the most common viral precipitants in the United States. There are probably strain differences in influenza that account for variations in RS severity of different epidemics.

Certain toxins are also implicated in RS. Reye's-like syndromes were noted with ingestion of hypoglycin (Jamaican vomiting sickness), aflatoxins (Thailand), and bonkrekate (Indonesia). Herbal remedies and fermented concoctions should raise suspicions about toxins. Aspirin use was *associated* with RS in the United States. Valproate and hopantenate (Japan) are other drugs associated with a Reye's-like syndrome.

The metabolic derangements in RS are all referable to the mitochondria. Inborn errors of amino, organic, and fatty acid metabolism also adversely affect mitochondrial metabolism, producing RS or Reye's-like illnesses. Thus, RS is now regarded as a mitochondrial encephalopathy. The precise sequence of metabolic events in RS remains unclear. This ambiguity exists because, just as some fundamental issues were being clarified, severe RS nearly disappeared. The insights we now have are hypotheses, largely untested because of the paucity of patients. Nonetheless, we have some general concepts.

Mitochondria are globally disturbed in RS, and many mitochondrial enzyme activities are reduced. Is this a fundamental impairment of biogenesis or a disruption of normally constituted mitochondria? An early event is depletion of carnitine. The rate of carnitine loss in the urine is very high and within several days would produce nearly total depletion. The associated high levels of acyl CoA could inhibit a variety of mitochondrial enzymes, thereby producing the secondary metabolic events (Table 2).

CONFOUNDING VARIABLES

A number of features of RS—given little attention in most reviews—confound our notions about treatment. Reye's syndrome has changed over the years—its incidence, severity, and response to therapy.

Incidence Variation

RS first reached medical consciousness as a discrete entity in 1963, though in retrospect, we can see it in earlier reports. Its incidence declined after 1985. Some in the United States have attributed this to reduced use of aspirin, but this notion does not explain some other observations. RS occurred (and receded in incidence) in countries where aspirin was little used. In countries where aspirin use is widespread, such as Japan, the incidence of RS also declined, despite a constant pattern of aspirin use. We are cognizant of similar long-term variations in other "parainfectious" syndromes, such as postencephalitic Parkinson's syndrome and streptococcal complications. These variations seem to reflect changes in the infectious agents between epidemics.

Severity Variation

RS is not the same each year. Some years it is mild, producing modest levels of coma and incapacity. In other

Table 1 Staging in Reye's Syndrome

Stage	Level of Consciousness	Respirations	Responses	Progress of Therapy
I	Lethargy, drowsiness	Normal	Normal	20% glucose
II	Disorientation, delirium	Hyperventilation	Agitation	Intubation
III	Obtundity	Hyperventilation	Decorticate posturing	Assisted ventilation
IV	Coma	Cheyne-Stokes respirations	Decerebrate posturing	Mannitol/glycerol, hyperventilation
V	Deep coma	Apnea	None, flaccidity	Consider withdrawing therapy

Table 2 Locus of Metabolic Derangements

Abnormality	Mechanism	Metabolic Site	Therapy
Hypoglycemia	Reduced gluconeogenesis, excessive glycolysis	Pyruvate carboxylase*	Hypertonic glucose, mitochondrial support (B vitamins, carnitine)
Hyperammonemia	Impaired urea cycle	N-acetylglutamate synthase*; ornithine transcarbamylase	Protein restriction, glucose, carnitine
Lactic acidosis	Excessive glycolysis (Crabtree effect) and impaired oxidative catabolism	Pyruvate dehydrogenase complex*	Restore oxidative metabolism (probable role of carnitine, B vitamins)
Elevated fatty acids	Excessive lipolysis; reduced oxidation	beta-Oxidation*	Restrict dietary fat; reverse catabolic state (glucose infusion)
Coagulopathy	Reduced protein synthesis	Coagulation cascade	Vitamin K, fresh-frozen plasma

*Affected by high acyl CoA esters.

years, the coma is deep. However, the level of coma does not tell the entire story.

Variable Response to Therapy

There have been years (e.g., 1976) when, though coma was deep—previously considered a grim prognostic indicator—full recovery was common. Treatments were not uniform at that time, and novel approaches were being attempted in different institutions. Lacking randomized studies, investigators concluded their new therapies were producing the recovery from deep levels of coma. That year we read rave reviews of barbiturate coma, exchange transfusion, and other strategies. Unbeknownst to these investigators, elsewhere physicians who used standard interventions were having similar good fortune. The next year, the novel therapies proved ineffectual: it was a bad year and deep coma correlated with poor outcome.

THERAPY

RS is a potentially fatal disorder. The critical neurologic events are the mitochondrial failure and its attendant cerebral edema; equally critical are the secondary compromise of vital cardiovascular and respiratory functions.

Initial Evaluation

Patients suspected of having RS on the basis of the clinical history, elevated liver enzymes, and ammonia, should be admitted to hospital. Deterioration can occur rapidly; monitoring should be frequent. The initial phase of RS provides the best opportunity for diagnosis of underlying causes. The workup also includes key factors for determining the severity of the metabolic derangements. Blood and urine samples are collected (Table 3). Samples for special metabolic testing are refrigerated until they can be transported to the appropriate laboratory. Computed tomography (CT) is helpful only in excluding other factors; in RS it reveals the small ventricles and effaced sulci associated with cerebral edema. Lumbar puncture carries an extra risk in RS and generally is not necessary. It reveals only increased

Table 3 Diagnostic Evaluation*

Confirm diagnosis and follow disease course
  Liver enzymes, liver biopsy
  Glucose
  Ammonia
  Free fatty acids
  Coagulation panel

Possible underlying causes
  Urine organic acids
  Urine and blood amino acids
  Urine and serum carnitine studies
  Salicylate level
  Biotinidase

Evaluate differential diagnoses
  CT
  Toxic screen
  Lead level
  Alpha$_1$-antitrypsin
  Urine orotic acid
  Bilirubin

Monitor for complications
  Blood gas monitoring
  Fluid and electrolyte monitoring
  Amylase
  Electrocardiography

*Blood/serum unless indicated.

pressure and glucose changes that parallel those in blood. Routine hematologic and chemical profiles are necessary on admission and daily thereafter.

Metabolic Therapy

Reversing the catabolic state is critical. Temperature should be normalized with acetaminophen or cooling blanket. Infusion of a 50 percent glucose bolus (1 g per kilogram) is used to reverse the initial hypoglycemia. Many subsequently utilize 10 percent dextrose because it requires a peripheral intravenous (IV). More aggressive therapy is indicated in RS. A constant central venous infusion of the "St. Louis" formulation is used: 20 percent glucose with 40 mEq sodium chloride, 15 mEq potassium acetate, 15 mEq potassium phosphate and one ampule of multivitamins per liter. When this is infused at 1600 ml per square meter, the serum glucose value will range between 250 to 350 mg per deciliter; this high level is desirable in RS, because it facilitates interruption of catabolic processes and reduces the use of proteins and fats as fuels. Glucose concentration of the infusate is adjusted as necessary to maintain this hyperglycemia. Carnitine (Carnitor) is also recommended, in doses of 100 mg per kilogram per day. IV carnitine is preferable but generally not available. Carnitine should be given early, before ileus develops, via nasogastric tube. Malate may also facilitate reduction of acyl CoA metabolites, but thus far it has only a limited track record with organic acidemias. Vitamin K, 1 mg IV or 5 mg IM daily, reverses coagulation abnormalities. B vitamins play many essential roles in mitochondria.

Intensive Care

RS is an ideal condition for intensive care unit (ICU) management: the critical elements are severe but all potentially reversible with aggressive management. Vital functions often require support, particularly ventilation. With onset of coma, elective intubation is desired. A T tube is sufficient initially. Ventilatory support is increased as the condition deteriorates. Posturing interferes with ventilator management and raises intracranial pressure; minimizing stimulation is indicated.

Intracranial Pressure

Cerebral edema is the life-threatening pathophysiologic event in RS. It is likely a mixture of angiogenic and cytotoxic edema, as both are precipitated by mitochondrial failure. The major issue is, however, cytotoxic edema. The main objective of treatment is reversing the critical metabolic events (as described). Other treatments are often needed, and effective: these include hyperventilation and the use of osmotic agents. Hyperventilation seeks to maintain the $Paco_2$ at 20 to 25 torr. Mannitol is commonly used in RS. Bolus mannitol doses of 0.25 to 3.0 g per kilogram treat acute deteriorations; constant infusions of 4 to 6 g per kilogram per day generally suffice in stabilized patients. Barbiturates lower metabolic demands and lower intracranial pressure in RS; however, barbiturates block mitochondrial respiration, and in some clinical trials produced a worse outcome in RS. Steroids have no proven benefit in RS.

The cerebral edema of RS often is not generalized. Brain*stem* swelling, associated with posturing and apnea, can occur with fundal venous pulsations and normal intracranial pressure monitor recordings. Recognition of these events requires clinical observation, an exercise that sometimes is discouraged in the ICU, where paralytic agents, sedation, and monitoring devices are emphasized. The monitor readings should not lull caregivers into inaction in the face of a deteriorating clinical picture.

Complications

Respiratory and circulatory compromise, the most common complications, are discussed above. A meta-

bolic *cardiomyopathy* may coexist and require specific therapy for congestive failure or arrhythmias. *Pancreatitis* can aggravate the metabolic derangements and produce significant abdominal and fluid management problems.

Recovery

Prompt metabolic therapy in stage I of RS generally carries an excellent prognosis. Further progression is not likely. In comatose patients, improvement generally occurs within 1 to 4 days. Metabolic therapy is withdrawn slowly over about a day.

FOLLOW-UP AND OUTCOME

The RS mortality rate varies between 5 and 20 percent, between epidemic years and various centers. When health care systems are slow to institute therapy, the mortality rate is 50 percent. If complications can be successfully managed in the intensive care setting, prognosis for survivors' neurologic function is excellent. Cognitive testing shows normal IQ, although some subtle educational problems may occur. Fortunately, RS recurrence is rare. During catabolic episodes, however, vigilance should be increased. It is to be hoped that altered mental status would trigger prompt intervention in the earliest stages that would interrupt the catabolic state and prevent progression. Recurrence suggests an underlying host metabolic disorder; because these are frequently recessively inherited, siblings are at similar risk and require more vigilance for early RS.

SUGGESTED READING

DeVivo DC. Reye syndrome. Neurol Clin 1985; 3:95–115.
Lovejoy FH, Smith AL, Bresnan MJ, et al. Clinical staging in Reye's syndrome. Am J Dis Child 1974;128:36–41.
Matsuishi T, Stumpf DA, Chrislip K. The effect of malate on mitochondrial propionate toxicity. Biochem Med Metabol Biol 1991;46:177–184.
NIH Concensus Conference. Diagnosis and treatment of Reye's syndrome. JAMA 1981;246:2441–2444.
Shaywitz BA, Lister G, Duncan CC. What is the best treatment for Reye's syndrome? Neurology 1986;43:730–731.
Stumpf DA, Parker WD, Angelini C. Carnitine deficiency, organic acidemias, and Reye's syndrome. Neurology 1985; 35:1041–1045.
Trauner DA. What is the best treatment for Reye's syndrome? Neurology 1986; 43:729.

PATIENT AND FAMILY RESOURCE

National Reye's Syndrome Foundation
Box 829
426 N. Lewis
Bryan, Ohio 43506
(800) 233-7393

HEPATIC COMA AND PORTAL-SYSTEMIC ENCEPHALOPATHY

MONROE COLE, M.D.
KEVIN D. MULLEN, M.B., F.R.C.P.I.

The syndrome of hepatic or portal-systemic encephalopathy is manifested mainly by an *alteration of consciousness,* usually on a background of chronic liver disease with portal-systemic shunting of blood. Such shunting occasionally occurs with a normal liver (Table 1). Portal-systemic shunting usually plays no role in the encephalopathy associated with acute hepatitis or fulminant hepatic failure.

Alteration of consciousness may vary from a mild confusional state to lethargy, stupor, or coma. If a reliable history is obtainable, the patient will have been noted, over the course of days or weeks (or sometimes hours if a catastrophic event such as gastrointestinal [GI] bleeding has occurred) to have decreased attention, decreased impulsion, slowed cognition, and alteration of behavior or personality, followed by more obvious evidence of confusion. Agitated confusion (delerium) is uncommon. Confusion may progress to lethargy, and eventually to coma. In some patients, however, mild to moderate confusion, alteration of personality, behavior or impulsion may simply persist, its severity fluctuating in relation to risk factors to be mentioned below. The deficits of higher cortical function may be so mild as to be virtually subclinical, depending on precision of historical data from family or employer and the finesse of the mental status examination. Certain psychometric tests such as the Reitan Trail Test, Digit Symbol Test, and Digit Copying Test, are employed in many hepatology clinics to reveal these "subclinical" patients. Other patients may develop the syndrome of chronic hepatocerebral degeneration.

Associated neurologic findings are dysarthria, incoordination, asterixis, grimacing, suck, grasp, and increased perioral reflexes. Tendon reflexes are exalted (except if peripheral neuropathy is present), plantar responses become extensor, and paratonic rigidity (*Ge-*

genhalten) is found on examination. Seizures may occur. If coma is sufficiently deep, it can mimic brain death. Neither asterixis nor the clinical picture is specifically diagnostic of *hepatic* encephalopathy in contradistinction to other metabolic encephalopathies.

Diagnosis is established on the basis of history and physical evidence of liver disease or portal-systemic shunting, plus the finding of one or more precipitating factors for hepatic encephalopathy (Table 2). Other causes of alteration of consciousness need to be considered. If no such cause is demonstrated and the patient responds to the therapeutic regimen outlined below, the diagnosis is established.

Although the exact role of ammonia metabolism in the pathogenesis of the syndrome may be argued, we are loathe to make the diagnosis, except with fulminant hepatic failure, unless we are able to demonstrate a serum arterial ammonia value greater than 120 μmol per liter. To obviate arterial puncture, an "arterialized" venous sample may be obtained by warming the patient's hand in 40°C water for 15 minutes before drawing blood from a distal vein. One of us (MC) continues to use a 1 hour postprandial (high-protein food such as hamburger) venous ammonia value in nonemergent clinical situations (ammonia tolerance test). Furthermore, most therapeutic measures are aimed at reducing the blood ammonia level to nearly normal.

THERAPY

The Stuporous or Comatose Patient

In our hospital we see a large population of patients who have severe liver disease. *Three simultaneous strategies are employed in all patients who come to our Emergency Department with known or suspected liver disease who exhibit significant diminution in alertness. (1) We rule out other causes of encephalopathy (Table 3). (2) A vigorous search for a precipitating cause of portal-*

Table 1 Conditions Associated with Portal-Systemic Shunts with Normal Liver Function Tests

Well-compensated cirrhosis
Surgical portal-systemic shunt
Congenital conditions: hepatic fibrosis, intrahepatic shunts, extrahepatic shunts
Splenic vein thrombosis
Portal vein thrombosis
Schistosomiasis
Idiopathic

Table 2 Precipitating Factors for Hepatic Encephalopathy

Nitrogen retention
　Gastrointestinal blood
　Constipation
　Excess dietary protein
　Azotemia

Electrolyte imbalance
　Hypokalemia

Systemic infection

Hepatic infection

Drugs
　Sedatives
　Narcotics
　Tranquilizers
　Valproic acid

systemic encephalopathy (Table 2) is undertaken. (3) We commence empirical therapy immediately (i.e., gut lavage, lactulose, and low-protein diet).

As the patient arrives, blood is immediately drawn for an 18-panel screen, full blood count, differential, platelet count, and coagulation studies. In addition to the blood tests, blood cultures are taken, one tube of serum is held for later toxicology study (both blood and urine are needed for toxicology), and another tube is saved in case studies such as a viral hepatitis serologic test are required later. This is particularly important if the patient subsequently requires massive transfusions. Any patient with signs of significant gastrointestinal hemorrhage is grouped and cross-matched for 2 to 4 units of packed red blood cells.

As we await the results of the blood tests, thiamine hydrochloride, 100 mg IV, is given routinely before commencement of a 5 percent dextrose in water infusion through a large-bore venous cannula. Concurrently, a nasogastric tube is placed and irrigated for signs of bleeding. If there is blood in the upper GI tract, ice water lavage is performed. A urethral catheter is inserted; recording of fluid input and output must be precise.

If the patient is febrile or if there are meningeal signs, lumbar puncture (LP) should be performed. Patients with advanced liver disease may be apyrexic or hypothermic. The diagnosis of meningitis should not be missed because of reluctance to do LP. We do not treat prolonged prothrombin time or diminished platelet count before a careful LP is performed by an experienced operator. When non-neurologists perform LP, they frequently neglect to record the opening pressure, a necessary item of the data. All body fluids obtained are examined and sent for culture.

Needless to say, at the same time that these measures are being made, a complete history and physical examination are obtained. Arterial blood gases and ammonia levels are also measured. Once the patient's condition is judged to be stable, a chest film and CT of the head are performed. The patient should be admitted to a medical intensive care unit.

Treatment should continue as follows:

1. Infuse with 5 percent dextrose and water at 50 cc per hour, unless the patient is hypovolemic, in which case fluid should be increased to 100 to 150 cc per hour.
2. Assess oxygenation; intubate if necessary.
3. If patient is hypotensive, infuse dopamine, 2 to 20 µg per kilogram per minute.
4. Transfuse with packed red blood cells if there is evidence of hemorrhage and the hematocrit is below 30 or there is hemorrhagic shock.
5. If there is evidence of GI bleeding, consult an endoscopist.
6. If there is blood in the GI tract it may be assumed that it is contributing to, or causing, the hepatic coma. To eliminate this protein excess, 30 to 45 g (45 to 60 ml) of lactulose should be administered via nasogastric tube thrice daily. Tap water enemas should be repeated until fluid runs clear. If the patient is not responding to therapy, and unless there is frank renal failure, metronidazole, 250 mg via nasogastric tube every 8 hours, or neomycin, 1 to 2 g every 6 hours, is added to the regimen. Neomycin is given by crushing the tablets and administering via nasogastric tube. (Our hepatology service prefers metronidazole.)
7. Sedatives should be interdicted. If the drug screen shows benzodiazepine metabolites, the specific benzodiazepine antagonist flumazenil should be administered, 0.2 mg IV over 30 seconds (Table 4).
8. Hypokalemia should be treated with potassium chloride, 15 to 40 mEq per liter, with monitoring of serum potassium every 30 to 60 minutes.
9. Hyponatremia (< 125 mEq per liter) is treated by water restriction. If the serum sodium value is less than 120 mEq per liter, furosemide, 0.5 mg per kilogram may be added. Because of reports attributing central pontine myelinolysis to rapid overcorrection of hyponatremia, correction should not proceed faster than 1.5 mEq per hour or 15 mEq per 24 hr.
10. A prolonged prothrombin time should be treated with vitamin K_1, 25 mg IM (*not* IV).

If the patient does not respond to treatment the usual explanation is (1) the wrong diagnosis has been

Table 3 Differential Diagnosis of Hepatic Encephalopathy

Diagnosis	*Procedure*
Drug toxicity	Urine screen, blood alcohol level
Meningitis	Lumbar puncture
Subdural hematoma	CT with and without contrast
Cerebral contusion	CT without contrast
Other metabolic encephalopathy	Chemistry screen, arterial gases, high sensitivity TSH, B-12, treatment with thiamine
Intracranial hemorrhage	CT, lumbar puncture
Other central nervous system (CNS) infection	VDRL test, screen for human immunodeficiency virus if risk factors warrant

Table 4 Drugs Used to Treat Hepatic Encephalopathy

Drug	Dosage	Use
Thiamine hydrochloride	100 mg/day IV 50 mg/day PO	Prevent Wernicke-Korsakoff syndrome
Dopamine	2–20 µg/kg/min (average dose)	Treat hypotensive shock
Lactulose	10–45 g t.i.d. PO (10 g = 15 ml)	Decrease colonic ammonia absorption
Neomycin sulfate	1–2 g q6h PO for 7–10 days	Decrease ammonia production
Metronidazole	250 mg t.i.d. PO for 5–7 days	Decrease ammonia production
Furosemide	20–40 mg or 0.5 mg/kg	Induce excretion of free water
Vitamin K_1	25 mg IM 10 mg PO	Correct prolonged prothrombin time
Flumazenil	0.2 mg IV over 30 sec; may use 0.2–0.5 mg/min (max. 3.0 mg)	Reverse benzodiazepine overdose

made (search for another) or (2) the patient is septic. A more vigorous search should be made for respiratory, urinary, peritoneal, bloodstream, or meningeal infection. Aminoglycosides should be avoided because of the enhanced risk of nephrotoxicity. Third-generation cephalosporins such as ceftriaxone or cefotaxime, but not moxalactam, cefoperazone, or cefamandole, should be used.

The Confused Patient

A patient who enters hospital for confusion and a patient emerging from coma are treated likewise. Lactulose, 10 to 45 g (15 to 60 ml), is administered thrice daily. The stool should be kept soft, but after the first days of treatment not diarrheal. If the patient is constipated, warm tap water enemas may be used. Digital removal of impacted feces is indicated. A retention enema of 150 ml warm mineral oil may be useful. Unless the confusion is mild and response to therapy rapid, metronidazole, 250 mg thrice daily, is given for 5 to 7 days. Alternatively, neomycin, 1 to 2 g, is given orally four times daily. Neomycin should be discontinued after 7 days.

The diet should be limited to 20 g of protein per day. The amount may be increased slowly to 50 g or more per day, depending on clinical response. The patient needs at least 2,000 calories per day. Multivitamins, thiamine supplements (50 mg per day), folic acid (3 mg per day), and vitamin K_1 (10 mg per day) should be continued. The patient and responsible caregiver should be referred to a dietitian for a specific diet plan, and they should be strongly encouraged to follow it. Compliance with the use of lactulose may be poor, but the patient should be encouraged to persevere.

Sedatives, tranquilizers, narcotics, and of course alcohol, should be interdicted. Electrolytes should be reasonably balanced and systemic or hepatic infection sought and treated.

Valproic acid and sodium valproate may cause hyperammonemia. We have seen a number of patients with the syndrome of ammonia encephalopathy in this setting. Some need not discontinue taking the anticonvulsant, because response to lactulose is gratifying.

Chronic Hepatocerebral Degeneration

Treatment is the same as for confused patients. Constipation should be prevented and the colonic contents acidified with lactulose, 15 to 50 ml per day, depending on clinical response and maintenance of at least one (preferably two) soft but not diarrheal stools per day. The diet should contain at least 2,000 calories, with 50 g of protein, per day. Episodes of acute hepatic encephalopathy, which often punctuate the course, should be treated as described above.

Other Causes of Hepatic Encephalopathy

Other hepatic encephalopathies mainly affect children. These include the inherited hyperammonemic syndromes secondary to urea cycle disorders and the Reye-Johnson syndrome. We have not personally treated any of these pediatric disorders and will not comment further about them.

Use of Flumazenil

A number of reports in the European literature address the beneficial effects of the benzodiazepine antagonist flumazenil in the treatment of hepatic encephalopathy. No controlled double-blind study has yet been reported. One of us (KM) used the drug in one patient with good results, but it was not clear whether the encephalopathy was due to exogenous benzodiazepines. Flumazenil is now available in the United States.

SUGGESTED READING

Ferenci P, Grimm G, Meryn S, et al. Successful long-term treatment of portal-systemic encephalopathy by the benzodiazepine antagonist flumazenil. Gastroenterology 1989; 96:240–243.

Grimm G, et al. Improvement of hepatic encephalopathy treated with flumazenil. Lancet 1988; 2:1392–1394.

Jones EA, moderator. The gamma-aminobutyric acid A (GABA$_A$) receptor complex and hepatic encephalopathy: Some recent advances. Ann Intern Med 1989; 110:532–546.

Mullen KD. Hepatic encephalopathy. In: Rector WG Jr, ed. Complications of chronic liver disease. St. Louis: Mosby–Year Book, 1992.

Raiford DS, Mitchell MC. Disorders of drug disposition. In: Rector WG Jr, ed. Complications of chronic liver disease. St. Louis: Mosby–Year Book, 1992.

Victor M, Adams RD, Cole M. The acquired (non-Wilsonian) type of chronic hepatocerebral degeneration. Medicine 1965; 44:345–396.

PATIENT RESOURCE

American Liver Foundation
998 Pompton Avenue
Cedar Grove, New Jersey 07009
(800) 223-0179

MITOCHONDRIAL ENCEPHALOMYOPATHY

DONALD R. JOHNS, M.D.

The mitochondrial encephalomyopathies are a diverse group of neurologic disorders associated with structural, biochemical, or genetic evidence of mitochondrial dysfunction. The description of the molecular genetic basis of these disorders has seen rapid progress since the first human mitochondrial DNA (mtDNA) deletion was discovered in 1988. These molecular genetic advances have had a profound impact on the diagnosis of the mitochondrial encephalomyopathies but to date have had less therapeutic impact. Here, I outline my current approach to the care and treatment of these patients.

MAJOR CATEGORIES OF MITOCHONDRIAL DISEASE

I first review selected diagnostic and nosologic features of some of the major categories of mitochondrial encephalomyopathy, with the caveat that many times the clinical presentation is partial or an overlap of syndromes that does not easily fit a single diagnostic category. Chronic progressive external ophthalmoplegia (CPEO) patients present with ptosis and symmetric weakness of extraocular muscles, usually in association with limb myopathy and a variable number of neurologic and somatic features (CPEO-plus). Kearns-Sayre syndrome is one well-defined category of CPEO-plus. Some 50 to 90 percent of CPEO patients, depending on the presence of other features (especially pigmentary retinopathy), exhibit a large mtDNA deletion in skeletal muscle.

The hallmark of the mitochondrial encephalomyopathy, lactic acidosis, and stroke-like episodes (MELAS) syndrome is stroke-like events that occur in the setting of prolonged focal seizures or severe vascular headache. Seizures are virtually always present, and the lactic acidosis may be mild and intermittent. Several of our

Table 1 Neurologic Manifestations of Mitochondrial Encephalomyopathy

Ptosis and ophthalmoparesis
Myoclonus
Seizures
Stroke-like episodes
Optic neuropathy
Sensorineural hearing loss
Pigmentary retinopathy (atypical)
Myopathy
Exercise intolerance and fatiguability
Peripheral neuropathy
Ataxia
Vascular headache
Developmental delay
Dementia

recent cases of MELAS syndrome were initially misdiagnosed as herpes simplex encephalitis. A number of neurologic manifestations common to many mitochondrial diseases are also seen in the MELAS syndrome (Table 1). Eighty percent of MELAS syndrome cases are due to a point mutation in the mitochondrial tRNA-leucine (UUR) gene at position 3,243 that can be readily detected in muscle, urine, and blood.

Myoclonic epilepsy and ragged red fibers (MERRF) is the third major mitochondrial encephalomyopathy whose molecular basis was identified. The major neurologic manifestations are myoclonic seizures and mitochondrial myopathy; the accompanying symptoms vary (see Table 1). MERRF is associated with a point mutation in the mitochondrial tRNA-lysine gene at position 8,344 that can be detected in muscle, urine, and blood.

Leber's hereditary optic neuropathy (LHON) is characterized by severe, subacute vision loss that is painless. Men are affected much more frequently than women (male-female ratio 2:1 or 3:1) and the majority of molecularly verified cases occur sporadically. There appears to be significant interplay between a genetic predisposition (mtDNA mutations) and environmental precipitating factors (especially alcohol and tobacco) in the pathogenesis of LHON. The differential diagnosis includes atypical optic neuritis and toxic-nutritional amblyopia. Several mtDNA mutations, which can be readily detected in blood, have been linked to LHON.

In addition to the disorders discussed above, a

number of novel mitochondrial disease phenotypes have been identified on the basis of mtDNA defects. The syndrome of peripheral neuropathy, ataxia, and typical retinitis pigmentosa (NARP) has been associated with an mtDNA point mutation in the adenosine triphosphatase 6 gene at position 8,993. Recently, this mutation, when present in a large proportion, has been linked to Leigh's disease. We have identified a family with acute optic neuropathy and myelopathy who exhibit point mutations in mtDNA tRNA-aspartate and cytochrome oxidase subunit II. A maternally inherited syndrome of mitochondrial myopathy and hypertrophic cardiomyopathy is associated with an mtDNA mutation in the tRNA-leucine (UUR) at position 3,260.

DIAGNOSTIC EVALUATION

Consideration of the possibility of a mitochondrial encephalomyopathy hinges on recognition of characteristic clinical features (see Tables 1 and 3), laboratory findings (Table 2), or a maternal pattern of inheritance. Skeletal muscle biopsy is the crucial diagnostic procedure, but a number of preliminary tests may precede it. Determination of the levels of lactate and pyruvate in blood and cerebrospinal fluid must be performed with technically correct collection and analysis procedures. These levels should be determined under consistent conditions, such as fasting or after a standardized exercise protocol. Nuclear magnetic resonance spectroscopy using phosphorus-31 can be used as a noninvasive method of assessing the status of high-energy phosphates in brain and skeletal muscle, but it is not routinely available.

Many of the mitochondrial encephalomyopathies have prominent neuro-ophthalmic manifestations, and referral to an experienced neuro-ophthalmologist may be invaluable. Nerve conduction studies may reveal evidence of peripheral neuropathy, and electromyography may detect non-inflammatory myopathy. Computed tomography (CT) or magnetic resonance imaging (MRI) may reveal previously unsuspected infarcts or basal ganglia calcification. Lumbar puncture may show an elevated level of cerebrospinal fluid (CSF) protein.

Skeletal Muscle Biopsy

Skeletal muscle biopsy provides material for morphologic, biochemical, and molecular genetic analysis.

Table 2 Laboratory Abnormalities in Mitochondrial Encephalomyopathy

Lactic acidemia
Ragged red fibers in skeletal muscle
Elevated cerebrospinal fluid (CSF) protein
Cerebral infarcts (posterior predominant, not in vascular territory)
Basal ganglia calcification
Myopathic potentials on electromyography
Axonal and demyelinating peripheral neuropathy on nerve
   conduction studies

Light microscopic studies should include the modified Gomori trichrome stain and a battery of oxidative stains (including succinate dehydrogenase, NADH, and cytochrome oxidase), to detect the hallmark ragged red fibers. Ultrastructural studies may reveal abnormal proliferating mitochondria and characteristic intramitochondrial inclusions.

Biochemical testing can confirm and localize a defect in oxidative phosphorylation. These studies may be performed on frozen tissue (enzymatic and spectrophotometric analyses), which can be shipped to a distant facility for analysis, or on fresh tissue (by oxygen electrode polarography, which can be performed on site only at a few highly specialized centers).

Molecular genetic analysis of mtDNA is the most specific testing available for the diagnosis of the mitochondrial encephalomyopathies, but it cannot be used as a screening method. These tests are all readily performed on skeletal muscle, and the pathogenetic mtDNA point mutations in MELAS syndrome, MERRF, and LHON can also be detected without resorting to biopsy (in blood and urine). Deletions of mtDNA are reliably detected only in muscle, by Southern blot analysis and the widely interspaced primer polymerase chain reaction method.

THERAPY

Detection and Correction of Comorbid Features

A number of signs and symptoms in the mitochondrial encephalomyopathies contribute significantly to their morbidity, and these should be rigorously pursued and corrected (Table 3). Seizures should be treated with carbamazepine or phenytoin if parenteral therapy is required; phenobarbital is avoided. Myoclonus may respond to clonazepam. Vascular headache in the proband or in oligosymptomatic relatives should be treated with calcium channel blockers (e.g., verapamil, sustained-release 120 to 480 mg per day). Ptosis surgery should be performed only by an experienced oculoplastic surgeon who is aware of the need for undercorrection, to avoid disabling exposure keratitis secondary to facial muscle weakness.

Virtually every organ system can be affected by mitochondrial encephalomyopathy, and referral to the appropriate specialist is warranted. Cardiology consultation can be particularly important, as the heart manifestations may be life threatening.

Avoiding Inappropriate Therapy

In addition to having direct therapeutic implications, establishing that the correct diagnosis is mitochondrial encephalomyopathy avoids inappropriate therapy for the wrong condition. For example, treatment for myasthenia gravis in chronic progressive external ophthalmoplegia or anticoagulation in the MELAS syndrome. Molecular genetic techniques may expedite the diagnostic workup and thereby avoid risks and complications of unnecessary procedures, such as angiography in the MELAS syndrome.

General Recommendations

Because energy metabolism is compromised in patients with mitochondrial encephalomyopathy, overexertion to the point of fatigue and exhaustion must be avoided. Patients are advised to avoid prolonged fasting and to eat frequent light meals. Fever is treated aggressively with acetaminophen, and aspirin is avoided. When antibiotic treatment is required, chloramphenicol and tetracycline should be avoided because of the toxicity to mitochondria.

Pharmacologic Therapy

Our knowledge of the specific pharmacotherapy of the mitochondrial encephalomyopathies is limited by several factors, including their variable natural history (especially MELAS syndrome) and their relative rarity. The availability of molecular genetics–defined cases may provide an appropriate study population for future clinical trials. Our current knowledge is dominated by anecdotal experience and clinical trials with small numbers of patients. Nevertheless, rational treatments have been based on our knowledge of oxidative phosphorylation and intermediary metabolism.

Pharmacologic therapy is aimed at circumventing the biochemical deficit and preventing the secondary deleterious effects (e.g., accumulation of reactive oxygen free radicals). Because one underlying principle is to avoid toxicity, many agents are naturally occurring compounds. Therapeutic monitoring can be accomplished by observing the clinical response, changes in the levels of lactate and pyruvate at rest and with standardized exercise, and by phosphorus-31 nuclear magnetic resonance spectroscopy.

The muscles of mitochondrial encephalomyopathy patients may be depleted of carnitine, especially if they suffer significant lactic aciduria. Repletion with L-carnitine, 2 to 3 g per day, is advocated if a low level of carnitine is documented in plasma or muscle.

Coenzyme Q_{10} (ubiquinone) has been used in a number of mitochondrial encephalomyopathy patients, in doses ranging from 60 to 300 mg per day (average 90 to 120 mg per day). The beneficial effects of coenzyme Q_{10} have been more prominent on skeletal muscle and cardiac muscle than on extraocular muscles. Large doses (300 mg per day) of coenzyme Q_{10} were used in conjunction with the oxidizeable substrate succinate, 6 g per day, to successfully treat a CPEO-plus patient. Coenzyme Q_{10} has been remarkably free of side effects, though some of our patients have complained of malodorous body secretions. Coenzyme Q_{10} does not readily cross the blood-brain barrier, and an analogue that achieves better central nervous system (CNS) penetration (idebenone) is not available in the United States.

Vitamin K_3 (menadione), an electron shuttle, has been used successfully in combination with vitamin C (ascorbate) to treat a patient with complex III disease, but menadione is no longer available in the United States. Cofactors of oxidative phosphorylation have been given in pharmacologic dosages, including riboflavin (vitamin B_2), 100 mg per day, and thiamine (vitamin B_1), 100 to 1,000 mg per day.

Free radical scavengers are used to allay the deleterious effects (e.g., lipid peroxidation) of excess free radicals that accumulate proximal to blocks in the electron transport chain. These include vitamin C (ascorbate), 2–4 g per day, vitamin E (tocopherol), 400 IU per day, and coenzyme Q_{10}, 60 to 300 mg per day. Dichloroacetate, which stimulates pyruvate dehydrogenase, has been used to treat lactic acidosis of diverse causes, including mitochondrial encephalomyopathy. In the United States, however, it is not available for routine use.

Corticosteroids are used in every neurologic condition for which effective therapy is not available, and the mitochondrial encephalomyopathies are no exception. Steroids have had "anecdotal success" in the treatment of MELAS syndrome but have had profoundly delete-

Table 3 Conditions Comorbid with Mitochondrial Encephalopathy

Condition	Detection Method	Treatment
Sensorineural deafness	Audiogram	Hearing aids
Cardiac conduction disease	Electrocardiography (ECG), Holter monitoring	Pacemaker
Diabetes mellitus	Hemoglobin A_1C	Insulin or diet
Cardiomyopathy	Echocardiogram	Medication
Hypoparathyroidism	Calcium, phosphate	Medication
Cataracts	Ophthalmic examination	Surgery
Episodic nausea and vomiting	Electrolytes	Repletion
Intestinal pseudo-obstruction	Radiography, endoscopy	
Renal disease	Blood urea nitrogen, creatinine Urine amino acids	Dialysis
Hepatic disease	Liver function tests	
Short stature	Measurement	

rious effects on a CPEO-plus patient. Impaired glucose tolerance is common in these diseases, and the glucose value must be monitored vigilantly during steroid therapy.

Genetic Counseling and Therapy

The "genetics" of the mitochondrial encephalomyopathies is complicated, owing to the genetic composition of oxidative phosphorylation complexes by nuclear DNA and mtDNA-encoded proteins that must interact in a very precise manner. Most cases of CPEO-plus are sporadic, so relatives are not at increased risk. Exceptional autosomal-dominant CPEO cases have been noted to be due to a defect in a nucleus-encoded factor involved in the maintenance of mtDNA fidelity. MERRF is maternally inherited, but there is a wide spectrum of clinical manifestations among maternal relatives. MELAS syndrome is also maternally inherited, but in any family only one or a few individuals tend to be overtly affected and most relatives have a partial, oligosymptomatic condition. LHON is strictly maternally inherited, but our extensive studies of molecular genetics–confirmed cases reveal that in most families only one person is affected. One powerful genetic counseling principle for maternally inherited disorders is the impossibility of paternal transmission: affected males can be confidently assured that they will not pass the condition to their offspring.

Our knowledge of the precise molecular basis of the mitochondrial encephalomyopathies is advancing rapidly, and ultimately this information may guide effective genetic therapy. In the interim, genetic systems such as the ρ^0 mtDNA-depleted cell lines may provide an important model in vitro in which to study the effects of pharmacologic agents on disordered oxidative phosphorylation.

SUGGESTED READING

Argov Z, Bank WJ, Maris J, et al. Treatment of mitochondrial myopathy due to complex III deficiency with vitamins K_3 and C: A ^{31}P-NMR follow-up study. Ann Neurol 1986;19:598–602.

Bresolin N, Bet L, Binda A, et al. Clinical and biochemical correlations in mitochondrial myopathies treated with coenzyme Q_{10}. Neurology 1988; 38:892–899.

Przyrembel H. Therapy of mitochondrial disorders. J Inher Metabol Dis 1987; 10:129–146.

Wallace DC. Diseases of the mitochondrial DNA. Ann Rev Biochem 1992; 61:1175–1212.

PATIENT RESOURCE

Muscular Dystrophy Association
3561 East Sunrise Drive
Tucson, Arizona 85718
(602) 592-2000

Molecular genetic testing of mitochondrial encephalomyopathies:
Donald R. Johns, M.D.
Johns Hopkins Hospital
600 N. Wolfe Street, Meyer 6-119
Baltimore, Maryland 21287-7619

INHERITED NEURODEGENERATIVE DISEASE OF CHILDHOOD

STEPHEN L. KINSMAN, M.D.
SAKKUBAI NAIDU, M.D.

Two major influences have dramatically enhanced our ability to search for and diagnose inherited neurodegenerative diseases: (1) increased awareness of the wide spectrum of presentations of these disorders through advancements in our knowledge of them, and (2) more widespread access to the biochemical and molecular biologic tools for diagnosing the disorders, even preclinically through carrier detection and prenatal diagnosis. These two influences have increased our appreciation that in some cases different metabolic conditions can present with common clinical manifestations, owing to involvement of similar neuroanatomic, cellular, and biochemical processes. For example, the metabolic disorders homocystinuria and Marfan's syndrome with ectopia lentis may show the same clinical manifestations, even though they result from different biochemical defects. We also now know that similar chemical abnormalities may lead to rather different phenotypes. Elevated levels of very long chain fatty acids [VLCFAs] are found in patients with generalized peroxisomal diseases and the X-linked form of adrenoleukodystrophy (ALD).

Increasing scientific knowledge of the biochemical pathways involved in inherited and noninherited neurodegenerative diseases will continue to become available and eventually will lead to improved treatments. It is the clinician's job to keep a high index of suspicion that a childhood neurologic disorder might be neurodegenerative. This is not always easy. Experience has taught us that many times the diagnosis of "static encephalopathy" should be accepted with caution. Careful history or serial neurologic examinations sometimes reveals a course of slow but progressive decline in neurologic function. When doubt exists, diagnosis of a neurodegenerative disease should be actively pursued. The hard task is to

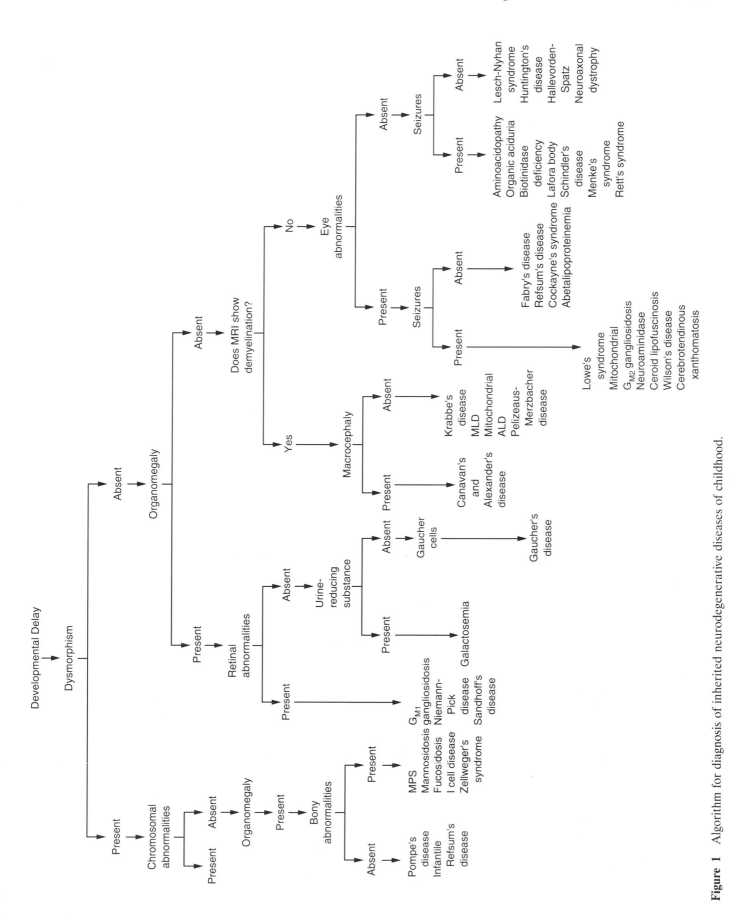

Figure 1 Algorithm for diagnosis of inherited neurodegenerative diseases of childhood.

Table 1 Ocular Abnormalities and Associated
Neurologic Disorders

Abnormality	Associated Neurologic Disorders
Kayser-Fleischer ring	Wilson's disease
Corneal opacity	Fabry's disease
	Zellweger's syndrome
	Mucopolysaccharidoses
	Lowe's syndrome
	Juvenile Gaucher's disease
	G_{M1} gangliosidosis
Cataracts	Galactosemia
	Zellweger's syndrome
	Lowe's syndrome
	Cerebrotendinous xanthomatosis
	Fabry's disease
Retinal pigmentary	Refsum's disease
degeneration	Mitochondrial abnormalities
	Zellweger's syndrome
	Neonatal adrenoleukodystrophy, infantile Refsum's disease
Cherry-red spot	G_{M1} gangliosidosis
	G_{M2} gangliosidosis
	Sandhoff's disease
	Neuraminidase deficiency with myoclonus
Macular degeneration	Ceroid lipofuscinosis
Optic atrophy	Leber's optic atrophy
	Metachromatic leukodystrophy
	Krabbe's disease
	X-linked ALD
	Canavan's disease
	Alexander's disease
	Pelizaeus-Merzbacher disease
	Neuroaxonal dystrophy
Glaucoma	Zellweger's syndrome
	Lowe's syndrome
	Homocystinuria

determine which biochemical, radiologic, and neurophysiologic tests are most appropriate for a given case. The choice of a laboratory test or tests is based on the suspected disorder and is dictated by the age of onset, presenting symptoms and signs, and the type of brain and peripheral nerve involvement. Correct diagnosis remains the critical element that allows the physician to draw on the growing array of therapeutic options. Currently there are few opportunities for empiric treatment; it must begin with an accurate diagnosis.

In order to help the clinician approach the problem of suspected neurodegenerative diseases of childhood we will (1) outline, using age-appropriate categories, clinical presentations that are helpful in focusing a diagnostic workup; (2) suggest important diagnostic tests used for evaluations, emphasizing screening tests when they are available; and (3) review the treatment strategies we use for various conditions. When suspicion of a neurodegenerative process exists, we advocate a vigorous biochemical workup to provide some information on prognosis, as well as genetic counseling, and increasingly to initiate therapy.

For this group of disorders, we suggest that tests be pursued in logical succession until, through the process of elimination, only a few biochemical tests remain to be done. It is then necessary to follow the biochemical assessment vigorously to establish the diagnosis and to provide a reasonable prognosis as well as genetic counseling for parents and siblings. The success rate of diagnosis is limited only by the current state of medical knowledge and the clinician's perseverance. A working guide is provided in Figure 1. Because eye changes reflect important associated abnormalities of the central nervous system, these are elaborated in Table 1. The biochemical abnormalities and mode of inheritance of a few of the neurodegenerative disorders are listed in Table 2. There are probably hundreds of neurodegenerative disorders, but only those for which we know a definitive treatment or treatment approach are considered here. Because certain disorders occur early and are associated with rapid progression and death, newborns and young infants should be distinguished from those who manifest illness later in life. Also, the medical management of the associated complications differs for the two groups.

NEWBORN PERIOD AND EARLY INFANCY

The clinical manifestations of neurodegenerative processes in the newborn period are often nonspecific and overlap with many non-neurologic conditions. For instance, poor feeding and lethargy, a common presentation of neonatal sepsis, can be the initial manifestation of various neonatal neurodegenerative conditions. Because some infants with metabolic disease are debilitated, infection may actually be an intercurrent illness.

Our greatest temptation as clinicians is to consider common presentations to be caused by common infections or other acute conditions. But we must remember that, collectively, the neurodegenerative diseases do account for a significant number of neurologically ill children and we will need to make these diagnoses from time to time. A family history of perinatal or infantile deaths should raise particular suspicion.

An important aspect of the neonatal diagnostic approach to the possibility of neurodegenerative disease is the vigorous attempt to establish a nondegenerative diagnosis, such as congenital infection or sepsis, to account for the presentation. Also, other metabolic disorders such as urea cycle defects, organic acidemias, and amino acidemia need to be seriously considered. It is our experience that several days are often lost while the diagnosis is assumed to be a common condition such as sepsis, when in fact a urea cycle defect exists and hyperammonemia is going untreated.

Disease Manifestations

Inherited neurodegenerative diseases of infants share common manifestations, which may include significant apathy, alteration in muscle tone, seizures, apnea, and respiratory distress. The following features provide initial guidelines for identification of a few of the disorders.

Table 2 The Biochemical Abnormalities and Mode of Inheritance of Neurodegenerative Disorders

Disease	Biochemical Defect	Mode of Inheritance
G_{M1} gangliosidosis		Autosomal-recessive
Type 1 (infantile)		
Type 2 (juvenile)	Beta-galactosidase	Autosomal-recessive
Type 3 (adult)		
G_{M2} gangliosidosis		Autosomal-recessive
Type 1 (Tay-Sachs)	Hexosaminidase A	
Type 2 (Sandhoff's)	Hexosaminidase A and B	
Type 3 (juvenile)	Hexosaminidase A (partial)	
Type 4 (adult)	Hexosaminidase A	
		Autosomal-recessive
Type 1 (previously A and B)	Sphingomyelinase	
Type 2 (previously C, D, E, and with sea-blue histiocytes)	Primary defect uncertain; secondary sphingomyelin storage	
Metachromatic leukodystrophy		Autosomal-recessive
Late infantile		
Juvenile	Arylsulfatase A	
Adult		Autosomal-recessive
Activator deficiency	Sphingolipid activator protein I	
Pseudodeficiency	Structural alteration of arylsulfatase A	
Gaucher's disease		Autosomal-recessive
Infantile		
Juvenile	Beta-glucosidase	
Adult		
Krabbe's disease		Autosomal-recessive
Infantile	Galactocerebroside beta-galactosidase	
Juvenile		
Adult		
Fabry's disease	Alpha-galactosidase	X-linked
Farber's disease	Acid ceramidase	Autosomal-recessive
Glycoproteinosis		Autosomal-recessive
Mannosidosis	Alpha-mannosidase	
Fucosidase	Alpha-fucosidase	
Aspartylglycosaminuria	Amidase	
Mucolipidosis I (cherry-red spot myoclonus)	Neuraminidase	
Mucolipidosis II (I cell disease)	N-acetyl glucosaminyl phosphotransferase	
Glycogenesis		Autosomal-recessive
Type II (Pompe's disease)	Alpha-glucosidase	
X-linked ALD	VLCFA	X-linked
Disorders of peroxisome biogenesis (e.g., Zellweger's syndrome)	VLCFA, plasmalogen synthesis, phytanic acid, bile acid intermediates	Autosomal-recessive
Canavan's disease	N-acetyl aspartic acid Aspartoacylase	Autosomal-recessive
Schindler's disease	Alpha-N-acetyl Galactosaminidase	Autosomal-recessive
Galactosemia	Galactose transferase	Autosomal-recessive
	Galactose kinase	
Lesch-Nyhan syndrome	Hypoxanthine-guanine Phosphoribosyl transferase	X-linked

Systemic Manifestations

Poor Feeding. Poor feeding results from lethargy and reduced muscle tone, which are common to many disorders, including aminoacidopathies, organic acidurias, lysosomal disorders, mitochondrial diseases with severe lactic acidosis, and peroxisomal diseases.

Vomiting. Vomiting is often persistent, particularly in conditions associated with protein intolerance after regular feeding, as well as in hyperammonemic syndromes, organic acidurias, galactosemia, phenylketo-nuria (PKU), Menkes' kinky hair disease, and Lesch-Nyhan syndrome.

Hypoglycemia. Hypoglycemia is a feature of some glycogen storage disorders but may be a concurrent abnormality in maple syrup urine disease, tyrosinemia, hypermethioninemia, methylmalonic acidemia, or congenital lactic acidosis.

Metabolic Acidosis. This feature of inherited neurodegenerative disease has a distressing generalized adverse effect on multiple systems and should prompt a search for organic acidurias, lactic acidosis, and glycogen storage diseases. Screening tests include serum amino acids, urine organic acids, serum ammonia, and serum glucose.

Body Changes

Dysmorphism. Although dysmorphism can be a feature of inherited neurodegenerative disease, chromosome aberrations and other known dysmorphic syndromes must be ruled out when making the diagnosis. In patients with the peroxisomal disorders, in particular Zellweger's syndrome, dysmorphic features are the rule. Others include mucopolysaccharidosis (MPS), G_{M1} gangliosidosis, I cell disease, and the oligosaccharidoses (mannosidosis, fucosidosis). Screening tests include plasma VLCFAs, urine spot test for mucopolysaccharides, and urine oligosaccharides.

Macroglossia. Macroglossia is seen with Pompe's disease and has also been described in G_{M1} gangliosidosis, I cell disease, hypothyroidism, and MPS.

Organomegaly. Organomegaly is not usually evident in most newborns with lysosomal disorders, although hepatomegaly may be present in severe forms of G_{M1} gangliosidosis and Wolman's disease (acid lipase deficiency). Many disorders, including glycogen storage disorders (types 1, 3, and 4) and most consistently, peroxisomal diseases and disorders such as methylmalonic aciduria, argininosuccinic aciduria, alpha$_1$-antitrypsin deficiency, tyrosinemia, hereditary fructose intolerance, and galactosemia, present in the neonatal or early infantile period with significant liver enlargement and abnormalities of liver function, including jaundice. As these disorders are also common features of intrauterine infections, those should be excluded by appropriate assay of blood titers (*Toxoplasma,* rubella virus, cytomegalovirus, and herpes simplex virus).

Abnormal Hair. Abnormal hair is a telltale sign of inherited neurodegenerative disease. The hair is sparse as well as kinky in Menkes' disease, rather pale and friable in argininosuccinicaciduria, and underpigmented in untreated PKU. Alopecia is associated with multiple carboxylase deficiency.

Nervous System Changes

Eye Abnormalities. In infantile and early juvenile presentations, abnormalities associated with the eye are particularly important, not only in terms of the symptoms they produce but because of their ability to help guide diagnostic thinking. We recommend complete eye examinations for any child suspected of having a neurodegenerative disease. An eye examination performed to establish evidence of chorioretinitis in support of intrauterine infection is essential. Cataracts are present in galactosemia, Lowe's disease, and sometimes in Zellweger's syndrome. Glaucoma is present in Zellweger's and Lowe's syndrome.

Seizures. Seizures are the most blatant evidence of central nervous system injury. Their occurrence is often overestimated in newborns. Once hypoxia and an electrolyte imbalance have been ruled out and seizures persist, other metabolic causes, such as the aminoacidopathies, organic acidurias, and peroxisomal diseases, should be strongly considered, as they often present with early seizures. It is important to identify pyridoxine dependency–induced seizures, primarily because they are treatable.

Abnormal Neuroimaging Findings. Metabolic and neurodegenerative diseases can demonstrate migrational abnormalities or white matter changes on computed tomography (CT) or magnetic resonance imaging (MRI) and have been associated with defects of structural brain development.

Treatment

As emphasized in the introduction, the first step in the management of an infant suspected of having a metabolic process is to establish its cause, so that appropriate treatment may be instituted. The management of the hyperammonemic disorders, aminoacidopathies such as maple syrup urine disease, PKU, organic acidurias, and mitochondrial disorders is beyond the scope of this chapter.

Acute Symptomatic Therapy

Hypoglycemia should be treated with 25 percent dextrose, 0.5 to 1 g per kilogram of body weight administered intravenously, and maintained at 0.5 g per kilogram per hour.

Seizures are controlled with phenobarbital, 20 mg per kilogram of body weight administered intravenously over 10 minutes, and if seizures persist, maintenance therapy is 3 to 4 mg per kilogram divided into doses taken intravenously, intramuscularly, and orally. Phenobarbital has an age-dependent half-life of 100 hours by 14 days and 20 hours by 28 days. The therapeutic range is 20 to 40 µg per milliliter, and if the blood level is 40 µg or more there is no therapeutic value in continuing phenobarbital. If seizures persist, phenytoin (Dilantin) may be added to the regimen in a dose of 20 mg per kilogram of body weight administered intravenously at a rate of 1 mg per kilogram per minute followed by 3 to 4 mg per kilogram per day. Early in the neonatal period, the age-dependent half-life is 104 hours, and 2 to 7 hours during subsequent weeks. The therapeutic range is 15 to 20 µg per milliliter. If seizures still are not controlled, diazepam may be added at 0.25 mg per kilogram administered intravenously, slowly over a 2 minute period and repeated as often as necessary. The half-life is 25 hours for preterm infants and 31 hours for term infants. Paraldehyde may be added in case of status epilepticus, in a single dose of 400 mg per kilogram administered intravenously or at 200 mg per kilogram per hour in a 5 percent dextrose solution; it can be maintained at 20 to 50 mg per kilogram per hour. The half-life is 18 hours; the therapeutic level is 100 to 200 µg per milliliter. As the half-life of these drugs is prolonged, repeated administration often is unnecessary. Blood levels should be followed in order to know whether more drug can be given if seizures continue (i.e., levels are still within or below the therapeutic range) or to identify levels that are above the therapeutic range and are contributing to coma symptoms.

Pyridoxine deficiency or dependency is established by giving 50 to 100 mg of pyridoxine intravenously during the electroencephalographic (EEG) examination. If the EEG shows the background activity to return to normal, pyridoxine therapy must be continued at 50 to 100 mg per day. If intrauterine seizures are suspected, the mother should be given a vitamin B_6 supplement of 100 mg per day. It is important to note that pyridoxine deficiency seizures can occur later in life, even beyond infancy.

Seizures and peculiar kinky and sparse hair are the key clinical features of Menkes' disease, which results from failure of copper absorption from the gut and copper transport in various tissues. It is an X-linked disease. No effective treatment is available, but according to Edwin Myer (personal communication, June 1989) attempts to increase the body's copper store with copper histidine, 500 μg per milliliter, in a daily dose of 0.5 ml given subcutaneously, beginning when the infant is 2½ months of age, have increased the serum copper level. When the infant is 10 months of age, hair color and quantity have been shown to improve, though the neurologic status does not. It seems possible that many of the adverse neurologic effects are established in utero. Because of the strict cell culture conditions required to assess labeled copper retention in amniotic cells after 24 hours, only a few laboratories attempt prenatal testing.

Hyperbilirubinemia in excess of 20 mg/dl or less in the presence of acidosis and prematurity, requires exchange transfusion. When levels of bilirubin appear to be rising early in the course of the illness, fluorescent lights alone may be beneficial.

Long-Term Therapy

For most patients with inherited neurodegenerative disease, long-term management consists of supportive care and palliation. In some patients, anticonvulsants may be required on a continuing basis; however, we discourage the use of multiple, large-doses of anticonvulsants, because of the high probability of central nervous system side effects. The degree of side effects needs to be frequently weighed against the level of seizure control. Poor swallowing requires nasogastric feeding, to be followed by gastrostomy with the Nissen fundoplication procedure, if necessary. This may also be required by patients with serious gastroesophageal reflux. Genetic counseling and prenatal testing are important components of family care and management. Symptoms of irritability and poor sleep require treatment with sedatives such as chloral hydrate, 10 to 50 mg per kilogram; pentobarbital, 5 mg per kilogram; or diphenhydramine, 2 to 3 mg per kilogram. When spasticity interferes with adaptive function or contributes to contractures, diazepam in doses of 0.5 to 10 mg may be given every 6 hours. Baclofen may be given alone or in conjunction with diazepam to alter muscle tone. The physician must be on the lookout for deterioration in oromotor function, which is manifested as increased drooling, dysphagia, and aspiration. Baclofen has the advantage of not producing sedative effects. It is added in gradually increasing doses of 5 to 20 mg every 6 hours. Dantrolene sodium in increasing doses of 12.5 mg twice daily to 25 mg every 6 hours has occasionally been helpful. Muscle spasms, which occur often in the leukodystrophies, can sometimes be blocked by bromocriptine in a dose of 1.25 mg twice daily to 5 mg every 4 hours, particularly if dystonia is an associated complication. Carbidopa 100/25 in a dose of one-half tablet per day to 1 tablet every 6 hours, or trihexyphenidyl, 2 mg twice daily to higher levels of 20 mg per day (depending on tolerance or effectiveness), have been tried, with some success. To emphasize again, drug interactions with anticonvulsants and sedative drugs are common; gastrointestinal and respiratory tract side effects should be monitored.

LATER-ONSET NEURODEGENERATIVE DISEASES

It is easier to recognize a progressive disease in patients older than 24 months of age, and with increasing age, the course is often less fulminant. Although at present most neurodegenerative diseases are incurable, many of the patients remain in a stable condition for prolonged periods and require prolonged supportive care (as described for neonates and infants). Case management of much needed patient and family services is also an important aspect of care, and the neurologist should make sure someone is providing this co-ordination service. Relief must be provided for symptoms such as seizures, poor feeding with malnutrition, dental problems, and spasticity. The identification of heterozygotes is essential for counseling parents on the risk of neurodegenerative disease in future offspring. Identifying heterozygotes has been particularly effective in Tay-Sachs disease. If a pregnancy is at risk, prenatal diagnosis by chorionic villus biopsy or amniocentesis is becoming available for an increasing number of disorders. For many of the diseases, parent support groups are available (names of some pertinent organizations are provided at the end of this chapter).

Lysosomal Diseases

Neufeld and her collaborators observed correction of the enzyme defect in mucopolysaccharidosis when skin fibroblasts from patients with the disorder were cocultured with normal skin fibroblasts. This triggered attempts to extend the phenomenon observed in vitro to treatment of patients with various lysosomal disorders. These ventures included the use of infusions of unfractionated plasma or white blood cells and the use of injections of purified enzymes from plasma, placenta, or the spleen. Subcutaneous implantation of fibroblasts and amniotic cells and organ transplants of spleen, liver, and kidney have also been attempted. Most of these procedures were not successful. Liver and kidney transplants have corrected failing function of these organs but in most instances have had no impact on overall metabolism. There is preliminary evidence that bone marrow transplantation (BMT) is of benefit for at least some of these disorders.

The aim of BMT is to provide normal white blood cells that will carry the required enzyme to the central nervous system. The technical problems with this procedure, the difficulty of obtaining an histocompatibility locus antigen (HLA)-matched donor, and the inherent risks of immunosuppression raise practical and ethical issues. Finally, because it takes time for transplanted cells to enter the nervous system, the treatment is not useful when deterioration is rapid, as it is in infantile forms of many neurodegenerative diseases. This mode of treatment has been successful in two patients with Wiskott-Aldrich syndrome. BMT has been performed for many of the forms of MPS, with variable results, some of them encouraging. BMT was extended to patients with metachromatic leukodystrophy and to a few with the juvenile form of Krabbe's disease. In patients with other conditions such as the Norrbottnian variant of Gaucher's disease, Niemann-Pick disease, Farber's disease, Lesch-Nyhan syndrome, glycogen storage disorder type II (Pompe's disease), and ALD, BMT has been attempted, with varying results, and in advanced cases the complications of transplantation have been distressing. The patients with the best outcome appear to be children who undergo the procedure early in the course of the illness and who have the least involvement of the central nervous system. Even with HLA-matched donors, the procedure has a 30 percent mortality rate, and its effectiveness in improving neurologic function remains to be established. Much of this is due to the complications of graft-versus-host disease. It is hoped that advances in immunology will reduce the morbidity and the mortality associated with this procedure. BMT may be viewed as a prelude to gene therapy. If after BMT a continuously increased level of enzyme could be shown to result in clinical improvement, this would provide strong impetus for new techniques that introduce the missing gene into the patient's own bone marrow–derived cells.

Of great practical value is the study of animal models that have lysosomal storage disease comparable to that of humans. The twitcher mouse is a model of the galactosylceramidase deficiency in Krabbe's disease. The transplantation of bone marrow from a normal animal into the twitcher mouse has resulted in prolonged survival, increased levels of the enzyme in visceral organs and the brain, and reduced levels of psychosin, the presumed toxic substance that accumulates in the brain. Globoid cells, which are the pathologic hallmark of the disease, gradually disappear, and foamy macrophages of donor origin are present in the brain, accompanied by extensive remyelination. Such favorable results are most encouraging and undoubt-edly provide new insights into the therapy of human disease states.

Considerable effort has also been directed at providing enzyme replacement therapy. The most successful results to date have come from Roscoe Brady and colleagues for the treatment of Gaucher's disease. Chemical modification of glucocerebrosidase (increasing the number of its mannose-terminated chains) has provided a means for making intravenously injected enzyme available to storage cells. They have demonstrated significant clinical gains, as evidenced by reduced hepatosplenomegaly and increased hemoglobin concentration, in their non-neuronopathic type I Gaucher's patients, but they are now beginning to study treatment of the neuropathic forms as well. Clinical trial doses for the intravenous use of mannose-terminated human placental glucocerebrosidase were 60 IU per kilogram per dose given over 1 to 2 hours every other week for 6 months. Patients may respond to smaller doses (see The New England Journal of Medicine 1992, Volume 327, pages 1632–1636, for a study using lower doses with no sacrifice of therapeutic effect). For further information on Ceredase please contact Genzyme (800-745-4447). Other storage diseases such as Fabry's disease and Niemann-Pick type B may also be amenable to this approach.

Peroxisomal Diseases

The generalized peroxisomal diseases (Zellweger's syndrome, neonatal ALD [NALD], and infantile Refsum's disease) are autosomal recessive and are marked by neonatal or early infantile onset with variable clinical progression. The X-linked form of ALD first is manifested after age 3 years, or sometimes even during adulthood. The diagnosis is based on clinical symptoms, the time of their first appearance, the mode of inheritance, and the demonstration of elevated levels of plasma VLCFAs. There is no established treatment or cure. In an attempt to ameliorate symptoms and prevent progression of illness, a dietary treatment that normalizes plasma levels of VLCFA is currently being tested. In cultured skin fibroblasts from ALD patients, the synthesis of VLCFAs was inhibited when the medium was rich in oleic acid. When ALD patients were tested with restricted intake of VLCFAs and increased intake of oleic acid to provide 60 to 75 percent of calories as fat, plasma VLCFAs were reduced 50 percent, though without significant clinical improvement. A new approach is being attempted with the addition of erucic acid to the diet mentioned above. This oil has a more powerful effect on fatty acid metabolism and has been shown to normalize plasma VLCFAs. Whether this will alleviate symptoms or prevent progression remains to be seen.

Phytanic acid is also elevated in the generalized peroxisomal diseases. As dietary restriction of phytanic acid results in considerable improvement in patients with Refsum's disease, this has also been attempted in some infants with NALD and infantile Refsum's disease, and it may help to stabilize the clinical status of some mildly affected patients.

Ceroid Lipofuscinoses

Ceroid lipofuscinoses are manifested in various forms. The *infantile* form (infantile neuronal ceroid lipofuscinosis [INCL] or Haltia-Santavouri form) often becomes symptomatic during the first year of life with microcephaly, hypotonia, myoclonic seizures, vision loss with macular degeneration, and ataxia. The diagnosis is based on a low-amplitude EEG and electroretinography (ERG) and on the demonstration of granular membrane-bound inclusions on electron microscopy of skin tissue. In the *late infantile* form (late infantile neuronal ceroid lipofuscinosis [LINCL] or Jansky-Bielschowsky form), onset usually occurs at age of 2 to 3½ years. Tonic-clonic and myoclonic seizures predominate, with vision failure, macular degeneration, retinal pigmentary changes, speech disturbance, and ataxia. Cortical atrophy on CT, low-amplitude ERG, and intracytoplasmic curvilinear bodies aid diagnosis. The *juvenile* form (juvenile infantile neuronal ceroid lipofuscinosis [JNCL] or Spielmeyer-Vogt form) begins at 5 to 6 years of age, with vision loss and clumping of retinal pigment, and macular degeneration. A few years later, insidious onset of behavior problems, mental decline, and seizures is followed by loss of speech, ataxia, and gait disturbance. Progressive deterioration of EEG findings and cortical atrophy occur. Diagnosis is established on the basis of an abnormal ERG and intracytoplasmic vacuoles with membrane-bound fingerprint-patterned inclusions in skin or rectal biopsy specimens. All of the diseases described above are transmitted in an autosomal-recessive manner. The *adult-onset* form (KUF), however, has been reported to have autosomal-recessive and autosomal-dominant forms, and it may be mistaken for Huntington's disease or Creutzfeld-Jakob disease because of the occurrence of behavioral disturbance, dementia, extrapyramidal signs, and in some patients, seizures. Considerable cortical atrophy is observed on CT; diagnosis is established by histologic examination of skin biopsy specimens and demonstration of ceroid lipofuscin accumulation in the cells.

Various therapies have been tried for this group of diseases, but none has been shown to be effective.

Wilson's Disease

Wilson's disease, or hepatolenticular degeneration, is transmitted as an autosomal-recessive trait and is characterized by reduced plasma ceruloplasmin and excessive copper deposition in tissues, notably brain and liver. Free serum copper is usually greater than 50 μg per deciliter (five times the normal level). It first manifests between ages 3 and 12 years with a slowly progressive dementia and early Parkinson's-like features, including tremor or cerebellar signs. Choreiform movements may cause confusion with Sydenham's chorea. Ocular motility may be affected, and seizures are common in the childhood-onset forms. Wilson's disease should be sought in patients who have a movement disorder and dysarthria, even if they have no history of psychiatric problems. Table 3 outlines current treatment strategies. The goal of treatment is to increase urinary copper excretion in order to achieve initial "decoppering," and then to prevent future accumulation of copper. It is important to direct treatment toward presymptomatic siblings of patients with Wilson's disease. Because they are at greatest risk (one chance in four) for Wilson's disease, they should routinely be screened.

Cerebrotendinous Xanthomatosis

Cerebrotendinous xanthomatosis is a form of normolipidemic xanthomatosis associated with dementia,

Table 3 Treatment of Wilson's Disease*

Medications†	Initial Decoppering‡	Lifelong Maintenance Therapy§	Side Effects
Penicillamine‖	Patient 10 years or older: 1 gm/day in 2–4 doses (may need to give up to 3 g); 25 mg pyridoxine daily	Same doses but less frequent monitoring	(Prevalence up to 20%)
	Patient younger than 10 years: 0.5–0.75 g/day in four doses (up to 500/mg/day); 25 mg pyridoxine daily		Urticaria, other rashes, fever, lymphadenopathy, bone marrow suppression, lupus-like syndrome, stomatitis
Triethylenetramine‖ hydrochloride (Trien)	Adults: 1 g/day in divided doses; 25 mg pyridoxine daily	Same doses but less frequent monitoring	Renal toxicity, bone marrow suppression, rashes
Zinc¶		50 mg zinc acetate t.i.d.	Very low toxicity

*Sometimes dietary (shellfish and liver) and water sources of copper must be assessed and consumption limited.

†Medications are most effective when taken between meals with water.

‡Goal of therapy is to increase copper excretion to approximately 3 g/day by titrating doses. Monitoring (see preceding footnote) should be weekly for the first 3 months.

§Goal of therapy is to eliminate copper accumulation by keeping free serum (nonceruloplasmin) copper <20 μg/dl. Monitoring can now be scheduled once every 3–12 months.

‖Monitoring should include serial neurologic examinations, complete blood counts with platelets, liver enzymes and bilirubin, abdominal examinations for hypersplenism, slit-lamp examinations, 24 hour urine copper, urinalysis, and free serum copper.

¶Zinc can be used for initial treatment of presymptomatic patients or as part of maintenance therapy in symptomatic patients.

pyramidal tract signs, cerebellar dysfunction, peripheral neuropathy, and tendon xanthomas. Seizures occur in a few patients. Menkes and associates reported the accumulation of cholestanol in the brain tissue of patients with this disorder. Salen reported that chenodeoxycholic acid excretion in bile was much reduced. The increased rate of synthesis of cholesterol precursors in bile and elevated tissue sterol concentrations are believed to be secondary to a block in chenodeoxycholic acid production with consequent loss of feedback inhibition. These authors, therefore, treated patients with chenodeoxycholic acid, 750 mg per day, and demonstrated remarkable improvements in cognitive function and pyramidal and cerebellar signs. Peripheral neuropathy was no longer detected, the EEG and brain stem auditory evoked response became normal, and CT findings improved. Plasma cholestanol levels declined, and abnormal bile acid synthesis was suppressed. In addition, the concentration of sterol and apolipoproteins A-I and B in cerebrospinal fluid declined.

Refsum's Disease

Refsum's is a rare autosomal-recessive disorder. An unusual 20-carbon, branched-chain fatty acid–phytanic acid that is of purely exogenous origin accumulates in blood and other tissues, owing to a deficiency of phytanic acid alpha-hydroxylase. The clinical features are cerebellar ataxia, peripheral neuropathy, retinitis pigmentosa, ichthyosis, nerve deafness, and nonspecific electrocardiographic changes.

Treatment consists of a diet low in phytanic acid. If carried out consistently, this can normalize plasma phytanic acid levels in 6 months. Hearing and retinal pigmentary changes are stabilized. Excessively high levels of phytanic acid can cause quadriparesis due to peripheral nerve involvement or cardiac arrhythmia. Under these circumstances, plasma exchange can bring about rapid improvement.

Abetalipoproteinemia

Abetalipoproteinemia is a lipoprotein deficiency inherited as an autosomal-recessive trait. Apolipoprotein B, which is present in chylomicrons and very–low density lipoproteins, is involved in the transport of triglycerides. In this disorder, apolipoprotein B is absent or markedly reduced. Abetalipoproteinemia is characterized by acanthocytosis, a striking abnormality in the shape of red blood cells. Associated fat malabsorption is present almost from birth and gives rise to steatorrhea. It is believed that this leads to a deficiency of vitamin E, which has been convincingly linked to the acquired neuromuscular abnormalities. Retinitis pigmentosa, sensory ataxia, and neuropathy develop gradually.

Treatment consists of restricting dietary intake of triglycerides, especially those containing long-chain fatty acids (C16–C24), and substituting the calories with protein and carbohydrate. Supplements of fat-soluble vitamins A and K are necessary for improved vision and coagulation. Vitamin E, 100 mg per kilogram per day, as a water-miscible or fat-soluble form over a prolonged period is reported to prevent progression of neuromuscular and retinal degeneration.

Multiple Carboxylase Deficiency

Multiple carboxylase deficiency can be caused by a dietary insufficiency of biotin, an abnormality of the biotin-recycling enzyme biotinidase, or a deficiency of the holocarboxylase synthetase apoenzyme. The brain normally does not recycle biotin and depends on receipt of a continued supply across the blood-brain barrier. Children with the disorder involving reduced activity of biotinidase suffer from an inability to liberate and recycle biotin during holocarboxylase turnover. An abnormality of holocarboxylase synthetase apoenzyme may also cause the disorder. In both conditions, symptoms begin by the second half of the first year of life and include seizures, ataxia, hypotonia, deafness, developmental delay, skin rash, and alopecia. It may be associated with metabolic acidosis and variable organic aciduria. In some patients, seizures may be the only presenting feature. Both enzyme deficiencies respond to biotin supplementation.

Isolated deficiencies of the mitochondrial biotin-containing carboxylases also occur. A decrease in brain pyruvate carboxylase results in a severe accumulation of lactate, early neurologic manifestations, and death. Other forms of isolated individual carboxylase deficiencies are propionicacidemia, caused by a deficiency of propionyl-coenzyme A carboxylase, and 3-methylcrotonyl-glycinuria (cat-urine odor), caused by 3-methylcrotonyl-coenzyme A carboxylase deficiency. These three disorders usually do not respond to biotin supplementation; however, protein restriction, avoidance of fasting, and general supportive measures during periods of metabolic stress are beneficial.

Treatment consists of 10 mg of biotin per day, which is 200 times the daily requirement.

Inherited Disorders of Cobalamin and Folate Metabolism

Hereditary defects in the intracellular metabolism of either cobalamin or folate can lead to neurologic dysfunction that is progressive. These disorders often present in infancy and childhood, although adult onset of symptoms has been reported. Symptoms and signs are attributable to white matter dysfunction, and MRI findings are frequently abnormal, with increased white matter signal. Seizures and cerebral ventricular dilatation are also reported frequently. Megaloblastic anemia is seen often, but not always.

These disorders are important to recognize because they are treatable. Diagnosis is made by demonstrating altered metabolites from these pathways, such as homocystinuria, methylmalonic acidemia, hypomethioninemia, and low cerebrospinal fluid concentration of S-adenosylmethionine. In cobalamin disorders, the serum vitamin B_{12} level is normal. In folate disorders, the red cell folate level is sometimes low. Details of how to diagnose and treat each specific disorder are beyond the scope of this chapter, and we refer the reader to Scriver and coworkers. Treatments include betaine, intramuscular hydroxycobalamin, L-methionine, and S-adenosylmethionine toluene sulphonate.

SUGGESTED READING

Adams R, Lyon G. Neurology of inherited metabolic diseases of children. New York: McGraw-Hill, 1982.
Brewer GJ, Yuzbasiyan-Gurkan V. Wilson disease. Medicine 1992; 71:139–164.
Opitz JM, Pullarkat RK, Reynolds JF, et al, eds. Ceroid lipofuscinosis: Batten disease and allied disorders. Suppl 5. New York: Alan R. Liss, 1988.
Scriver CR, Beaudot AL, Sly WS, Valle D, eds. The metabolic basis of inherited disease. Vols 1 and 2. New York: McGraw-Hill, 1989.

PATIENT RESOURCES

United Leukodystrophy Foundation
2304 Highland Drive
Sycamore, Illinois 60178
Telephone: (815) 895-3211

International Rett Syndrome Association
9121 Pascataway Road #2B
Clinton, Maryland 20735
Telephone: (301) 856-3334

Batten Disease Support and Research Association
2660 Parsons Avenue
Columbus, Ohio 43207
Telephone: (800) 448-4570

National Tay-Sachs and Allied Diseases Association
2001 Beacon Street, Suite 204
Brookline, Massachusetts 02146
Telephone: (617) 277-4463

National Organization for Rare Disorders (NORD)
Box 8923
New Fairfield, Connecticut 06812
Telephone: (203) 746-6518

Wilson's Disease Association
Box 75324
Washington, D.C. 20013
Telephone: (703) 636-3003; (703) 636-3014

National Gaucher Foundation
1424 K Street NW, 4th Floor
Washington, D.C. 20005
Telephone: (202) 393-2777

Lowe's Syndrome Association
222 Lincoln Street
West Lafayette, Indiana 47906
Telephone: (317) 743-3634

National Center for the Study of Wilson's Disease
5447 Palisade Avenue
Bronx, New York 10471
Telephone: (212) 892-5119

National MPS Society
17 Kramer Street
Hicksville, New York 11801

NUTRITIONAL DISEASES

SUBACUTE COMBINED DEGENERATION

JOHN LINDENBAUM, M.D.

DEFINITION

Cobalamin (vitamin B_{12}) deficiency of the nervous system is a chronic progressive disorder usually characterized first by impairment of sensation. Paresthesias in the extremities, ataxia of gait, or both symptoms are the initial and chief complaints in 90 percent of patients. Impairment of vibratory sensation, proprioception, and cutaneous touch and pain sensation (in various combinations) are the most common neurologic findings. In a minority of patients, however, other symptoms or signs predominate, including muscle weakness, memory loss, mood disorder, personality change, confusion, psychosis, anosmia, decreased visual acuity, orthostatic hypotension, impotence, urinary urgency and frequency, or urinary or fecal incontinence. The debate continues as to whether the sensory deficits that are typically seen early in the disorder reflect predominant involvement of peripheral nerve or the posterior columns of the spinal cord. In advanced cases, cortical spinal tract involvement ensues, with hyperreflexia, abnormal reflexes, and, ultimately, spastic paraparesis. The term *combined system disease* has often been reserved for patients with cortical spinal tract manifestations. These never occur in cobalamin deficiency without concomitant sensory deficits. Because the treatment does not vary with the extent of involvement of the nervous system, I discuss the management of all neurologic disorders caused by deficiency of the vitamin in this chapter.

Cobalamin deficiency of the nervous system almost always develops in a patient who has a disorder in the absorption of the vitamin. About 80 percent of patients have the adult form of pernicious anemia, the result of chronic atrophic gastritis. In others the underlying disorder of the gastrointestinal tract may be jejunal diverticulosis, tropical sprue, or resection of the stomach or ileum. Approximately 2 percent of patients develop cobalamin deficiency of the nervous system as a consequence of less severe forms of atrophic gastritis than that typically seen with pernicious anemia; these patients lack gastric acid and pepsin, although intrinsic factor secretion is still adequate and the Schilling test result is normal. Nonetheless, because of impaired acid peptic digestion of food they cannot liberate cobalamin from animal proteins to which it is bound in the diet. This is the syndrome of *food cobalamin malabsorption*. The importance of this newly recognized disorder is that the Schilling test cannot be used to rule out underlying cobalamin deficiency as a cause of nervous system damage. The Schilling test is also normal in those unfortunate dentists and anesthetists who habitually abuse nitrous oxide and develop neurologic disorders identical to those seen in cobalamin deficiency, owing to inactivation of the vitamin by the anesthetic.

RECOGNITION

Since the nervous system damage eventually becomes irreversible in neglected or mistreated patients, early recognition is crucial. In some patients, the manifestations of cobalamin deficiency are predominantly neurologic, in others predominantly hematologic. In many patients with mild or severe neurologic damage, abnormalities of the blood are remarkably slight. The hematocrit is normal in more than one quarter of cases; when present, anemia is often mild. The mean cell volume (MCV) is also normal in approximately 25 percent of patients, even in the absence of intercurrent iron deficiency. In such cases, after cobalamin therapy, the initially normal MCV may fall significantly, to a lower level but within the normal range, indicating that the MCV was actually above the usual baseline value for that patient.

With the widespread availability of automated blood counting, including the MCV, and radioassays for serum cobalamin, in current practice patients are increasingly seen during earlier stages of cobalamin deficiency. It is increasingly unusual to see the florid textbook neurologic and hematologic manifestations of cobalamin deficiency. Patients who present with cortical spinal tract signs are much less common today than those with only sensory deficits. One of the most common hematologic findings is an elevated MCV associated with normal hematocrit value, white blood cell count, and platelet count, and very minor changes on the blood smear. Most busy clinical laboratories miss the occasional hypersegmented neutrophil or macro-ovalocyte that may be found on careful examination of the blood smear. Serum LDH and serum billirubin are normal in the majority of persons who have neurologic involvement.

In most patients, the *serum cobalamin* value is low (< 200 pg per milliliter); however, in 5 percent the serum cobalamin is normal (typically in the lower end of the normal range, 200 to 350 pg per milliliter), so a normal serum level does not rule out deficiency. A more serious problem with the serum cobalamin is its lack of specificity. Approximately 50 percent of patients with nervous system disorders whose serum cobalamin value is low do not prove to be deficient in the vitamin by any other criterion; these patients' neurologic disturbance does not respond to cobalamin therapy and is due to another cause. Because of these difficulties in diagnosis, serum assays for the metabolites that accumulate when cobalamin-dependent reactions are blocked (*methylmalonic acid* and *total homocysteine*) are extremely useful for confirming the diagnosis of cobalamin deficiency. Because of their high specificity, these tests are likely to replace the Schilling test in most patients as confirmation of cobalamin deficiency. They are currently available in several national commercial laboratories. If both metabolites are normal, cobalamin deficiency is virtually ruled out. If these tests are not available, however, a therapeutic trial of cobalamin (see below) should always be considered in a patient with a neurologic disorder that is consistent with that of cobalamin deficiency.

Lack of cobalamin is common. The prevalence of pernicious anemia in the general population may be of the order of at least one in 100. It should be expected, therefore, that deficiency of the vitamin is frequently superimposed on other common disorders such as diabetic neuropathy, alcoholism, or Alzheimer's disease. Not every patient with hematologic or biochemical evidence of cobalamin deficiency and a disorder of the nervous system has a neurologic response to cobalamin therapy, even though hematologic abnormalities resolve. These patients do not necessarily have irreversible neurologic damage due to cobalamin deficiency, but they often have another underlying disorder of the nervous system.

CHOICE OF COBALAMIN PREPARATION

Cyanocobalamin (vitamin B_{12}), the most widely used cobalamin preparation, appears to be completely safe. There is no dose-related toxicity. The very rare anaphylactic reactions that have been reported are attributable to the preservatives used. A quite acceptable alternative to cyanocobalamin is hydroxycobalamin, which is widely used in Europe. Because hydroxycobalamin is better retained in the body than cyanocobalamin, maintenance therapy can be given at less frequent intervals. It has not been widely used in the United States, however, perhaps because it is somewhat more expensive than cyanocobalamin or because of concern raised by reports of

patients who developed antibodies to transcobalamin II while receiving this agent. Although these antibodies may cause prolonged elevation of the serum cobalamin level, they do not appear to be associated with failure of therapy. There is no longer any role for injections of liver extract.

Folic acid is sometimes mistakenly given along with vitamin B_{12} to treat cobalamin deficiency. There is no indication for its use in this setting, except in the emergency treatment of patients with megaloblastic anemia pending results of serum cobalamin and folate tests or other studies. Long-term use of folic acid in the treatment of cobalamin deficiency should be condemned, even if it is administered along with cyanocobalamin. Patients may neglect to receive the parenteral injections and continue to take the oral folic acid, thereby exposing themselves to the risk of neurologic damage.

ROUTE OF ADMINISTRATION

Cyanocobalamin or hydroxycobalamin can be given intramuscularly or subcutaneously. Recently, there has been renewed interest in the reintroduction of oral cyanocobalamin preparations for treatment of pernicious anemia. Studies done in the 1960s showed that, if given in doses of 1,000 µg daily, oral cyanocobalamin is as effective in maintaining hematologic and neurologic remission and a normal serum cobalamin level as monthly parenteral therapy. A tiny fraction of these very large oral doses can be absorbed by a non–intrinsic factor–dependent mechanism. Smaller oral doses are unreliable for preventing relapse. For a number of reasons, oral formulations were never widely used in the United States, although a large series of patients in Sweden have been successfully managed with such preparations. At this time, we lack adequate data to recommend oral treatment of cobalamin deficiency. Further studies are needed of currently marketed oral preparations to establish their bioavailability and efficacy. The only nonexperimental situation in which I currently use oral cyanocobalamin is in the rare patient who develops deficiency due to strict vegetarianism in the absence of any gastrointestinal disorder; such persons can be treated with as little as 50 µg cyanocobalamin daily.

DOSAGE

The therapy of the patient with cobalamin deficiency of the nervous system can be divided into two phases: (1) *immediate* and urgent correction of the presenting disorder, which should include full repletion of body stores of the vitamin, and (2) long-term *maintenance* treatment. There are numerous recommendations for immediate therapy. The often expressed opinion that some patients with cobalamin deficiency of the nervous system require much larger doses of the vitamin than those with anemia alone is anecdotal and not based on convincing observations. Indeed, it is well-documented that the nervous system disorder responds well to tiny doses of cyanocobalamin. Some authorities also argue that, since most of a large parenteral dose of cyanocobalamin is excreted in the urine, it is wasteful and unnecessary to give large amounts. Therefore, doses of the range of 30 to 100 μg are frequently recommended. No controlled studies have compared various doses of the order of 30 to 1,000 μg, however. There is also tremendous variation from patient to patient in the amount of cobalamin that needs to be given to replete body stores and in the rate at which deficiency recurs if vitamin treatment is interrupted after remission is achieved.

Given these considerations, I believe that a most important goal in the immediate treatment of cobalamin deficiency is to saturate body stores and to prevent subsequent relapse as long as possible, in the event that patients discontinue maintenance therapy at some later time, as approximately 10 to 20 percent of patients do. Even though a larger percentage of the dose will be excreted in the urine when 1,000 μg is given, the body retains a larger total amount of cobalamin than when smaller doses are injected. I therefore regularly use 1,000 μg of cyanocobalamin (1 ml of a 1 mg per milliliter preparation) as the unit dose for both immediate and maintenance therapy. I see no advantage in using a smaller dose.

There is no relationship between the frequency and intensity of immediate therapy and the rate and extent of neurologic remission. Patients treated with only a single intramuscular dose of 1,000 μg of cyanocobalamin may go into complete (although temporary) hematologic and neurologic remission.

IMMEDIATE THERAPY

In a series of 35 patients whose cobalamin treatment for pernicious anemia was interrupted, we observed that the interval before clinical relapse was significantly longer for those who had previously received at least 12 mg of cyanocobalamin. Based on these empiric observations, I currently give twelve 1 mg doses of cyanocobalamin as initial therapy for cobalamin deficiency. The schedule of these injections is not important and can be tailored to the convenience of the patient. For example, if he or she is to be hospitalized for 12 days or longer, the entire series of 12 injections can be given during that hospitalization, daily or every other day. On the other hand, if the patient is an outpatient and has neurologic abnormalities, I give one injection a week for 12 weeks. Once the entire series of twelve 1 mg injections is given, the patient can be switched to a maintenance regimen.

MAINTENANCE THERAPY

The most widely used maintenance schedules in this country call for monthly injections. Monthly dosing is not based on solid data. In fact, in the 35 patients who interrupted their maintenance cobalamin therapy and went without treatment for long periods, the mean time to relapse was more than 5 years. No patient showed any clinical sign of relapse within 21 months of interrupting maintenance therapy. Similarly, the median time to develop megaloblastic anemia following total gastrectomy in patients reported in the literature is of the order of 5 to 6 years. These clinical observations suggest that monthly injections are unnecessary. Over the past 15 years we have conducted trials of maintenance treatment with cyanocobalamin every 2, 3, or 6 months in patients with pernicious anemia. None has shown any symptoms of relapse, even on the 6 month regimen over periods of observation of more than 5 years, with the exception of one patient who developed a feeling of loss of balance while walking if she received cyanocobalamin more frequently than every 4 months. (There are no objective neurologic findings, and her gait appears normal.) However, although patients treated as infrequently as every 6 months have no complaints, they often have a low serum cobalamin level, elevated concentrations of methylmalonic acid and total homocysteine in the serum, and very slight hematologic abnormalities, indicating that they are in a borderline state of deficiency. Although there are no apparent clinical consequences to these abnormalities, in theory it is undesirable to keep patients in borderline nutritional status. Therefore, I currently recommend maintenance therapy with 1 mg of cyanocobalamin every 2 or 3 months. In England and elsewhere in Europe, a maintenance schedule of 1 mg of hydroxycobalamin every 3 months has been widely used and found satisfactory. No relapses have been reported on this every-3-months regimen.

Patients or family members can be taught to administer subcutaneous or intramuscular cyanocobalamin at home, thus decreasing the cost and nuisance of visits to a clinic or physician's office several times a year. Alternatively, a visiting nurse can provide the service.

RELAPSES

More important than specific dosing recommendations and intervals is prevention of relapse as the result of all too frequent interruptions of maintenance therapy. It should be made absolutely clear to the patient that relapse is inevitable after cessation of treatment, although the time to recurrence is quite variable (of the order of 2 to 12 years, although I do not inform patients that they may be able to go as long as a decade without treatment). It is very advisable to speak with someone close to the patient and give that person exactly the same message. The importance of follow-up visits, which I recommend be annual, lies not in the need to see a neurologist or an internist for any particular reason but mainly to ensure that there is continuing compliance.

Relapses after interruption of maintenance therapy tend to be mimetic. Patients who have had neurologic manifestations at the initial presentation of cobalamin deficiency are more likely to have neurologic symptoms on relapse than those whose nervous system was spared at the time of first presentation with megaloblastic anemia. Neurologic symptoms may be noticed by the patient who has interrupted maintenance therapy even before the serum cobalamin is subnormal or there are clear-cut hematologic abnormalities. The mimetic nature of recurrences is, however, by no means invariable. A patient who first presented with megaloblastic anemia without neurologic dysfunction is still at risk for neurologic damage if cyanocobalamin maintenance therapy is interrupted.

NEUROLOGIC EXACERBATIONS DURING EARLY THERAPY

It has long been axiomatic that although treatment with vitamin B_{12} may not reverse all neurologic deficits, the disorder does not progress during cobalamin therapy. In terms of long-term outcome this is basically correct, although in about 2 percent of patients transient exacerbation of neurologic symptoms occurs during the first month of therapy, most often worsening of the intensity and geographic extent of pre-existing paresthesias. Tingling and numbness may spread proximally in a striking fashion during the first week of injections. In two patients, we have also seen an acute psychosis during the first 12 to 72 hours after beginning vitamin B_{12}. It is uncertain whether the psychosis was related to therapy or was in some way a consequence of hospitalization. The mechanisms underlying these exacerbations are obscure; however, they have been seen only during the first 1 to 4 weeks after beginning cobalamin therapy and in each instance were followed by sustained, long-term neurologic improvement.

An apparent exacerbation has been reported during therapy in some patients whose tendon reflexes in the lower extremities were initially absent and became hyperactive during treatment. This has been interpreted as an indication of return of peripheral nerve function, which unmasks underlying cortical spinal tract degeneration.

RESPONSES TO THERAPY

Virtually all patients seen in modern practice with neurologic damage show some improvement in response to cobalamin therapy. These responses are frequently not complete, however. In about 50 percent of a large series of patients followed for an average of 3 years there were no residual neurologic signs or symptoms. The remaining patients had apparently permanent neurologic deficits, although in every instance they felt better and almost all showed substantial improvement in their neurologic status over that before therapy.

Two factors are strongly predictive of residual neurologic deficits. One is the duration of neurologic symptoms before treatment. Those who have had symptoms for more than a year are significantly more likely to have residual neurologic dysfunction. A much stronger predictor of post-treatment neurologic impairment, however, is the degree of dysfunction before therapy. Patients with minimal neurologic deficits are most likely to have complete clearing of symptoms and signs; those with extensive neurologic disease are more prone to be left with permanent residua. A weaker prognostic indicator is the hematocrit value. Curiously, the higher the hematocrit the more likely it is that the patient will have extensive neurologic deficits at presentation and residual damage after prolonged therapy. This is consistent with the view that in some patients cobalamin deficiency predominantly involves the nervous system and in others the bone marrow.

These generalizations, however, should not obscure the striking variability in patient responses and the dramatic reversal in some instances of advanced neurologic damage. In the majority of patients paresthesias clear completely or are markedly improved after therapy, as are coordination and joint position sense. Abnormalities in cutaneous sensation (touch and pain) return to completely normal in most cases. Muscle weakness and tenderness often clear rapidly. Urinary frequency, urgency, and incontinence usually improve or disappear. Absent knee jerks reappear almost invariably. In about 50 percent of patients absent ankle jerks return. Approximately half of those who have abnormal reflexes such as extensor plantar responses experience improvement or clearing. A positive Romberg's sign usually becomes negative or substantially less impressive. Most patients who are bedridden or unable to walk without assistance show substantial improvement. Fewer than 10 percent of patients have serious long-term disability (e.g., inability to walk unassisted).

For many patients, improvement in symptoms is greater than in signs. For example, even after a decade of maintenance therapy it is common to have a permanent, residual deficit in vibration sense, though it is less extensive than before treatment. Such a patient may be completely free of neurologic symptoms and merely exhibits an abnormality on the neurologic examination.

The responsiveness of disorders of cerebral function is also variable. Most acute psychoses and disturbances in mood completely resolve after cobalamin therapy. The improvement in cerebral function may be striking and rapid during the first month. This is true in many patients with dementia. In others, cognitive function shows no improvement whatsoever and continues to deteriorate slowly during therapy. In these patients, cobalamin deficiency most likely was not the underlying cause of the mental impairment but coexisted with another disorder such as Alzheimer's disease. Another pattern of response that we have seen frequently is transient improvement in cognitive function over a period of months followed by long-term deterioration. Here, cobalamin deficiency of the nervous system has most likely been superimposed on slowly progressive Alzheimer's disease. One cannot predict, therefore, whether any individual patient's cognitive function will improve. The shorter the duration of impairment, however, the more likely a response will occur.

RATE OF RESPONSE

Neurologic improvement is often rapid and commences during the first 2 weeks of cobalamin therapy; however, in a significant minority of patients, no response is noted during the first 4 to 6 weeks, and this often casts doubt on the validity of the diagnosis. Clear-cut neurologic improvement occurs, however, during the second and third months of treatment. If no response is noted within 3 months of intensive cobalamin therapy such as that recommended above, the physician can be confident that no improvement will occur later. This usually does not indicate that the patient has suffered irreversible damage to the nervous system due to cobalamin deficiency. Rather, the diagnosis is wrong and the patient has another neurologic disorder.

Although some response is seen within 3 months, patients frequently continue to show improvement during the first 6 to 12 months of cobalamin treatment. About 90 to 95 percent of the return of neurologic function that will ultimately occur is seen during the first 6 months. A few patients, however, continue to exhibit objective improvement during 1, 2, or even 3 years of cyanocobalamin replacement.

SUGGESTED READING

Healton EB, Savage DG, Brust JCM, et al. Neurologic aspects of cobalamin deficiency. Medicine 1991; 70:229–245.

Lindenbaum J, Healton EB, Savage DG, et al. Neuropsychiatric disorders caused by cobalamin deficiency in the absence of anemia or macrocytosis. N Engl J Med 1988; 318:1720–1728.

Lindenbaum J, Savage DG, Stabler SP, Allen RH. Diagnosis of cobalamin deficiency: II. Relative sensitivities of serum cobalamin, methylmalonic acid, and total homocysteine concentrations. Am J Hematol 1990; 34:99–107.

Rundles RW. Prognosis in the neurologic manifestations of pernicious anemia. Blood 1946; 1:209–219.

Savage D, Lindenbaum J. Relapses after interruption of cyanocobalamin therapy in patients with pernicious anemia. Am J Med 1983; 74:765–772.

PERIPHERAL NERVE DISORDERS

ACUTE GUILLAIN-BARRÉ SYNDROME

THOMAS E. FEASBY, M.D.

Guillain-Barré syndrome (GBS) is an acute, and often frightening, paralytic disease. Affected persons have the potential for excellent recovery but also a significant mortality rate. Two new treatments, plasma exchange and intravenous (IV) immunoglobulin, have improved the outcome. Accurate diagnosis, careful monitoring, good intensive care unit (ICU) care, and active rehabilitation are the essentials of management.

DEFINITION AND DIAGNOSIS

GBS is an acute, inflammatory, demyelinating disease of the peripheral sensory and motor nerves and nerve roots. It usually presents with distal numbness or weakness, which progresses, often in an "ascending" fashion, to peak, on average, in 12 days (range 1 to 30). The weakness is usually roughly symmetric and more prominent than the sensory signs, which may be limited to distal loss of vibration sensation, especially in mild cases. Facial weakness occurs in about 40 percent of cases and is helpful in excluding from diagnostic consideration spinal cord compression. Respiratory failure requiring ventilation happens in 30 percent of cases, and involvement of bulbar or extraocular muscles in about 10 percent. Tendon reflexes almost always are lost. The bladder is seldom affected.

Several laboratory tests may assist in diagnosis. The cerebrospinal fluid (CSF) protein value is usually raised, especially by 7 days after onset of symptoms, but there are usually fewer than 10 leukocytes per cubic millimeter. Findings of nerve conduction studies are always abnormal. Early in the illness, distal motor latencies may be prolonged but the most characteristic abnormality is conduction block which is indicative of demyelination in motor nerves. Later, slowing of conduction velocity, dispersion of motor nerve compound action potentials, and abnormalities of sensory conduction are often seen.

Many diseases can simulate certain aspects of GBS, but usually only a few merit serious consideration, and often the diagnosis is made easily on clinical grounds. The most important disorder to exclude is spinal cord compression. This is usually easy in the absence of upper motor neuron findings, reflexes and a sensory level, and in the presence of cranial nerve signs and typical nerve conduction abnormalities. When in doubt, spinal cord imaging may be necessary. Acute myasthenia gravis occasionally may mimic GBS, but a careful sensory examination often excludes this diagnosis. Acute intermittent porphyria should be excluded with a porphyrin screen. Poliomyelitis is a consideration in some countries. The clinical picture usually includes fever and meningismus without sensory symptoms or signs; it is often asymmetric, and the CSF shows significant pleocytosis.

MANAGEMENT

Patient management is complicated and demanding. Though only two treatments have been shown to specifically alter the course of the disease, many less specific measures help to manage or avoid the complications that frequently accompany GBS.

Specific Treatments

Plasma exchange (PE) was the first treatment shown to speed recovery from the neurologic deficits of GBS. Although the effect is neither immediate nor dramatic, it has been proven in two large and several smaller randomized clinical trials. PE is used frequently in children and in the Miller Fisher variant of GBS, but proof of its effectiveness in these situations is not available.

PE should be given as soon as possible to all GBS patients who are unable to walk unassisted. Those whose disease progresses slowly and who consult a physician before they are so disabled should be observed for further progression before PE is instituted. PE should not be started in patients seen 3 weeks after onset, unless there is clear evidence of continued clinical progression. The total amount of plasma to be removed in 4 or 5 exchanges over 8 to 10 days is about 250 cc per kilogram of body weight. A continuous-flow machine should be used; 5 percent albumin is the replacement fluid. More intensive PE regimens (e.g., daily treatments) are not recommended, as they may increase the chance of a relapse. The rate of relapse after PE is 10 to 15 percent, and it usually occurs within 3 weeks of the initial treatment. These patients usually improve further following a repeat course of two PEs.

PE is usually safe and well-tolerated. Good peripheral venous access is desirable, but a subclavian line can be utilized. Hypotensive episodes may be more frequent in GBS patients treated with PE, but these can usually be managed with fluid infusion. Infection is, theoretically, a risk.

Intravenous immunoglobulin (IVIG) has been used recently in several autoimmune diseases, including acute and chronic demyelinating neuropathies. A recent Dutch study of IVIG for GBS suggested that it was at least as effective as PE. Current studies are re-examining this and comparing these treatments with the combination of PE and IVIG.

IVIG is safe and is more convenient to use than PE, although it is expensive. A dose of 0.4 g per kilogram is given daily for 5 days by infusion pump. Rarely, allergic reactions and minor hypotensive episodes have been reported. It is particularly useful in centers where PE is not available.

I mention steroids here only to discourage their use. A recent large randomized trial showed that large doses of methylprednisolone were not effective in GBS.

General Treatment

The management of patients with GBS is often very complicated, and good general medical and nursing care are crucial to the outcome. During the early progressive phase, careful observation is essential and hospitalization is mandatory, probably even for mild cases. The patient's vital capacity (VC) should be checked regularly, even hourly if necessary. Intubation is usually necessary when the VC reaches about 1 liter, but the patient must be watched for signs of respiratory fatigue or bulbar incompetence, which may necessitate earlier intubation. Cardiac monitoring must be done during the progressive stage of GBS and during ventilation, to detect potentially dangerous cardiac arrhythmias. Subcutaneous heparin, 5,000 units every 12 hours, should be given as prophylaxis against deep venous thrombosis.

The 30 percent of GBS patients who require ventilation are subject to other complications. Most develop a pulmonary infection, which requires prompt appropriate antibiotic treatment, good bronchial toilet, and vigorous chest physiotherapy. Nursing in a private room adjacent to the ICU can minimize nosocomial infections and improve the psychological environment. Autonomic instability is common, producing hypertension, hypotension, and arrhythmias. Hypertension, the most common problem, usually requires no treatment. Systolic pressure greater than 200 mm Hg may need treatment, but this should be done cautiously, lest marked hypotension result. The safest agents are beta-adrenergic blockers given in medium-sized doses. Postural hypotension can be treated by supine positioning. Supine hypotension usually responds to volume expansion, but pressor agents are sometimes needed. Sinus tachycardia, the commonest arrhythmia, usually requires no treatment. Bradyarrhythmia is cause for more concern. It may be provoked by suctioning or repositioning. Atropine may be necessary, and occasional patients have required a pacemaker.

Pain is an underestimated problem in GBS. Low back pain often occurs early in the illness, and pain on straight leg raising is an early sign. Persistent limb pain, usually in the proximal legs or buttocks, occurs in about 50 percent of patients. This is usually a deep, aching, constant pain that can be very troubling; it can be dysesthetic. It is important to discuss this pain with patients and to provide treatment. It responds best to narcotic analgesics. Occasionally, this type of pain persists many months.

Poor communication frequently complicates the management of GBS. At the time of diagnosis, each patient deserves a frank discussion of the nature of the disease and its treatment. This should include a discussion of the prognosis, both for recovery and for respiratory failure, including the need for ventilation. Patients deal with ventilation and the ICU much better if they know what to expect. I have found the booklet entitled *Guillain-Barré Syndrome* published by The Guillain-Barré Syndrome Support Group International (see Patient Resources) to be very useful for patients. I give a copy to the patient and to relatives at the time of diagnosis. This provides comprehensive information about all facets of the disease and its treatment.

Later in the disease, communication is a problem for patients who are ventilated and in the ICU. Speech is impossible, and the weakness is often profound. Because most of the patients in an ICU are either very sick or unconscious, there is a tendency on the part of ICU personnel to think that GBS patients do not need to communicate. On the contrary, these patients can see, hear, think, and remember. Communication with them is vital. The care givers and the family need to be instructed about this. A letter board, which displays the letters of the alphabet in rows, can be used to allow the patient to pick out letters and put together words and sentences. This is essential to the patient's psychological and physical well-being. Another psychological aid that is sometimes helpful is a visit to an acutely ill GBS patient in the ICU from a recovered GBS patient.

Physiotherapy and good positioning are necessary during the paralytic phase of GBS. The joints and muscles must be kept mobile and supple by passive movements. This helps to prevent contractures and deep venous thrombosis. Care should be taken with positioning to avoid pressure on exposed peripheral nerves. A footboard helps prevent contractures of the Achilles tendon, and wrist splints can prevent contractures at the wrists.

Once the acute phase of GBS is over, a graduated

program of active rehabilitation can begin. For severely affected patients this starts after discharge from ICU. Gradual strengthening of the muscles eventually leads to assisted ambulation in parallel bars and in the pool. Drop foot splints may be helpful at this stage, and some patients must use them indefinitely.

COURSE AND PROGNOSIS

The outlook for GBS patients has brightened considerably with the development of modern ICU respiratory management and newer antibiotics. Plasma exchange and IVIG have improved the prognosis even more.

It is important for both the physician and the patient to know the natural history of the illness and its prognosis. The mean time from onset to peak disability in GBS is about 12 days, and 90 percent of patients reach this point by 3 weeks. About 75 percent make a full neurologic recovery, 10 percent have minor signs and symptoms, 10 percent will have more significant problems such as marked foot drop, and the mortality rate should be less than 5 percent. In more severe cases it is too early to measure outcome even 1 year after onset, because improvement can continue much longer.

Recent studies have provided some useful prognostic guidance. Older age is a negative prognostic factor. As a group, children may do better than adults. Patients who require artificial ventilation fare less well. Rapid onset of disability has been thought by some to be a sign of poor outcome. This seems to be true for those who become severely disabled in the first week. All patients should submit to nerve conduction studies and electromyography within the first few days. The finding of very low distally evoked compound muscle action potentials (< 20 percent of the lower limit of normal) is a poor sign for recovery. This likely correlates with the degree of axonal degeneration.

SUGGESTED READING

Hughes RAC. Guillain-Barré syndrome. Berlin: Springer-Verlag, 1990.
Ropper AH, Wijdicks EFM, Truax BT. Guillain-Barré syndrome. Philadelphia: FA Davis, 1991.
Van der Meche FGA, et al. A randomized trial comparing intravenous immune globulin and plasma exchange in Guillain-Barré syndrome. N Engl J Med 1992; 236:1123–1129.

PATIENT RESOURCES

The Guillain-Barré Syndrome Foundation International
Box 262
Wynnewood, Pennsylvania 19096
(215) 667-0131

The Guillain-Barré Support Group of Canada
111 Lock's Street
Petersborough, Ontario
K9J 2Y5

The Muscular Dystrophy Association
810 Seventh Avenue
New York, New York 10019

The Muscular Dystrophy Association of Canada
150 Eglinton Avenue E, Suite 400
Toronto, Ontario, M4P 1E8
(416) 488-0030

CHRONIC INFLAMMATORY DEMYELINATING POLYRADICULONEUROPATHY

EVA L. FELDMAN, M.D., Ph.D.
ZACHARY SIMMONS, M.D.

Chronic inflammatory demyelinating polyradiculoneuropathy (CIDP) is a chronic progressive or relapsing disorder of the peripheral nervous system. The average yearly incidence probably is less than that for acute inflammatory demyelinating polyradiculoneuropathy (AIDP, or Guillain-Barré syndrome; 0.6 to 1.9 cases per 100,000 population). Because of its prolonged course, the prevalence of CIDP is probably greater than that of AIDP. CIDP occurs at all ages and in both sexes, although men appear to be affected more frequently than women. There is no known geographic predilection. An antecedent event such as an upper respiratory tract infection, vaccination, or surgery is identified in the history of 20 to 30 percent of patients, in contrast to the much higher incidence (approximately 60 to 70 percent) in AIDP. A variety of underlying systemic disorders, including systemic lupus erythematosus, human immunodeficiency virus (HIV) infection, paraproteinemias, Castleman's disease, diabetes mellitus, and demyelinating disorders of the central nervous system (CNS) may occur in association with CIDP. Most cases are idiopathic, however, and are not associated with other systemic illnesses.

IDIOPATHIC CIDP

Evaluation and Diagnosis

The initial symptoms are most commonly distal sensory disturbances or weakness. Muscle weakness often begins distally and ascends, but there is much variability. Most patients ultimately note proximal as well as distal weakness. Although a period of progression of at least 4 weeks is required for CIDP, peak impairment may occur a year or longer after onset of symptoms. Difficulty chewing or swallowing is rare. Examination reveals symmetric proximal and distal limb weakness and may demonstrate sensory loss. There is hyporeflexia or areflexia. In contrast to AIDP, cranial nerve involvement is uncommon. Facial, oropharyngeal, and extraocular muscle involvement occurs in fewer than 15 percent of patients. Respiratory failure and autonomic dysfunction are very uncommon.

The diagnosis of CIDP should be confirmed by a battery of diagnostic tests. Screening hematologies and blood chemistry studies, antinuclear antibody (ANA), hepatitis screen, HIV titer, and serum protein electrophoresis and immunoelectrophoresis are used to identify associated systemic disorders. Porphyria and heavy metal poisoning can be excluded by analysis of urine samples. Cerebrospinal fluid (CSF) is obtained for protein, glucose, cell count, and a VDRL test. The CSF protein value is generally elevated, and there should be fewer than 10 mononuclear leukocytes per cubic millimeter (albuminocytologic dissociation). Electrodiagnostic evaluation is particularly helpful, and we believe the following criteria are suggestive of primary demyelination as seen in CIDP: conduction velocity less than 75 percent of the lower limit of normal in two or more motor nerves, distal latency exceeding 130 percent of the upper limit of normal in two or more motor nerves, evidence of unequivocal temporal dispersion or conduction block on proximal stimulation, consisting of a proximal-distal amplitude ratio less than 0.7 in one or more motor nerves, and an F-response latency exceeding 130 percent of the upper limit of normal in one or more nerves. If at least three of these four criteria are present and isolated nerve entrapment can be ruled out, it is highly likely that a primarily demyelinating polyneuropathy is present. In our experience, approximately 60 percent of patients with the clinical diagnosis of CIDP meet these criteria. Needle electromyography (EMG) reveals abnormal spontaneous activity in most patients.

Disorders that mimic CIDP can include hexacarbon abuse, porphyria, diphtheria, arsenic or lead intoxication, uremic polyneuropathy, diabetic polyradiculoneuropathy, and meningeal carcinomatosis. Features that cast doubt on the diagnosis include persistent marked asymmetrical or weakness, persistent bowel or bladder dysfunction, CSF pleocytosis (>50 mononuclear cells per cubic millimeter), polymorphonuclear cells in the CSF, and a distinct sensory level.

Therapy

Therapy can be divided into four categories: (1) oral immunosuppressive therapy, (2) plasma exchange, (3) intravenous gamma globulin therapy, and (4) supportive care and rehabilitation. Frequently, a combination of therapies is indicated because of the severity and progression of the disease. An algorithm for the treatment of CIDP is shown in Figure 1.

Oral Immunosuppressive Therapy

Corticosteroids are of demonstrated benefit in CIDP in both controlled and uncontrolled trials. Many prednisone treatment protocols exist. We most frequently use oral prednisone as the initial treatment for these patients, beginning with a daily dose of 1 mg per kilogram (usually 60 to 100 mg daily for adults). Patients are monitored monthly for evidence of hypertension, hyperglycemia, or electrolyte imbalance. They are cautioned about the hyperphagia, agitation, and sleep disturbances that may accompany even short-term prednisone use and are counseled about long-term side effects of this drug, such as osteoporosis and cataract formation.

Patients take large oral doses of prednisone, if it is tolerated, until there is significant clinical improvement or 2 months has elapsed. Prednisone is then tapered off to an every other day schedule, decreasing the alternate-day dose by 10 mg every 2 weeks until the patient is taking 10 mg on the alternate day. Next, the alternate-day dose is decreased by 5 mg every 2 weeks until the patient takes nothing on the alternate days. The patient is then maintained on a 1 mg per kilogram alternate-day schedule for 1 to 3 months. A second prednisone taper is started if the patient has regained normal or nearly normal strength. This is achieved by decreasing the alternate-day dose by 5 mg every 4 weeks until the alternate-day dose is 40 mg, then decreasing the alternate-day dose by 2.5 mg every 4 weeks until reaching an alternate-day dose of 20 mg. At that point, we decrease the alternate-day dose by 2.5 mg every 2 to 4 months until the alternate-day dose is 10 mg. Patients are maintained on that dose unless the disease completely resolves, in which case an attempt may be made to very slowly taper the patient off prednisone, which may or may not be successful (see "Prognosis" below).

We frequently use azathioprine as a prednisone-sparing agent, particularly for patients who are intolerant of prednisone or for whom the side effects of prednisone are considered particularly high risk. We may also use it as a second-line drug for patients who fail to improve with prednisone. An initial dose of 1 mg per kilogram per day is administered for 2 weeks, and, if tolerated, the dose is then increased to 2 to 3 mg per kilogram per day. Total white blood cell count and liver function tests initially are monitored every 2 weeks for 3 months, then monthly thereafter. The dose is cut in half if leukopenia or lymphopenia (total white blood cell count less than 3,000 or total lymphocyte count less than 500) develops or if the serum glutamic-oxaloacetic transaminase or serum glutamic-pyruvic transaminase value exceed two times normal. Azathioprine is discontinued if these abnormalities persist or worsen. Approximately 30 percent of our elderly patients develop an azathioprine-induced influenza-like illness (nausea, vomiting, fever, chills), which resolves with discontinu-

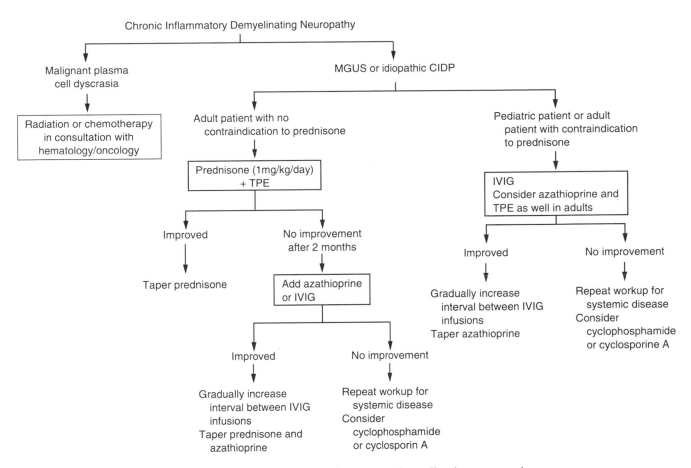

Figure 1 Treatment of chronic inflammatory demyelinating neuropathy.

ation of the drug. It takes at least 4 to 6 months for the full therapeutic effect of azathioprine to be realized.

Cyclosporin A, cyclophosphamide, and other immunosuppressive medications are used infrequently at our institution.

Plasmapheresis

A single double-blind study and a large body of anecdotal evidence suggest that patients with CIDP improve with therapeutic plasma exchange (TPE, or plasmapheresis). When beginning prednisone therapy in a patient with newly diagnosed CIDP, we suggest a series of five exchanges of one plasma volume (approximately 40 to 50 ml per kilogram) each, over a period of 7 to 14 days, for a total volume exchange of 200 to 250 ml per kilogram using a continuous-flow TPE machine. Two-thirds of our patients can undergo TPE via peripheral venous access. Some patients, however, require placement of a central venous catheter because of poor peripheral access. We use a Shiley double-lumen catheter and either a subclavian or femoral vein route. Patients who require placement of a central venous catheter are hospitalized during the course of their TPE.

Intravenous Gamma Globulin

Uncontrolled trials appear to show that some patients with CIDP respond to intravenous gamma globulin (IVIG) therapy. We use IVIG to treat CIDP in adult patients when prednisone or TPE is contraindicated or unsuccessful. In addition, we have found IVIG to be especially useful in children, because the side effects of traditional immunosuppressive therapy are avoided and TPE is difficult because of low body weight and limited peripheral venous access. A loading dose of 2 g per kilogram is given, usually over a 2 day period. Maintenance therapy is begun at 1 g per kilogram as a single intravenous dose, and is given at 2 weeks and 4 weeks after initial therapy and then at monthly intervals. The medication is generally well-tolerated: headache, chills, flushing, and low-grade fever are reported during the infusion in fewer than 10 percent of cases. These symptoms usually respond to a reduction of the infusion rate. Premedication with diphenhydramine and aspirin or acetaminophen may also be used. It has been our experience that patients who respond to IVIG therapy do so within the first month. A multicenter controlled trial of IVIG for treatment of CIDP is now under way.

Supportive Care and Rehabilitation

Patients with CIDP usually are not ill enough to require hospitalization, though those with severe weakness may require admission for nutritional or respiratory support. Although some CIDP patients recover quickly, the majority have a slow, progressive recovery over many months, or even years. Early consultation with occupational and physical therapists has proved useful for our patients. Splints for both the hands and feet help prevent contractures and allow for increased stability. Occupational therapists are particularly helpful in providing devices and strategies that permit patients to continue their activities of daily living.

DYSPROTEINEMIC NEUROPATHY

A group of patients exists in whom there is a type of acquired demyelinating polyradiculoneuropathy that differs from CIDP only in its association with a paraproteinemia. Affected patients may have a variety of malignant plasma cell dyscrasias or a monoclonal gammopathy of undetermined significance (MGUS). The incidence of neuropathy in patients with MGUS is unknown. Approximately 35 percent of our patients with MGUS and an associated neuropathy have an IgM paraprotein, whereas 55 percent have IgG, and 10 percent IgA. Neuropathy is quite common in association with other plasma cell dyscrasias. Clinical evidence of neuropathy occurs in approximately 3 to 5 percent of patients with typical osteolytic multiple myeloma, and 30 to 40 percent have evidence of neuropathy on electrodiagnostic or morphologic studies. Neuropathy occurs in 40 to 50 percent of patients with osteosclerotic myeloma and in approximately 15 percent of patients with primary systemic amyloidosis.

Evaluation and Diagnosis

Patients with an MGUS can present with a progressive sensorimotor polyneuropathy accompanied by electrodiagnostic evidence of demyelination, such as that seen in idiopathic CIDP. In our experience, IgG MGUS clinically resembles idiopathic CIDP. Patients with an IgM MGUS often are less weak than patients with idiopathic CIDP but are significantly impaired owing to severe sensory loss. Less commonly, MGUS can be associated with a distal axonal polyneuropathy. Of our patients with polyneuropathy and MGUS, 56 percent had a demyelinating polyneuropathy and 44 percent axonal neuropathy. The neuropathy of osteolytic multiple myeloma is clinically more diverse than that associated with MGUS. In addition to a CIDP-like picture, it may present as a mild sensorimotor axonal polyneuropathy or a pure sensory neuropathy. Patients with osteosclerotic myeloma develop a neuropathy that resembles CIDP, both clinically and electrodiagnostically. The neuropathy of primary systemic amyloidosis is predominantly a painful, small fiber neuropathy with prominent autonomic symptoms and superimposed me-

dian mononeuropathies at the wrists. Diagnosis is best made by rectal or sural nerve biopsy, which are reported to yield positive findings 70 and 90 percent of the time, respectively. This neuropathy should not be classified as a form of CIDP because it is primarily axonal.

We screen all patients who present with a progressive polyneuropathy for monoclonal proteins using serum protein electrophoresis (SPEP) and immunoelectrophoresis (IEP). If the SPEP and IEP findings are negative, we proceed to immunofixation (IF) of both serum and urine. We have found this to be important, because small monoclonal spikes may be obscured in the SPEP and because patients with normal SPEPs and IEPs can excrete monoclonal light chains into the urine, which are only found on IF. If a monoclonal protein is present, we suggest patients undergo radiologic skeletal survey and bone marrow biopsy. We take biopsy specimens from all suspicious bone lesions as well as "benign" bone lesions in patients with MGUS and a demyelinating polyneuropathy who do not respond to conventional (prednisone, TPE) therapy. Two of our CIDP-MGUS patients who did not respond to conventional therapy had bone lesions that were considered radiographically "benign" but that, on biopsy, were found to be plasmacytomas.

Therapy

We treat all patients with MGUS and an associated demyelinating polyneuropathy with prednisone, TPE, azathioprine, and/or IVIG, as outlined above for CIDP. In our experience, those patients who have IgG MGUS respond well, like those with idiopathic CIDP. In contrast, patients with an IgM monoclonal protein, many of whom have elevated titers of antibodies to myelin-associated glycoprotein, often have a poorer response to therapy. The poorer response is in keeping with our clinical impression that sensory deficits in patients with demyelinating polyneuropathy respond less well to therapy than motor deficits. Patients with MGUS and an axonal polyneuropathy typically are elderly and have minor neurologic deficits that do not warrant immunosuppressive therapy.

Patients with a neuropathy associated with a lymphoproliferative disorder are treated under the direction of a hematologist/oncologist according to standard protocols. Thus, patients with multiple myeloma are treated with monthly bursts of melphalan and prednisone. Those with osteosclerotic myeloma receive radiation therapy to solitary lesions, which often improves the neuropathy. Those with multiple lesions are treated with chemotherapy, though improvement in the neuropathy is rare. The neuropathy of amyloidosis does not improve with treatment of the amyloidosis.

LONG-TERM PROGNOSIS FOR IDIOPATHIC CIDP AND CIDP WITH PARAPROTEINEMIA

Patients with CIDP may have a monophasic, relapsing and remitting, or chronic progressive course. Those with idiopathic CIDP most commonly have a monophasic or relapsing/remitting course and their long-term outlook is good: at last follow-up approximately three-fourths have mild disability, if any. Many patients suffer relapse when their immunosuppressive therapy is completely discontinued, however, and require maintenance with low dose of immunosuppressive therapy indefinitely. A few patients (3 to 6 percent) die as a direct result of their illness, and the remainder have more severe deficits. The long-term outcome of patients with CIDP and MGUS is not as well-studied. Although those with IgG MGUS would be expected to have a long-term prognosis similar to that for idiopathic CIDP, those with IgM MGUS typically have primarily sensory deficits and a chronic progressive course and show little improvement with therapy.

SUGGESTED READING

Cook D, et al. High-dose intravenous immunoglobulin in the treatment of demyelinating neuropathy associated with monoclonal gammopathy. Neurology 1990; 40:212–214.
Dyck PJ, et al. Prednisone improves chronic inflammatory demyelinating polyradiculoneuropathy more than no treatment. Ann Neurol 1982; 11:136–141.
Dyck PJ, et al. Plasma exchange in chronic inflammatory demyelinating polyradiculoneuropathy. N Engl J Med 1986; 314:461–465.
Dyck PJ, et al. Plasma exchange in polyneuropathy associated with monoclonal gammopathy of undetermined significance. N Engl J Med 1991; 325:1482–1486
Van Doorn PA, et al. Intravenous immunoglobulin treatment in patients with chronic inflammatory demyelinating polyneuropathy. Arch Neurol 1991; 48:217–220.

BRACHIAL NEURITIS

DAVID R. CORNBLATH, M.D.
VINAY CHAUDHRY, M.B., B.S., M.R.C.P. (UK)

Brachial neuritis is a well-recognized clinical syndrome characterized by acute onset of proximal upper extremity pain, usually around the shoulder girdle, followed rapidly by lower motor neuron paralysis of shoulder girdle and upper extremity muscles. Initial reports of this syndrome appeared in the medical literature in the 1940s, and the papers of Parsonage and Turner (1948 and 1957) clearly established it as a recognizable clinical entity. Other names used to describe this syndrome are neuralgic amyotrophy, Parsonage-Turner syndrome, brachial plexus neuropathy, and acute brachial radiculitis. The disorder is rare: the annual incidence in Rochester, Minnesota is 1.6 per 100,000 population.

CLINICAL FEATURES

Brachial neuritis occurs mainly in men between age 30 and 60 years. In almost all patients, the first symptom is a deep, aching pain in and around the shoulder girdle. The pain is often very severe and is made worse by movement of the arms but not by coughing, sneezing, or moving the neck. One to fourteen days after the onset of pain, rapid onset of flaccid weakness is noted. The weakness usually coincides with lessening of the pain, though not always. Muscle atrophy develops within 2 to 3 weeks.

Many authors have commented on the puzzling distribution of weakness in this syndrome. In most patients, weakness is patchy and involves muscles of the shoulder girdle and upper extremity. The serratus anterior, deltoid, both spinati, biceps, and triceps are the most frequently involved muscles, whether in isolation or in various combinations. The symptoms are usually unilateral, although as many as 25 percent of patients shows bilateral involvement on electromyography (EMG) (see below). For reasons that remain unclear, the right side is more frequently affected than the left. In some patients, selective weakness can occur in the distribution of a single root, trunk, cord, or peripheral nerve, although when one or more muscles in that distribution are spared, localization of the lesion to a single site is difficult. In other patients, individual nerves are affected in isolation. The most frequently affected individual nerves are the long thoracic, axillary, suprascapular nerve, radial, anterior interosseous branch of the median nerve, and, rarely, the phrenic nerve.

Despite the severe weakness, sensory abnormalities are surprisingly minor. The most commonly reported sensory loss is in the distribution of the axillary nerve. Diminished sensation may also be found in the radial and median nerve distributions. Also reported are paresthesias in the shoulder girdle or upper extremity that do not conform to known anatomic distributions. A radicular pattern of sensory loss is never found. Muscle stretch reflexes are diminished or absent, depending on the degree of weakness.

DIFFERENTIAL DIAGNOSIS

Given the clinical presentation of this disorder, the differential diagnosis is extensive. The main concern is neoplastic infiltration of the brachial plexus, but with the advent of advanced imaging, computed tomography, or magnetic resonance imaging of the upper lung and brachial plexus, these disorders should be readily diagnosed. A rare condition, hereditary liability to brachial plexopathy, should be sought in the family history.

Early diagnosis may be difficult, owing principally to two clinical features. First, patients may present before the onset of weakness, when pain is the only complaint. At that time, the differential diagnosis includes mainly orthopaedic or rheumatic disorders. It is when weakness appears that neurologic disorders are considered. Second, the weakness may not conform to the anatomic distributions of roots, plexuses, or peripheral nerves; this confounds neuroanatomic diagnosis.

When the illness affects only the phrenic or the anterior interosseus nerves, serious diagnostic confusion can result. We have seen patients with isolated anterior interosseous nerve palsies whose problem was initially diagnosed as nerve entrapment and who underwent unnecessary surgical releases. A carefully taken history and electrodiagnostic studies usually correct the confusion. Isolated diaphragmatic weakness due to phrenic nerve palsy from brachial neuritis can be even more confusing. These patients usually undergo extensive pulmonary evaluation, including imaging of the thorax and bronchoscopy. Myasthenia may be considered in the differential diagnosis. In these cases, brachial neuritis becomes a diagnosis of exclusion.

LABORATORY EVALUATION

Electrodiagnostic studies provide diagnostic and prognostic information and are particularly helpful in differentiating lesions in roots, trunks, cords, or peripheral nerves. Especially important is recording sensory nerve action potentials (SNAP) and comparing them to those from the contralateral limb. With plexus or peripheral nerve disorders — that is, processes that affect nerves distal to the dorsal root ganglia — both sensory and motor evoked amplitudes are smaller than those of the unaffected nerve. In contrast, SNAP amplitudes are normal in root lesions. Routine evaluation of suspected brachial neuropathy includes bilateral sensory and motor nerve conduction studies, particularly of the affected nerves, comparing values from affected and unaffected limbs. In comparing motor or sensory evoked amplitudes from side to side we regard as significant any difference greater than 50 percent. In addition, recording of less commonly studied sensory nerves, such as the medial or lateral antebrachial cutaneous nerves, can be helpful in localization. The combination of these motor and sensory studies increases the probability of a correct diagnosis. In brachial neuritis, EMG reveals denervation potentials and initially variable degrees of loss of functioning motor units. The change in functioning motor units ranges from an absence of voluntary motor units to only a slight reduction in the number of voluntary motor unit potentials. Also helpful in confirming the diagnosis and recognizing the widespread nature of the problem is EMG evaluation of ostensibly normal muscles, as these may also show subtle evidence of denervation. In many patients, especially those who apparently have only a single affected nerve, performing EMG on the opposite limb is useful, as some patients also exhibit subtle changes of denervation in the opposite limb.

Cerebrospinal fluid (CSF) examination is unremarkable in most patients, though rare patients may show mild pleocytosis or a mild increase in CSF protein, or both. Other routine clinical laboratory studies are generally normal.

Nerve or muscle biopsy is almost never indicated. In patients who have undergone biopsy, marked axonal degeneration in the radial sensory nerve and denervation changes in muscle have been described.

ETIOLOGY

The cause of brachial neuritis is unknown. Frequently, the patient notes a "virus-like" syndrome that antedated the pain and weakness. In addition, brachial neuritis is encountered after trauma, operations, and childbirth, and it has been linked to prior vaccination. These epidemiologic observations are similar to those in the Guillain-Barré syndrome, which is thought to be an autoimmune or postinfectious disorder. Thus, one could conceptualize brachial neuritis as one end of the spectrum of postinfectious, autoimmune, monophasic neuropathies, of which Guillain-Barré syndrome and Bell's palsy are included; however, modern pathophysiologic correlative studies of brachial neuritis are still lacking.

THERAPY

Since the cause is unknown, there is no specific treatment for the weakness and wasting, so treatment is supportive. Occupational and physical therapy remain mainstays and are useful for all patients with functional deficits.

In the early stages, pain management is required. Immobilization of the arm often helps, because movement around the shoulder girdle makes the pain worse. A good range of passive movement at the shoulder joint should, however, be maintained as soon as the pain is relieved, to avoid the possibility of frozen shoulder. Nonsteroidal anti-inflammatory drugs (NSAIDs) may suffice for mild pain, although most patients need short-term treatment with narcotic analgesics. We use ibuprofen, 600 mg every 4 to 6 hours. If no relief is obtained by 24 hours, acetaminophen in combination with codeine or with oxycodone should be used at 4- to 6-hour intervals.

Although there is no evidence that corticosteroids alter the prognosis of the disease, they are helpful in pain management during the acute phase. For patients whose disease does not respond to NSAIDs, or where side effects such as sedation, dizziness, nausea, constipation, respiratory depression, and addiction are conflicting factors, we recommend prednisone, 60 mg per day, which is rapidly tapered off over 2 weeks.

PROGNOSIS

The prognosis is good. In series with long-term follow-up, 90 percent of patients make a full recovery, thanks to collateral reinnervation by the motor units that survive the initial attack. If, however, at the peak of the illness, EMG reveals no voluntary motor units in muscle, the prognosis is poor, as recovery must then occur solely by axonal regrowth, usually an incomplete process. Recurrence rates reported in the literature range from 3 to 14 percent. In recurrent cases, the possibility of hereditary recurrent brachial neuropathy should be considered.

SUGGESTED READING

England JD, Sumner AJ. Neuralgic amyotrophy: An increasingly diverse entity. Muscle Nerve 1987; 10:60–68.

Parsonage MJ, Turner JWA. Neuralgic amyotrophy: The shoulder-girdle syndrome. Lancet 1948; i:973–978.

Subramony SH. AAEE case report #14: Neuralgic amyotrophy (acute brachial neuropathy). Muscle Nerve 1988; 11:39–44.

Turner JWA, Parsonage MJ. Neuralgic amyotrophy (paralytic brachial neuritis) with special reference to prognosis. Lancet 1957; ii:209–212.

BELL'S PALSY AND HERPES ZOSTER OTICUS

JOHN K. NIPARKO, M.D.
DOUGLAS E. MATTOX, M.D.

The patient with acute facial palsy suffers both functional impairment (reduced facial motion) and the emotional impact of a skewed facial appearance. An acute facial palsy can substantially alter the quality of life, and acute disorders of the facial nerve pose a clinical challenge to health professionals from a wide variety of disciplines.

Centuries of investigation of facial nerve disorders have generated controversies that have often been lively, and not infrequently heated. Although Sir Charles Bell resolved many questions about patterns of facial innervation, Bell's palsy, the disorder named after him, continues to generate substantial debate and study. Despite decades of expanded insights into Bell's and other acute facial palsies, no clear consensus has yet emerged on many aspects of their causation, evaluation, and management. In this chapter we summarize our approach to evaluating and managing two common acute facial palsies, Bell's palsy and herpes zoster oticus.

DEFINITION OF DISORDERS

Bell's Palsy

No cause can be found for approximately two-thirds of acute facial palsies. The clinical diagnosis of Bell's palsy is appropriately applied to such cases. Bell's palsy is an acute, unilateral paresis or paralysis of the face in a pattern consistent with peripheral nerve dysfunction. Typically, its onset and evolution are rapid (< 48 hours) and may be associated with other acute cranial neuropathies. Pain or numbness affecting the ear, mid-face, and tongue, as well as taste disturbances, are common. Recurrence of Bell's palsy occurs in about 10 percent of patients. Recurrences appear more likely in patients who have a family history of Bell's palsy or diabetes.

Herpes Zoster Oticus

Herpes zoster oticus (Ramsey-Hunt syndrome) is a syndrome of acute peripheral facial palsy associated with otalgia and varicelliform lesions that accounts for approximately 10 percent of acute facial palsies. The lesions may involve the external ear, the ear canal, or the soft palate. Hearing loss, dysacusis, and vertigo reflect extension of the infection to involve the eighth nerve. Other cranial nerves (V, IX, and X) and cervical branches (2, 3, and 4) with anastomotic communications with the facial nerve may be involved as well.

INCIDENCE AND RISK FACTORS

Age and gender influence the likelihood of contracting Bell's palsy. It rarely occurs in patients younger than 10 years, but thereafter the incidence increases with age. Females in their teens and twenties have a predilection for the disorder, whereas among adults there is nearly equal distribution by sex (a slight male predominance in older groups).

The risk posed by diabetes mellitus for developing Bell's palsy remains undetermined, although most series suggest heightened susceptibility. Pregnancy also predisposes to Bell's palsy, particularly in the third trimester. Pre-eclampsia contributes further to the risk.

Recent clinical observations have suggested that immunodeficiency confers a greater risk of Bell's palsy and herpes zoster oticus. Cranial neuropathies, including facial palsy, have been observed in patients with human immunodeficiency viral (HIV) infection, often in association with a symmetric polyneuropathy. Neuropathies may appear at any stage of HIV infection: early after initial infection, as part of the chronic illness characterized by the acquired immunodeficiency syndrome (AIDS), or with AIDS-related meningitis.

Facial palsy associated with the conditions noted above is not necessarily Bell's palsy. These patients should be evaluated as completely as those who do not carry these risk factors, with the notable exception of omitting radiologic studies during pregnancy.

CLINICAL EVALUATION

Differential Diagnosis

The diagnosis of Bell's palsy is applied to cases of acute peripheral palsy *only after the exclusion* of traumatic, neoplastic, infectious, metabolic, and congenital causes. Strict attention to the evaluation, particularly the history and otoscopic and neurologic findings, may distinguish acute facial palsy from true Bell's palsy. Many of us are familiar with patients who have been rendered a grave disservice by a careless evaluation that missed a treatable or life-threatening cause of a facial palsy.

Next to Bell's palsy, the most common causes of acute, peripheral facial paralysis are trauma, herpes zoster oticus, bacterial infection, perinatal factors, and neoplastic involvement of the nerve. An acute facial palsy due to trauma or infection often presents with characteristic findings that are diagnostic. In contrast, differentiating neoplastic involvement of the facial nerve from Bell's palsy frequently poses a dilemma. A facial palsy produced by a neoplasm may differ only subtly from Bell's palsy. Experience indicates that the prevalence of sudden facial palsy is approximately 25 percent in patients found to have neoplastic involvement of the nerve, a surprisingly high incidence given the slow growth and good encapsulation of most tumors (schwannomas and neurofibromas) responsible for the

palsy. The following historical and clinical features suggest that a neoplasm may be responsible for facial palsy:

- Progression of a facial palsy over 3 weeks or longer
- No return of facial function within 6 months of onset of paralysis
- Failure to resolve an incomplete paresis within 2 months
- Facial hyperkinesia antecedent to the palsy
- Associated dysfunction of regional cranial nerves
- Prolonged otalgia or facial pain
- A mass in the middle ear, ear canal, digastric region or parotid gland
- Recurrent ipsilateral palsy

Although Bell's palsy may recur, a recurrent palsy should prompt an exhaustive search for tumor. Delayed or failed diagnosis of a neoplasm carries potential consequences of extension into the labyrinth and cranial fossas and diminished opportunity for effective reanimation.

The onset of a facial palsy in childhood is frequently obscured by the excellent tone of aponeurotic tissues and skin, and thus their ability to suspend the middle and lower portions of the face. Consequently, childhood facial nerve disorders are often referred to as "asymmetric crying facies."

The diagnostic approach to a facial palsy in a child is influenced by observations that although Bell's palsy is the most common childhood facial palsy, it accounts for a substantially smaller proportion of palsies than in adults. For instance, a clinically or radiographically identifiable cause can be found for 20 percent of adult palsies initially diagnosed as Bell's palsy, whereas this prevalence often exceeds 50 percent in series of childhood palsy. Facial palsies in patients younger than 18 years are most likely due to Bell's palsy and trauma, though infection, congenital causes, and neoplasms account for larger proportions than in adults.

Radiologic Evaluation

Radiologic evaluation is dictated by historical and clinical findings. Imaging studies are intended to exclude a neoplasm or other pathologic process based in the central nervous system, temporal bone, or parotid gland.

Magnetic resonance imaging (MRI) is the most sensitive method of imaging the intratemporal segment of the facial nerve and extends to include the entire intracranial (pontine, cerebellopontine angle, intracanalicular) and extratemporal segments of the nerve.

Before MRI was available, the diagnosis of Bell's palsy was established when the clinical presentation, taken in the context of historical features and physical findings, failed to reveal other disease. MR-based observations, however, suggest that the diagnosis of Bell's palsy may be positively established in some cases. Gadolinium-DTPA enhancement of the affected facial nerve has been observed in cases of Bell's palsy. Enhancement is often diffuse, in contrast to the focal enhancement produced by neoplasms. The appearance of the facial nerve on MRI should be evaluated for intensity, homogeneity, distribution of enhancement, and whether the nerve is displaced. Contralateral comparison is required, and care should be taken not to mistake enhancing mucosa or fat for the facial nerve. Although contrast-enhanced MRI detects neoplasms and other pathologic changes with good sensitivity, its utility in positively diagnosing Bell's palsy is limited when background enhancement is prominent.

Natural History

Our counseling of patients with acute facial palsy relies heavily on the known natural history of the disorder. The course of Bell's palsy varies along a continuum: from early, complete recovery to a debilitating course of nerve degeneration with permanent motor dysfunction. In the majority of Bell's palsy cases, spontaneous and complete recovery occur. Of particular concern, however, is nerve impairment that produces severe sequelae.

Suboptimal motor regeneration can result in mild paresis, which is manifested as epiphora, nasal obstruction, and oral incompetence. Persistent dysgeusia, ageusia, and dysesthesias may result from involvement of sensory components. Substantial nerve degeneration, followed by impaired or aberrant reinnervation, can produce synkinesis, residual weakness, and facial spasm and tics. These sequelae are classified as severe, because they frequently produce facial asymmetry and substantial functional impairment.

Although studies of the natural history of Bell's palsy vary somewhat in their findings, some patterns have been observed across studies:

1. Approximately one-third of Bell's palsy patients demonstrated varied levels of preserved facial function (paresis or incomplete paralysis). The remaining patients demonstrated complete clinical paralysis. Patients who do not advance to complete paralysis enjoy an excellent prognosis for full recovery of facial function; few of these patients demonstrate long-term sequelae.
2. All patients who develop complete paralysis exhibit some recovery, although the extent of the recovery varies. Complete return of function is highly likely for patients who demonstrate signs of recovery within the first 6 weeks after onset of paralysis. This is the course for the majority of patients with complete paralysis. The remaining patients with complete paralysis showed evidence of recovery 2 months or more after onset of the paralysis and they are likely to develop more severe sequelae.

These observations suggest that the longer the interval before recovery begins, the greater is the likelihood of severe residua. Overall, the spontaneous course of a paralysis produced by Bell's palsy is associated with inadequate nerve regeneration producing obvious sequelae in about 20 percent of patients, about half of whom report resultant disturbance of their lifestyle.

The prognosis for recovery of facial function with herpes zoster oticus is less favorable than that associated with Bell's palsy. In the majority of cases of herpes zoster oticus recovery is incomplete, and about one-third of all patients suffer major sequelae.

Facial Nerve Testing

In the initial evaluation of patients with acute facial paralysis, we aim to determine the cause of the paralysis; subsequently, using facial nerve testing, we evaluate the prognosis for recovery. Early determination of the prognosis for recovery may guide treatment to minimize nerve injury and optimize regeneration.

Because the clinical presentation of a facial paralysis does not distinguish between simple conduction block and axonal disruption, testing procedures designed to define the extent of nerve injury are used.

Topognostic test batteries (tear, stapedial reflex, taste, and salivary flow), as initially conceived, were intended to determine the level of facial nerve injury. Early findings that suggested that more proximal levels of dysfunction correlated with higher risk of degeneration and incomplete recovery have not been replicated. Topognostic modalities produce inconsistent information on the level of neural injury, probably because these tests are subject to vagaries produced by "skip" lesions of the nerve that affect the motor, sensory, and autonomic portions differently.

Because of the uncertainties inherent in topognostic testing, electrophysiologic responsiveness has emerged as the measure of choice for assessing nerve conductivity and the risk of nerve fiber degeneration. Ideally electrophysiologic testing provides an index of severity of injury to the nerve as a whole by reflecting the proportion of motor fibers that have progressed beyond first-degree injury.

Electrophysiologic tests that are commonly used indirectly assess the severity of injury to the intratemporal facial nerve. Given the skull encasement of this segment of the nerve, electrical stimulation proximal to the site of conduction blockade is possible only when the nerve is activated intracranially. For this reason, the ability of a nerve to propagate an impulse is assessed distal to the stylomastoid foramen. Even in the presence of severe neural injury, conduction distal to a lesion continues until its axoplasm is consumed and wallerian degeneration ensues. This process requires 48 to 72 hours to progress from intratemporal to extratemporal segments, thus rendering results of electrical stimulation tests "false-normal" during this period. Routine electrophysiologic tests, therefore, fail to detect nerve conduction instantaneously, thus delaying differentiation of neuropraxia from degeneration.

Nerve Excitability Testing

Minimal excitability testing with the Hilger nerve stimulator provides a readily accessible method of facial nerve assessment. The test reflects the elevated thresholds for neuromuscular stimulation produced by axonal disruption and degeneration. The lowest stimulus intensity that consistently excites all branches on the uninvolved side establishes the normal threshold. A 2 to 3.5 mA difference between the uninvolved and involved sides is reported to suggest impending denervation.

This test offers technical advantages: the necessary equipment is portable and it uses minimal stimulation, which is comfortable for the patient. It does have an element of subjectivity, because it relies on visual detection of the response. In addition, current levels at threshold for peripheral branches are likely to selectively activate large nerve fibers (which have lower thresholds) and those fibers closer to the stimulating electrode, thereby excluding some motor fibers from the assessment. Excitability testing is best utilized as a screening method to identify patients who need further evaluation.

Electromyography

Although previous reports suggest a role for early electromyography (EMG) in prognosticating functional recovery, potential pitfalls of early EMG testing may mislead the examiner. Sparse residual motor units that suggest a favorable outcome may be evident early on, despite severe injury to large portions of fibers at risk for degeneration. Subclinical motor activity detected by the EMG can, however, complement the use of evoked EMG in the early phase of a clinical paralysis, as discussed below.

Substantial axonal loss and impaired reinnervation yield fibrillation potentials as long as postsynaptic membranes remain electrically active. With loss of this electrical activity, EMG recordings are silent and insertional activity is absent. Conversely, successful reinnervation generates high-frequency polyphasic potentials that increase in amplitude and duration and replace fibrillation potentials. In cases of protracted paralysis, we use longitudinal EMG evaluations to detect reinnervation or persistent degeneration.

Evoked Electromyography

Evoked electromyography (EEMG) assesses the facial motor response to a supramaximal stimulus. EEMG technique records the compound muscle action potential (CMAP) with surface electrodes placed in the nasolabial fold (Fig. 1). Responses are analyzed to compare optimal peak-to-peak amplitudes between the normal and the involved side. Waveforms can be graphically displayed for quantitative analysis and printed for the medical record.

Patients with incomplete paralysis due to Bell's palsy invariably recover normal or nearly normal function and do not require EEMG evaluation. The reappearance of

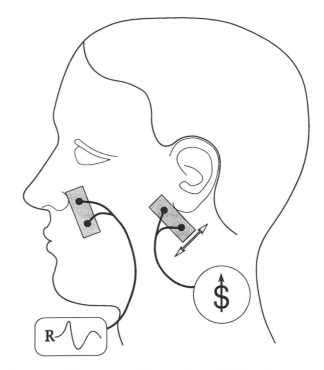

Figure 1 Illustration of the surface EEMG stimulus and recording technique. The orientation of the stimulating electrode is adjusted to produce a maximal biphasic (CMAP) response recorded at the nasolabial fold.

clinical movement within 3 to 4 weeks after onset also predicts an excellent prognosis for functional recovery.

When used in a timely fashion, reductions in the EEMG responses on the affected side are thought to reflect the percentage of motor fibers of the facial nerve that have undergone degeneration. Facial EEMG is most reliable during that initial phase of accelerated denervation—in the first 2 to 3 weeks following onset of paralysis due to Bell's palsy or herpes zoster oticus. When neuropraxic fibers become "deblocked," either in the recovery phase or, later, as axons regenerate peripherally, stimulated nerve fibers discharge asynchronously. Because regenerated fibers do not discharge in synchrony, the response is disorganized and consequently diminished. This phenomenon imposes a time constraint on the reliability of EEMG testing that must be considered when interpreting test results, and EMG sampling of voluntary motor activity is required to detect visually imperceptible facial function.

More recent clinical trials support the early findings of Fisch and Esslen (1972), indicating that EEMG provides an accurate prognostic guide early in the course of facial paralysis. These trials indicate that for more than 50 percent of paralyzed patients whose CMAP amplitude was reduced 90 percent or more spontaneous return of facial function was less than satisfactory. When results demonstrated less than 90 percent denervation (> 10 percent in CMAP amplitude relative to the normal side), recovery was uniformly excellent.

Repeated testing on an every-other-day basis is

recommended to detect ongoing degeneration beyond the 90 percent critical level. The time course of reduced electrical excitability (velocity of denervation as demonstrated by repeated testing) and the degree of degradation of the CMAP response (the nadir of the response) appear to be most useful in predicting the ultimate level of spontaneous recovery. The earlier the response drops to 10 percent or less than normal, the worse the prognosis.

Electrophysiologic testing with EEMG is now recognized to be the most straightforward and accurate means of determining the prognosis of recovery from Bell's or herpes zoster oticus facial paralysis; however, accurate results depend on an evaluation that incorporates historical and physical findings determined prior to testing, as well as careful administration of the test and interpretation of results. For many of electrophysiologic tests it has not been possible to establish a clear correspondence between response profiles in the acute phase of paralysis and functional outcome. With EEMG testing, however, it now appears possible to identify with greater precision early on those patients who are at increased risk for permanently impaired facial function.

TREATMENT

Our approach to managing Bell's palsy is based on current understanding of the pathophysiology underlying this disorder. Studies of the intratemporal facial nerve suggest that Bell's palsy and herpes zoster oticus most often result from impaired facial nerve conduction in the temporal bone, particularly at the meatal foramen, where the facial nerve enters the temporal bone. The most time-honored hypotheses of the genesis of Bell's palsy hold that impaired neural conduction follows disturbances in microcirculation and demyelinization resulting from immune-mediated injury.

Emerging evidence for a viral cause of Bell's palsy is based on virologic cultures, serologic tests and, more recently, ultrastructural and PCR-based findings of herpes simplex virus (HSV) in nerve biopsy specimens. The HSV and varicella-zoster virus (VZV) are both DNA viruses of the herpesvirus group and their ultrastructural features are only subtly different. Although differences in their biologic behavior suggest that neuritis resulting from the respective viruses should have distinctive clinical features, infections from HSV and VZV may mimic one another. Moreover, HSV, mumps, and cytomegalovirus infections may produce a clinical picture resembling herpes zoster oticus, and VZV neuritis may occur in the absence of a rash *(zoster sine eruptione)*. HSV and VZV infections may thus remain indistinguishable by their clinical presentation.

The postulated mechanisms of nerve injury underlying Bell's palsy are not necessarily distinct processes. Rather, they may sequentially and synergistically mediate the pathologic process. Although inflammation and ischemia appear to dominate the early pathophysiologic events, neural blockade and degeneration, and subsequent fibroblastic response, assume major importance later in the sequence. Given the confinement of the nerve trunk within the meatal foramen, it is likely that compression at this site is a determinative event in the genesis of these palsies triggered by viral infection.

Glucocorticoids

In many cases, guidelines and indications for steroid treatment are empirical. Such guidelines apply to the use of steroids in the treatment of Bell's and of other facial palsies where benefit is uncertain. Nonetheless, the pharmacologic effects of steroids make them attractive agents for ameliorating symptoms associated with the acute phase of disorders such as Bell's palsy and herpes zoster oticus, and theoretically for improving the likelihood of full recovery.

Our goal in the initial treatment of an acute facial paralysis is to induce effective anti-inflammatory control with steroids. In order to provide such control, the inflammatory process should be treated with consistent, pharmacologic levels, beginning as soon as possible. Once the inflammatory process is checked and the stimulus for inflammation removed, therapy can be discontinued; though abrupt withdrawal may be followed by rebound disease activity. To prevent such rebound, withdrawal is achieved by tapering off the daily glucocorticoid dose—over 10 to 14 days seems reasonable.

The optimal glucocorticoid dosage regimen for treating inflammatory neuritis depends on the time course of the underlying disease process. The duration of accelerated inflammation associated with viral neuropathy is difficult to estimate. As discussed above, two viruses that are frequently associated with facial palsy are HSV and VZV, which have incubation periods of approximately 3 and 14 days, respectively. Although duration of the active phase of these infections is impossible to establish, the typical electrical profiles of progression of the palsy in patients with Bell's palsy and herpes zoster oticus point to reasonable conclusions. The acute phase of the infection, as measured by the evoked electrical response and progression of the palsy, peaks in 5 to 10 days for Bell's palsy and 10 to 14 days for herpes zoster oticus. Because lesions induced by these infections in other organs generally heal in 1 to 2 weeks, it seems certain that accelerated inflammation of the facial nerve with these viruses would normally be confined to this period.

These considerations suggest the following strategy for steroid treatment of Bell's palsy and herpes zoster oticus: oral prednisone, 1 mg per kilogram per day in three doses for 7 to 10 days. The daily dose should then be tapered to zero over 10 days. Theoretically, this dosing regimen maximizes anti-inflammatory activity while minimizing side effects.

Side effects that are likely to be manifested during short-term steroid treatment include hyperglycemia, fluid and electrolyte disturbances, gastrointestinal irritation, and central nervous system effects, including psychotic breaks. An adverse effect of glucocorticoid administration that deserves special consideration is heightened susceptibility to infection. Although this effect on host resistance has been demonstrated in experimental trials, typical schedules of glucocorticoids (1 mg per kilogram per day prednisone or its equivalent) given for 3 weeks or less are rarely associated with such susceptibility. The risk of steroid-induced dissemination of viruses is of particular concern when treating acute facial palsies of viral origin. With steroid therapy beyond 1 month and in immunosuppressed patients the risk of dissemination of virus is significant. Otherwise, clinical experience suggests that the risk of this complication is minimal.

Reported trials of steroid treatment of Bell's palsy suggest that steroids:

- May reduce the risk of denervation if initiated early
- May prevent or lessen synkinesis
- May prevent progression of incomplete paralysis to complete paralysis
- May hasten recovery
- Prevent autonomic synkinesis (crocodile tears)

Theoretically, steroids may provide similar benefits in treating herpes zoster oticus. In addition, steroids are claimed to reduce postherpetic neuralgia in other VZV neuritides.

Antiviral Therapy

Antiviral chemotherapy is a new adjunct for treating acute facial palsy of viral origin. Based on its spectrum of activity and low toxicity, acyclovir (acycloguanosine), a synthetic purine nucleoside analogue, has found clinical use in treating these disorders.

Preliminary reports suggest that acyclovir may mitigate neurologic deficits produced by herpes zoster oticus. Intravenous acyclovir, 10 mg per kilogram every 8 hours for 7 days, appears to produce substantially greater functional return in patients treated within the first 72 hours after onset of paralysis. Moreover, acyclovir treatment has been associated with early recovery of facial nerve function and reversal of sensorineural hearing loss associated with herpes zoster oticus in response to early administration of the drug. Given the high incidence of nerve degeneration associated with this disorder, these results appear promising.

The use of acyclovir for treating Bell's palsy is currently under evaluation. In light of support for HSV's being the pathogen, such an approach is attractive. We currently administer intravenous acyclovir if the paralysis is complete and the patient presents early after onset of the palsy.

Nerve Decompression

As anatomic and electrophysiologic studies have located the site of lesion in Bell's palsy at the meatal foramen, procedures for surgical intervention have focused on decompressing this region of the nerve when the chances for complete recovery with medical therapy alone are deemed poor. The meatal foramen is most easily approached via the middle cranial fossa. The middle cranial fossa approach to the labyrinthine and geniculate segments of the facial nerve facilitates direct meatal foramen decompression with minimal risk to the labyrinth. It also permits direct stimulation of the facial nerve proximal to the meatal foramen, enabling verification of the site of impairment if complete loss of response to electrical stimulation has not yet occurred. Intraoperative stimulus trials typically reveal severely attenuated response (if any) proximal to the foramen, whereas stimulation distal to the foramen evokes potentials of substantially greater amplitude (Fig. 2).

Prospective study of Bell's palsy cases stratified by EEMG has suggested that nerve decompression via the middle fossa approach enhances recovery in cases when evoked response amplitude is no more than 10 percent that of the normal side. This criterion was based on the observation that approximately one-half of patients whose disease progressed to a nadir of 90 to 100 percent degeneration within 2 weeks of the onset of the paralysis

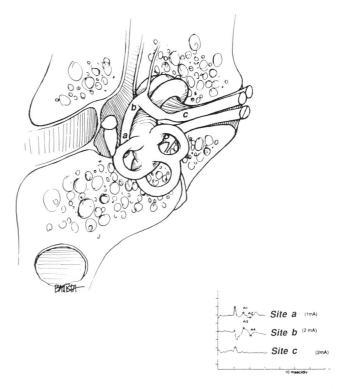

Figure 2 EEMG records of direct stimulation of the facial nerve during nerve decompression. Stimulation trial was performed via the middle cranial fossa approach that exposed the tympanic *(site a),* perigeniculate *(site b),* and meatal *(site c)* segments of the facial nerve. Responses were obtained with intramuscular electrodes placed in the nasolabial fold. Stimulation of the nerve proximal to the decompressed meatal foramen *(site c)* failed to evoke substantial motor unit potentials.

demonstrated permanent, unsatisfactory recovery of facial function. All patients who underwent decompression when degeneration reached 90 percent demonstrated satisfactory return of facial movements. The 90 percent rate of satisfactory outcome with surgery compared favorably with the 50 percent chance of satisfactory return noted in unoperated patients matched by EEMG profile.

Eye Care

The dry, unprotected eye is a potential complication of any complete facial paralysis. The "windshield wiper" effect of the eyelids is lost, and diminished parasympathetic input reduces lacrimation. Schirmer's tear test provides a practical guide for assessing tear production and the need for adjunctive eye care. Aggressive management is necessary to enhance eye protection and avoid corneal drying. We often employed some or all of the following measures to maintain hydration of the cornea and reduce the risk of abrasion:

- Strict avoidance of eye patching (unopposed third nerve function typically opens the eyelids despite the tightest of patches).
- Tear substitutes prescribed for daytime use. An agent with long retention time and high affinity for corneal epithelium is preferred.
- Ocular lubricants (ointments) are advised for night-time use or when artificial tears fail to provide adequate protection during waking hours. These preparations typically blur vision.
- Added support to the lower eyelid can be obtained with (Steri-Strip) taping to elevate the lower lid and improve apposition to the inferior cornea.
- External shielding with eyeglasses reduces the risk of injury and drying due to exposure to air currents. Humidification can be further enhanced by covering the eye with Saran wrap sealed to the orbital rim with a gel.

Surgical procedures are necessary in cases of prolonged paralysis associated with ectropion or when conservative measures fail adequately to hydrate the cornea. We manage such cases with an approach that utilizes upper lid loading with gold weights, with or without lower lid shortening and canthopexy.

Postreinnervation blepharospasm may be so severe as to require botulinum toxin injection. While most patients experience relief of the spasm, the average duration of maximum improvement is only 3 to 4 months. Orbicularis oculi neurectomy or myectomy is occasionally necessary.

Electromyographic Rehabilitation

EMG rehabilitation is occasionally useful for managing patients with synkinesis and hyperkinesis following facial nerve recovery from Bell's palsy or herpes zoster oticus. This form of sensory feedback training is most frequently utilized when the pattern of reinnervation produces inability to separate mouth movement from eye closure. This produces involuntary eye closure on smiling. Muscle retraining with EMG feedback has produced subjective improvement in very motivated patients.

SUGGESTED READING

Dickens JRE, Smith JT, Graham SS. Herpes zoster oticus: Treatment with intravenous acyclovir. Laryngoscope 1988; 98:776–779.

Fisch U. Surgery for Bell's palsy. Arch Otolaryngol 1981; 107:1–11.

Hughes GB. Practical management of Bell's palsy. Otolaryngol Head Neck Surg 1990; 102:658–663.

Jackson CG. Facial nerve paralysis: Diagnosis and treatment of lower motor neuron facial nerve lesions and facial paralysis. Presented at the American Academy Otolaryngology–Head Neck Surgery Foundation, Washington, DC, 1986.

Mattox DE, ed. Management of facial nerve disorders. Otolaryngol Clin North Am 1991; 24:479–756.

Mattox DE. Clinical Disorders of the Facial Nerve. In: Cummings CW, Frederickson JM, Harker LH, et al, eds. Otolaryngology–Head and Neck Surgery. St. Louis: Mosby–Year Book, 1992; 3217–3232.

Niparko JK, Kileny PR, Kemink JL, et al. Neurophysiologic intraoperative monitoring: II. Facial nerve function. Am J Otol 1989; 10:55–61.

MEDIAN NERVE COMPRESSION

THOMAS M. BRUSHART, M.D.

CARPAL TUNNEL SYNDROME

Carpal tunnel syndrome (CTS) is the final common pathway for a variety of pathophysiologic processes. Only when these processes have been ruled out should the disease be treated as idiopathic. The carpal tunnel is bounded by bone, joint, and ligament; it contains tendon, synovium, and blood vessels, in addition to the median nerve. Alteration of the size or shape of these structures by mechanical or systemic factors diminishes the space available for the median nerve and result in CTS.

The volume of the carpal tunnel itself may be diminished by fracture of the radius or by either fracture or subluxation of the carpal bones. Osteoarthritis of radiocarpal or intercarpal joints may project osteophytes into the canal, and ganglia may arise from affected joints, further compromising the space available for the median nerve. This commonly occurs when arthritis affects the trapeziometacarpal joint at the base of the thumb. If the history suggests post-traumatic or osteoarthritic compromise of the carpal canal, anteroposterior (AP), lateral, and carpal tunnel x-ray views of the wrist should be obtained. Trapeziometacarpal arthritis is demonstrated by the "grind" test—axial compression and circumduction of the first metacarpal to elicit painful crepitus in the joint—and is confirmed by radiography of the thumb base. Infrequently, carpal tunnel volume may be diminished by amyloidosis, causing thickening of the transverse carpal ligament, which forms the palmar boundary of the canal.

CTS more often results from disease affecting the contents of the carpal canal. The synovium surrounding the flexor tendons may become inflamed in response to repetitive activity; this occasionally causes visible swelling just proximal to the ulnar side of the volar wrist crease, and more often results in palpable crepitus in this area on flexion and extension of the digits. Synovitis in the canal is a common feature of rheumatoid arthritis (RA), so much so that every patient with RA should be screened for signs and symptoms of CTS. Flexor synovitis may also be seen in association with other forms of inflammatory arthritis, such as gout. Carpal tunnel symptoms, which are brought on rapidly by hand activity, should arouse suspicion of an abnormal muscle in the canal or of a persistent median artery. Both increase in size with activity, compressing the median nerve. If these abnormalities are present, rapid, repetitive digital flexion and extension should reproduce the patient's symptoms. Generalized swelling in the canal may be associated with hypothyroidism, pregnancy, menopause, or diabetes; the latter is also associated with a peripheral neuropathy that may increase nerve susceptibility to compression. Less common space-occupying lesions in the canal include tumors such as multiple myeloma, bleeding (in hemophiliacs), and abnormal swelling of the nerve itself in macrodactyly.

Increasingly often, the patient's treatment cannot begin without definition of the relationship between the onset or worsening of symptoms and the nature of work activities. The Centers for Disease Control has formulated guidelines to aid in making this determination. For CTS to be considered work related, the job must include one or more of the following activities: (1) frequent, repetitive use of the same or similar hand or wrist motions, (2) regular tasks that require generation of high forces by the hand, (3) regular or sustained tasks that require abnormal hand position, (4) regular use of vibrating hand tools, and (5) frequent or prolonged pressure over the wrist or base of the palm. I find it difficult to ascribe the initial cause of CTS to a work activity, especially repeated generation of force, unless the activity has been pursued for several years and involves predominantly the symptomatic hand. More often, the patient's history indicates that carpal tunnel symptoms are brought on by work activity and relieved by rest, especially a weekend or vacation. The implica-

tions of this distinction between work-caused and work-related CTS varies according to state workmen's compensation law: in Maryland, both situations are covered; in Virginia, neither.

Treatment of CTS is based on staging of the disease and understanding the pathophysiology of each stage. Most patients' CTS can be readily classified as mild, moderate, or severe. In mild CTS, there is intermittent compromise of epineurial blood flow; axonal transport may be decreased, but there are no structural changes in the nerve. Patients present with intermittent numbness and paresthesias, corresponding to the periods of ischemia. Symptoms have usually been present for less than 1 year. Physical examination reveals minimal sensory abnormalities if any, and no weakness or thenar atrophy. Electrical testing discloses minimally increased latency of 1 to 2 msec, and no fibrillations in the abductor pollicis brevis (APB). Moderate CTS is characterized by persistent compromise of intraneural circulation, with epineurial and intrafascicular edema. Constant pressure on the nerve may result in demyelination, especially of the more superficial fibers. Patients complain of constant numbness and paresthesias. Sensory thresholds are increased, as determined by testing with Semmes-Weinstein monofilaments, two-point discrimination may be increased or normal, and there is often weakness, but rarely atrophy, of the APB. Electrical testing usually detects increased motor latency greater than 1 msec and, occasionally, fibrillations. Severe CTS results from long-standing endoneurial edema and fibrosis with demyelination and axonal degeneration. Patients complain of persistent, often profound, loss of sensory function, weakness, and marked interference with hand function. Physical examination reveals elevated two-point discrimination and thenar atrophy, often with inability to actively abduct the thumb from the palm. On electrical testing there is marked prolongation of motor latency, sensory conduction often is not obtainable across the wrist, and fibrillations are expected in the APB.

When CTS has been diagnosed and staged, underlying causes must still be identified and treated before a standard treatment regimen can be instituted. Malunion of previous wrist fractures and intercarpal fractures or subluxations, may require independent surgical treatment. Osteoarthritis may respond to splinting and a course of anti-inflammatory medication. A small, hand-based splint to immobilize the first metacarpal during stressful use of the hand is particularly helpful for patients with trapeziometacarpal arthritis and carpal tunnel complaints. Flexor synovitis often results from work activities, and every effort should be made to understand the specific hand positions used, the stresses involved, and the frequency of the activity. Employers are often willing to modify a work position or job description to avoid more costly lost time or surgical treatment. Typists usually benefit from lowering the keyboard to lap level, to avoid positions of wrist flexion, and the placement of a foam wrist pad at the proximal edge of the keyboard. Assembly line workers may perform the same forceful wrist motion in an awkward position several thousand times a day. Rotating through different positions with different upper extremity demands and taking frequent breaks often lessen their symptoms. Occasionally the machinery or tools can be simply modified to avoid a particularly harmful wrist activity. For example, butchers working with straight-handled knives spend much of their day in a position of marked ulnar wrist deviation with variable flexion. Modifying knives by placing the handle at right angles to the blade allows most work to be done with the wrist in neutral position. As a general principle, those with work-related flexor synovitis benefit from splinting the wrist in neutral position while working and taking anti-inflammatory medications. Flexor synovitis may also result from systemic diseases such as RA, which should be under optimal medical management by a rheumatologist for at least 6 months before surgery is considered. Other systemic causes of CTS, such as diabetes and hypothyroidism, should also be well-controlled, independently of treatment for CTS. Hypothyroidism often responds dramatically over a period of several months, eliminating the need for surgery. Finally, any mass that appears to be causing median nerve compression in or near the carpal tunnel should be evaluated in the routine manner.

Treatment of isolated, mild CTS begins with a 1-month course of splinting the wrist during sleep in neutral or slight dorsiflexion. The cross-sectional area of the carpal tunnel increases by approximately 15 percent when the wrist is dorsiflexed from neutral, and decreases by approximately 10 percent when it is flexed. These alterations in cross-sectional area are correlated with changes in pressure in the canal. In normal subjects, the pressure in the carpal tunnel is 2 to 3 mm Hg, and it increases to 30 mm Hg with wrist flexion. Patients with CTS, in contrast, may have resting pressure up to 30 mm Hg with the wrist in neutral, and pressures up to 90 mm Hg with the wrist flexed. The wrist often falls into a position of flexion during sleep because the volar, grasping muscles exert greater resting force than the dorsal, positioning muscles. Splinting prevents wrist flexion, and the attendant increase in carpal tunnel pressure that results from a decrease in available volume.

If the patient with mild CTS is not significantly relieved by a 1 month course of splinting, I proceed with cortisone injection of the carpal tunnel. The procedure is first described to the patient, who is instructed to hold the hand immobile throughout the injection. Significant nerve injury may result from unanticipated withdrawal of the hand while the needle is in place. Similarly, the patient is instructed to report any paresthesias and localize them as accurately as possible. After sterile preparation of the volar wrist, a 25-gauge needle is introduced from proximal to distal, at a 45 degree angle to the skin, parallel to the long axis of the forearm. The skin puncture should be 1 cm proximal to the proximal wrist crease, at a point midway between the palmaris longus tendon on the radial aspect and the flexor carpi ulnaris tendon on the ulnar aspect. The palmaris longus

tendon is identified by asking the patient to forcefully compress the tips of the thumb and little finger while flexing the wrist; the flexor carpi ulnaris becomes prominent with resisted wrist flexion in ulnar deviation. As the needle is advanced, it passes through the resistant dermis to a layer of underlying fat, which offers little resistance. The transition between fat and the relatively unyielding transverse carpal ligament is clearly palpable, and increased pressure is required for further progress. When the 2 to 3 mm of transverse carpal ligament has been traversed, the needle pops into the carpal canal. Paresthesias encountered in the superficial fatty layer result from contact with the ulnar nerve and are avoided by placing the needle 2 to 3 mm radial; those encountered for the first time when the needle pierces the carpal canal result from contact with the median nerve and are avoided by replacement of the needle in a more ulnar position. When the needle is within the carpal canal, and no paresthesias results from a further 1 to 2 mm advance, 1 cc of Kenalog (10 mg per milliliter) is injected. If paresthesias are encountered on two successive needle placements, I usually abandon the attempt. Steroid should never be injected into the nerve, as this may result in severe, irreparable damage.

Between 40 and 50 percent of patients with mild CTS remain asymptomatic for 1 year after a course of splinting and steroid injection. Those whose repetitive work activities are a continuing irritant to the flexor tendons are less likely to benefit. If relief is significant but only transient, patients often request repeat injection; however, I am reluctant to offer more than three injections per year. CT injection may offer dramatic relief to women with moderate or even severe CTS symptoms in the third trimester of pregnancy. Unfortunately, many obstetricians advise their patients to avoid CT injection, in spite of the absence of evidence linking third trimester CT injection to the development of fetal abnormalities. Relief for a period of at least 6 months after injection correlates very well with a successful outcome from carpal tunnel release (CTR), should it eventually become necessary. Injection of the CT may also be helpful diagnostically. For instance, a patient may have more than one area of suspected nerve compression. If CT injection provides dramatic relief of symptoms, treatment can be focused in this area while the other areas of potential compression are merely observed. If no relief is obtained and electrodiagnostic studies show only mild CTS, attention should be focused proximally.

Other forms of conservative treatment may be used for patients with mild CTS who obtain little or only transient relief from injection. Vitamin B_6, 50 mg daily, occasionally provides relief when combined with splinting. Patients should be cautioned that 3 months of consistent therapy will be necessary before the success of treatment can be evaluated. Larger doses may cause peripheral neuropathy themselves, and should be avoided. If swelling of the involved hand is a prominent complaint, potassium sparing diuretics may also be useful.

Moderate CTS is usually treated surgically. CTR is conveniently performed under local anesthetic, and is relatively safe for even older patients with severe medical problems. Surgical release of the transverse carpal ligament results in a 25 percent increase in the volume of the carpal canal and immediate reduction of pressure on the median nerve. The procedure should not include "internal neurolysis" or excision of a portion of the epineurium with surgical separation of the individual nerve fascicles. This procedure was initially advocated to release constricting scar within the nerve, but it has been found in prospective studies to be of no benefit, and in some cases harmful. Similarly, Guyon's canal should not be released in patients in whom ulnar distribution numbness accompanies CTS, but who have no evidence of a focal ulnar nerve lesion. Their symptoms resolve with CTR alone, possibly because CTR secondarily changes the contour of Guyon's canal from triangular to oval, increasing its volume and the space available to the ulnar nerve.

Although CTR is a brief outpatient procedure, postoperative recovery is often prolonged. Strength usually recovers to 75 percent of normal by 2 months, but an additional month is required before full strength is regained. Recently, endoscopic CTR has been advocated in an attempt to return patients to work more rapidly. A small arthroscope and cutting tools are introduced into the carpal canal through an incision at the wrist crease. The transverse carpal ligament is sectioned from within, but the overlying palmar fascia and skin are not violated. For many patients, return to work is indeed accelerated; however, the risk of neural injury with this procedure is significant. Many question whether this risk, compared to the safety of open CTR, is justified by the benefits of more rapid return to work.

Severe CTS is also treated surgically, but deficits of both sensory and motor function must be addressed. In addition to release of the transverse carpal ligament, a tendon transfer should be considered to restore thumb opposition. This additional procedure can also be performed with local anesthesia. Most simply, the palmaris longus tendon (vide supra) can be elongated with palmar fascia during the CTR and rerouted to the distal first metacarpal, to replace the function of the atrophic abductor pollicis brevis muscle. Patients should be aware that the wrist and thumb will be immobilized for 3 weeks to allow the transfer to heal.

PROXIMAL MEDIAN NERVE COMPRESSION

In some patients, the diagnosis of CTS may be incomplete or inaccurate. These patients may have additional areas of median nerve compression proximal to the carpal tunnel or an isolated proximal compression presenting with signs and symptoms similar to those of CTS. Evidence of proximal median compression should thus be sought in any patient with median nerve symptoms or findings that suggest "atypical" CTS. Although proximal compression syndromes are usually discussed as separate entities, their presentations have been shown to overlap significantly as larger numbers of cases are presented. I thus prefer to treat them as a group, basing treatment on the severity of the lesion and tailoring it secondarily to the anatomic location.

The pathophysiology of proximal median compression differs from that of CTS. Whereas the median nerve is subjected to a diffuse increase in pressure in the CT, proximal entrapment usually results from focal pressure. Structures already present become enlarged as a result of trauma, repetitive motion, or muscle hypertrophy and press on the nerve from one side. These structures include normal anatomic variants, such as a fibrous arcade where the nerve passes beneath the origin of the flexor digitorum sublimis, or true anatomic abnormalities, such as the ligament of Struthers originating from a supracondylar spur of the humerus. The findings of proximal median compression, especially those affecting predominantly the anterior interosseous nerve, may also be produced by neuralgic amyotrophy (Parsonage-Turner syndrome); however, shoulder girdle pain (and eventually weakness) usually set this cause apart from the more common anatomic compressions.

Proximal median compression may be classified into three categories, depending on the severity of the lesion. Mild compression is characterized by aching pain that often is increased by activity. Intermittent sensory loss may occur, but muscle strength is maintained. Moderate compression results in similar symptoms, but with the addition of muscle weakness. Severe compression is accompanied by muscle paralysis.

Discrete sites of proximal median nerve compression include, from proximal to distal, the ligament of Struthers, the bicipital aponeurosis, the pronator teres, and the origin of the sublimis muscles. The ligament of Struthers is a rare anatomic abnormality that originates from a bony spur 2 to 3 inches proximal to the medial epicondyle of the humerus, and it serves as the origin for an accessory head of the pronator teres muscle. A palpable spur, often tender and readily visualized on radiographs, and a Tinel's sign over the adjacent median nerve confirm the anatomic diagnosis. The bicipital aponeurosis (lacertus fibrosus) extends distally and medially from the distal biceps tendon, fanning out over the median nerve and brachial artery. Compression in this area is suggested by a focal Tinel's sign and the production of pain on tightening the aponeurosis. The latter is accomplished by resisting elbow flexion and wrist supination, starting from a position of elbow extension and wrist pronation. Compression by or just proximal to the pronator teres is again suggested by a focal Tinel's sign. If the pronator is involved directly, muscle spasm often forms a painful mass adjacent to the compression site. Pain is increased by resisted pronation in a position of elbow extension to maximally stretch the pronator across the elbow joint. There may also be anomalous fascial bands in this area that compress predominantly the anterior interosseous components of the nerve and that are not specifically identified by provocative testing. The most distal area of potential compression results from passage of the nerve beneath a firm, fascial arcade, which often borders the origin of the sublimis muscles. Resisted sublimis flexion of the middle finger (achieved by holding the other digits extended to block profundus function) causes sharp pain as the nerve is scissored by the taut muscle origin.

Mild compression of the median nerve may occur at any of the sites mentioned. In designing a treatment plan, attention should be focused initially on the identification of repetitive work or leisure activities that worsen the symptoms. These activities are most likely to involve repetitive pronation-supination movements, and they should be modified or eliminated. With relatively mild symptoms, activity modification and a 1 month course of anti-inflammatory medication is often helpful. If the symptoms are more disabling or persist in spite of initial treatment, I splint the affected extremity and interdict its use in work activities. Splinting is designed to relax the structure compressing the median nerve. If this is the bicipital aponeurosis, the elbow is splinted in a position of flexion with the wrist in supination. Conversely, the pronator teres is relaxed by splinting the elbow in flexion and mild pronation. The sublimis muscle does not cross the elbow, so the wrist alone is splinted in a neutral or slightly flexed position (if there are no signs of CTS). If 4 to 6 months' conservative treatment fails to resolve proximal median compression, many patients elect to tolerate their symptoms rather than undergo surgery. Those whose lifestyle or work activity is affected more dramatically usually request surgical relief. In these patients the more common areas of compression are all explored, leaving the median nerve free from the proximal elbow to the mid-forearm.

The initial treatment of moderate proximal compression is similar to that described above, but the indications for surgical intervention vary according to the symptoms. Weakness in the distribution of the anterior interosseous nerve usually reflects compression by or adjacent to the pronator teres. Patients with significant weakness but few sensory changes and little pain, commonly described as "anterior interosseous syndrome," often improve after several months of conservative treatment. Surgery is recommended only if no recovery is observed in the first 4 to 6 months and if there is a pressing need for the muscle function that has been compromised. Compression at the same level, or at the bicipital aponeurosis or sublimis origin, can also produce an entirely different complex of symptoms and findings, the so-called pronator syndrome. These patients are most troubled by chronic pain and sensory abnormalities. They are more apt to require surgery for moderate compression, as their other symptoms are often significantly disabling by the time weakness is noted.

Severe compression is initially treated conservatively, often using a strong anti-inflammatory such as Indocin, or even a short course of steroids, in addition to splinting. If paralysis has not improved after 6 weeks, surgical exploration is strongly recommended to minimize the risk of permanent paralysis.

SUGGESTED READING

Gelberman RG. Operative nerve repair and reconstruction. Philadelphia: JB Lippincott, 1991.

PATIENT RESOURCES

Carpal Tunnel Syndrome (pamphlet)
American Society for Surgery of the Hand
3025 South Parker Road, Suite 65
Aurora, Colorado 80014-2911

Carpal Tunnel Syndrome (booklet)
Krames Communications
1100 Grundy Lane
San Bruno, California 94066-3030

VASCULITIC NEUROPATHY

JOHN T. KISSEL, M.D.
JERRY R. MENDELL, M.D.

CLASSIFICATION

By definition, *vasculitis* is a condition characterized by inflammation and necrosis of blood vessel walls. The clinical vasculitis syndromes represent a heterogeneous group of diseases. We have found the following classification scheme (Table 1) to be clinically useful in the management of these patients, since it has important implications for treatment and prognosis and also indicates which disorders are more likely to be associated with peripheral nerve involvement.

Systemic necrotizing vasculitis (group 1) includes a diverse group of potentially life-threatening disorders that affect multiple organ systems. Small- and medium-sized arteries are involved by the vasculitic process. The peripheral nerve is commonly affected in all of the conditions included in this group.

Hypersensitivity vasculitis (group 2) involves small vessels, including capillaries, arterioles, and venules. Cutaneous manifestations dominate the picture; peripheral nerve and other organ systems may be involved, but much less often. The term hypersensitivity vasculitis

Table 1 Classification of Vasculitic Neuropathy

Group 1: Systemic necrotizing vasculitis
  Classic polyarteritis nodosa
  Allergic angiitis and granulomatosis (Churg-Strauss disease)
  Wegener's granulomatosis
  Vasculitis associated with connective tissue disease
  Overlap syndromes

Group 2: Hypersensitivity vasculitis
  Henoch-Schönlein purpura
  Serum sickness
  Vasculitis associated with infections
  Drug-induced vasculitis
  Vasculitis associated with malignancy

Group 3: Giant cell arteritis
  Temporal arteritis
  Takayasu's arteritis

Group 4: Localized vasculitis
  Isolated angiitis of the peripheral nervous system (nonsystemic
    vasculitic neuropathy)
  Isolated angiitis of the central nervous system

implies exposure to an antigen that may be exogenous or endogenous. Removal of the offending antigen, when this is possible, may reverse the process.

Giant cell arteritis (group 3) involves the large and medium-sized arteries, frequently branches of the carotid artery (particularly the temporal artery and retinal vessels) and the aortic arch and its branches. Temporal arteritis and Takayasu's arteritis are the two clinical syndromes that comprise this group. Mononuclear cells and giant cell formation represent the characteristic tissue reaction in this type of vasculitis. Involvement of peripheral nerve in this group is unusual but has been reported.

Localized vasculitis (group 4) refers to disorders confined to the nervous system. In the peripheral nervous system the condition is called isolated peripheral nerve vasculitis or non-systemic vasculitic neuropathy. The pathologic features observed in the nerve are identical to those of group 1 vasculitides, but clinically patients have no other organ involvement. Clinical manifestations are restricted to the peripheral nerve, although nonspecific symptoms such as malaise, arthralgias, and less often fever, may be present. In our experience, and that of others, isolated peripheral nerve vasculitis has a better prognosis for recovery than the neuropathy complicating any of the systemic necrotizing vasculitides (group 1).

Isolated angiitis of the central nervous system represents an entity clearly distinct from all other forms of vasculitis, and it is not discussed further here. The prognosis is said to be poor, but early diagnosis and treatment have been reported to be effective in some patients.

DIAGNOSIS

The most distinctive clinical pattern of neuropathic involvement of vasculitis is a true multiple mononeu-ropathy in which motor and sensory findings are limited to the distribution of one or more nerves. This restricted distribution, however, occurs in a minority of patients; most have overlapping multiple mononeuropathies. The pattern of individual nerve involvement is obscured by the extent of the process, and the involvement of multiple nerves in one extremity produces more contiguous findings. Careful clinical examination facilitated by electrophysiologic testing usually demonstrates that multiple individual nerves are involved. In some cases, the multifocality of the damage in the proximal nerve trunks reaches a point at which summation of findings produces the clinical picture of a distal, symmetric sensorimotor polyneuropathy.

A definitive diagnosis of vasculitis rests on the histologic demonstration of transmural inflammation and segmental vessel wall necrosis in a biopsy-accessible organ. In peripheral nerve vasculitis, a tissue diagnosis can be expected in at least 80 percent of cases. Selection of the appropriate nerve for biopsy is based on clinical and electrophysiologic evidence of involvement of a specific cutaneous nerve that is accessible for biopsy. In the lower extremity, either the sural or superficial peroneal nerve can be easily approached. The superficial peroneal nerve offers the advantage of simultaneous muscle biopsy through a single incision from the adjacent peroneus brevis muscle. This is important, because vasculitis is more frequently demonstrable in the peroneus muscle than in the superficial peroneal nerve, even in patients with "isolated" peripheral nerve vasculitis. In occasional patients with selective upper extremity involvement, biopsy of the superficial radial nerve may be required.

The laboratory evaluation of patients with suspected systemic vasculitis should be directed toward identification of multiple organ system involvement, especially in kidneys and lungs. No single serologic study is diagnostic of vasculitis, except, possibly, antineutrophil cytoplasmic antibodies, which are very suggestive of Wegener's granulomatosis. Other findings that can be supportive of vasculitis include an accelerated erythrocyte sedimentation rate, positive rheumatoid factor, cryoglobulinemia, hepatitis B antigenemia, and eosinophilia. Serologic tests for lupus, including an antinuclear antibody as well as anti–double-stranded DNA titers, can be useful in specific instances. The presence of extractable nuclear antigens (SS-A, SS-B, RNP) can suggest Sjögren's syndrome or a mixed connective tissue disease.

THERAPY

The classification scheme outlined above provides a valuable framework on which to base therapeutic decisions. Although the exact regimen used for vasculitis must be individualized on the basis of severity, extent, and tempo of involvement, there is general agreement that patients in group 1 should be treated with a combination regimen of corticosteroids and a cytotoxic agent (usually cyclophosphamide), whereas patients in

Table 2 Treatment of Peripheral Nerve Vasculitis

Group 1: Peripheral nerve vasculitis with systemic necrotizing
    vasculitis
      Initiate treatment with daily prednisone, 1.5 mg/kg, and
      cyclophosphamide, 2 mg/kg
      Maintain cyclophosphamide at 2 mg/kg for 1 year
      Switch to alternate-day prednisone with signs of neuro-
      logic improvement and slowly taper prednisone after
      maximum improvement

Group 2: Peripheral nerve vasculitis with hypersensitivity vasculitis
      Remove inciting agent when identified
      Treat with prednisone for limited time (<3 months) if
      necessary

Group 3: Peripheral nerve vasculitis with giant cell arteritis
      Treatment identical to that for temporal arteritis (i.e.,
      daily prednisone monotherapy at dose of 1.5 mg/kg/day
      for 3–5 months followed by slow taper, as above)

Group 4: Isolated peripheral nerve vasculitis
      Initiate treatment with daily prednisone, 1.5 mg/kg, and
      cyclophosphamide, 2 mg/kg
      Taper cyclophosphamide after demonstrating unequivocal
      neurologic improvement
      Maintain prednisone for at least 6 months

groups 2 and 3 are usually managed with steroids alone (Table 2). Some patients with a hypersensitivity vasculitis (group 2) can be treated solely by removing or suppressing an identifiable inciting antigen (such as an exogenous drug, infectious agent, or malignancy), whereas others require corticosteroids. For patients in group 4 with isolated peripheral nerve vasculitis, we suggest a modified approach to immunosuppressant therapy because of the lack of systemic organ system involvement and the better prognosis.

Peripheral Nerve Vasculitis with Systemic Necrotizing Vasculitis

For patients with peripheral neuropathy complicating systemic necrotizing vasculitis, we institute therapy with cyclophosphamide, 2 mg per kilogram per day, and prednisone, 1.5 mg per kilogram per day, both given orally. Prednisone is given mornings as a single daily dose for 4 weeks and then on alternate days at the same dose, 1.5 mg per kilogram. Although rare patients require more prolonged daily steroid treatment, we have found that most receive equal efficacy with fewer side effects from alternate-day therapy. In fulminant cases, when neurologic involvement is extensive, we initiate treatment with an intravenous methylprednisolone "pulse" regimen. Our protocol is to give 1 g of methylprednisolone intravenously every other day for six doses; oral prednisone therapy then follows, as outlined above.

With combination drug therapy for vasculitis, both prednisone and cyclophosphamide are continued until significant improvement occurs and the clinical condition stabilizes, after which prednisone can be *slowly* tapered. We recommend decreasing by 5 mg every 2 weeks, until the dose is 20 mg and then decreasing by 2.5

mg every 2 weeks. This usually extends the total prednisone course to approximately 1 year. During the prednisone taper, fatigue and arthralgias may occur as part of a steroid withdrawal syndrome. These symptoms can easily be confused with an exacerbation of the underlying vasculitis. Temporarily stopping the tapering process while carefully monitoring the patient's neurologic status for signs of deterioration usually clarifies the cause of these symptoms. Cyclophosphamide should be continued 12 months in large doses; tapering can be achieved in 25 mg decrements every 2 weeks.

If symptoms relapse either during tapering or after discontinuation of medication, reinstitution of combination drug therapy is required, following the guidelines established for new patients. We discourage the practice of increasing immunosuppressive drugs in small increments; such an approach is less effective in our experience.

Careful monitoring of side effects is crucial. We strongly advise the use of single dose, alternate-day therapy in an attempt to minimize the devastating side effects of prednisone. In addition, dietary restriction is important. Well-motivated patients can avoid the major side effects of fluid retention, cushingoid appearance, weight gain, hyperglycemia, and hypertension if they adhere to a low-sodium (4 g), low–simple sugar, calorie-restricted diet. Older patients are advised to take vitamin D, 50,000 units orally, twice weekly to increase gastrointestinal calcium absorption. In addition, we recommend at least 1 g of calcium supplementation per day, usually in the form of an over-the-counter calcium-containing antacid tablet. Blood pressure and serum potassium should be monitored every 4 weeks. Prednisone-induced hyperglycemia usually occurs in the first few weeks of treatment. Ocular examinations to assess lens clarity and intraocular pressure should be performed every 6 months. Although many physicians suggest the routine addition of H2 receptor antagonists, we have not found this necessary unless patients have a history of peptic ulcer disease or symptoms of dyspepsia. The occasional patient who develops emotional lability and depression while taking steroids may need antidepressant medication. Osteonecrosis of the femoral head has been an uncommon steroid-induced manifestation in our patients, but it must be considered when any patient develops persistent hip pain while taking corticosteroids. The potential for this serious and debilitating side effect of steroids must always be discussed with patients prior to treatment.

Patients taking cyclophosphamide should have a complete blood count monthly. The cyclophosphamide dose is adjusted to maintain a leukocyte count greater than 3,000 per cubic millimeter and an absolute neutrophil count greater than 1,000 per cubic millimeter. Hemorrhagic cystitis occurs in approximately 15 percent of patients on cyclophosphamide. Oral hydration (at least 8 glasses of water per day) is recommended as prophylaxis. In addition, patients are advised to take cyclophosphamide early in the day to avoid prolonged exposure of the bladder to cyclophosphamide metabolites during sleep. Urinalysis should be performed monthly for microscopic hematuria. Gross hematuria necessitates stopping the drug until bleeding subsides and restarting the cyclophosphamide at a reduced dose (1.5 mg per kilogram per day). Microscopic hematuria requires reducing the dose while maintaining treatment. Alopecia, nausea, and vomiting are not significant problems with oral dosing. Opportunistic infections are always a concern with immunosuppressive therapy, and the slightest hint of infection must be investigated expeditiously and aggressively in these patients.

The purine analogue azathioprine, 2 mg per kilogram per day, is our drug of choice for patients who cannot tolerate cyclophosphamide; it is used in an analogous fashion to cyclophosphamide. In addition to leukopenia, the principal side effect of azathioprine is an influenza-like systemic reaction characterized by fever, nausea, vomiting, diarrhea, and anorexia. This allergic-type reaction occurs in about 10 percent of patients, and in our experience always precludes further use of the drug. We have challenged patients on repeated occasions and have not observed tolerance for the drug, even at one-fourth the initial dose. If liver enzyme values are elevated the dose of azathioprine should be reduced to 1.5 mg per kilogram and titrated to lower doses if necessary.

No accurate serologic test, including the erythrocyte sedimentation rate, consistently reflects the activity of vasculitis. For patients with vasculitic neuropathy, clinical evaluation of motor strength and sensory function are the methods for documenting response to immunosuppressive therapy. Increased muscle strength in proximal muscles represents the earliest sign of improvement. Distal muscles require more time for recovery, because nerve regeneration proceeds at a rate of only approximately 1 inch per month. Patients who show continuing signs of functional improvement can be tapered from medications; cyclophosphamide is stopped after 1 year.

Isolated Peripheral Nerve Vasculitis

As experience in patients with isolated peripheral nerve vasculitis (group 4, nonsystemic vasculitic neuropathy) has grown, it has become clear that many patients in this group do not have a life-threatening process but are prone to relapsing disease. For patients without signs of multiple–organ system involvement we do not feel compelled to recommend cyclophosphamide treatment for 1 year. At the start of treatment, prednisone and cyclophosphamide are given in doses identical to those recommended for systemic necrotizing vasculitis. In contrast to our approach for patients in group 1, however, we taper cyclophosphamide after demonstrating unequivocal neurologic improvement in response to treatment. This approach often allows us to stop cyclophosphamide after 3 to 6 months. Prednisone is always maintained for a minimum of 6 months.

Peripheral Nerve Vasculitis Complicating Giant Cell Arteritis

Rarely, peripheral nerve vasculitis can be seen with temporal arteritis. The treatment for this condition parallels that for treating the temporal artery manifestations; corticosteroids are given in a daily regimen, but cyclophosphamide is not indicated.

Physical Therapy

Although physical and occupational therapy are important treatment modalities in all patients with vasculitic neuropathy, they are particularly important for patients who suffer extensive axonal damage and severe neurologic compromise. An aggressive therapy program aimed at maintaining range of motion, minimizing atrophy (both due to disuse and the effects of steroids), preventing contractures, and optimizing strength and function within the limits of the nerve damage should therefore be instituted as soon as feasible and continued throughout the recovery period.

SUGGESTED READING

Dalakas M. Pharmacologic concerns of corticosteroids in the treatment of patients with immune-related neuromuscular diseases. Neurol Clin 1990; 8:93–118.

Haynes BF, Allen NB, Fauci AS. Diagnostic and therapeutic approach to the patient with vasculitis. Adv Rheumatol 1986; 70:355–368.

Hunder GG, Arend WP, Bloch DA, et al. The American College of Rheumatology 1990 criteria for the classification of vasculitis. Arthritis Rheum 1990; 8:1065–1144.

Kissel JT, Mendell JR. Vasculitic neuropathy. Neurol Clin 1992; 10:761–781.

Kissel JT, Rammohan KW. Pathogenesis and therapy of nervous system vasculitis. Clin Neuropharmacol 1991; 14:28–45.

ATAXIC NEUROPATHIES

JOHN W. GRIFFIN, M.D.

OVERVIEW OF THE DIAGNOSTIC APPROACH

In this chapter I focus on the ataxic neuropathies. The first step in evaluating a patient with gait ataxia is to determine whether the process is likely to be cerebellar or sensory in origin, or whether another problem (frontal lobe disease, hydrocephalus, vestibular disease, among others) is mimicking or amplifying these major possibilities (Table 1). Multiple factors may contribute and produce confusing pictures, especially in elderly persons. The strongest evidence of a sensory ataxia is Romberg's sign — losing balance with the eyes closed but not with the eyes open. If the patient does not develop marked instability when standing normally with the eyes closed, the task can be made more difficult by asking him or her to stand in the tandem position (keeping in mind that some normal persons and many patients with cerebellar disease have difficulty with eyes open or closed). If Romberg's sign is positive, the next question is whether the tendon reflexes are present (or exaggerated) or absent. In some disorders, particularly vitamin B_{12} deficiency, myelopathic sensory loss may be associated with mild neuropathy, so that the ankle reflex may be depressed or absent but the active reflexes at the knee and the extensor plantar reflexes point to spinal cord disease. Similar confusion can occur in patients with combined lumbar radiculopathy and cervical spondylosis, and in patients with Friedreich's ataxia and other spinocerebellar degenerations, in which sensory ataxia is associated with corticospinal tract degeneration and with features of cerebellar disease, including dysarthria and eye movement abnormalities. In general, the eye movements — particularly nystagmus and macrosaccadic oscillations — and dysarthria provide the most reliable means of recognizing cerebellar disease clinically when there is a question of neuropathic sensory ataxia, cerebellar involvement, or both.

Once it is determined that the disorder appears to be sensory ataxia, the possibilities are disease of the sensory nerves or of the dorsal columns. The difficulties in making the clinical distinction between these possibilities on the basis of gait and sensory neuron testing are to be expected, because the primary sensory neuron is involved in both peripheral and cord sites. The keys to differential diagnosis of the sensory ataxias are: first, to determine whether the process involves the peripheral process of the sensory neuron or its central process; if the latter, to distinguish between disease of the dorsal roots (reflexes should be lost) and dorsal columns (reflexes should be present or exaggerated); and finally, to determine the nature of the responsible cellular lesion (neuronal loss, axonal loss, demyelination).

Electrodiagnosis is an essential aid. Figure 1 provides a differential decision tree; from this scheme it is clear that the major branch points are determined by the electrodiagnostic results. For example, three groups have normal sensory nerve action potentials: myelopathies with predominant dorsal column involvement (such as subacute combined degeneration associated with vitamin B_{12} deficiency) that can masquerade as neuropathies; dorsal radiculopathies, such as tabes dorsalis, in which only the central process of the primary sensory neuron and not the peripheral portion is involved; and hysteria with astasia-abasia and a factitious gait ataxia.

A small but distinctive group of neuropathies produce gait ataxia. Within this group the causes are diverse, but most produce a similar clinical picture. The treatments vary with the cause, so accurate diagnosis of the cause is the cornerstone of therapy. All the disorders to be considered here produce loss of kinesthesia and joint position sense, with the consequent clinical manifestations of gait ataxia, rombergism, pseudoathetosis of the outstretched hands in the absence of visual control, and defects in localization of limbs in space, associated with loss of tendon reflexes but preservation of strength. A unifying concept is that all these disorders produce loss of sensibility from muscle and joint receptors in both short and long nerves. The underlying lesion that produces these deficits is most frequently loss of sensory neurons in the dorsal root ganglia (sensory neuronopathy). Less frequently, demyelination, distal axonal degeneration, or selective loss of dorsal root fibers with preservation of the sensory neurons and their peripheral processes can be invoked.

Generalized loss of the sensory nerve action potentials with preservation of the motor amplitudes and velocities suggests diffuse degeneration of the primary sensory neurons, of the type seen in the *sensory ganglionitis syndromes (sensory neuronopathies).*

Table 1 Differential Diagnosis of Acquired Ataxic Neuropathy

Immune-mediated disorders
  Sensory ganglionitis
    Carcinomatous sensory neuropathy
    Sensory neuropathy associated with sicca syndrome
    Idiopathic sensory neuronopathy
  Demyelinating neuropathies
    Guillain-Barré syndrome
      Rare primary manifestation
      Residua in severe typical cases
      Miller Fisher syndrome
    Rare cases of chronic inflammatory demyelinating
      polyneuropathy
    Some cases of IgM k gammopathies

Infectious disorders
  Tabes dorsalis
  Diphtheritic polyneuropathy
  Rare manifestation of human immunodeficiency virus
    (HIV)–related sensory neuropathy

Toxic disorders
  Vitamin B_6
  Cis-platinum
  Metronidazole
  Vacor

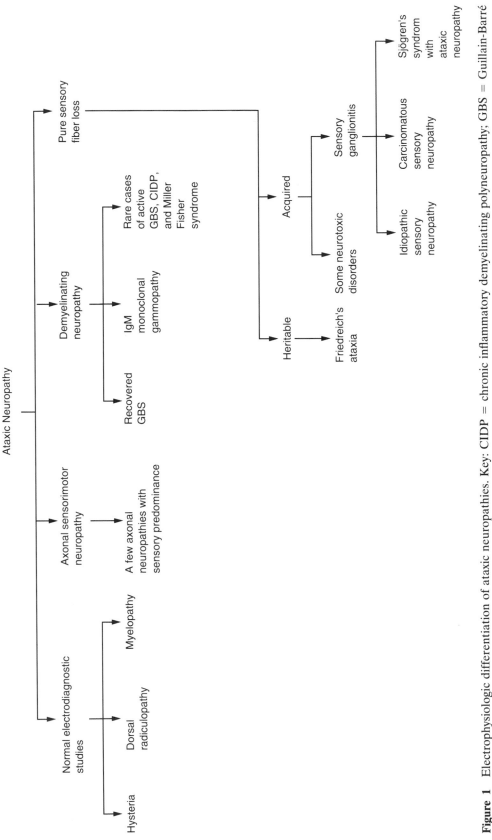
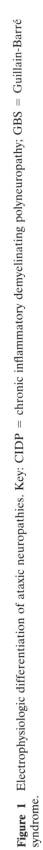

Figure 1 Electrophysiologic differentiation of ataxic neuropathies. Key: CIDP = chronic inflammatory demyelinating polyneuropathy; GBS = Guillain-Barré syndrome.

These disorders are characterized by inflammatory destruction of the sensory neurons with consequent loss of the nerve fibers in both the central and peripheral branches. Their electrodiagnostic pattern contrasts with that seen in the usual *axonal* or *dying back* neuropathies, in which length-dependent fiber vulnerability results initially in loss of the longest sensory and motor fibers, with relative preservation of shorter fibers. In these disorders the sural sensory potentials may be reduced or absent at times when the sensory potentials in the arms are relatively normal. In addition, distally predominant denervation is usually found in the legs. Although such distally predominant degeneration of long axons is the most prevalent pathologic picture in peripheral neuropathies in general, it is less commonly the sensory neuropathy among the ataxic neuropathies.

The nerve conduction studies in demyelinating neuropathies are also easily distinguished from the sensory neuronopathies. In demyelination there are reduced conduction velocities, usually out of proportion to the reductions in the evoked amplitudes. Often, even though the clinical deficits appear to be predominantly sensory, evidence of motor fiber demyelination, with slowing or conduction block, can usually be found. Among the disorders that produce this picture a small number of cases of Guillain-Barré syndrome (GBS) and of chronic inflammatory demyelinating polyneuropathy (CIDP), the distinctive but uncommon disorder named for Miller Fisher, and the immunoglobulin M (IgM) paraproteins that have reactivity against an epitope of the myelin-associated glycoproteins (MAG) and other nerve glycolipids and glycoproteins.

SENSORY GANGLIONITIS SYNDROMES

Three disorders are included under the designation sensory ganglionitis: ataxic neuropathy associated with Sjögren's syndrome, idiopathic sensory neuronopathy, and carcinomatous sensory neuropathy. All share the pathologic features of lymphocytic infiltration of dorsal root ganglia and destruction of sensory neurons. However, as indicated in Table 2, there are clinical differences that allow suspicion of the correct diagnosis in the clinic.

Ataxic Neuropathy With Features of Sjögren's Syndrome

This recently recognized disorder is the most frequent cause of ataxic neuropathy diagnosed at Johns Hopkins (Fig. 2). The ocular and other features of Sjögren's syndrome are often minor, and the neuropathy is usually the presenting manifestation. Some patients do have xerophthalmia and dry mouth sufficient to diagnose sicca syndrome before the neurologic symptoms develop. Conversely, reviews of the neuropathic consequences of typical Sjögren's syndrome have shown that the ataxic neuropathy is rare, whereas multiple mononeuropathies and axonal sensorimotor neuropathies are frequently encountered. The ataxic neuropathy patients thus form a distinct subgroup of the Sjögren's patients. The salient point is that ataxic neuropathy associated with features of Sjögren's syndrome is a syndrome that can readily be recognized by clinical and laboratory testing; its pathophysiologic relationship to more usual manifestations of Sjögren's syndrome awaits better understanding of the pathogenesis.

The laboratory features useful in recognizing this syndrome are positive Schirmer and rose bengal tests, inflammation of the minor salivary glands on lip biopsy, and a markedly abnormal antinuclear antibody titer, with or without the Ro or La reactivity often associated with Sjögren's syndrome.

The neurologic examination is dominated by the loss of kinesthesia. In the legs, this is reflected as Romberg's sign. In the upper extremities a useful test is to ask the patient to find the thumb of one hand with the index finger of the other without visual guidance. In normal persons this is a prompt, secure movement. In patients with loss of kinesthesia the moving hand must search for the thumb. In the most severe cases, so much touch sensibility is lost that the patient may not recognize when contact is made. The fingers and arms demonstrate pseudoathetosis — slow, writhing movements of the fingers and hands. Pseudoathetosis is easiest to see with the arms outstretched, but in severe cases it can be recognized in the hands at rest.

Autonomic dysfunction is common. A characteristic abnormality is the development of Adie's pupils, unilaterally or, more often, bilaterally. In one case, a unilateral Adie's pupil predated development of symptomatic Sjögren's syndrome and subsequent ataxic neuropathy

Table 2 Sensory Ganglionitis Syndromes

Feature	Sicca Syndrome	Idiopathic	Carcinomatous
Female predilection	Marked	Modest	Absent
Course	Variable, acute to chronic	Variable, acute to chronic	Subacute
Progression	Variable, may stabilize or improve	Variable, may stabilize or improve	Progressive
Fiber predilection	Large fiber, kinesthetic loss	Large fiber, kinesthetic loss	More global
Associated central nervous system involvement	Usually none	None	Cerebellar involvement
Serologic studies	ANA$^+$, Ig ↑	Normal	Normal
Antineuronal nuclear antibody	−	−	+
Cerebrospinal fluid	Normal	Normal	↑ cells, protein
Nerve biopsy	Inflammation, large fiber loss	Large fiber loss	More global fiber loss

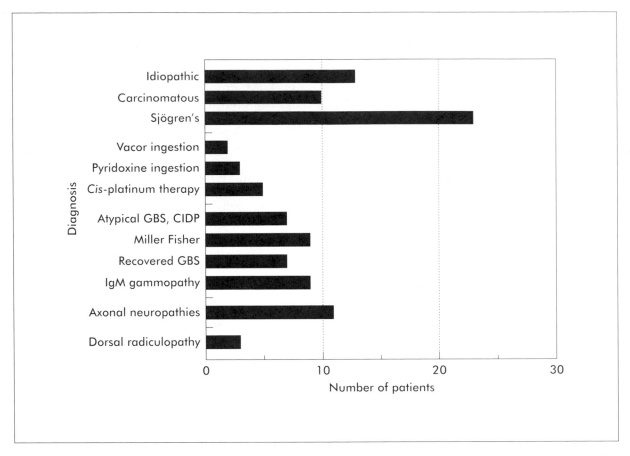

Figure 2 Numbers of patients with acquired ataxic neuropathies evaluated at Johns Hopkins, 1981–1989. The first three rows, the sensory ganglionitis syndromes, were the most frequent diagnoses. Key: CIDP = chronic inflammatory demyelinating polyneuropathy; GBS = Guillain-Barré syndrome.

by 24 years. As the ataxic neuropathy began, this patient developed an Adie's pupil in the second eye.

The histologic appearance is remarkable for a variable degree of neuronal loss and marked lymphocytic infiltration of the ganglia and dorsal roots. In cutaneous sensory nerves, large myelinated fibers are lost. Small myelinated and unmyelinated fiber densities are relatively preserved. Several nerve biopsy specimens have had small perivascular inflammatory cuffs around epineurial vessels.

Therapy

In general, attempts at immunotherapy have proved disappointing. In most patients, oral and intravenous corticosteroids, cyclophosphamide, and azathioprine have had no obvious effect on the course of the disorder, although a slowing of the progression cannot be excluded. Most patients received their initial therapy at a time when SNAPs were markedly reduced or absent, making the likelihood of recovery low. Rare patients with relatively preserved SNAPs stabilize or improve after treatment with intravenous methylprednisolone and oral azathioprine.

Idiopathic Sensory Neuronopathy

This category, one of the most frequent causes of acquired ataxic neuropathy, includes patients with acute, subacute, and chronic disease courses. The acute form is particularly dramatic: devastating sensory loss develops over a few days. The spinal fluid protein value may be elevated. In the more chronic forms, it is usually normal. Results of other laboratory tests are normal and useful principally in excluding Sjögren's syndrome and cancer. Pathologic studies have been rare, but the results have been similar to the findings in Sjögren's syndrome with sensory ganglionitis.

The prognosis is highly variable, but in time the majority of patients with this disorder are able to return to their previous career. The role of therapy is uncertain; most patients have received corticosteroids at some point, and some authors have suspected that such therapy may minimize progression. In acute cases, I use oral prednisone for 10 days with a rapid taper. More important are reassurance, gait training and safety instruction, as described below.

Carcinomatous Sensory Neuropathy

While the sensory neuronopathy associated with underlying lung, breast, ovary, or other carcinomas has a pathologic basis similar to the other two disorders described, the clinical manifestations are often sufficiently different to suggest the diagnosis. The initial symptom is often neuropathic pain. In contrast to most painful neuropathies in which the pain is most intense in the feet, the hands, and in some cases the face, are often severely affected. The spinal fluid is frequently abnormal, with either pleocytosis or elevated protein. Often there is evidence of CNS involvement such as dementia, cerebellar dysfunction, or myelopathy. The sensory loss is more global, as reflected in nerve biopsies showing loss of small myelinated and unmyelinated fibers as well as large myelinated fibers. Finally, a significant proportion of patients have antineuronal antibodies directed against a 37 kD nuclear antigen (anti-Hu antibodies). Patients who present with subacute sensory neuronopathy require meticulous examination for underlying carcinoma.

The course is usually inexorable, although occasionally the disease stabilizes. Early discovery of the neoplasm can be life saving, but it only infrequently results in improvement in the neurologic disorder. Immunosuppressive therapies have had disappointing results, and at this time I recommend no drug therapy other than that indicated for the cancer. Control of the neuropathic pain is often difficult and may require opiates.

IMMUNE-MEDIATED DEMYELINATING NEUROPATHIES

Predominantly sensory neuropathies in which demyelination is the underlying lesion occur in several settings. Rarely, GBS and CIDP present with predominantly sensory manifestations. A related but distinctive disorder, the Miller Fisher syndrome, is characterized by ataxia, areflexia, and internal and external ophthalmoplegia with little or no weakness. That this is a demyelinating neuropathy has been inferred from electrophysiologic findings of temporal dispersion, and from the occasional patients who go on to develop more typical motor involvement or paralysis. Recently, a high frequency of antibodies against $GD1_q$ has been recognized in this disorder. An easily diagnosed group is comprised of persons who recover from severe but otherwise typical GBS but who often are left with sensory loss and ataxia; this presumably reflects the recovery of strength by regeneration of motor fibers coupled with the inability of degenerated dorsal root fibers to regenerate into the spinal cord.

Another disorder with underlying demyelination includes patients with benign monoclonal gammopathies and IgM paraproteins. These paraproteins share reactivity directed against a sulfated glycoconjugate. This epitope is found in some nerve glycolipids, but it was initially recognized because it is also in the MAG. The disorder associated with "anti-MAG" antibodies usually progresses slowly (over years); in addition to sensory loss, a rapid tremor is frequently noted. The paraprotein can be found bound to involved myelin sheaths, and characteristic pathologic changes occur in animals injected with the human IgM. These findings suggest that the IgM itself causes the nerve damage and that lowering the level of the paraprotein should be beneficial. Although some data indicate some benefit from plasmapheresis, the results are not impressive. In view of the age of most of the patients, the slow pace of progression, and the expense, I do not use plasmapheresis or cytotoxic agents in these patients. In these latter cases, in addition to SNAPs suggesting demyelination, motor conduction studies have shown clear-cut evidence of demyelination, despite the apparent absence of motor symptoms.

NEUROTOXIC CAUSES OF SENSORY NEURONOPATHY

Pyridoxine intoxication should be sought in patients with ataxic neuropathies. The history of exposure needs to be specifically sought; patients may not consider their vitamin supplements as noteworthy, yet vitamin B_6 is ingested as a "health food" in 500 to 1,000 mg capsules. Doses as low as 200 mg per day taken for long periods appear to be sufficient to induce gait ataxia and numb feet. These smaller doses are typical of the levels often suggested by physicians for treating premenstrual or carpal tunnel symptoms. Affected patients often have uncomfortable dysesthetic symptoms. Signs of large fiber loss and gait ataxia are the major clinical manifestations. Patients usually improve after stopping B_6, which suggests that the pathology, at least in milder cases, is distal axonal degeneration of primary sensory neurons. The therapy is therefore self-evident.

Cis-platinum is an effective chemotherapeutic agent for a number of solid tumors, including ovarian carcinoma, but neurotoxicity, ototoxicity, and nephrotoxicity limit its use. Neurotoxicity is clearly dose dependent, and dysesthesias often precede more severe sensory loss. The frequency with which neurologists are called to see such patients is declining as dosage guidelines have evolved. Still, occasional patients who require the agent develop neurotoxicity. The clinical picture includes loss of proprioceptive and vibratory sensibility, and loss of tendon reflexes, usually beginning at the ankles. Ataxia with pseudoathetosis frequently develops, but at least moderate recovery can be anticipated after the drug is discontinued. *Taxol,* a microtubule-stabilizing agent useful in cancer chemotherapy, also can produce an ataxic neuropathy.

Vacor, a phenylnitrourea rodenticide, was widely used 10 years ago as an alternative to warfarin. Introduced in the hopes that it might be less toxic to humans and large animals, it proved to be popular for suicide attempts. Vacor produces a distinctive clinical picture of abdominal pain and hyperglycemia due to toxin-induced pancreatic necrosis, followed by sensory and autonomic neuropathy. Although it should be encountered very rarely now, it is important because there is a specific antidote that is effective when given early: large doses of nicotinamide prevent, and even reverse, the toxic manifestations.

DORSAL RADICULOPATHIES

A small but intriguing group of conditions is distinguished by the combination of sensory ataxia, areflexia, preserved SNAPs, and normal or nearly normal cutaneous nerve on examination of biopsy tissue. Although no pathologic confirmation is available, the combined clinical, electrodiagnostic, and histologic features suggest that such patients may have a disease that selectively involves the dorsal roots proximal to the ganglia. Tabes dorsalis can also be regarded as a form of dorsal radiculopathy with kinesthetic loss. Tabes patients have a characteristic loss of pain sensibility and are predisposed to sustain painless injuries in addition to their ataxia. I have followed a patient with severe ataxia and normal SNAPs who proved to have the acquired immunodeficiency syndrome (AIDS), and this possibility should be considered in such patients.

The differential diagnosis of the constellation of findings that suggest dorsal radiculopathy must include hysteria and myelopathies with dorsal column involvement such as subacute combined degeneration.

GENERAL THERAPEUTIC STRATEGIES FOR ATAXIC NEUROPATHIES

In all of these disorders the most important principles are *avoidance of falls and injuries* and *continuation of supervised walking.* For these disorders, a committed physical therapist is invaluable. In my view, the best therapy is continued walking. The ability of profoundly "deafferented" patients to "relearn" and compensate for the sensory deficits is remarkable. Conversely, falls, and the attendant time in bed, represent major setbacks, and it often takes months for the patient to return to the preinjury level of function. Reviewing safety in the home includes a floor plan of the house and special attention to the location of steps and the layout of the bathroom. Handrails and, in the bathroom, grab rails mounted in the joists of the wall are essential. Patients are well advised to accept assistance and to use stable walkers when appropriate. Younger patients compensate and recover function more quickly and completely than older patients, but an optimistic prognosis is realistic for most persons with acquired sensory neuropathies.

SUGGESTED READING

Asbury AK. Sensory neuronopathy. Semin Neurol 1987; 7:58–66.

Griffin JW, Cornblath DR. The ataxic neuropathies. In: Sluga E, Budka H, eds. Sensory neuropathies. Berlin: Springer-Verlag, 1993 (in press).

Griffin JW, Cornblath DR, Alexander E, et al. Ataxic sensory neuropathy and dorsal root ganglionitis associated with Sjogren's syndrome. Ann Neurol 1990; 27:304–315.

Sterman AB, Schaumburg HH, Asbury AK. The acute sensory neuropathy syndrome: a distinct clinical entity. Ann Neurol 1980; 7:354–358.

Thomas PK, Ochoa J. Clinical features and differential diagnosis. In: Dyck PJ, Thomas PK, Griffin JW, et al., eds. Peripheral neuropathy. 3rd ed. Philadelphia: W.B. Saunders, 1993:749.

FAMILIAL NEUROPATHIES

THOMAS O. CRAWFORD, M.D.
J. DAVID THOMPSON, M.D.

Our understanding of the specific genetic and cellular pathogenesis of many of the familial peripheral neuropathies has begun to expand rapidly in recent years. Unfortunately, this progress has not yet extended to any form of specific therapy. Despite the lack of definitive treatments the functional status of many patients can be substantially altered by supportive therapy. Moreover, careful and appropriate counseling is important to minimize the individual and familial distress that often accompany the diagnosis.

DIAGNOSIS

The most common familial neuropathy, Charcot-Marie-Tooth disease type I (CMT-I) is dominantly inherited with complete penetrance though potentially discordant severity within the family. Diagnosis rests on the demonstration of peroneal muscle weakness and atrophy, enlarged nerves, and symmetrically slow nerve conduction velocities in two or more generations. In some persons the deficits may be so subtle as to be unknown: in this case taking the family history often requires individual physical examinations. In unusual or isolated cases sural nerve biopsy is indicated to demonstrate the characteristic monotonous onion bulb formations without noteworthy active demyelination or remyelination. The recent finding of a specific region of duplication on chromosome 17 in most families with CMT-I will undoubtedly soon spawn a commercial blood test useful for the diagnosis of unusual patients or those without available family.

Two other dominantly inherited disorders may cause the peroneal muscle atrophy syndrome. The first, Charcot-Marie-Tooth type II, has a similar phenotype but normal or nearly normal nerve conduction velocities with diminished compound muscle action potential and sensory nerve action potentials. The other, distal spinal muscular atrophy, is similar to CMT-II but spares sensory function and sensory nerve action potentials. Some recessive disorders may have phenotypic similarities. The most common, Friedreich's ataxia, may have comparable peroneal muscle atrophy with pes cavus, but in addition has more profound sensory and cerebellar ataxia with other distinctive neurologic, cardiac, and orthopaedic features.

GENERAL SUPPORTIVE CARE

Most inherited neuropathies are not directly associated with neuropathic pain, although pain sensibility is usually spared and associated orthopaedic problems may be painful. Many patients complain of diffuse leg and foot aching at the end of the day, especially after strenuous activity. This may be the result of cumulative ligament strain with distal weakness. Pain of this sort can usually be palliated with over-the-counter analgesics; rarely tricyclic antidepressants (amitriptyline) may be necessary. Proper shoes, with adequate sole cushioning, are important.

An associated problem is frequent ankle sprains. Most patients with weak ankles do not need to be told to forego high-heeled shoes. The type of surface most often associated with falling may determine the best therapy. Patients with weak ankles who stumble on irregular ground may benefit from articulated ankle-foot orthoses (AFOs), which provide medial and lateral ankle support but allow dorsiflexion and plantar flexion for a more normal gait. The patient with foot drop who occasionally "catches a toe" while indoors may want to change to smooth-soled shoes that are less likely to grab the floor. With more severe foot drop, a standard AFO is appropriate. To be effective the AFO must extend over the entire calf: short AFOs or supramalleolar orthoses (SMOs) provide no more support than high-topped shoes or boots.

The potential for missing focal nerve entrapment syndromes may be increased in patients with mild generalized polyneuropathy. Carpal tunnel syndrome and ulnar entrapment may be more common in patients with nerves enlarged by onion bulb formation. A high degree of suspicion and careful electrophysiologic examination through the entrapped area is necessary for the diagnosis. Surgical intervention is generally indicated if symptoms agree with electrophysiologic findings. Wheelchair-bound patients should be carefully positioned, with trunk supports if necessary, to thwart weight bearing on the elbows and consequent ulnar nerve compression. Available space within the spinal canal may be effaced when nerve roots are much enlarged, causing symptoms of spinal claudication, a cauda equina syndrome, myelopathy, or root compression. Generally, these rare complications should respond to surgical decompression.

Role of Therapy

In general, the role of physical and occupational therapy is to maintain function through stretching and light-load exercise, provide appropriate assistive devices, and encourage a sense of self-reliance. These goals can usually be met with routine but infrequent visits. In many cases, a home evaluation by a therapist reveals ways that independent functioning can be enhanced that may not have been suspected otherwise. Examples of such devices include grab bars, high toilets with lateral or transfer supports, tub access aids, lever "doorknobs," and stair ramps or climbers. Patients with limited hand use benefit from built-up handles on utensils, hair and toothbrushes, dressing aids, and jar and can openers. The number of different devices that may be helpful is very large: a good idea is to lend patients a catalogue of self-help aids to review with a therapist.

Many patients have difficulty writing. Because many light-duty jobs require some form of written communication, attention to assistive written communication devices is particularly important and cost effective. This emphasis is appropriate even for children before significant disability appears, as all patients should be encouraged to learn typing and computer skills well. Typing by patients with Friedreich's ataxia is often limited by unsteadiness of the hands at the keyboard. This problem is easily addressed by fashioning detachable Velcro bracelets that stick to a Velcro-covered wrist rest placed in front of the keyboard.

Orthopaedics

The orthopedic problems of patients with familial neuropathies can be characterized as (1) frequent progressive foot deformity and disability, (2) scoliosis of variable incidence (common in Friedreich's ataxia, uncommon in CMT disease), and (3) occasional hand disability. The orthopaedic deformities and disabilities of familial neuropathies present a spectrum of clinical involvement that varies with the severity of the specific disorder and the age at onset. In general, orthopaedic deformities are more common, more severe, and more progressive when neurologic disease progression takes place during the years of skeletal growth than after skeletal maturity.

Pes cavus, the presence of pronounced arch or excessive plantar flexion of the first ray, occurs by the second or third decade in most patients with CMT disease. Although pes cavus is the most readily recognized of the foot deformities of CMT (Fig. 1), it is characteristically accompanied by other foot deformities, including foot equinus, heel varus, and claw toe. AFOs can retard the development of foot equinus when

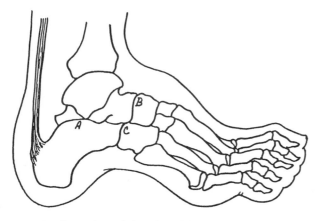

Figure 1 Cavus foot deformity with *(A)* subtalar joint, *(B)* talonavicular joint and *(C)* calcaneocuboid joint.

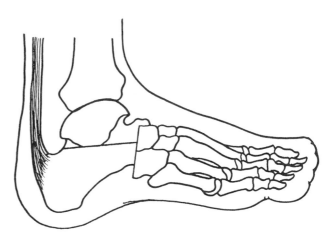

Figure 2 Triple arthrodesis with bone resection and correction of deformity.

they are used before deformity is fixed. In contrast, shoe inserts do not retard deformity, but for some patients they can lessen the pressure, discomfort, and problems of wearing shoes.

Patients who develop significant but dynamic deformity before skeletal maturity may be most advantaged by operative tendon transfers that redirect the posterior tibial and extensor hallucis longus tendons to new insertion sites. This balances the deforming forces across the foot to prevent or significantly retard the development of fixed deformity. When fixed deformity and disability develop, triple arthrodesis (resection of bone to correct deformity and fusion of the subtalar, talonavicular, and calcaneocuboid joints; Fig. 2) improves foot position and stability, but the prevalence of long-term good or excellent results is only 25 to 40 percent. Pseudoarthrosis (15 percent) and secondary degenerative changes in the ankle and midfoot (25 to 60 percent) are significant later complications.

Scoliosis has been reported in 10 percent of CMT patients, though only a minority require spine fusion as treatment. The scoliosis of CMT is comparable to idiopathic scoliosis in age of onset, types of curves, risk of progression, response to brace treatment, and need for spine fusion.

Hand weakness and atrophy are common but infrequently cause serious disability. Rarely, hand procedures such as opponensplasty (tendon transfers for improved thumb abduction or opposition) are indicated to improve function.

The most common orthopaedic manifestations of Friedreich's ataxia are scoliosis and pes cavus. Scoliosis affects 90 percent of patients, is usually progressive, and responds little to bracing. Early spine fusion (when curvature has reached as little as 35 degrees in the upright spine) should be considered, because steady progression is usual and delay increases operative risks as most patients also have advancing cardiomyopathy.

The pes cavus of Friedreich's ataxia may contribute

to the gait disorder, but ataxia is usually the most significant problem. Operative procedures similar to those for CMT are indicated when the foot deformity significantly limits ambulation.

The ataxia can be partially compensated with AFOs (standard or articulated) along with ambulation aids (single-point or quad canes, crutches, walkers). Truncal bracing may produce some improvement in overall functioning by stabilizing the trunk, which in turn steadies the hand.

Counseling

Patients with CMT-I or -II should be advised that they can expect to have a normal life span. Most remain productive throughout, although many need to make adjustments to maintain function. Expectations about the course of the disease are naturally shaped by the experiences of affected older members of the family. While this is a useful start, the variable severity of the neuropathy within a family means such experience may be falsely alarming or reassuring. A better predictor of an individual's future function is his or her present function, the rule being that changes are generally slow but steady.

One experience common to many who care for families with CMT and other chronic neurologic disorders is how poorly the degree of neurologic impairment predicts the degree of independent functioning. Our experience suggests that the presence or absence of a good sense of perspective on the neurologic problems is an equally good, or more important, predictor. The primary goal of physical and occupational therapy should be to promote good judgment about the functional significance or insignificance of a neurologic deficit. Factors in the doctor-patient relationship may play an important role in the patient's self-definition of disability. If the physician encounter is focused predominantly on the lack of primary treatments, the need to secure disability entitlements, or by perceived physician indifference to comorbid problems, the indirect message is that CMT is a relentless and disabling disease. Alternatively, if the physician is perceived as realistic but enthusiastic, with a focus on solutions to specific obstacles, the indirect message encourages personal ambition and responsibility. (Curiously, the actual physician work product—e.g., a prescription for a walker or disability papers—may be the same in either case.)

These issues of self-definition are most important to children when important features of self-image are formed. All children, sick and well, experiment with the sick role at times and through this define their own personal limits for withdrawal from activity. Most children with CMT are not handicapped but are perceived as unathletic or clumsy. To seek refuge in a chronic sick role solves the child's short-term social concern for "saving face" but may encourage a long-term sense of disability. Parents, teachers, therapists, and physicians thus confront the difficult task of fostering an accurate but productive self-image.

This problem is especially apparent in school. The twin perils of overprotection and underidentification of disability should be recognized. On the one hand, bureaucratic concerns sometimes insulate children with a neurologic diagnosis, however mild. On the other, children with CMT may appear more able bodied than they are. The notion of some that weak or clumsy children need to "try harder" may not fit those with deficits related to sensation as well as weakness. In general, children with CMT should participate in physical education with their peers, although they may experience problems with certain running or jumping activities. Direct communication with teachers can help much. It is virtually impossible to prescribe accurately the correct level of school activity. Instead, it is important to share these problems of assessment with parents, teachers, administrators, and therapists; sanction (in writing) the use of their best judgment; and promote communication between them. All concerned, including the children themselves, should be encouraged to tolerate, learn from, and adjust to the inevitable errors of assessment as they occur.

The recent finding of a DNA test for many patients with CMT-I raises the possibility of early prenatal diagnosis and selective abortion of an affected fetus. Separate from the complex and controversial issues raised by this use of genetic information, there is also significant potential for the misuse of genetic information. Decisions about terminating a pregnancy are based partly on impressions of the severity of the disease, which may be determined by the most visible, and hence most impaired, CMT-affected persons. A more broadly assessed impression of CMT suggests it is a less severe condition. Most persons with CMT consider it more a mild, persistent problem than a handicap. Genetic counselors thus need to help potential parents to develop a clear understanding of both the probability of meaningful impairment as well as the probability of inheritance.

RARE DISEASES WITH SPECIAL CONCERNS

Abetalipoproteinemia

Children with vitamin E deficiency due to abetalipoproteinemia (Bassen-Kornzweig disease), cholestasis, or chronic liver disease are at risk for developing a peripheral neuropathy mixed with features of posterior column and cerebellar deficits. If recognized prior to age 3 years, many of these neurologic problems can be minimized. Vitamin E given as tocopherol polyethylene glycol succinate (Liqui-E, available in health food stores) is better than Aquasol E because it is better absorbed by these patients. The best measure of tissue vitamin E is adipose vitamin E level; the best serum test is the vitamin E–total serum lipid ratio. Breath ethane tests may be a better assay of biologic vitamin E availability in patients with abnormal serum lipids. In many patients the neuropathy may progress despite adequate vitamin E therapy, presumably because of multiple other dietary deficiencies.

Refsum's Disease

The progression of symptoms of Refsum's disease (peripheral neuropathy, deafness, and vision loss due to retinitis pigmentosa) can be retarded with careful dietary restriction of phytanic acid. Phytanic acid is found in leafy green vegetables and the meat or milk of ruminant animals; it is low in fish, chicken, and corn. Other disorders of phytanic acid metabolism (identified by serum phytanic acid levels above 3.0 μg per milliliter) may also be aided with strict dietary control.

Hereditary Sensory Autonomic Neuropathy

Rare patients with hereditary sensory autonomic neuropathy, leprosy, or another severe sensory neuropathy may have ulcers or excessive corns and calluses on the soles of the feet. If these are not aggressively treated, they can lead to severe foot deformity through chronic infection. Treatment is directed toward fastidious foot care, extreme attention to shoe fit, and avoidance of trauma by wearing shoes full time while awake. Even more rare are patients with mutilating disorders of the digits, often associated with repeated paronychia. Similar attention to hand care is indicated, with padded gloves and built-up utensils, pens, and keys to avoid all risk of trauma.

Fabry's Disease

The peripheral neuropathy of Fabry's disease is unusual in that small fibers are particularly involved and paroxysms of burning pain from the hands and feet are common. Treatment consists of anticonvulsant doses of phenytoin or carbamazepine.

SUGGESTED READING

Alexander IJ, Johnson KA. Assessment and management of pes cavus in Charcot-Marie-Tooth disease. Clin Orthop 1989; 246:273–280.
Cady RE, Babechko WP. Incidence, natural history and treatment of scoliosis in Friedreich's ataxia. J Pediatr Orthop 1984; 4:673–676.
Charcot-Marie-Tooth disorders: Pathophysiology, molecular genetics, and therapy. Neurol Neurobiol 1990; 53.

PATIENT RESOURCES

Muscular Dystrophy Association
810 Seventh Avenue
New York, New York 10019
Telephone: (212) 586-0808

The MDA is a nonprofit national organization that provides funds for patient care, education, support, and research. Patients with Charcot-Marie-Tooth are eligible for services; those with other diagnoses may not be eligible. Local chapters in the United States are easily found in phone directories or through the national office.

Charcot-Marie-Tooth Association
Crozer Mills Enterprise Center
601 Upland Avenue
Upland, Pennsylvania 19015
Telephone: (215) 499-7486

The Charcot-Marie-Tooth Association primarily provides education, sponsorship of patient conferences, and local physician referral.

NEUROMUSCULAR JUNCTION AND MUSCLE DISEASES

MYASTHENIA GRAVIS

DANIEL B. DRACHMAN, M.D.

Myasthenia gravis (MG) is an autoimmune disorder of neuromuscular junctions, characterized by weakness and fatigability of skeletal muscles. Typically, the extraocular and eyelid muscles are affected early, producing symptoms of diplopia and ptosis. The limb muscles are often weak, with proximal muscles (deltoids, triceps, and iliopsoas) affected more than distal muscles. Life-threatening weakness of the muscles of respiration and swallowing may occur; the patient is then said to be in *crisis*. Neuromuscular *fatigue,* manifested by increased weakness on repeated muscle use and improvement after rest, is characteristic of MG. The outlook for patients with MG has improved much; if properly treated, more than 90 percent can return to full, productive lives. However, the ultimate goal of a cure has not yet been reached; most patients must continue to take medications despite the risks of adverse side effects. At present, four methods of treatment are available: (1) enhancement of neuromuscular transmission (anticholinesterase [anti-ChE] agents), (2) surgical thymectomy, (3) immunosuppression, and (4) plasmapheresis to deplete circulating antibodies.

Rational treatment of MG requires an understanding of the pathogenesis of the disease. The basic abnormality in MG is a reduction of acetylcholine receptors (AChRs) at neuromuscular junctions, which results in impairment of neuromuscular transmission, and hence weakness and muscle fatigue. Antibody-mediated autoimmune mechanisms play a key role in this process; anti-AChR antibodies are detectable in the sera of more than 80 percent of patients with MG. These autoantibodies act to decrease the number of available AChRs by several well-described mechanisms. Though anti-AChR antibodies are clearly implicated in the pathogenesis of MG, their absolute serum concentration does not correspond closely with the patient's clinical

status. However, in a given patient, treatment-induced reduction of anti-AChR antibody levels usually parallels clinical improvement.

Although anti-AChR antibodies are produced by the B lymphocytes, the factors that trigger the autoimmune response are not yet known. The complex relationship of the thymus to MG suggests that this organ may play an important role in the origin and maintenance of the autoimmune response in MG.

EVALUATION OF PATIENTS

The diagnosis of MG usually commits the patient to medical or surgical therapy that entails significant risks. Therefore, before initiating treatment of the myasthenic patient, it is essential (1) to establish the diagnosis unequivocally (Table 1), (2) to search for associated conditions that may influence the choice of treatment (Table 2), and (3) to assess the patient's baseline strength, in order to evaluate the effectiveness of subsequent therapy. The most useful objective tests are those of forward arm abduction time and vital capacity.

Since the natural course of MG is variable, it is

Table 1 Diagnosis of Myasthenia Gravis

History
  Weakness in characteristic distribution
  Fluctuation and fatigue: worse with repeated activity, improved by rest
  Effects of previous treatments
Physical examination
  Ptosis, diplopia
  Motor power survey: quantitative testing of muscle strength
  Forward arm abduction time
  Vital capacity
  Absence of other neurologic signs
Laboratory testing
  Anti-AChR radioimmunoassay: >80% positive; definite diagnosis if positive; negative result does not exclude MG
  Edrophonium chloride (Tensilon) 2 mg + 8 mg IV: highly probable diagnosis if *unequivocally* positive
  Repetitive nerve stimulation: decrement of >15% at 3 Hz; highly probable
  Single fiber electromyelography: blocking and jitter, with normal fiber density; confirmatory, but not specific
  For ocular or cranial MG: exclude intracranial lesions by CT or MRI

This chapter also appeared in Lichtenstein LM, Fauci AS, eds. Current Therapy in Allergy, Immunology, and Rheumatology, 4th ed. St. Louis: Mosby–Year Book, 1992.

Table 2 Disorders Associated With Myasthenia Gravis

Other autoimmune disorders: lupus erythematosus, rheumatoid arthritis, thyroiditis, skin disorders, family history of autoimmune disorder
Conditions that may exacerbate MG: hyperthyroidism or hypothyroidism, occult infection, medications (aminoglycoside antibiotics, penicillamine, antiarrhythmics)
Disorders that may interfere with therapy: tuberculosis, diabetes, ulcer disease, hypertension, asthma, osteoporosis
Recommended laboratory tests
    Lupus erythematosus preparations, antinuclear antibody, rheumatoid factor, antithyroid antibodies
    Thyroid function tests
    Pulmonary function tests
    Tuberculin test
    Chest radiography
    Fasting blood sugar
    MRI or CT of mediastinum
    Bone densitometry in older patients

difficult to evaluate the effects of treatment on the basis of a weekly or monthly office visit. Therefore, I ask patients to keep regular records throughout the day, emphasizing the specific myasthenic features that are most pronounced, such as limb weakness, diplopia, ptosis, and so on. A subjective scale (E = excellent; G = good; F = fair; and P = poor) is useful. Patients also keep timed records of medications taken.

THERAPY

Anticholinesterase Agents

Anti-ChE agents continue to be used first for treatment of most patients with MG. They prolong the action of acetylcholine (ACh) released at neuromuscular junctions and thereby enhance neuromuscular transmission. Pyridostigmine bromide (Mestinon) is the most widely used anti-ChE drug. Its action begins within 10 to 30 minutes, reaches a peak at about 2 hours, and declines gradually thereafter. The initial dosage is usually 60 mg (1 tablet) every 4 hours during the day. The dosing schedule is then readjusted to meet the patient's individual needs, based on the recorded evaluations at the time of peak action (usually about 2 hours) and the time immediately preceding the next dose. For example, if weakness occurs just before successive doses, the interval between doses may be shortened. If the effect at the peak time is insufficient, the dose may be increased by 30 or 60 mg. The maximum useful dosage of pyridostigmine rarely exceeds 120 mg every 3 hours. The dosage requirement may depend on the time of the day; some patients require larger doses in the late afternoon or early evening. If there is difficulty in chewing or swallowing, medication should be given 30 to 45 minutes before meals. A sustained-release preparation (Timespan) containing 90 or 180 mg of pyridostigmine is available but should not be used for daytime

treatment because of variable absorption. It may be useful at bedtime, if the patient experiences weakness at night or in the early morning.

Ephedrine is sometimes helpful as an adjunct to anti-ChE medication and is thought to enhance ACh secretion from cholinergic terminals. The usual dose is 25 mg two or three times a day. If it causes agitation or insomnia, the dose may be reduced or the evening dose omitted entirely.

The most common side effect of anti-ChE treatment is diarrhea, which can be controlled with diphenoxylate hydrochloride with atropine sulfate (Lomotil) or loperamide hydrochloride (Imodium), taken once or twice a day. Excessive amounts of anti-ChE medication may rarely cause increased weakness that is reversible after decreasing or discontinuing treatment. Anti-ChE treatment should be used with care in patients with asthma, as it may increase bronchospasm.

Although anti-ChE medication benefits most patients, the improvement is often incomplete. In general, its effectiveness is usually greatest when treatment is begun, but later becomes less helpful in most patients. Therefore, a majority of patients require further therapeutic measures, as described in the following sections.

Thymectomy

More than 75 percent of patients with MG have thymus abnormalities. "Hyperplasia" is present in 85 percent of these cases, with microscopic evidence of germinal centers and in some cases, gross enlargement. The remaining 15 percent have thymomas. The thymus is frequently removed surgically from myasthenia patients, either to prevent further spread of a thymoma or for its beneficial effect on myasthenic weakness.

Surgery is indicated for the removal of a thymoma, since these tumors may spread locally and become invasive, though they rarely metastasize. Magnetic resonance imaging (MRI) or computed tomography (CT) of the mediastinum is helpful in detecting thymomas, although the scan cannot distinguish between a tumor mass and thymic hyperplasia. An anterior mediastinal mass in a myasthenic patient over age 40, or progressive enlargement of the thymic shadow on repeated scanning in a patient of any age, is strongly suggestive of a neoplasm and should lead to surgery. The tumor and the remaining thymus gland should be removed as completely as possible. If the thymoma cannot be completely removed or if it is invasive, nonferromagnetic marker clips should be placed at the tumor site during surgery and postoperative irradiation should be carried out. Some patients become weaker following removal of a thymoma and require further immunosuppressive treatment (see following).

Surgical thymectomy has gained increasing acceptance during the past decade as a treatment for generalized MG. Remission occurs in approximately one-third of patients following thymectomy, and lesser degrees of improvement occur in another 50 percent. I recommend thymectomy for patients with generalized weakness who are past the age of puberty and younger than 50 years. These limits are not absolute. Prepubertal children or adults over 50 years of age may be considered candidates for thymectomy if their myasthenia is poorly controlled by medication. Thymectomy should be performed in institutions where there is extensive experience, not only with the surgery but also with the preoperative and postoperative management of myasthenia patients. Under these circumstances, the mortality rate for the procedure is now essentially that of anesthesia.

Preoperative preparations should aim to optimize the patient's strength, but immunosuppressive agents should be avoided if possible, because of the increased risk of infection. Anti-ChE medication is optimized. If the patient is weak, with a vital capacity less than 1.5 to 2 L, plasmapheresis should be carried out before surgery to provide improvement in strength during the perioperative period (see following). The surgical approach should remove as much of the thymus as possible. A sternum-splitting incision allows exploration of the anterior mediastinum and the adjacent space extending up to the neck, with removal of all thymic tissue and related fat. Postoperatively, myasthenic patients should be admitted to an intensive care unit prepared to meet their specific needs.

Because the requirement for anti-ChE medication may be somewhat decreased after thymectomy, I give anti-ChE medication intravenously in a dose equivalent to three-fourths the patient's previous optimal dose for the first 2 days after surgery. For each 60 mg of oral pyridostigmine, I substitute 0.75 mg of neostigmine (Prostigmin) administered intravenously by constant infusion pump over the same time period. For example, if the patient was receiving 60 mg of pyridostigmine every 4 hours, an infusion containing 0.75 mg of neostigmine is given over each 4-hour period. After 1 to 2 days, oral medication is resumed and the dosage adjusted as before. Pulmonary physiotherapy, including deep breathing exercises and intermittent positive-pressure breathing are used postoperatively to avoid atelectasis. The patient should be carefully watched for signs of infection. Fever continuing 2 days after surgery should be considered presumptive evidence of infection and treated promptly with antibiotics.

The benefits of thymectomy are usually experienced on a delayed time scale of months to years following surgery. In the meantime, other therapeutic measures as described may be needed.

Immunosuppressive Treatment

Immunosuppressive treatment should be considered for any patient whose myasthenia is not satisfactorily controlled by anti-ChE medications, thymectomy, or both. The definition of satisfactory control usually depends on the patient; some are satisfied to live with moderate degrees of generalized weakness, whereas for others even mild ptosis or diplopia may interfere with their ability to function effectively.

Adrenal glucocorticoids are the most widely used immunosuppressive agents for the treatment of MG. They produce improvement in the great majority of patients with all degrees of muscle weakness, from diplopia to severe respiratory involvement. Glucocorticoid treatment should be considered in the early stages following thymectomy, before the beneficial effects of thymectomy occur. Following removal of a thymoma, I usually use glucocorticoid treatment because of the improved results obtained. Older male patients seem to respond particularly well to glucocorticoid treatment. Diplopia, which often fails to improve on anti-ChE medication, can usually be corrected by glucocorticoid treatment.

Relative contraindications for glucocorticoid therapy include hypertension, ulcer disease, diabetes, chronic infection, osteoporosis, and obesity, although these problems can usually be circumvented by appropriate medical measures. Long-term treatment with glucocorticoids requires continued medical attention by an experienced physician; patients who cannot or will not be followed medically should *never* be given prolonged glucocorticoid treatment.

Before initiation of steroid therapy, the anti-ChE medication should be adjusted optimally. Patients with significant generalized weakness are hospitalized for initiation of glucocorticoid therapy, whereas those with mild MG may be treated on an outpatient basis. Since large doses of glucocorticoids may exacerbate weakness during the early stages of treatment, I use a gradually increasing dosage schedule. Prednisone is begun at a dose of 15 to 20 mg per day and increased by about 5 mg every second or third day until the patient attains a satisfactory clinical response or reaches the level of 50 mg per day. The rate of increase must be guided by the patient's response. Exacerbation of weakness is a signal to lower the dose of prednisone or to proceed more slowly in increasing the dose. Close observation of the patient and good daily records are essential in managing this phase of prednisone treatment. About 90 percent of myasthenic patients improve with glucocorticoid treatment. The clinical effect usually begins within 2 to 6 weeks, although maximal benefit may not be realized until 6 months to 1 year or longer. Side effects of glucocorticoid can be minimized by the use of alternate-day treatment. Accordingly, when the patient has shown definite improvement, usually 2 to 3 months after beginning treatment, the dosage is gradually shifted toward an alternate-day schedule. The amount given on the *on* day is increased by 5 mg, whereas that on the *off* day is decreased by the same amount until an alternate-day regimen is established. Some patients must take a small dose of prednisone on the *off* day to prevent fluctuations in strength.

Glucocorticoid treatment must be continued indefinitely in nearly all patients, although the dose may be reduced. The goal is to establish the *minimal dose* required by each patient, not to eliminate all medication. The minimal dosage usually ranges from 10 to 100 mg every other day, and must be established by trial and error for each patient. The tapering of glucocorticoid medication is a slow process, since the consequences of lowering the dose too far may not be apparent for several months. A common error in treatment of myasthenic patients is to lower the dose of prednisone too quickly or to too low a level.

Prednisone can produce adverse side effects in some patients, including cataracts, osteoporosis, aseptic necrosis of bone, reduced resistance to infection, ulcer disease, hypertension, exacerbation of diabetes, increased appetite and obesity, and salt and fluid retention. Treatment with prednisone requires consistent follow-up for all these potential problems. Patients should be encouraged to notify their physician at the first sign of infection or unexplained symptoms of any kind. Glucocorticoid-treated patients should be followed with routine measurement of blood pressure, blood sugar and serum electrolyte levels, and periodic chest radiographs, as well as ophthalmologic evaluation for cataracts and glaucoma. To minimize the risks of osteoporosis, especially in older patients, I recommend moderate exercise and treatment with vitamin D, 50,000 U twice a week, and calcium, 1 g per day (in the form of calcium lactate or calcium gluconate).

Other Immunosuppressive Drugs

Azathioprine (Imuran) is effective in many patients, though its beneficial effects may take 6 months or longer to appear. It is useful in patients for whom glucocorticoids are contraindicated, whose response to glucocorticoids is insufficient, or as an adjunct to permit the gradual reduction of glucocorticoid dosage.

The usual dose of azathioprine is 2 to 3 mg per kilogram per day, or 125 to 300 mg for adult patients. For obese patients, the dose depends on the total body weight (not the lean body mass). A test dose of approximately 50 mg per day should be given daily for the first week. If this is well tolerated, the dose is gradually raised, while complete blood counts and liver function tests are followed. In patients who are not receiving glucocorticoids, the dose of azathioprine can be increased until the white blood count decreases to approximately 3,000 per cubic millimeter. This measure cannot be used in patients receiving prednisone because of the glucocorticoid-induced leukocytosis, but a lymphocyte count below 1,000 per cubic millimeter is a useful alternative measure in this situation. An increase in the mean corpuscular volume of red blood cells above 100 is also indicative of a positive azathioprine effect.

One side effect of azathioprine that precludes its use is an acute idiosyncratic reaction of fever and myalgia, which occurs in about 10 percent of patients. Leukopenia and alterations in hepatic function may also be seen. If the transaminase level increases above three times the normal range, the azathioprine dose should be reduced. Prolonged use of immunosuppressive agents in patients who have had organ transplants may predispose to the development of malignancies, but this has not been reported in myasthenic patients treated for many years with azathioprine.

Cyclosporin A (CsA) has recently been used alone or in conjunction with prednisone in the treatment of MG. Its benefit is similar to that of azathioprine, but it acts more promptly, usually within 1 to 3 months. CsA is usually begun at a daily dose of 5 mg per kilogram, taken in two divided doses (morning and evening) with a fat-containing meal. Adjustment of dosage is based on periodic measurement of serum "trough levels" of CsA determined in the morning before the drug is taken. The appropriate serum level depends on the method of assay, and standards for the clinical laboratory should be consulted for recommended values. The most important adverse side effect is nephrotoxicity, and the dose of CsA should be reduced if serum blood urea nitrogen and creatinine levels increase. Other side effects include hypertension, headache, hirsuitism, and hepatotoxicity. As with all immunosuppressive drugs, the dosage of CsA should be gradually tapered once satisfactory clinical response has been attained. At present, the high cost of CsA limits its availability for some patients.

Cyclophosphamide has also been used in some patients whose MG is refractory to other immunosuppressive drugs. However, its toxic side effects, including increased risk of late development of malignancy, limits its application.

Plasmapheresis

Plasmapheresis removes antibodies and other circulating factors from the serum of myasthenic patients and has proven of short-term benefit in appropriate patients. In general, plasmapheresis is useful in getting the patient over a difficult period (e.g., before thymectomy, during a myasthenic crisis, or in conjunction with the initiation of immunosuppressive therapy in order to improve the clinical status quickly). The effect of plasmapheresis is temporary. It is occasionally helpful for maintaining the rare refractory patient who does not respond to the other methods outlined previously. Plasmapheresis is expensive and entails risks of hypotension, thromboembolism, and hypocalcemia. In our large group of myasthenic patients, plasmapheresis is needed only a few times each year.

Immunoglobulin

Intravenous immunoglobulin has been used in patients with a variety of autoimmune diseases including MG. Its effectiveness is variable, but may be dramatic. It may be used in place of plasmapheresis or may be given periodically to help maintain improvement in some refractory patients. The usual dose is 400 mg per kilogram IV daily on 5 successive days. The effect of intravenous immunoglobulin may last weeks to several months. It may be used to advantage when plasmapheresis is not available because of lack of equipment or limitations of venous access. Disadvantages of intravenous immunoglobulin are the inconsistency of response in different patients, and its high cost.

MYASTHENIC CRISIS

When assistance with the vital functions of respiration or swallowing are required, the myasthenic patient is said to be in crisis. Fortunately, modern treatment has made myasthenic crisis an uncommon problem. Any myasthenic patient who complains of dyspnea or dysphagia should be admitted to the hospital immediately. If the vital capacity falls below 25 percent of normal (or roughly 1 L), the patient should be transferred to an intensive care unit well versed in respiratory support techniques. Intubation should be carried out only if spontaneous respirations are insufficient. Total management of the patient's vital functions must be undertaken, and nutrition and fluid and electrolyte balance must be carefully maintained. The goal of management is to restore the patient to independent function as quickly as possible.

Special attention must be given to the following areas of care.

Infection

Infection of any sort is particularly hazardous for myasthenic patients for several reasons: (1) infection and fever may exacerbate the weakness of MG and indeed may have precipitated the crisis in the first place; (2) the patient's respiratory muscle weakness makes recovery from pneumonia difficult; and (3) many myasthenic patients are receiving immunosuppressive agents; even those not immunosuppressed are very vulnerable to infection and should be treated for infection *immediately and vigorously.* The most common error in the management of a myasthenic crisis is to wait too long before initiating antibiotic therapy. If infection is strongly suspected, appropriate cultures should be obtained, and empiric therapy should be begun based on the best information available from Gram's stain and experience with the organisms prevalent in the institution. Although the aminoglycoside antibiotics are known to have adverse effects on neuromuscular transmission, they may be used when necessary to treat infections in myasthenic patients. The method of treatment of infection in MG is analogous to that used for oncology patients receiving chemotherapy.

Ventilation

Myasthenia patients in crisis cannot ventilate adequately. Artificial respiration must be provided by an expert in ventilator management. Maintenance of a clear airway by repeated gentle suction, pulmonary physiotherapy, and periodic inflation of the lungs should be used to prevent atelectasis and pulmonary infection. Incentive spirometry should be avoided in myasthenia patients because it may cause fatigue of the respiratory muscles.

Specific Treatment for Myasthenia Gravis

Measures that may improve the patient's strength should be used in an attempt to end the crisis as promptly as possible. This is one of the prime indications for plasmapheresis. Glucocorticoids may also be helpful in this situation, but in the presence of infection, they should be used with caution. Because the patient is already on a respirator, there is no advantage in gradually increasing the dose of prednisone; a quicker response can be obtained by starting with large-dose prednisone treatment (50 to 80 mg per day). If the patient requires constant mechanical ventilation, anti-ChE agents may be withdrawn for 48 to 72 hours. This "drug holiday" may result in an enhanced response to anti-ChE medication when later it is restarted.

OCULAR MYASTHENIA GRAVIS

In some myasthenic patients, weakness is confined to the extraocular muscles and lids. Anti-ChE medication often does not succeed in correcting diplopia. Thymectomy is usually reserved for patients with generalized weakness, though a recent study reports improvement in patients with purely ocular symptoms. If the symptoms are troublesome, glucocorticoids are usually effective in correcting diplopia. In many instances, only a small maintenance dose of prednisone is required to maintain correction of diplopia.

NEONATAL MYASTHENIA GRAVIS

Approximately one of six infants born to a mother with MG develops transient weakness during the neonatal period. Weakness of sucking and crying, impairment of swallowing and respiration, and in some instances, generalized weakness, may begin at birth or within 1 to 3 days postnatally and persist for up to 3 weeks. Neither the mother's clinical status nor laboratory tests can predict which mothers may have clinically affected infants; therefore, it is advisable for deliveries to be carried out in an institution where specific care for the myasthenic neonate is available. Although it is difficult to perform in the neonate, repetitive nerve stimulation is useful to establish the diagnosis of MG. The treatment of neonatal MG consists of anti-ChE medication. Pyridostigmine syrup (4 to 10 mg) may be given orally or by nasogastric tube if necessary every 4 hours as long as it is needed. Intravenous neostigmine, 0.05 to 0.1 mg every 3 to 4 hours may be given by infusion pump. The weakness improves spontaneously, and care should be taken to avoid overmedication.

ADDITIONAL CAUTIONS

If surgery is necessary for an intercurrent problem and oral medication must be discontinued, anti-ChE medication can be given by intravenous infusion pump at a full equivalent dose (i.e., 1 mg neostigmine IV substituted for each 60 mg of oral pyridostigmine bromide). If the patient has been receiving prednisone before surgery, parenteral glucocorticoids (hydrocortisone or methylprednisolone) are given during the 2 to 6 days following surgery in a daily dose equivalent to the "on" day dose of oral prednisone.

Curare-like drugs should never be used in myasthenic patients. Certain other drugs should be used with caution in patients with MG, including aminoglycoside antibiotics (see previous mention), procainamide, quinine, quinidine, and beta-adrenergic blocking agents.

Myasthenic patients should be urged to contact their physicians immediately if they develop fever, sore throat, or infection of any sort.

No limitations on activity are prescribed. The effects of overexertion are reversible, and the myasthenic patient will usually establish a comfortable level of activity for himself or herself.

SUGGESTED READING

DeBaets MH, Oosterhuis HJGH, Toyka KV, eds. Myasthenia gravis. Vol 25. Basel: Karger, 1988.

Drachman DB (ed.). Myasthenia gravis. Biology and treatment. Ann NY Acad Sci 1987; 505:1.

Drachman DB. Biology of myasthenia gravis. Ann Rev Neurosci 1981; 4:195.

Oosterhuis HJGH. Myasthenia gravis. Edinburgh: Churchill-Livingstone, 1984.

Seybold ME. Myasthenia gravis. A clinical and basic science review. JAMA 1983; 250:2516.

LAMBERT-EATON MYASTHENIC SYNDROME

KATHLEEN M. McEVOY, M.D., Ph.D.

Lambert-Eaton myasthenic syndrome (LES) is a rare disorder of neuromuscular transmission characterized by fluctuating muscle weakness, hyporeflexia, and autonomic dysfunction. The disease was first recognized as a distinct clinical entity in 1957, when the clinical and electrodiagnostic features were described by Eaton and Lambert. LES is autoimmune mediated and is often associated with small cell lung carcinoma or with other organ-specific autoimmune disorders. Distinction from the more common myasthenia gravis (MG) is usually possible on clinical, electrophysiologic, and serologic grounds, but in some cases the two may coexist. LES is often debilitating but rarely life threatening. The response to treatment is generally less favorable than that of MG.

LES occurs most commonly in older persons but may begin in young adulthood or even childhood. Both sexes are affected approximately equally, though the paraneoplastic form is probably more common in males and the primary autoimmune form in females. The total number of LES patients in the United States may be less than one thousand.

CLINICAL AND LABORATORY FEATURES

Muscle weakness is the chief feature of LES, and in essentially all cases is most pronounced in the hip girdle and proximal lower extremities. Axial muscles, shoulders, arms, and legs are frequently involved to a lesser degree. Oropharyngeal and ocular muscles are usually only mildly affected, if at all, in contrast to MG. Edrophonium (Tensilon) enhances strength less dramatically than in MG, if at all. On examination, muscle strength may be noted to facilitate or to improve initially with sustained or repeated activity, again in contrast to MG where early fatiguability is seen.

Deep tendon reflexes are reduced or absent, and these too may facilitate after brief exercise of the muscle or repeated tapping of the tendon. Autonomic dysfunction typically is confined to cholinergic mechanisms, including dryness of the mouth, impotence in males, and loss of normal sweating. Significant noradrenergic dysfunction raises the question of a separate paraneoplastic dysautonomia.

Well over half of newly diagnosed LES cases prove to be paraneoplastic, though the malignancy (almost always small cell lung cancer) may not be diagnosed for several years. Symptoms tend to develop more quickly in paraneoplastic cases, often over a period of a few weeks, as compared to the usually insidious onset of primary autoimmune LES.

Many LES patients, including those with underlying cancer, have other organ-specific autoimmune disorders in addition to LES. These include Hashimoto's thyroiditis, pernicious anemia, vitiligo, premature ovarian failure, and other members of the so-called thyrogastric cluster of autoimmune disorders.

The muscle weakness of LES is due to a defect of neuromuscular transmission. The elegant microphysiologic studies of Lambert have proven that the defect is presynaptic and due to impaired release of acetylcholine from the motoneuron terminal. Repeated activation of the motoneuron transiently increases acetylcholine release enough to increase strength.

The impaired release of acetylcholine in LES results from antibody-mediated dysfunction of voltage-gated calcium channels (VGCC) in the motor nerve terminal membrane. This reduces the calcium uptake and thus inhibits acetylcholine release. Similar events occur at autonomic nerve terminals. VGCC in small cell carcinoma cells provides the antigenic stimulus for the development of LES in patients with underlying malignancy.

Though LES may be strongly suspected on clinical grounds, the diagnosis rests on the electrophysiologic findings. These serve to support the clinical diagnosis and to exclude the most likely imitators, MG and myopathy.

The resting compound muscle action potential amplitude (CMAP) is low in muscles involved by LES, in contrast to MG where the routine nerve conduction studies are normal. With 2 Hz repetitive stimulation there is a decrement in the resting CMAP, as is also seen in MG. A striking finding is observed in LES after brief exercise or with rapid repetitive stimulation (20 to 50 Hz). These maneuvers produce a marked increase or facilitation of the resting CMAP, to at least twice and sometimes more than 10 times its baseline value. This is the electrophysiologic correlate of the facilitation of muscle strength and reflexes that may be seen on examination.

Antibodies directed at VGCC are detectable in the serum of about 50 percent of LES patients. The rate of seropositivity is about 75 percent in cancer-associated cases, and 30 percent in those without evidence of cancer, so a positive finding increases the suspicion of underlying malignancy. Other autoantibodies are frequently detected in the serum of LES patients, reflecting their tendency to develop autoimmune diseases, as noted above.

THERAPY

Delineation of the electrophysiologic and immune mechanisms of LES has laid the groundwork for rational and effective therapy. The response to treatment in LES is generally slower and less complete than in MG. Avenues of therapy include treatment of the underlying tumor, drugs to improve neurotransmission, and immunosuppression. A combined approach is usually required for optimal control (Fig. 1).

Cancer must be suspected whenever a new case of LES is discovered. Diagnosis of LES typically precedes cancer detection, sometimes by as much as four years. A diligent search for malignancy must be conducted in patients with new-onset LES, especially smokers and those who exhibit rapid onset and progression of symptoms. The presence of other autoimmune disorders does not rule out an underlying malignancy. The initial search for malignancy in a smoker or a patient with rapid onset and progression of symptoms should include bronchoscopy and computed tomography (CT) of the chest with contrast medium. If these findings are negative, CT should be repeated in 2 to 3 months, then every 3 to 4 months for the first year and every 6 months for the next 3 years. If new symptoms raise clinical suspicion, bronchoscopy should be repeated. For nonsmokers with LES of insidious onset, yearly CT of the chest for 4 years should suffice.

Eradication or even temporary control of the underlying malignancy may induce partial or complete remission of LES. Return of LES symptoms may herald tumor recurrence, but in some cases tumor may recur without an increase in LES disease activity. Small cell lung carcinoma may be treated with surgery, radiation, or chemotherapy, alone or in combination, depending on the extent and location of disease in each patient. Despite the opportunity for earlier cancer detection, LES patients fare no better with respect to their cancer than those without LES.

Because of the delay in detection of underlying malignancy, treatment for the LES is often necessary long before the tumor is even diagnosed. The pathophysiologic mechanisms of disease are identical in the primary and paraneoplastic forms of LES, and the treatments described below are effective for both. Though immunosuppression might theoretically impair the body's ability to suppress growth of the tumor, this does not appear to alter the long-term outcome.

Since the electrophysiologic defect in LES is due to impaired release of acetylcholine from motor and autonomic nerve terminals, effector function may be enhanced by drugs that increase the availability of acetylcholine in the synaptic space, either by promoting its release or by preventing its subsequent breakdown.

Drugs that promote release of acetylcholine are directly suited to treating the electrophysiologic defect of LES. Guanidine is effective in this regard and does increase strength in LES, but its toxicity limits its usefulness. Aminopyridines also increase acetylcholine release. These potassium channel blockers prolong the duration of the action potential, thus prolonging activation of VGCC, enhancing calcium uptake, and therefore acetylcholine release.

4-Aminopyridine is effective in LES but crosses the blood-brain barrier well and is quite epileptogenic in the dose range required for neuromuscular efficacy. 3,4-Diaminopyridine (3,4-DAP) is probably more potent at the neuromuscular junction and penetrates the blood-brain barrier less well, resulting in less convulsant activity.

Clinical experience with 3,4-DAP has shown it to be effective in increasing strength and ameliorating autonomic symptoms in patients with both primary and paraneoplastic LES. Electrophysiologic parameters, quantitative strength testing, and subjective and objective measures of patients' functional abilities all improve significantly with treatment. Mildly affected patients do well on 3,4-DAP alone. Supplemental pyridostigmine may be used to enhance the effects of 3,4-DAP in patients with moderate weakness. More severely affected patients will likely benefit from the addition of immunosuppressive therapy.

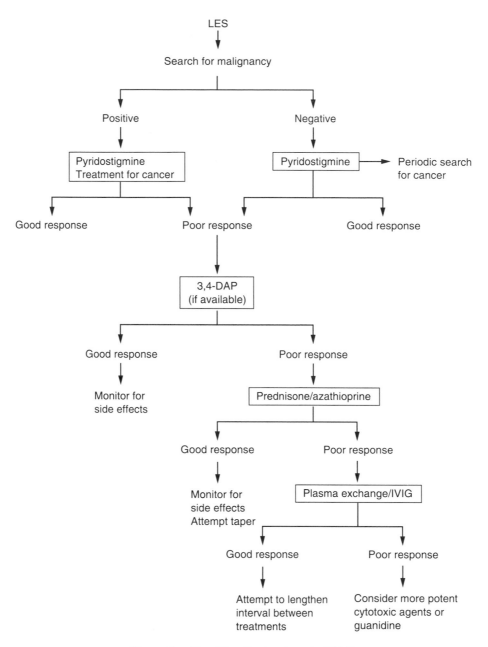

Figure 1 Algorithm for treatment of LES.

The effects of a dose of 3,4-DAP typically last 4 to 6 hours, so four or five divided doses usually give a smooth effect through the day. Most patients do well on doses in the range of 10 to 15 mg five times per day or 20 mg four times a day, but some can tolerate only much smaller doses. For this reason, it is best to start with a small dose such as 5 mg three times a day, and to increase slowly, first to four or five times per day, then by 5 mg per dose every 4 or 5 days, until maximum therapeutic benefit is attained without undue side effects. Eighty milligrams per day is quite effective for most patients. With 100 mg or more per day the risk of seizures may be increased.

3,4-DAP is generally tolerated well, but mild and dose-related side effects are seen in many patients, including perioral (and sometimes digital) paresthesias after doses, epigastric distress if the drug is taken on an empty stomach, and insomnia after bedtime doses. After 3 or 4 days on a recently increased dose, some patients develop a subjective sense of weakness and malaise, which resolves with dose reduction though therapeutic benefit is sustained.

The only serious side effect yet to be observed with 3,4-DAP is seizures, which have been observed in two patients taking larger doses of the drug (100 mg per day). The chance of seizures thus appears to be about 2 to 4 percent, and they may appear after many months of treatment. Anticonvulsants may be given with 3,4-DAP to control these. No cardiac conduction defects have been documented to be caused by 3,4-DAP, but this is a theoretical possibility.

In summary, 3,4-DAP is effective in relieving the motor and autonomic symptoms of LES and generally is tolerated well. Patients with a possible predisposition to seizures or with cardiac conduction defects probably should not be treated with this medication. Thus far, 3,4-DAP has not been approved for general use, and it is available only through experimental protocols.

Acetylcholinesterase inhibitors such as pyridostigmine bromide (Mestinon) prevent breakdown of acetylcholine and confer at least modest benefit for many LES patients. This safe and available form of treatment is a reasonable first line of therapy. The dose may be gradually increased from 30 mg three times per day to 60 or 90 mg three or four times per day, increasing the dose as long as increasing benefit is obtained. Side effects of abdominal cramps and diarrhea are usually easily controlled with atropine or Imodium.

Guanidine, which enhances acetylcholine release, may be considered as a last resort for patients with severe weakness who cannot tolerate or have failed to respond to all other available treatments. Initial oral doses of 1 to 2 mg per kilogram four to six times per day may be increased as needed and as tolerated every 3 to 4 days, to a maximum dose of 50 mg per kilogram per day. Close clinical observation is essential with frequent blood testing for renal, hematologic, and hepatic function. Side effects are frequent and severe, including renal dysfunction, bone marrow suppression, hepatic toxicity, cardiac arrhythmia, tremor, ataxia, paresthesias, confusion, and psychosis. Death has been reported.

Immunosuppressive treatment is helpful in LES but is generally slower to take effect and less effective than in MG. If despite treatment with pyridostigmine (and 3,4-DAP if available) and treatment of malignancy, a patient is significantly disabled, immunosuppression may be indicated.

Corticosteroids are effective in LES, but the onset of benefit is often so gradual that patients may not be aware of it until the drug is discontinued and the effect vanishes. Initial doses of prednisone, 60 to 80 mg per day, may become effective within a few weeks, and dosage then might be converted to 100 to 120 mg every other day, to minimize side effects. After 2 to 3 months the dose may be tapered slowly, as tolerated, to about 30 mg every other day over several months, and further as long as symptoms do not recur. Patients must, of course, be made aware of the numerous possible side effects of steroid treatment, and continued medical follow-up of patients during treatment is essential. Treatment is usually required indefinitely, as LES does not tend to remit spontaneously. Thus, a steroid-sparing agent is desirable.

Azathioprine has proven effective in treatment of LES, alone or especially in combination with corticosteroids. The onset of effect is even slower than with steroids—6 months or more—and maximal benefit may not be attained for more than 18 months. The initial dose of 50 mg per day may be increased at weekly intervals over 3 to 4 weeks to a total dose of 2 to 2.5 mg per kilogram of body weight per day in two or three doses. Dividing the dose further may improve tolerance in persons prone to gastrointestinal upset from azathioprine. Blood testing, including a complete blood count with platelets and liver enzymes, should be done weekly for the first month, monthly for the first year, and at least quarterly thereafter as long as the patient is taking azathioprine.

Before instituting therapy, the physician may wish to check serum levels of red blood cell thiopurine methyltransferase (rbc TPMT), as a measure of the patient's capacity to metabolize thiopurine drugs. One in three hundred persons is homozygous for a deficiency in this enzyme, and thus at high risk to develop life-threatening bone marrow suppression after even just a few doses. Even those with normal TPMT levels must be followed-up with regular blood testing. Azathioprine cannot be taken concurrently with allupurinol.

In patients who are unable to metabolize azathioprine, the white blood cell count may drop precipitously, necessitating immediate withdrawal of the medication and close medical observation. If it remains above 3000 with an adequate neutrophil count, the dose usually need not be adjusted. If it falls below 3000 but not below 2500, halving the dose of azathioprine may allow recovery of bone marrow function. A white count below 2500 usually necessitates discontinuing azathioprine, though it may sometimes be reinstituted in smaller doses.

Hepatic toxicity, if it is to occur, is usually an early complication, often in the first week. As many as 10 percent of patients are unable to tolerate azathioprine because of a serum sickness syndrome or other specific sensitivity. After some months on azathioprine the red blood cell mean corpuscular volume typically increases, reflecting the metabolic effects of the drug. While increased risk of hematologic malignancies has been attributed to azathioprine in some special patient populations, there is no convincing evidence in patients with autoimmune diseases.

Addition of azathioprine to corticosteroid therapy may allow continued reduction of corticosteroid doses, and sometimes discontinuation. As noted above, corticosteroid therapy in combination with azathioprine is more effective than either alone. Nonetheless, immunosuppressive therapy rarely achieves complete remission of symptoms. Supplementation with pyridostigmine (or 3,4-DAP, if available) may be helpful and should be tried.

Plasma exchange is effective, but again less dramatically so than in MG, and, as in that disorder, the effects last only a few weeks. The peak effect may be expected two weeks after a course of 5 to 15 exchanges; little if any benefit remains after 6 weeks' time. As in MG, maintenance therapy with plasma exchange every few weeks may be considered in refractory cases, but is expensive, invasive, and fraught with complications.

Intravenous immunoglobulin (IVIG) has been anecdotally reported to be of benefit in LES and other autoimmune neuromuscular disorders. Its efficacy as compared to plasma exchange or other immunosuppressive treatments remains to be defined.

Some cases of LES are refractory to the usual treatments. Although LES is rarely fatal it can produce ventilatory failure and death. Even in non–life-threatening cases the disability may be marked. Once the usual means of treatment have failed, more potent immunosuppressives and cytotoxic agents or guanidine may be indicated. In such cases the disability and potential benefits of treatment must be carefully weighed against the potential risks of treatment.

Patients with LES should avoid or use with caution drugs that may interfere with neuromuscular transmission, including succinylcholine, *d*-tubucurarine, aminoglycoside antibiotics, beta- and calcium channel blockers, quinine, quinidine, and procainamide. Magnesium salts and intravenous contrast dye have also been reported to increase weakness. Many other drugs have been reported to worsen symptoms, and patients should be observed closely after the addition of any new medication. Systemic illness or a hot, humid environment often exacerbates LES symptoms. Patients should receive regular influenza and pneumonia vaccinations.

SUGGESTED READING

Chalk CH, Murray NM, Newsom-Davis J, et al. Response of the Lambert-Eaton myasthenic syndrome to treatment of associated small-cell lung carcinoma. Neurology 1990; 40:1552–1556.

McEvoy KM. Treatment for Lambert-Eaton myasthenic syndrome. In: Lisak RP, ed. Handbook of myasthenia gravis and myasthenic syndromes. Marcel Dekker, in press.
McEvoy KM, Windebank AJ, Daube JR, Low PA. 3,4-Diaminopyridine in the treatment of Lambert-Eaton myasthenic syndrome. New Engl J Med 1989; 321:1567–1571.
Newsom-Davis J, Murray NM. Plasma exchange and immunosuppressive drug treatment in the Lambert-Eaton myasthenic syndrome. Neurology 1984; 34:480–485.

PATIENT RESOURCES

Muscular Dystrophy Association
3300 East Sunrise Drive
Tucson, Arizona 85718
Telephone: (602) 529-2000
Information on nerve and muscle diseases including LES, research, and patient care clinics.)

Myasthenia Gravis Foundation
53 West Jackson Boulevard
Suite 909
Chicago, Illinois 60604
Telephone: (312) 427-6252
(Information about local chapters and disorders of neuromuscular transmission including LES.)

National Organization for Rare Disorders
P.O. Box 8923
New Fairfield, Connecticut 06812-1783
Telephone: (203) 746-6518
(Clearing house for information about rare disorders including LES, research, available treatments, patient care.)

MAJOR MUSCULAR DYSTROPHIES

GEORGE KARPATI, M.D., FRCPC

The muscular dystrophies are progressive diseases of skeletal plus or minus cardiac muscles due to a defect of a nuclear gene. This review focuses on Duchenne muscular dystrophy (DMD), myotonic dystrophy (MyD), and fascioscapulohumeral dystrophy (FSH).

In principle, therapeutic approaches to these diseases may be divided into four categories: (1) correction of the deleterious effects of the gene defect by introducing normal alleles of the gene that suffered the mutation, (2) replacement of the missing (or defective) protein product of the gene in question by normally functioning molecules, (3) modification (usually by pharmacologic agents) of the metabolic and/or physiologic characteristics of the muscle fibers (and/or of the

organism) in order to reduce their susceptibility to damage or destruction as a result of the gene defect, and (4) palliative measures to minimize the inconvenience or suffering from the progressive skeletal and/or cardiac muscle fiber loss.

Currently, only items in categories 3 and 4 have practical application. Prevention of the diseases by appropriate genetic counseling or prenatal detection can also be considered an important aspect of the management, but these measures are not discussed in this article.

DUCHENNE MUSCULAR DYSTROPHY

DMD is caused by various types of mutations of a 2.4 megabase gene at locus Xp21 (on the short arm of the X chromosome). The gene normally codes for a 427 kd rod-shaped cytoskeletal protein that is situated on the cytoplasmic aspect of the plasma membrane. Its putative function is mechanical reinforcement of the plasmalemma of muscle fibers. In DMD, its absence causes recurrent segmental necrosis of muscle fibers. Although regeneration is active, it cannot replace all necrotic segments, and as a result a progressive loss of muscle fibers supervenes. This causes severe atrophy and weakness of all limb, neck, and trunk muscles. Eventually, respiratory and cardiac insufficiency supervene and cause death, usually by age 20 years unless supportive measures are instituted.

The possible therapeutic approaches to DMD are discussed under the four headings indicated in the Introduction.

Strategies for Introducing Normal Alleles of the Dystrophin Gene into Skeletal Muscle Fibers

In principle, this goal may be achieved by three methods: (1) heterologous myoblast transfer (HMT), (2) gene replacement, or (3) autologous myoblast transfer (AMT). Because all these procedures are still in the experimental stage, only brief comments will be made.

In HMT, suspensions of normal, viable, fusion-competent, and contamination-free cultured myoblasts are injected into the patient's muscle. The myoblasts are obtained usually from the father or from an unaffected sibling. Because of risk of immunorejection, some form of immunosuppression is used, at least for a period of time. Some of the injected myoblasts fuse with the host muscle fibers, and thus their nuclei become myonuclei of the host fibers. If enough donor myoblasts fuse with the DMD host fibers, the normal dystrophin genes (in the myonuclei derived from the injected myoblasts) may give rise to enough dystrophin to protect a given fiber segment from damage or necrosis. Myoblast transfer appears to be feasible and safe in DMD, but its efficiency so far has proven poor. In the injected DMD muscles, little or no dystrophin has been found, and the force generation of muscle has not significantly improved as compared to sham-injected control muscles of the same patient up to 1 year after injection. The reasons for the poor efficiency are not quite clear. Efforts are under way to improve the "take" of the myoblasts by creating abundant regeneration in the injectable muscle and reducing the impediments to myoblast mobility posed by the extracellular matrix.

Gene replacement therapy consists of the introduction of artificially engineered dystrophin gene constructs, either as naked DNA or by viral targeting. In the genetically dystrophin-deficient mouse model (mdx), intramuscular injections of large amounts of plasmids carrying either the full length dystrophin cDNA (13.9 kb) or a partial cDNA (a "minigene" of 6.5 kb) driven by a viral promoter gave rise to some dystrophin-positive muscle fibers generated by the expression of the injected genes that were taken up by an unknown mechanism into the host fibers. The same result has been achieved with similar gene constructs that were recombined with a replication-defective human adenovirus vector. The number of muscle fibers that acquire dystrophin after injection of artificial gene constructs is relatively few, and thus the efficiency of this procedure still falls below what would be expected from an efficient therapeutic modality. Efforts are under way to increase the efficiency of these procedures in experimental animals. Only when this is achieved can human trials be contemplated with some form of gene replacement therapy.

In AMT, the patient's own myoblasts are removed and in a culture they are transfected by a normal dystrophin gene construct. Those myoblasts that acquired normal dystrophin alleles by this manipulation can be selected and reinjected into the muscles of the same patient. The advantage of AMT over HMT is that in the former immunosuppressive therapy is not necessary. This approach still suffers from the poor efficiency of myoblast transfer in general.

Replacement of Dystrophin

Dystrophin is a large cytoskeletal molecule with complex attachments to the plasma membrane and the internal cytoskeleton of the muscle fibers. For these reasons there is no realistic expectation that dystrophin could be replaced by intramuscular injections, even if large quantities of the pure molecule were available.

Pharmacologic Approach

In recent years, reliable evidence has been presented that prednisone, 0.75 mg per kilogram per day orally, produced significant beneficial effects in DMD patients. Strength and functional ability were significantly improved in all age groups tested. The beneficial effects were noted as early as 10 days and were sustained up to 2 years while the medication was continued.

The drawback for prednisone treatment was side effects, the particularly troublesome ones being weight gain and stunted growth. A newer analogue of prednisone, deflazacort, has fewer side effects than prednisone, and its effectiveness in DMD is presently being tested in a large clinical trial. If it proves to be as effective as prednisone, it could for the time being become the drug of choice for treatment of DMD.

The biochemical or cellular or molecular basis of the beneficial effects of glucocorticoids in DMD is unknown. It is probably not simply an immunosuppressive effect, as azathioprine has no beneficial effect. Glucocorticoids may stimulate the expression of an autosomally coded dystrophin analogue (dystrophin-related protein), which could possibly compensate, in part, for dystrophin deficiency. Another possibility is that glucocorticoids may rescue some regenerating myotubes from a naturally occurring (programmed) death.

Which DMD patients should get glucocorticoids? When is the treatment to be started? Presently, firm recommendations are hard to give. Theoretically, treatment could be started as soon as the diagnosis is made in all reliably confirmed cases of DMD (but not BMD), particularly if deflazacort proves to be effective and becomes available. Currently, it is clear that glucocorticoids do not represent definitive treatment for DMD. Nevertheless, they appear to be the agent of choice for preventing severe deterioration in DMD boys until a more definitive treatment becomes available.

Palliative Treatment

Muscle Stretching

As soon as the diagnosis is made, regular stretching of certain muscle groups by the parents should be encouraged to prevent or minimize troublesome contractures. Particular attention is to be directed to the iliotibial bands, hip flexors, hamstrings, and ankle dorsiflexors. Since plantar flexor contractures are particularly prone to occur, light night splinting should be encouraged early, which is tolerated well even by very young children.

Bracing

Ambulation fails around 8 to 10 years of age. The ambulation period may be prolonged by 1 or 2 years with the use of long-legged braces to stabilize the knee joints.

Tenotomies

Despite stretching and night bracing, contractures often develop at various sites in the lower extremities. Contractures pose a problem for walking, sitting, and overall care. They can also negate the use of walking braces. Percutaneous tenotomies can help with minimal morbidity and without necessitating long-term limb immobilization.

Wheelchair Seating

When the DMD patient spends most of his time in a wheelchair, there is the risk of progressive thoracolumbar scoliosis. This can be minimized or delayed by proper, preferably custom-molded, seating with adequate back support. A thoracolumbar spinal orthotic device or body jacket is not useful. Careful monitoring of spine alignment is essential. Scoliosis of more than 30 percent is usually an indication for some form of corrective surgery, as long as the child is no longer in the active growth phase. Spinal fixations are major invasive procedures, but they make patients' lives much more comfortable and prevent the life-threatening chest deformities that could compromise cardiopulmonary function.

Respiratory Support

In the terminal phases of DMD, respiratory insufficiency sets in, causing much subjective discomfort. The effects of respiratory insufficiency can be worse at night when there is natural hypoventilation. This can be alleviated by providing external mechanical ventilation through a mask. No tracheostomy is recommended. If respiratory support is required during the day, a portable ventilator attached to the wheelchair can be used. Mechanical respiratory devices should be used only if the

topic is carefully discussed and agreed upon by the family.

The most efficient delivery of all these measures to the DMD patient is made possible by the co-operative efforts of an expert team consisting of physiotherapists, occupational therapists, orthopaedic surgeons, orthotists, pediatricians, neurologists, teachers, and social workers working closely with the family.

Treatment of Cardiac and CNS Manifestations

Symptomatic cardiomyopathy develops only in later stages and can cause congestive cardiac failure. This should be treated by the usual measures. Cardiac transplantation is not justified.

Approximately 30 percent of DMD patients have a nonprogressive mental deficit that often requires special education.

MYOTONIC DYSTROPHY

MyD, a multisystem progressive disease, is transmitted as an autosomal dominant trait and tends to exhibit more severe clinical phenotypic expression in subsequent generations. However, there is marked variability of the severity of the clinical phenotype, even among siblings.

Clinically, the most prominently affected tissues are skeletal muscles, heart, the endocrine system, and the ocular lens. Skeletal muscle involvement manifests in two ways, myotonia and progressive wasting and weakness of limb muscles, trunk and respiratory musculature, and some craniobulbar muscles.

The gene defect consists of a variable length expansion of a trinucleotide (CTG) repeat in the noncoding 3' region of a gene on the long arm of chromosome 19. In normal persons, there are 5 to 27 tandem CTG trinucleotide repeats, whereas in MyD patients the number ranges anywhere from 50 to several thousand. The extent of the expansion of the trinucleotide repeat roughly correlates with the severity of the clinical phenotype. This mutation creates a highly unstable region of the gene. It is still unclear how this mutation subverts the function of the gene, which apparently codes for a form of protein kinase A.

Skeletal Muscle

For some patients myotonia may be functionally disabling even though there is not much muscle weakness. This is usually the most troublesome in the hands (grip myotonia), but it can also occur in the muscles of the jaw, neck, tongue, and legs. Symptomatic treatment of myotonia is unsatisfactory, as the physiologic basis of membrane instability giving rise to myotonia is still unknown. Procainamide, quinine, or phenytoin provides only very slight improvement in most cases and may precipitate or aggravate cardiac problems. We have found prednisone, 10 mg orally, very useful in producing marked reduction of myotonia for about 2 to 3 hours, but prolonged use of glucocorticoids is not recommended because of inevitable side effects. Muscle weakness is currently not amenable to treatment. Foot drop can be controlled by braces. Respiratory insufficiency may be alleviated by breathing exercises and postural drainage, as well as prompt treatment of infections. Intermittent use of a respirator, as described for DMD, is rarely indicated. Some clinical and biochemical improvement has been reported from the use of anabolic steroids; however, this modality is still in the experimental stage.

Dysphagia is rarely severe enough to warrant cricopharyngotomy. This situation sharply contrasts with that in oculopharyngeal dystrophy.

The prospects for myoblast transfer and gene replacement therapy in MyD are unclear, even if otherwise these procedures become efficient. This is because of the fact that with a dominantly inherited disease the number of normal gene copies required for a normal clinical phenotype may be quite large and unattainable by these procedures.

Heart

The most common cardiac problems—tachyarrhythmias and, less often, congestive failure—are treated by the usual methods. A pacemaker can be used for second-degree heart block or trifascicular conduction defects. Cardiac transplantation is not recommended.

Eye

Posterior capsule cataracts are treated surgically when vision obscuration so indicates. Eyelid ptosis rarely requires tarsorrhaphy; indeed, tarsorrhaphy may result in incomplete closure of the eyelids and risk of corneal ulcers.

Endocrine System

Diabetes mellitus is managed in the routine manner. Besides testicular atrophy, there are no other stigmata of hypogonadism that warrant androgenic hormone replacement therapy.

Congenital Myotonic Dystrophy

In the newborns of some mothers with MyD, severe muscular hypotonia and weakness, dysphagia, and respiratory insufficiency can be present at birth. If other causes can be ruled out, congenital MyD is diagnosed. Because the symptoms tend to improve 4 to 6 weeks postnatally, vigorous support, in the form of feeding by gavage and even mechanical ventilation, is justified.

FASCIOSCAPULOHUMERAL DYSTROPHY

There are several phenotypes of FSH. The most common one is an autosomal dominant form with onset during the second decade of life. There is considerable variability in the severity of the clinical phenotype, ranging from mild involvement of facial and scapular musculature to severe wasting and weakness of limb and trunk muscles, which is the result of a progressive course. The gene has been localized to chromosome 4 (q35), but it has not been cloned.

Apart from physiotherapy for limb muscle weakness few other measures may be used to mitigate the inconvenience of muscle weakness; this includes foot drop braces and body corset to stabilize the thoracolumbar spine. Because limitation of arm abduction is an early feature that limits the activities of daily living, it is of special importance. The failure of abduction is often due to an insufficiency of the scapular fixator muscles. A surgical procedure of using fascia to keep the scapulas on the rib cage on attempted abduction can increase the abduction angle significantly (at least temporarily) in selected patients.

In the inflammatory type of FSH, corticosteroids had been used, which may help with the pain in the shoulder region, but they have no significant effect on the progression of the disease.

SUGGESTED READING

Acsadi GY, Dickson G, Love DR, et al. Human dystrophin expression in mdx mice after intramuscular injection of DNA constructs. Nature 1992; 352:815–818.

Angelini C, Pegoraro E, Perini F, et al. A trial with a new steroid in Duchenne muscular dystrophy. In: Angelini C, Danieli GA, Fontanari D, eds. Muscular dystrophy research: From molecular diagnosis toward therapy. New York: Elsevier, 1991:173.

Aslanidis C, Jansen G, Amemiya C, et al. Cloning of the essential myotonic dystrophy region and mapping of the putative defect. Nature 1992; 355:438–551.

Burrow KL, Coovert DD, Klein CJ, et al. Dystrophin expression and somatic reversion in prednisone-treated and untreated Duchenne dystrophy. Neurology 1991; 41:661–666.

Buxton J, Shelbourne P, Davies J, et al. Detection of an unstable fragment of DNA specific to individuals with myotonic dystrophy. Nature 1992; 355:547–548.

Cwik VA, Brooke MH. Recent advances in diagnosis and treatment of Duchenne muscular dystrophy. Curr Opin Orthoped 1992; 3:218–223.

Fenichel GM, Florence J, Pestronk A, et al. Prednisone slows strength decline in Duchenne muscular dystrophy: Two-year observation. Neurology 1991; 41(suppl 1):166.

Fenichel GM, Mendell JR, Moxley RT, et al. A comparison of daily and alternate-day prednisone therapy in the treatment of Duchenne muscular dystrophy. Arch Neurol 1991; 48:575–579.

Griggs RC, Karpati G, eds. Myoblast transfer therapy. New York: Plenum, 1990.

Griggs RC, Moxley RT, Mendel JR. The Clinical Investigation of Duchenne Dystrophy Group: Prednisone in Duchenne dystrophy: A randomized controlled trial defining the time course and dose response. Arch Neurol 1991; 48:383–388.

Griggs RC, Moxley RT, Pandya S. Randomized, controlled trial of prednisone and azathioprine in Duchenne dystrophy. Neurology 1991; 41 (suppl 1):166.

Harley HG, Brook JD, Rundle SA, et al. Expansion of an unstable DNA region and phenotypic variation in myotonic dystrophy. Nature 1992; 355:545–546.

Harper PS. Myotonic dystrophy. 2nd ed. London: WB Saunders, 1989.

Hoffman EP, Brown RH Jr, Kunkel LM. Dystrophin: The protein product of the Duchenne muscular dystrophy locus. Cell 1987; 50:509–517.

Karpati G. Approaches to the introduction of normal alleles into skeletal muscle fibers for therapeutic purposes in Duchenne muscular dystrophy. In: Kakulas BA, Howell J McC, Roses AD, eds. New York: Raven, 1992; 223.

Mendell JR, Moxley RT, Griggs RC, et al. Randomized double blind six month trial of prednisone in Duchenne's muscular dystrophy. N Engl J Med 1989; 320:1592–1597.

Quantin B, Perricaudet LD, Tajbaksh S, Mandel JL. Adenovirus as an expression vector in muscle cells in vivo. Proc Natl Acad Sci USA 1992; 89:2581–2584.

Rossiter B, Stirpe N, Caskey T. Report of the MDA gene therapy conference, Tucson, Arizona, Sept. 27-28, 1991. Neurology 1992; 42:1413–1418.

Sarfarazi M, Wijmenga C, Upadhyaya M, et al. Regional mapping of facioscapulohumeral muscular dystrophy gene on 4Q35. Combined analysis of an international consortium. Am J Hum Genetics 1992; 51:396-403.

Sklar R, Brown RH. Methylprednisolone increases dystrophin levels by inhibiting myotube death during myogenesis of normal human muscle in vitro. J Neurol Sci 1991; 101:73–81.

Wolff JA, Malone RW, Williams P, et al. Direct gene transfer into muscle in vivo. Science 1990; 247:1465–1468.

Worton RG, Gillard EF. Muscular dystrophy, molecular genetics. Encyclopedia of Human Biology 1991; 5:191–205.

Zubrzycka-Gaarn EE, Bulman DE, Karpati G, et al. The Duchenne muscular dystrophy gene product is localized in the sarcolemma of human skeletal muscle fibers. Nature 1988; 333:466–469.

PATIENT RESOURCES

Voluntary Health Agencies Dedicated to Providing Support for Patients with Neuromuscular Disease

Muscular Dystrophy Association Inc, USA (National Office)
3561 East Sunrise Drive
Tucson, Arizona 85718
Telephone: (602) 529-2000
Fax: (602) 529-5300

Muscular Dystrophy Association of Canada,
150 Eglinton Avenue East, Room 400
Toronto, Ontario, M4P 1E8
Telephone: (416) 488-0030
Fax: (416) 488-7523

Association Française Contre les Myopathies
13 Place de Rungis
75013 Paris
Telephone: (1) 45-65-13-00
Fax: (1) 45-80-37-36

European Alliance of Muscular Dystrophy Associations
Lt. Gen. van Heutszlaang
NL-3743 JN Baarn
The Netherlands
Telephone: (31) 2154-18400
Fax: (31) 2154-21616

POLYMYOSITIS

ANDREA M. CORSE, M.D.
RALPH W. KUNCL, M.D., Ph.D.

The inflammatory myopathies are a diverse group of muscle disorders that have distinct pathogenic mechanisms. Included among the inflammatory myopathies are polymyositis, dermatomyositis, inclusion body myositis, and inflammatory myopathy associated with human immunodeficiency virus (HIV), among others. Polymyositis and dermatomyositis are the most common of the inflammatory myopathies. The annual incidence of polymyositis and dermatomyositis is 0.5 to 1.0 per 100,000. The cause of these two distinct clinical entities is unknown; however, an autoimmune mechanism is generally accepted.

DIAGNOSIS

Polymyositis is defined by the following clinical, laboratory, electrophysiologic, and pathologic criteria.

Weakness

Muscle weakness is proximal, symmetric, generally worse in the legs than in the arms, and has a subacute or chronic course. Difficulty climbing stairs, rising from a chair, and washing hair are frequent complaints. The neck muscles are often involved, resulting in difficulty raising the head off a pillow or keeping the head erect (head ptosis). About 15 to 20 percent of patients suffer dysphagia. Respiratory musculature can be affected, and respiratory insufficiency may even be a presenting feature. Facial weakness is rare, and ocular muscles are spared.

Creatine Kinase

Serum creatine kinase (CK) activity is a sensitive though nonspecific test for polymyositis and dermatomyositis; over 85 percent of patients have an elevated level. The levels can be 50 times the normal value. Conversely, the absence of elevated serum muscle enzymes does not exclude the diagnosis. As many as 15 to 20 percent of patients with polymyositis or dermatomyositis do not have elevated serum muscle enzymes at the time of diagnosis. Serum aldolase activity is not useful. Historically, its use preceded use of CK, but aldolase is less sensitive and adds no additional information.

Electromyography

Electromyography (EMG) is abnormal in the great majority of patients with polymyositis or dermatomyositis, though not in all. EMG demonstrates brief-duration, small-amplitude, polyphasic voluntary motor unit potentials and increased spontaneous activity, including fibrillations, positive sharp waves, and complex repetitive discharges. The increased spontaneous activity may be most evident or occur earliest in paraspinal muscles.

Biopsy

The most specific diagnostic test for polymyositis and dermatomyositis is muscle biopsy, which must demonstrate necrosis, regeneration, and *primary* inflammation. The key feature, primary inflammation, consists predominantly of lymphocytes and macrophages surrounding and invading non-necrotic myofibers.

Exclusion of Mimicking Diseases

History and biopsy must distinguish conditions that clinically mimic polymyositis and dermatomyositis, including drug-induced myopathy; sarcoid myopathy; HIV-associated inflammatory myopathy; inclusion body myositis; bacterial (pyomyositis), viral, and parasitic inflammatory myopathies; eosinophilic fasciitis; metabolic myopathies such as acid maltase deficiency; and, rarely, myasthenia gravis or muscular dystrophy with inflammation.

Pathologic confirmation of polymyositis and dermatomyositis should be attempted prior to initiation of therapy. The biopsy should be performed by a physician familiar with the specifications of muscle processing, to ensure the highest diagnostic yield. Proximal muscles (quadriceps, deltoid, biceps) with mild or moderate weakness are most appropriate for biopsy; muscles recently studied by EMG should be avoided, to prevent misdiagnosis of artifactual inflammation associated with needle trauma. Cylindrical pieces of muscle tissue should be obtained for snap freezing in 2-methyl butane for histochemical analysis and metabolic enzyme assays (if indicated after histochemical review), as well as for routine formalin fixation and paraffin sectioning. In addition, a stretched, clamped, thin piece of muscle fixed in glutaraldehyde should be obtained for possible electron microscopy. Repeat muscle biopsy is occasionally indicated in the case of treatment failure, to confirm the diagnosis, to evaluate for inclusion body myositis, or to distinguish disease progression from steroid myopathy.

In the setting of polymyositis or dermatomyositis, further evaluation for coexisting collagen vascular disease or systemic cancer is indicated. The diagnosis of a malignancy can precede or follow the diagnosis of polymyositis or dermatomyositis by years. The risk of associated malignancy is greatest with dermatomyositis. We perform an evaluation for malignancy (including stool for occult blood, mammography, pelvic examination, and chest computed tomography) in all adult patients with polymyositis and dermatomyositis at the time of diagnosis and repeat a malignancy screen periodically. The most commonly associated tumors occur in the lung, gastrointestinal tract, pancreas, breast and ovary. In dermatomyositis, for example, the risk of cancer of the ovary is increased 17 fold, as reported in a recent article by Sigurgeirsson and colleagues.

It is important to note that significant muscle pain or tenderness occurs *infrequently* (prevalence 25 percent) with polymyositis or dermatomyositis. Muscle cramps are more frequently a feature of denervating diseases than of primary myopathy.

PATHOGENESIS

Polymyositis

An autoimmune pathogenesis of polymyositis and dermatomyositis is implied by their association with other autoimmune disorders, the presence of inflammatory cells on muscle biopsy, and the response to immunotherapy. Both humoral and cell-mediated mechanisms are implicated. At present, no autoantibody has been identified with a clear pathogenic role in polymyositis. The only autoantibody with any specificity is the Jo-1 antibody, directed against histidyl-tRNA synthetase, which is present in at least 50 percent of patients with the syndrome of polymyositis in combination with autoimmune interstitial lung disease. Autoreactive lymphocytes, predominantly activated CD8 (cytotoxic-suppressor) T cells, are a characteristic feature of polymyositis. Although the precise antigenic target recognized by the cytotoxic T cells has yet to be identified, the antigen appears to be associated with the major histocompatibility complex (MHC)-I antigen expressed on abnormal myofibers in polymyositis.

Dermatomyositis

Dermatomyositis is not polymyositis with a rash. Their clinical and pathologic features are distinct. Dermatomyositis often presents more acutely and is more frequently associated with systemic disease. Characteristic skin features in dermatomyositis include an erythematous dermatitis most commonly involving the neck, upper trunk, and extensor surfaces of the proximal interphalangeal and metacarpophalangeal joints, elbows, and knees; Gottron's nodules; nailbed infarcts; a heliotrope (lilac) discoloration of the upper eyelids; and periorbital edema. Distinctive pathologic findings in dermatomyositis are perifascicular myofiber atrophy, necrosis, and regeneration, as well as evidence of vasculopathy with reduced myofiber capillary number and deposition of complement membrane attack complex within the intramuscular microvasculature. These findings support an immune-mediated vascular pathogenesis in dermatomyositis.

THERAPY

Immunotherapy is the mainstay of treatment of polymyositis and dermatomyositis, based on the presumed autoimmune pathogenesis (Table 1). There has never been an adequate controlled clinical trial of any immunotherapy for either polymyositis or dermatomyositis. Nonetheless, based on case reports and the available uncontrolled clinical trials, the consensus is that immunotherapies are effective.

Untreated, polymyositis and dermatomyositis almost invariably have a chronic, progressive course. Spontaneous remissions are rare. With treatment, more than two-thirds of patients exhibit enough response to avoid functional disability. The success of therapy should be assessed on the basis of functional gains and quantitative muscle testing. Serum CK activity is a crude indicator of disease activity and, in isolation, should not guide therapy.

Corticosteroids

Corticosteroids are the initial drugs of choice, despite their frequent side effects, for the treatment of polymyositis and dermatomyositis. We institute treatment with prednisone at a single daily dose of 1 mg/kg until a stable clinical response is achieved or for a period of 2 to 3 months, whichever comes first. The dosage is then gradually adjusted to an alternate-day regimen over 6 to 8 weeks by increasing the "on" day dose by 10 mg and decreasing the "off" day dose by 10 mg per week toward a regimen of 100 to 120 mg on alternate days. Further gradual tapering of the "on" day dose is attempted, decreasing by 10 mg monthly to 50 mg, followed by 5 mg monthly to 25 mg, then 2.5 mg monthly as tolerated. Polymyositis does not require divided daily doses of prednisone, which severely increases steroid toxicity. The goal of therapy is to use the least prednisone necessary to control the disease.

The patient, internist, and treating neurologist must join efforts to prevent and detect adverse effects related to corticosteroid therapy as early as possible. The more common adverse effects of corticosteroid treatment include weight gain, gastrointestinal distress, hypertension, glucose intolerance, osteoporosis, avascular necrosis, and cataracts. Children's growth rate can be retarded.

We routinely place a tuberculin skin test prior to instituting corticosteroid therapy. Once therapy is begun, patients are followed regularly (frequently monthly) for weight and blood pressure monitoring, quantitative and functional strength assessment, and routine laboratory tests, including serum electrolytes and glucose. Biannual ophthalmoscopic examination is advised. We follow an empiric strategy for prevention of corticosteroid-induced osteoporosis in all patients. Calcium supplementation (calcium carbonate, 1,000 to 1,500 mg per day) begins at the start of prednisone

Table 1 Immunosuppressive Treatment of Polymyositis

Drug	Usual Adult Dose	Time to Onset of Improvement	Time to Maximal Improvement	Unique Toxicity Monitoring
Prednisone	1 mg/kg/day	2–8 wk	3–6 mo	Weight, blood pressure, fasting glucose, electrolytes, ophthalmoscopy, bone density, vitamin D, urine Ca^{2+}
Azathioprine (Imuran)	2–3 mg/kg/d PO (100–250 mg daily)	3–12 mo	1–2 yr	Complete blood count (CBC), differential, MCV, platelets, liver functions
Methotrexate	0.2 mg/kg once weekly IV, increasing weekly by 5 mg up to 0.7 mg/kg once weekly IV, to either tolerance or effectiveness (max. 40–50 mg) Alternatively, 5–10 mg once weekly PO, increasing gradually every 3–6 weeks by 5 mg, up to 15–50 mg/wk	1–3 mo	2–5 mo	CBC, differential, liver functions & biopsy (see text), diarrhea, mouth ulcers, fetal death
Cyclosporine (Sandimmune)	5 mg/kg/d PO, divided b.i.d. (125–200 mg b.i.d.)	2–12 wk	4–6 mo	Blood pressure, K^+, blood urea nitrogen, creatinine, cyclosporine level (12 hr trough) by radioimmunoassay, amylase
Intravenous immunoglobulin	2 g/kg IV, divided over 5 successive days	Unreported	Unreported	Anaphylaxis, fluid overload

therapy. A 24 hour urinary calcium level is checked every 6 months. If hypercalciuria is detected, initiation of a thiazide and potassium-sparing diuretic (e.g., amiloride-hydrochlorothiazide) is recommended to reduce calcium clearance. Vitamin D replacement (ergocalciferol, 50,000 units 1 or 2 times weekly) is initiated if the serum 25-OH vitamin D level is less than 40 ng per milliliter. Especially for post-menopausal women, bone densitometry is suggested before therapy.

Steroid myopathy can follow long-term corticosteroid therapy. It is rare in doses equivalent to less than 25 mg of prednisone per day. There may be no specific clinical, laboratory, or electrophysiologic clues that distinguish between worsening of polymyositis or dermatomyositis and steroid myopathy; though steroid myopathy does not elevate serum CK activity. For steroid myopathy, a therapeutic trial of dose reduction should result in clinical improvement, usually within 8 weeks.

After institution of prednisone therapy, occasional patients show improvement in strength within a few days. Most patients who are going to respond to prednisone do so within 3 to 6 months. An adequate trial of high doses of steroids lasts at least 6 months. If prednisone provides no quantitative improvement in muscle strength, if relapses recur with lower steroid doses, or if corticosteroid toxicity outweighs the benefit, a steroid-sparing intervention is required. Most commonly, steroid therapy is continued and a second immunosuppressive agent is added for combination therapy. If steroid toxicity is severe, prednisone can be tapered as an alternative immunosuppressive therapy is initiated. Included among the conditions that do not respond to steroids is the syndrome of inclusion body myositis, a morphologically distinctive vacuolar inflammatory myopathy most commonly seen in older men. Patients often appear to have had polymyositis for several years. On histologic examination, inclusion body myositis is characterized by autophagic vacuolar inclusions, intranuclear and cytoplasmic intermediate filamentous inclusions, and inflammation. Inclusion body myositis is generally unresponsive to therapy.

Azathioprine

No adequate studies are available that can recommend one nonsteroidal immunosuppressive treatment over another as second-line therapy for polymyositis or dermatomyositis. We most frequently use azathioprine, a purine analogue, which has proven efficacy in many other autoimmune diseases. Azathioprine is generally well tolerated orally and has less hepatotoxicity than methotrexate. The primary disadvantage of azathioprine is the slow onset of action. Though the initial beneficial response can be seen in 3 months, it may not be apparent for as long as 12 months.

Azathioprine is instituted at a dose of 50 mg daily for 1 week. The dosage is increased by 50 mg per week toward a dose of 2 to 3 mg per kilogram per day. Weekly monitoring of complete blood count with differential and serum transaminase values is performed until a maintenance dose is determined. The target dose is one that demonstrates biologic activity of the drug: a white blood cell count of 3,000 to 4,000 per cubic millimeter and an MCV greater than 100. Concurrent treatment with steroids results in drug-induced leukocytosis; in that case, a relative lymphocyte count of 5 to 10 percent is the appropriate target. Once a stable dose is established, patients are followed every 2 months, and laboratory studies should include complete blood count (CBC) with differential, platelets, and serum transaminase values.

The most common side effect of azathioprine is gastrointestinal distress. This improves with divided dosing after meals (two to three times daily), dose reduction, or the addition of sucralfate. Potential adverse effects of azathioprine include leukopenia, anemia, thrombocytopenia, and elevation of serum transaminase values (two- to 10-fold). Both the hematologic and hepatic effects are reversible following reduced doses or temporary discontinuation of the azathioprine; later re-establishment of dose is usually possible. Ten percent of patients develop a hypersensitivity reaction consisting of abdominal discomfort, influenza-like symptoms, fever, and, rarely, rash. If these symptoms occur, further use of azathioprine is not an option. Relative contraindications to the use of azathioprine include existing liver disease and bone marrow depression. Dose reduction is necessary with concurrent use of allopurinol. As with all immunosuppressants, azathioprine therapy carries a small increased risk of susceptibility to infections and of neoplasia.

A number of uncontrolled studies have reported 60 to 70 percent efficacy of azathioprine in the treatment of polymyositis and dermatomyositis. We consider an adequate trial of azathioprine to be at least 12 months.

Methotrexate

Methotrexate, a folic acid antagonist, is an alternative immunosuppressive agent used to treat polymyositis or dermatomyositis. Relative disadvantages of methotrexate compared to azathioprine are twofold. First, there is the potential for insidious, irreversible hepatotoxicity, including necrosis and cirrhosis, and, more rarely, the potential for possibly fatal hypersensitivity pneumonitis in a very small percentage of patients. Second, unlike azathioprine, which is used frequently in the management of myasthenia gravis, neurologists are less familiar with the use of methotrexate, which is not commonly used to treat other autoimmune neurologic disorders.

Methotrexate can be administered orally, intramuscularly, or intravenously. We initiate therapy with an oral dose of 5 to 10 mg once weekly; this is increased every 3 to 6 weeks by 5 mg until a beneficial response is obtained or adverse effects develop. The usual dose range is 15 to 25 mg weekly. The maximum dose is 50 mg weekly. Intravenous therapy begins with a single dose of 0.2 mg per kilogram. The weekly dose is gradually increased by 5 mg per week to 0.7 mg per kilogram weekly. The maximum IV dose is 40 to 50 mg weekly. The onset of beneficial results can occur within 1 to 3 months.

The most common side effects include oral ulcers, gastrointestinal disturbance, and fever. The most serious possible adverse effects are hepatotoxicity, bone marrow suppression, and hypersensitivity pneumonitis. The risk of hepatotoxicity is greater for patients who have pre-existing liver disease, who daily consume more than 60 ml of ethyl alcohol, who are obese or have diabetes mellitus, who are of advanced age, or who take methotrexate daily. Most though not all patients with methotrexate-induced hepatotoxicity demonstrate abnormal liver function tests.

Before beginning therapy with methotrexate a CBC and serum transaminase, alkaline phosphatase, and bilirubin values are obtained. Liver biopsy is not routinely performed unless risk factors are present. CBC is checked weekly until a stable dose is established. Thereafter, CBC and liver function tests are followed at least every 2 months. Total cumulative methotrexate dose is recorded, and liver biopsy is considered for all patients after each 1.5 g of methotrexate received. Methotrexate is not metabolized and is excreted in the urine. Creatinine clearance should be followed routinely every 2 months.

Cyclosporine

Our experience with the use of cyclosporine in the treatment of polymyositis and dermatomyositis is limited. For other autoimmune diseases (e.g., myasthenia gravis) cyclosporine is an effective immunomodulator. It is particularly potent in inhibiting the production of soluble cell mediators such as interleukin 2, thus blocking the proliferation of helper T cells and blocking the development of cytotoxic lymphocytes. Since T cell–mediated muscle damage is thought to be important in the pathogenesis of polymyositis, it seems most likely that cyclosporine would be effective in the management of that disease. There has been limited published experience with cyclosporine treatment in polymyositis. Leuck and coworkers reported on four patients with inflammatory myopathy that was refractory to conventional treatment with prednisone and azathioprine and that apparently responded to cyclosporine and prednisone. In each case, benefits appeared within weeks and substantial functional improvements occurred within months; the dosage was 2 to 6 mg per kilogram per day in two doses. In all patients there was significant steroid sparing. A double-blind, placebo-controlled randomized trial of cyclosporine as sole therapy in polymyositis is needed.

Cyclosporine is initiated at a dose of 5 mg per kilogram in two doses taken with meals. Maintenance dosage is determined by the serum cyclosporine trough (12 hour) levels and side effects. Serum levels should be obtained every 2 weeks until a stable dose is obtained. The specific therapeutic drug level range varies, depending on laboratory assay techniques. The dose is adjusted by 0.5 mg per kilogram per day not more often than once a month.

The most serious adverse effect of cyclosporine is nephrotoxicity, which appears to be dose dependent and potentially reversible upon dose reduction. Signs of nephrotoxicity include increasing BUN followed by increasing creatinine. Nephrotoxicity is increased in patients with pre-existing renal disease (creatinine value greater than 1.3 mg per deciliter) and in the presence of other nephrotoxic drugs, especially nonsteroidal anti-inflammatory drugs. Additional potential adverse effects of cyclosporine include hypertension and elevated serum potassium levels. Cyclosporine is extensively metabolized in the liver by the P_{450} system, so hepatic dysfunction or concurrent administration of other drugs so metabolized can cause dramatic changes in the elimination of cyclosporine. Several drug interactions must be recognized, therefore, to use cyclosporine safely. Cyclosporine is excreted in the bile; this is responsible for the interaction with lovastatin to produce toxic myopathy.

The length of an adequate cyclosporine therapeutic trial is not known. Case reports indicate a generally rapid response within weeks.

All the nonsteroidal immunosuppressive therapies discussed above carry potential risk of teratogenicity. The possible benefits of these immunosuppressive regimens in patients of childbearing age must be carefully weighed against the potential risks.

Human Immunoglobulin

A most recent alternative treatment in polymyositis and dermatomyositis is human immunoglobulin (HIG) therapy, either alone or in combination with other immunosuppressive regimens. HIG has proven efficacy and safety in the treatment of other immune-mediated disorders such as immune thrombocytopenic purpura. Data on the use of HIG in polymyositis, dermatomyositis, myasthenia gravis, chronic inflammatory demyelinating polyneuropathy, and other autoimmune neurologic conditions involves small numbers of patients, though the results are promising. Standard dosage is 2 g per kilogram intravenously divided over 3 to 5 successive days. Repeat administration appears necessary, generally every 2 months. Mild transient side effects include headache, fever with rigors, diarrhea, and fluid overload. Relative contraindications include immunoglobulin A deficiency and renal insufficiency. Reversible acute renal failure has been reported in two patients with baseline creatinine levels greater than 1.3 mg per deciliter. A major disadvantage to HIG therapy is its cost: $5,000 to $27,000 for a single 2 g per kilogram treatment.

Other Immunosuppressive Therapies

Occasional reports of therapeutic benefit are mixed with disappointing effects for cyclophosphamide, chlorambucil, plasmapheresis, thymectomy, hydroxychloroquine, antilymphocyte globulin, total body irradiation, and total lymphoid irradiation.

REHABILITATION

Rehabilitation therapy, including physical and occupational therapy, can provide valuable contributions to the treatment of patients with polymyositis and dermatomyositis. Range of motion, stretching, and isometric exercise regimens are important therapeutic maneuvers to reduce the risk of contractures, reduce potential side effects of steroid therapy (osteoporosis), and increase endurance. Swimming is frequently recommended as recreational exercise. In addition, patients should be evaluated for assistive devices. Self-care aids such as long-handled comb, pick-up devices, and an elevated seat for the commode can dramatically ease activities of daily living and restore independence.

SUGGESTED READING

Bohan A, Peter JB. Polymyositis and dermatomyositis. N Engl J Med 1975; 292:344–347; 403–407.
Dalakas M. Polymyositis and dermatomyositis. Boston: Butterworths, 1987.
Dalakas M. Polymyositis and dermatomyositis, and inclusion body myositis. N Engl J Med 1992; 325:1487–1498.
Lueck C, Trend C, Swash M. Cyclosporine in the management of polymyositis and dermatomyositis. J Neurol Neurosurg Psychiatry 1991; 54:1007–1008.
Sigurgeirsson B, Lindelof B, Edhag O, Allander E. Risk of cancer in patients with dermatomyositis or polymyositis. N Engl J Med 1992; 326:363–367.

PATIENT RESOURCE

Patients with polymyositis and dermatomyositis qualify for services provided by The Muscular Dystrophy Association (MDA). Educational information is available, and newsletters keep patients informed on many aspects of the disease. Many local chapters offer support groups and financial assistance for medical care. Additional information can be obtained from the headquarters:

The Muscular Dystrophy Association
3561 East Sunrise Drive
Tucson, Arizona 85718
602-529-2000

METABOLIC MYOPATHIES

RONALD G. HALLER, M.D.
JAMES P. KNOCHEL, M.D.

Metabolic myopathies include *acquired* muscle injury or weakness attributable to systemic disorders or toxins and *inherited* errors of muscle metabolism. In the former, removal of the toxin or correction of the underlying systemic disorder corrects the myopathy. The management of these disorders is covered well in general textbooks of neurology and internal medicine and is not considered further here. Instead, we will focus on inborn metabolic errors, in particular those that affect muscle energy metabolism.

PATHOPHYSIOLOGY OF DISORDERS OF MUSCLE ENERGY METABOLISM

Impaired phosphorylation of adenosine diphosphate represents the fundamental lesion in disorders of muscle energy metabolism. The result is a deficient rate of adenosine triphosphate synthesis relative to utilization, with accumulation of fatigue-promoting hydrolysis products of adenosine triphosphate and related metabolites in circumstances in which the affected pathway normally provides an important contribution to energy production. Increased degradation of muscle adenine nucleotides may accompany this imbalance between muscle energy supply and demand, leading to increased serum uric acid, sometimes associated with gout. Additional factors that may contribute to the pathophysiology of these disorders include depletion of crucial metabolites or cofactors secondary to the enzymatic block; accumulation of toxic metabolites proximal to the block; and dysregulation of preserved metabolic pathways due to altered cellular patterns of regulatory metabolites. Similarly, altered levels of metabolites that normally signal muscle energy demand may alter the regulation of oxygen delivery, ventilation, and neuroendocrine responses to exercise. Finally, the expression of the metabolic defect in other tissues (e.g., central nervous system [CNS], heart, liver) may complicate metabolic myopathies and influences treatment strategies.

GENERAL TREATMENT STRATEGIES: MANAGEMENT OF MYOGLOBINURIA

The ideal therapy of metabolic myopathy would replace the defective gene to permit normal synthesis of the missing enzyme. Currently, this is not a therapeutic option. In disorders associated with deficiency of specific cofactors, dietary supplements of these cofactors may improve enzyme kinetics and reduce or eliminate symptoms. For muscle energy defects, strategies to optimize energy production via preserved metabolic pathways in the muscle cell and to avoid exercise or dietary factors that engage defective pathways are used to improve energy availability and to prevent accumulation of toxic metabolites or depletion of crucial cofactors.

Recurrent acute muscle injury is a major complication of muscle defects that impair glycolysis or lipid metabolism. The first goal of therapy of these disorders is to avoid rhabdomyolysis and myoglobinuria. If significant muscle injury occurs, however, the next important goal is to minimize the complications of myoglobinuria. We advise patients subject to recurrent myoglobinuria to obtain orthotolidine test tape (e.g., Hemastix), which sensitively detects the presence of urinary heme protein (including myoglobin) even when the urine is not grossly pigmented. The suspicion of myoglobinuria or persistent muscle pain should motivate the patient to avoid further exertion, to increase fluid intake, and to promptly seek medical attention to minimize complications of myoglobinuria (Table 1).

Hospital evaluation is warranted for patients whose creatine kinase (CK) level is 25,000 IU per liter within 6 hours of injury (CK level typically peaks 12 to 24 hours after injury and subsequently declines approximately 50 percent every 48 hours), whose creatinine–urea nitrogen ratio in serum exceeds 0.2, whose serum uric acid value is 9, or who has demonstrable myoglobin in the urine. Acute renal failure occurs in approximately 25 percent of patients with severe rhabdomyolysis. The likelihood of this complication increases in patients with volume depletion and shock; thus, the importance of adequate fluid replacement (normal saline or half normal saline in dextrose) to maintain renal perfusion. Intravenous mannitol, 25 g, and furosemide, 200 mg, may be required to maintain urine output. Persistent oliguria (urine flow less than 20 ml per hour) despite correction of hypotension and the use of mannitol and furosemide, suggests acute tubular necrosis. Further volume replacement in this setting risks pulmonary edema. Such patients often require early and aggressive hemodialysis.

Hyperkalemia due to release of intracellular potassium from necrotic muscle may cause life-threatening cardiac arrhythmias or even cardiac arrest, particularly in the setting of renal failure. The effect of hyperkalemia is potentiated by hypocalcemia, a common complication of rhabdomyolysis attributable to deposition of calcium salts in injured muscle. The electrocardiogram is more valuable than serum potassium values per se to assess hyperkalemic cardiotoxicity. Emergent treatment of hyperkalemia includes intravenous glucose and insulin, calcium salts, and hyperventilation to promote cellular uptake of potassium. Oral or rectal disodium polystyrene sulfonate is useful but acts more slowly. Hemodialysis may be required.

MUSCLE GLYCOGEN STORAGE DISEASES

Acid Maltase Deficiency

Acid maltase deficiency is a generalized enzyme defect that blocks lysosomal degradation of glycogen but does not affect the energy-yielding process of glycogenolysis. A fatal infantile form of the disease (Pompe's disease) is associated with hypotonia and cardiopulmonary failure. Childhood and adult forms of the enzyme deficiency are characterized by progressive myopathy in which there is often early impairment of respiration, owing to involvement of the diaphragm. The childhood disorder may mimic muscular dystrophy, and the adult form may resemble myositis or limb girdle dystrophy. A high-protein diet—20 to 30 percent of daily calorie intake (2 to 2.5 g per kilogram per day for adults; 4 to 5 g per kilogram per day for children)—combined with regular exercise has been reported to be of benefit. Regular pulmonary function testing with institution of ventilatory support when necessary is an important component of managing the disease.

Glycogen Debrancher Deficiency

Debrancher deficiency (oligo-1,4-glucantransferase and alpha-1,6-glucosidase deficiency; Forbes-Cori disease) is a generalized enzyme defect that blocks glycogenolysis at branch points in the glycogen molecule, so

Table 1 Major Complications of Rhabdomyolysis and Myoglobinuria

Complication (Mechanism)	Management
Acute renal failure (toxic effect of myoglobin, potentiated by hypovolemia)	Maintain urine output with mannitol, furosemide; hemodialysis
Hyperkalemia (release of intracellular potassium, renal compromise)	Glucose + insulin; calcium; potassium-binding resins; hemodialysis
Hypocalcemia (deposition of calcium salts in injured muscle), potentiates cellular effects of hyperkalemia	No specific treatment of hypocalcemia; treat hyperkalemia as above
Hyperphosphotemia	No specific treatment
Hemorrhage (related to disseminated intravascular coagulation, thrombocytopenia, fibrinolysis, capillary injury)	Fresh-frozen plasma
Adult respiratory distress syndrome	Artificial ventilation
Compartment syndrome (muscle injury, swelling)	Fasciotomy may be required

that only the terminal chains of glycogen are accessible for hydrolysis by glycogen phosphorylase. The disease is usually a benign disorder of childhood associated with hepatomegaly and fasting hypoglycemia (attributable to the block in hepatic glycogenolysis). Because the block in muscle glycogenolysis is incomplete, symptoms of exercise intolerance typically are less prominent than in phosphorylase and phosphofructokinase (PFK) deficiencies, and muscle cramps and myoglobinuria are not features of the disorder. The most common neuromuscular feature is progressive weakness. Management includes adequate dietary carbohydrate to counter the propensity to develop hypoglycemia, frequent feedings, and a diet high in protein (e.g., 50 to 55 percent carbohydrate, 25 percent protein, 20 to 25 percent fat). Oral, uncooked cornstarch is absorbed slowly and effectively maintains blood glucose levels when administered every 6 hours.

Myophosphorylase Deficiency (McArdle's Disease)

McArdle's patients experience lifelong premature exertional fatigue and are subject to exertional muscle pain, contractures, and rhabdomyolysis when muscle energy demands exceed supply. Later in life, McArdle's patients may develop fixed weakness.

The main therapeutic aims in McArdle's disease are to improve exercise tolerance and to reduce the frequency and severity of muscle injury. Success hinges on efforts to avoid patterns of activity that require glycogen as an energy source and to promote the utilization of preserved energy pathways—especially lipid oxidation—to meet muscle energy needs (Table 2). Glycogen has anaerobic and oxidative functions. Anaerobic glycogenolysis can support rates of energy turnover more than twice that achieved by oxidative metabolism, and it is necessary to fuel intense exercise and when oxygen delivery is blocked. No substitute for anaerobic glycogenolysis exists. To avoid muscle injury, it is therefore necessary for patients to avoid ischemic or isometric exercise such as heavy lifting and arm wrestling.

Glycogen also fuels pyruvate-dependent oxidative metabolism, and glycogen unavailability makes muscle dependent on the availability of blood-borne oxidative fuels. This is exemplified by the *second wind* phenomenon, in which exercise tolerance improves and the rate of muscle oxidative phosphorylation is augmented when the availability of blood-borne oxidative substrate (particularly free fatty acids and glucose) to muscle is increased. The mobilization, delivery, and cellular transport of blood-borne substrates are sluggish in comparison with the availability of glycogen-derived pyruvate, so the oxidative energy deficit is apparent in the transition from rest to exercise. Also, maximal rates of oxidative phosphorylation able to be achieved by blood-borne fuels are low compared with that achieved with pyruvate. Warming up before engaging in any sustained activity improves substrate availability by increasing muscle blood flow and facilitating substrate mobilization.

A diet rich in protein and adequate in carbohydrate is recommended for McArdle's disease. Protein requirements are increased by the ongoing muscle injury and increased muscle regeneration that are typical of this condition. Also, amino acids provide a potential alternative oxidative fuel for skeletal muscle. When combined with a program of regular exercise, a high-protein diet was found to improve exercise capacity significantly.

Dietary carbohydrate sufficient to maintain hepatic glycogen stores is desirable, because glucose utilization and hepatic glycogenolysis are increased during exercise in McArdle's disease. The immediate effect of a

Table 2 Regulation of Substrate Utilization by Skeletal Muscle

Substrate for Skeletal Muscle	Activities, Conditions That Increase Substrate Use by Muscle	Interventions That Promote Substrate Storage or Decreased Use
Muscle glycogen	Transition from rest to exercise; near maximal aerobic exercise (aerobic glycogenolysis); ischemic, isometric exercise (anaerobic glycogenolysis); poor physical conditioning (reduced capacity to oxidize lipid)	Recent carbohydrate meal, especially after exercise; submaximal exercise (i.e., exercise that can be fueled by lipid); good physical conditioning (enhanced ability to oxidize lipid)
Adipose tissue → free fatty acids	Diet: fasting, high fat diet; prolonged, submaximal exercise; warm up exercise; conditioning: regular aerobic exercise (increases enzymes involved in fat metabolism)	Recent carbohydrate meal
Liver glycogen → blood glucose	Fasting, reduced carbohydrate intake; prolonged exercise; depletion of muscle glycogen	Recent carbohydrate meal

Key: Arrow indicates adipose tissue is the source of the free fatty acids which is the substrate used by muscle.

carbohydrate meal may be to reduce exercise capacity, owing to homeostatic mechanisms that maintain blood glucose in a narrow range and the corresponding reduction in plasma fatty acids levels. *Intravenous* glucose raises blood glucose levels, increases glucose transport into muscle, and augments exercise capacity, but it is useful primarily in a hospital. Glucagon increases hepatic glycogenolysis and may improve exercise capacity in the short term, but indications for chronic treatment are unproven.

Long-chain free fatty acids (FFAs) represent the dominant available oxidative fuel in glycolytic defects, but a high-fat diet has not provided consistent benefits. Epinephrine increases exercise capacity by augmenting lipolysis and increasing muscle blood flow. A medium-chain triglyceride (MCT) diet increases medium-chain fatty acids, which are preferentially oxidized in liver to ketones, which can be oxidized by skeletal muscle. MCT oil supplements may improve exercise tolerance, but some patients experience nausea, diarrhea, and meager improvement in exercise capacity, if any.

Regular *aerobic* exercise, by promoting mitochondrial biogenesis and increasing the activity of rate-limiting oxidative enzymes, increases fat oxidation and reduces the requirement for carbohydrate utilization to supply muscle energy needs. Conditioning exercise must be undertaken with caution, as overexertion may precipitate muscle injury. We prescribe "low-level" exercise (approximately 50 percent of maximal) performed for 20 to 40 minutes, three or four times per week. Because exercise tolerance often varies in the course of a given exercise session owing to patterns of substrate mobilization, exercise intensity should be varied accordingly. Heart rate is a good objective index of relative exercise intensity that the patient can monitor with a pulsemeter (preferably) or by timing the pulse. Serum CK should be monitored to ensure that the exercise program is not producing increased muscle injury.

The most devastating acute consequence of McArdle's disease is massive exertional muscle injury with myoglobinuria. It is crucial to recognize muscle injury that is sufficient to cause myoglobinuria, so that appropriate treatment can be instituted (see Table 1). The major long-term consequence of McArdle's disease is muscle weakness. A likely mechanism is recurrent muscle injury, which ultimately exceeds the regenerative capacity of skeletal muscle. Muscle magnetic resonance imaging sensitively identifies focal muscle injury and decreased mass. For patients with focal muscle atrophy, special attention should be given to eliminating patterns of exercise that promote muscle injury; to measures to augment substrate availability and improve the capacity to oxidize available substrates; and to providing adequate dietary protein to promote protein synthesis.

Muscle Phosphofructokinase Deficiency (Tarui's Disease)

Symptoms of PFK deficiency are similar to those of myophosphorylase deficiency. Patients experience pre-mature muscle fatigue and are subject to exertional pain, cramping, and nausea, and to recurrent exertional myoglobinuria. Fixed muscle weakness associated with muscle atrophy and fatty replacement are common with advancing age.

Substrates available for working muscle are more limited in muscle PFK deficiency than in myophosphorylase deficiency, as the metabolic defect blocks utilization of glucose as well as glycogen. As a result, patients are heavily dependent on lipids to meet muscle energy requirements. Muscle oxidative metabolism and exercise capacity are augmented (second wind) by increased availability of FFAs. In contrast, exercise capacity dramatically drops when fatty acid levels are reduced by a carbohydrate meal or intravenous glucose. This state of severe deficiency of oxidative substrate has been termed *the out of wind effect.* An additional feature of muscle PFK deficiency is the presence of a partial enzyme defect in red blood cells, with resulting compensated hemolytic anemia.

Treatment is similar to that for McArdle's disease: attempt to optimize substrate availability by warming up before exercise; engaging in regular aerobic training to improve the capacity to oxidize fatty acids; avoiding ischemic, isometric exercise; and instituting prompt treatment of acute muscle injury with myoglobinuria (see Table 1).

Distal Blocks in Muscle Glycogenolysis

With rigorous exercise, patients with deficiency of phosphoglycerate mutase, phosphoglycerate kinase, or lactate dehydrogenase experience muscle pain, cramping, and rhabdomyolysis with myoglobinuria. The block in glycogenolysis is incomplete in these disorders, and pyruvate-dependent oxidative metabolism is apparently relatively preserved compared to myophosphorylase and muscle PFK deficiencies. This implies that oxidative metabolism may be less dependent on blood-borne substrates and thus that major fluctuations in exercise tolerance are less prominent. Recommendations for management include warming up before exercise, regular aerobic exercise to promote lipid oxidation by muscle, strict avoidance of rigorous exercise, and prompt treatment of any episodes of myoglobinuria.

LIPID DISORDERS

Carnitine Palmitoyl Transferase Deficiency (CPT II Deficiency)

Hepatic and muscle forms of carnitine palmitoyl transferase (CPT) deficiency have been described: the hepatic form is attributable to deficiency of CPT I, the muscle form to deficiency of CPT II. The muscle form of the disease usually becomes symptomatic in the second decade of life or later and is manifested as recurrent muscle fatigue, pain, and myoglobinuria triggered by metabolic challenges such as fasting and prolonged exercise, which normally require fatty acid oxidation as a major source of muscle energy production. Exertional muscle cramps are not a feature of the disorder, and patients are not subject to muscle injury during brief bouts of intense exercise or during the transition from rest to exercise, as is the case in muscle glycolytic defects. The metabolic defect promotes glycogen depletion, because the glycogen-sparing effect of fatty acid oxidation is lacking. Effective treatment consists of maintaining adequate muscle glycogen stores by eating a high-carbohydrate diet, having regular meals, and avoiding prolonged exercise. Prompt medical attention should be sought to reduce the risk of acute tubular necrosis should prolonged muscle pain or pigmenturia occur.

Carnitine Deficiency

Primary carnitine deficiency is attributable to impaired cellular carnitine transport and is associated with cardiomyopathy or myopathy. Oral carnitine supplements, L-carnitine 100 mg per kilogram per day in divided doses, may effectively reverse symptoms even when only a modest (but apparently critical) increase in cellular carnitine level can be achieved.

Secondary carnitine deficiency is more common and occurs as a consequence of metabolic defects involving the oxidation of organic acids, especially beta-oxidation defects at the level of medium-, long-, or short-chain acyl coenzyme A (acyl CoA) dehydrogenases. The majority of reported cases have involved infants or children who exhibit systemic symptoms of aketotic hypoglycemia (owing to the coexisting metabolic defect in liver) and episodes resembling Reye's syndrome, with or without symptoms of muscle weakness or fatigability. Metabolic crises are triggered by the mobilization of fatty acids in response to fasting or infection, leading to the accumulation of toxic levels of organic acids behind the metabolic block. Pregnancy may also be a risk factor in precipitating metabolic crises. Carnitine depletion occurs through the action of carnitine acyl transferases, which convert accumulated acyl CoA esters to acylcarnitines, which diffuse from the cell and are excreted by the kidney. Treatment—designed to prevent or reduce fatty acid mobilization—consists of a high-carbohydrate, low-fat (less than 20 percent of dietary calories) diet and frequent feedings. L-Carnitine replacement, 100 mg per kilogram per day in divided doses, counters carnitine depletion, promotes the formation of relatively nontoxic acyl carnitines from more toxic acyl CoA esters, and may increase the ratio of free to esterified CoA.

Multiple acyl CoA dehydrogenase deficiency due to impairment of a riboflavin-dependent reaction common to straight and branched-chain acyl CoA molecules commonly is associated with carnitine depletion and a lipid myopathy in which skeletal muscle weakness and fatigability are prominent features. Of great importance is the fact that some of these patients respond to pharmacologic doses of riboflavin (up to 100 mg three times per day) with dramatic reversal of clinical symptoms. Additional therapeutic measures include

L-carnitine replacement to counter secondary carnitine deficiency. These patients are subject to life-threatening, Reye's syndrome–like metabolic crises triggered by metabolic stresses that lead to fatty acid mobilization. Strict maintenance of carbohydrate intake with a low-fat, high-carbohydrate diet is crucial.

Deficiency of long- and short-chain hydroxyacyl CoA dehydrogenases have been recognized and other beta-oxidation defects likely will be identified. It seems likely that the principles of treatment for these disorders will be similar to those for other lipid defects: avoid lipid mobilization, ensure carbohydrate availability, and supplement with carnitine.

MITOCHONDRIAL DISORDERS

Muscle Respiratory Chain and Related Defects

Mitochondrial defects involving the Krebs cycle (fumarase deficiency, succinate dehydrogenase deficiency) and abnormal coupling of adenosine diphosphate phosphorylation to oxygen uptake (Luft's disease) have been described, but the most common mitochondrial myopathies are associated with respiratory chain abnormalities. The clinical presentation in these disorders is heterogeneous. Major manifestations of muscle involvement include infantile hypotonia, weakness, and lactic acidosis; severe exercise intolerance and easy fatigability; and variable fixed weakness, often involving the extraocular muscles. Additionally, infantile or childhood encephalomyopathies have been identified in which CNS (e.g., seizures, ataxia, stroke-like episodes) and muscle symptoms coexist. Clinical syndromes include mitochondrial encephalomyopathy, lactic acidosis and stroke (MELAS), myoclonus epilepsy with ragged red fibers (MERRF), and Kearns-Sayre syndrome, in which ophthalmoplegia, retinal pigmentary degeneration, heart block, and variable CNS features are associated.

Rapid progress has been made in clarifying the molecular basis of these disorders. Deletions of mitochondrial DNA, which codes for some peptide subunits in respiratory chain complexes I, III, IV and V, have been identified in many patients with progressive external ophthalmoplegia, including virtually all patients with Kearns-Sayre syndrome. Mitochondrial DNA point mutations have been identified in patients with MERRF and MELAS. Nuclear genomic defects have been identified on the basis of inheritance pattern or suspected on the basis of selective respiratory chain enzyme defects. Depletion or deficiency of mtDNA has been found to underlie some mitochondrial myopathies.

Unfortunately, progress in treatment of these disorders has lagged and remains largely anecdotal and empirical. In some cases, the metabolic block may be at least partially bypassed. The Krebs cycle intermediate *succinate* donates electrons to complex II, and in vitro is capable of supporting mitochondrial respiration in the presence of inhibitors of complex I. Thus, succinate, 2 to

6 g per day, may benefit patients with selective or predominantly complex I defects. No side effects have been reported in the small number of patients so treated. In a patient with a selective defect involving complex III of the electron transport chain, exercise intolerance responded to treatment with menadione (vitamin K_3), 20 to 80 mg per day, and ascorbate (vitamin C), 4 to 5 g per day. The therapeutic benefit may relate to the ability of menadione to act as an electron acceptor from complex I of the respiratory chain and for ascorbate to function as an electron donor to complex IV, thus bypassing the site of the metabolic block in complex III. Potential side effects of menadione include hemolysis in persons who are deficient in glucose-6-phosphate dehydrogenase and depression of hepatic function.

Coenzyme Q is a component of the respiratory chain that receives electrons from complex I and II and donates electrons to complex III. Oral supplementation of ubiquinone (CoQ_{10}), 100 to 150 mg per day, has been reported to be of benefit in some patients with Kearns-Sayre syndrome, in some patients with selective complex I defects, and in patients with apparent deficiency of CoQ. Evidence of clinical effectiveness has included improved endurance with reduced levels of blood lactate after standard exercise tests and improved strength of limb or respiratory muscles. In addition to correcting deficiency of the cofactor, CoQ may improve mitochondrial function by antioxidant effects. Administration of riboflavin, 100 to 300 mg per day, was associated with improved exercise capacity in a patient with a defect in complex I. The mechanism of benefit is unclear, but flavin mononucleotide and flavin adenine dinucleotide, the physiologically active forms of riboflavin, serve as cofactors in respiratory flavoproteins found in complex I and II of electron transport.

The accumulation of potentially toxic peroxides and related free radicals as a consequence of the block in electron transport is a possible mechanism of muscle injury in respiratory chain defects. Treatment with *antioxidants* such as vitamin E *(tocopherol),* 400 to 800 IU per day; *ascorbate,* 1 to 4 g per day; or *ubiquinone* may therefore be justified. Glucocorticoids (e.g., prednisone, prednisolone) have been reported to benefit some patients, possibly owing to their capacity to inhibit phospholipases, which mediate lipid peroxidation.

Lactic acidosis present at rest or with minor exercise is a typical feature of respiratory chain defects and is attributable to impaired oxidative metabolism and consequently increased demand of anaerobic glycogenolysis to meet skeletal muscle energy needs. *Dichloroacetate,* which activates pyruvate dehydrogenase and thus increases entry of pyruvate into mitochondria, has been administered to alleviate lactic acidosis in a variety of clinical settings, including mitochondrial myopathy. Thiamine is a cofactor of pyruvate dehydrogenase and in doses of 200 mg per day has been reported to reduce lactic acidosis in patients with mitochondrial myopathy.

Respiratory chain defects result in secondary blockade of specific steps in beta oxidation. Low muscle carnitine levels have been reported in some patients with electron transport defects, presumably related to the accumulation of these unmetabolized fatty acids. This provides a rationale for treatment with *L-carnitine* and for institution of a relatively *low-fat diet,* similar to the management recommended for beta-oxidation defects.

Immunohistochemical differentiation of the invariably fatal form infantile cytochrome oxidase deficiency (mtDNA-encoded subunit II is present) from a benign, reversible form of the disease (subunit II initially is absent) is crucial, to ensure provision of appropriate medical care in the benign condition until reversal of the enzyme defect.

SUGGESTED READING

Fernandes J, Leonard JV, Moses SW, et al. Glycogen storage disease: Recommendations for treatment. Eur J Pediatr 1988; 147:226–228.

Gregersen N. Riboflavin-responsive defects of β-oxidation. J Inher Metab Dis 1985; 8(suppl 1):65–69.

Haller RG, Lewis SF. Glucose-induced exertional fatigue in muscle phosphofructokinase deficiency. N Engl J Med 1991; 324:364–369.

Penn AMW, Lee JWK, Thuillier P, et al. Melas syndrome with mitochondrial tRNA ^Leu(UUR) mutation: Correlation of clinical state, nerve conduction, and muscle 31P magnetic resonance spectroscopy during treatment with nicotinamide and riboflavin. Neurology 1992; 42:2147–2152.

Shoffner JM, Wallace DC. Oxidative phosphorylation diseases—disorders of two genomes. Adv Hum Genet 1990; 19:267–330.

Slonim AE, Goans PJ. Myopathy in McArdle's syndrome, improvement with a high-protein diet. N Engl J Med 1985; 312:355–359.

Tanaka K, Coates PM, eds. Fatty acid oxidation: Clinical, biochemical and molecular aspects. New York: Alan Liss, 1990.

PATIENT RESOURCE

Muscular Dystrophy Association
3300 East Sunrise Drive
Tucson, Arizona 85718
Telephone: (602) 529-2000
Fax: (602) 529-5300

PAINFUL NEUROPATHIES

MARCO PAPPAGALLO, M.D.

Any pathologic condition that affects the peripheral (PNS) or central nervous system (CNS) pain pathway may bring on a painful state that is appropriately termed neuropathic pain. The pathophysiology of pain in peripheral neuropathy is complex and is currently the object of an intensive study. The prevailing idea is that the underlying disease activates or alters the nociceptor afferents (A delta and C fibers). These small fibers can be affected at the distal nerve endings or more proximally at the root-trunk level. An inflammatory process affecting the nerve root may in fact cause neuropathic pain by activating the small fibers known as nervi nervorum; for example, this mechanism may contribute to the pain often experienced in the Guillain-Barré syndrome. Although impaired by the underlying primary disease, the injured afferent fibers remain in a state of prolonged regeneration. In painful diabetic neuropathy, the presence of regenerating unmyelinated fibers has been correlated with neuropathic pain. In this state, the C fibers may become ectopic "pain generators." Hyperexcitability may arise from the accumulation of some of the transported membrane-bound proteins (such as those making the sodium channels) at the site of the nerve ending. This hyperexcitability might be sustained by the accumulation of alpha-adrenergic receptors in the regenerating nociceptors. Finally, ongoing ectopic activity of nociceptors may initiate a central pain mechanism in the dorsal horn, which clinically manifests itself as secondary hyperalgesia. The chronic pain that arises from these pathophysiologic changes is the major object of treatment for many patients.

DIAGNOSIS

The possible causes of painful neuropathy are numerous (Table 1). It is essential to establish a diagnosis of the underlying disease. An understanding of the complex pathophysiology helps the clinician develop a logical treatment plan. Clinical experience has suggested a division between sympathetically maintained pain (SMP), producing causalgia and related syndromes, and sympathetically independent pain (SIP). SMP has been associated with a multitude of pathologic conditions. Most often, it follows a partial nerve injury, but sometimes the inciting event cannot be identified. The typical SMP syndrome is characterized by distal, severe, burning pain in a single extremity associated with exquisite hyperalgesia to light touch and cold stimuli. In contrast, typical SIP syndromes are seen with generalized neuropathies and are

Table 1 Causes of Painful Neuropathy

Neuropathy	Cause
Focal neuropathy (SIP, SMP?)	Diabetes mellitus
	Ischemic microangiopathy:
	Polyarteritis nodosa, rheumatoid arthritis, systemic lupus erythematosus
	Arterial: Trauma, surgery, thrombosis, embolism
	Post-traumatic neuroma
	Entrapment neuropathy
	Carcinomatous disease
	Nerve tumors (neurofibroma)
	Herpes zoster
	Idiopathic causes (Parsonage-Turner brachial plexopathy)
Generalized neuropathy (SIP, SMP?)	Diabetes mellitus
	AIDS
	Alcoholism and malnutrition
	Paraneoplastic
	Myeloma
	Amyloid
	Acute inflammatory polyneuropathy (Guillain-Barré syndrome)
	Toxicity: Arsenic, thallium, isoniazid, metronidazole, cisplatin, high-dose pyridoxine, hydralazine, nitrofurantoin, disulfiram
	Hereditary disease: Fabry's disease (sex-linked recessive), dominantly inherited sensory neuropathy
	Hypothyroidism (?)
	Uremia (?)
	Idiopathic causes

characterized by paroxysmal pain, paresthesias, and spontaneous burning pain. These are occasionally associated with tactile hyperalgesia and rarely with cold hyperalgesia. Sensory and motor neurologic deficits may be present in the neuropathic pain syndromes. The clinical features of the patient's pain help distinguish between sympathetically maintained and sympathetically independent neuropathic pain syndromes.

SMP remains overdiagnosed and much less common than SIP, but it is useful to rule out an SMP mechanism in many patients. Recently, the response to intravenous phentolamine has been advocated as an adjunctive means of differentiating the two. If the clinical history and the examination are suggestive of SMP, the patient should undergo the intravenous phentolamine test. This test is performed in a blinded fashion. Such a protocol is conducive to identifying placebo responders and is more specific than sympathetic nerve block. If the response to the intravenous phentolamine test is positive (i.e., pain is improved or relieved), the treatment plan will include sympatholytic agents, and possibly sympathectomy. The treatment of SMP is extensively discussed in a separate chapter.

MANAGEMENT OF NEUROPATHIC PAIN

Most painful neuropathies seem to involve sympathetically independent pain. The treatment of chronic sympathetically independent neuropathic pain remains a challenge in clinical practice. Assuming that the best efforts are being made to control and treat the primary disease, the management of pain is the major task of the clinician. The treatment plan should include a sequence of pharmacologic trials. The drug administration route can be oral, intravenous, or transcutaneous. The clinical experience has established the usefulness of the following drugs (Table 2): tricyclic antidepressants (TCAs), antiepilepsy drugs (AEDs), local anesthetics, capsaicin, and opioids. In order to carry out the proper pharmacologic trial, the clinician is required to know the pharmacokinetics and pharmacodynamics of each drug and how to manage drug-related side effects. In some cases, monitoring of drug serum levels is needed. The

Table 2 Pharmacologic Treatment of Neuropathic Pain

Tricyclic antidepressants	Topical agents
Amitriptyline	Lidocaine
Nortriptyline	Capsaicin
Desipramine	
	Opioids
Antiepilepsy drugs	Morphine
Carbamazepine	Oxycodone
Phenytoin	Hydromorphone
Clonazepam	Methadone
	Levorphanol
Oral local anesthetics	Fentanyl (patch)
Mexiletine	

response of the patient should be followed by rating scales for pain intensity, pain relief, and functional activity. The overall algorithm for pharmacologic treatment is shown in Figure 1.

Alternative treatment options include neural stimulation techniques such as spinal cord stimulation (SCS) and transcutaneous electrical nerve stimulation (TENS).

Tricyclic Antidepressants

Traditional hypotheses of the action of the TCAs involve inhibition of norepinephrine and serotonin uptake. These two bioamines seem to play a major role in the endogenous pain-modulating system. The potential interactions of TCAs with central, and possibly peripheral, pain mechanisms are complex and not yet defined. Amitriptyline is the TCA most extensively studied and used, and its analgesic effect has been documented in diabetic painful neuropathy. However, amitriptyline is also the TCA with the highest incidence of side effects. In patients with a compromised cardiovascular system (conduction disturbances, orthostatic hypertension), nortriptyline is the TCA of choice. In patients with a history of urinary retention, angle-closure glaucoma, or severe constipation, desipramine, the TCA with the least anticholinergic effect, should be used. In these settings, or when patients complain prominently of sedation and dry mouth, desipramine is preferred over amitriptyline.

The TCA is usually given at bedtime. Amitriptyline and nortriptyline may cause nightmares, and desipramine may cause insomnia. If these side effects develop, the TCA should be given in the morning.

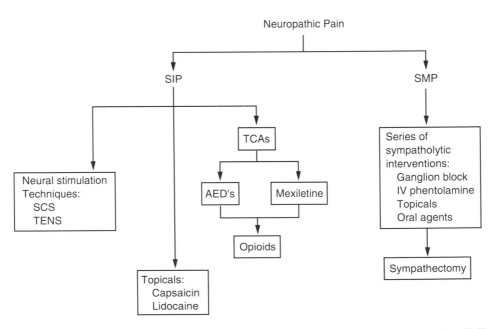

Figure 1 Treatment algorithm for neuropathic pain. Key: SIP = sympathetically independent pain; SMP = sympathetically maintained pain; SCS = spinal cord stimulation; TENS = transcutaneous electrical nerve stimulation; TCAs = tricyclic antidepressants; AEDs = antiepilepsy drugs.

Confusion and memory impairment are more common with amitriptyline, and the medication should be switched to desipramine or nortriptyline if they appear.

Oral doses of TCA should start at 10 to 25 mg at bedtime and be increased twice weekly by 10- to 25 mg increments. According to the limiting side effects, the total daily dose should be in the range of 75 to 150 mg and should be maintained for at least 3 weeks. Between the titration and the maintenance time, a period of 6 weeks may be required for a proper trial with the TCAs.

If, at the end of the 6 week period, analgesia has not been obtained, the TCA plasma level should be determined to ensure that oral absorption or noncompliance does not represent a limiting factor for the pharmacologic trial. The plasma level of amitriptyline plus its metabolite nortriptyline should be between 100 and 200 ng per deciliter. The level of nortriptyline by itself may vary from 50 to 150 ng per deciliter. The level of desipramine should be between 125 and 300 ng per deciliter. If the plasma levels of these TCAs are low, the dose can be increased and the trial should proceed accordingly. If the plasma levels are optimal and no analgesia has been obtained, a second drug should be introduced.

Antiepilepsy Drugs

Except for the management of trigeminal neuralgia, the AEDs are considered second choice agents for trials of neuropathic pain control. The traditional view directs attention at the AED action in stabilizing nerve membrane and in suppressing neuronal paroxysmal discharges at multiple levels, from the peripheral nerve/DRG neuron up to the CNS. Carbamazepine and phenytoin have similar actions in blocking sodium channels. Clonazepam instead would decrease the excitability of the central pain-signaling neurons secondary to the ongoing nociceptive input. Clonazepam may induce neuronal hyperpolarization through an increase of chloride conductance.

We recommend carbamazepine in an initial dose of 100 mg twice daily. The dose will be increased to a total of 800 mg per day or until limiting side effects occur. The most frequent side effects are dizziness, drowsiness, nausea, and vomiting. These side effects, which are often particularly prominent in older patients, can be minimized by initiating the treatment with small doses. Adverse reactions such as skin rash or leukopenia warrant discontinuation of the treatment. Baseline and follow-up complete blood counts are recommended. Between titration and maintenance, a period of 3 weeks is usually recommended for a proper trial with carbamazepine. If no analgesia has been obtained, the carbamazepine plasma level should be determined and the dose increased accordingly. If the plasma level was found to be in the optimal range, carbamazepine should be tapered off quickly and discontinued.

The second AED to try is clonazepam, which should be started at a dose of 0.25 mg per day in two doses. Drowsiness is the principal side effect, but it tends to subside quickly. Other side effects include hypotonia and ataxia. If tolerated, clonazepam can be increased to 0.5 to 1 mg twice daily. Between titration and maintenance, a proper trial with clonazepam may require 3 weeks. If no analgesia has been obtained, the AED and the TCA should be tapered off and discontinued.

Local Anesthetics

Local anesthetics block nerve conduction by inactivating the membrane sodium channels. Small nerve fibers, such as nociceptors, seem to be more susceptible than most of the large fibers to low concentrations of anesthetics. Mexiletine, an oral local anesthetic, blocks the neuronal membrane sodium channels and so may act in the same way as carbamazepine and phenytoin. Whether the patient should start taking mexiletine if a proper trial with carbamazepine has failed is debatable; however, a rational way to proceed would be to have the patient undergo a prognostic intravenous lidocaine test. Lidocaine can be infused in a dose of 5 mg per kilogram over 1 hour. The infusion should be performed in a blinded fashion and before giving lidocaine, normal saline should be given for 15 to 30 minutes, in order to establish a baseline level of pain intensity and to rule out a possible placebo response. Pain intensity and pain relief assessment are performed throughout the intravenous testing.

If a consistent positive response of more than 50 percent pain relief is obtained, a trial with oral mexiletine can be recommended. Caution should be exercised in patients with pre-existing sinus node dysfunction or intraventricular conduction abnormalities. Lidocaine and mexiletine are contraindicated for patients with second- or third-degree atrioventricular block. Mexiletine can be started at a dose of 150 mg per day PO and increased by 150 mg increments every 3 or 4 days. Mexiletine can be adjusted up to a total dose of 10 mg per kilogram per day, which can be given in three doses. There is a high incidence of side effects such as nausea, vomiting, altered taste, dizziness, co-ordination difficulties, tremors, and tinnitus. The drug should be given with food or antacids. Unfortunately, the side effects are so prominent that very often the medication has to be discontinued. Between titration and maintenance, a trial with mexiletine may require 3 weeks.

Opioids

Increasing attention has recently been given to the use of opioids in the management of neuropathic pain. The opioids act directly at the spinal level by blocking nociceptive inputs and supraspinally by inhibiting the central pain-signaling neurons. Analgesia seems to be derived mainly from the activation of the kappa receptors (spinal cord) and of the mu receptors (supraspinal CNS). In our experience, satisfactory long-term pain management is possible in patients who have failed TCA and AED trials. The opioids recommended for a formal trial are listed in Table 2.

Several factors are crucial in determining a successful result by using opioids. It has been said that opioid responsiveness is a continuum. Upward dose adjustment is necessary until unmanageable side effects are seen or until successful analgesia (at least 50 percent pain relief) and improvement in daily function are obtained. Among the neuropathic pain patients there is variability in terms of predisposition to side effects and analgesic response. There is also variability among the different opioids in producing successful analgesia and intolerable side effects when used on the same patient. Our clinical experience with opioids has established that addiction and tolerance to the analgesic effects are rare events. These observations are consistent with those in patients who suffer cancer pain. In our institution, the following strict guidelines must be followed before a neuropathic pain patient may be started on the opioid trial.

1. A history of substance abuse or significant personality disorder should be considered a contraindication. The opioid trial will be discontinued if any evidence of aberrant drug-taking behavior is noted. The patient should be followed by a single physician, preferably one trained in pain management.
2. The opioid trial can be considered when a specific diagnosis of the patient's pain has been made and when TCA, AED, or other drug trials have failed.
3. We titrate the opioid dose, aiming for 50 percent pain relief or significant improvement of the patient's physical and social function. The initial dose adjustment may require several weeks (1 month on average). Throughout the trial, pain relief, pain intensity, and level of function should be assessed. Pain relief can be expressed as a percentage and pain intensity on a scale of 1 to 10, ten being the worst pain ever suffered. The level of function can be simply assessed by using a 10 cm line as a visual analog scale. One end of the line would be equivalent to the patient's best activity performance prior to the onset of the painful disease. The other end of the line would be equivalent to the patient's worst performance while affected by the pain. Using this visual analog scale, the comparison of the overall level of function or of specific activities (e.g., walking, cleaning, shopping, reading) before and during the opioid treatment can be made. While using opioids, not only analgesia should be assessed but also improvement in the patient's physical and social function. A formal test of the patient's cognitive function before and during the trial may be indicated. In fact, it should be assessed whether the pain itself or the drug affects and lowers the patient's attention span and mental acuity.
4. In order to enhance the patient's compliance and to achieve a steady level of analgesia throughout the day, slow-release opioid preparations and around-the-clock dosing are recommended. Slow-release morphine, such as MS Contin, can be given every 8 to 12 or every 24 hours. Fentanyl can be slowly delivered by a skin patch that is changed every 72 hours. Oxycodone and hydromorphone can be formulated in a slow-release preparation by a compounding pharmacy and they can be given every 6 to 8 hours. *Careful drug titration is necessary when using the compounded drug preparations.*
5. Patients should be informed of opioid-related side effects before the beginning of the trial. *The most important factor for a successful result is the capable management of opioid side effects.*

Major Side Effects of Opioids

Tolerance. Drug tolerance is defined as the need for larger doses to produce the same effect, but clinical experience has shown that tolerance to opioid analgesic effect is uncommon. On the contrary, the need for an increased dose to maintain analgesia arises when the underlying disease progresses. Patients with stable disease can be maintained on the same dose. It should be noted that if the patient's daily physical activity increases, the level of pain may increase proportionally. A dose adjustment is then necessary. This situation occurs when a treated patient who feels comfortable at rest finally becomes more active. True tolerance to the sedative and euphoric side effects, to nausea and urinary retention, may develop more commonly than tolerance to analgesia. This constitutes a positive phenomenon, because it allows titration of the opioid in order to achieve satisfactory pain relief.

Physical Dependence. Physical dependence consists of an abstinence syndrome following sudden drug withdrawal. In the management of chronic pain, physical dependence does not constitute a concern as long as the patient is informed and warned against suddenly stopping the drug. The use of a mixed agonist-antagonist opioid must be avoided.

Addiction (Psychological Dependence). Addiction consists of abnormal drug-seeking behaviour. There is usually a past or current history of alcohol or illicit drug abuse for recreational purposes. Patients who are prone to develop addiction behave inconsistently. They state that they obtain no benefit from the opioid but at the same time they show an overwhelming concern for its procurement. Extensive clinical experience in the cancer patient population and observations reported in several surveys as well as in our experience, have shown that the prevalence of addiction to therapeutic opioids is probably less than 0.01 percent. It is important to stress the notion that patients who take opioids on a regular basis are not addicted. The opioid is necessary to maintain the pain relief and to improve the patient's quality of life.

Respiratory Depression. Respiratory depression is rare when opioids are properly prescribed. It will not occur unless the opioids have induced severe sedation and profound analgesia. Aiming at 50 percent pain relief during the opioid titration leaves a large enough margin of safety to avoid this severe adverse side effect. Careful titration is required for patients with significant pulmonary disease. Tolerance develops.

Nausea and Vomiting. Opioids can cause an increase in vestibular sensitivity, stimulation of the medullary chemoreceptor trigger zone, and gastroparesis. Tolerance may develop in several days. Hydroxyzine, transdermal scopolamine, metoclopramide, or prochlorperazine may be useful, alone or in combination, to counteract these side effects. If nausea and vomiting persist and are unmanageable, a trial with a different opioid must be considered. Severe epigastric pain secondary to biliary tract spasm can be caused by opioids, in particular by morphine. It is a rare event with the oral preparations, and it can be relieved by sublingual nitroglycerin. Tolerance to this side effect may develop; otherwise a different opioid is recommended.

Constipation. Tolerance usually does not develop. Prophylactic use of senna and docusate sodium is recommended. If constipation is unmanageable, trial with a different opioid is required.

Sedation. Tolerance may develop within a few days. Small doses of pemoline, 18.75 mg every morning, can be used in some situations to ameliorate opioid-induced sedation. If it is unmanageable, a trial with a different opioid might be required.

Euphoria. Euphoria rarely occurs with slow-release oral preparations. Tolerance quickly develops.

Confusion. Confusion is common in patients with underlying mild dementia or encephalopathy. Tolerance usually develops. A trial with a different opioid might be necessary. Organic hallucinosis has been reported.

Urinary Retention. Urinary retention is quite infrequent. Tolerance usually develops. The dose of opioid can be decreased and slowly adjusted upward again.

Myoclonus. Reassurance is the best treatment; otherwise, a very small dose of Klonopin (0.25 mg per day) is recommended. If myoclonus remains refractory, a trial with different opioid is required.

Pruritus, Flushing, Hypotension, Sweating, Rhinorrhea, and Headaches. Some or all of these side effects can be due to the release of histamine, which can produce vasodilatation, increased capillary permeability, itch, and stimulation of exocrine glands. The release of histamine seems to be mediated through a nonopioid receptor mechanism. Trials with nonsedating H1 or H2 antagonists are recommended. Headaches can also respond to nonsteroidal anti-inflammatory drugs. If these side effects remain unmanageable, a trial of a different opioid is necessary. It should be noted that pruritus is more common with intraspinal opioids. In this case, pruritus seems to have a central mechanism and it is easily controlled by small doses of naloxone.

Allergy. Immune-mediated allergic reaction is an extremely rare event. A trial of a different opioid is an option.

A proper trial of an opioid may require 4 to 6 weeks. For instance, MS Contin can be started at 15 to 30 mg per day. The patient should be given a prescription for Atarax, 25 mg per day, to be taken with the MS Contin if nausea develops. The patient should be also given Senokot-S, 1 tablet once or twice a day, for constipation. The dose of the opioid will be titrated upward, aiming for 50 percent pain relief. The patient should be followed closely through phone conversations at least twice a week for the first 3 weeks of treatment. The smallest dose of opioid should be used with elderly patients. Methadone and levorphanol should be used with caution. With these two medications, the duration of analgesia is about 4 to 6 hours, but the half-life of elimination is much longer (12 to 100 hours for methadone; 12 to 16 hours for levorphanol). Drug accumulation may result in delayed toxicity.

Topical Agents

It can be assumed that for some painful neuropathies the pain generators are located in the skin of the symptomatic areas, in which case treatment of the affected skin with topical agents would be a rational approach. Topical agents obviate some of the major systemic side effects of oral therapy. Moreover, the topical agents may have a synergistic effect when used in combination with oral agents. In cases of painful neuropathy affecting a relatively limited skin area and characterized by intense hyperalgesia to light touch, high-concentration lidocaine ointment can be used successfully. The stratum corneum is the limiting barrier to transcutaneous drug absorption. Lidocaine in a concentration higher than 10 percent is added to a vehicle that has a hydrating and mildly keratolytic effect. The patient applies a thin layer of the lidocaine ointment to the symptomatic areas. No more than 3 to 5 cc of the ointment should be applied per day. Applying an occlusive plastic film over the ointment promotes transcutaneous absorption of lidocaine by increasing skin hydration. After a few days, analgesia or anesthesia may develop. If no effect is seen, the lidocaine concentration can be slowly increased. The lidocaine serum level should be checked weekly, until the maintenance dose is achieved. The keratolytic agent can cause skin peeling, and it will be withdrawn from the ointment once analgesia or anesthesia has been obtained. These topical local anesthetic preparations can be formulated by a compounding pharmacy.

Capsaicin is a neurotoxin that has been shown to cause analgesia to painful heat, but not to painful mechanical stimuli. It appears that capsaicin in doses used clinically may selectively deactivate the heat transduction mechanism of the nociceptors. It is possible that in some neuropathic pain states the heat-sensitive nociceptors may play a pathogenic role. Capsaicin, 0.075 percent, can be applied four times a day for 4 weeks. If no benefit is derived, the ointment can be discontinued. Because of the initial intolerable burning sensation, and because frequent daily applications are required, the use of capsaicin is associated with poor patient compliance, and it appears to be useful topically in a very few patients.

In conclusion, topical agents can be used concurrently with TCAs, AEDs, or opioids. The lidocaine ointment is recommended for painful neuropathies associated with marked tactile hyperalgesia.

Neurostimulation Techniques

Spinal cord stimulation trial should be considered when the neuropathic pain affects essentially the patient's lower extremities and when results of pharmacologic management is unsatisfactory. The contemporary technique consists of a multi-electrode device inserted percutaneously and placed epidurally over the lower thoracic segments of the spinal cord. The spinal cord stimulator has been successfully used in chronic pain syndromes secondary to arachnoid fibrosis and characterized by radicular, lower extremity pains.

A trial with the TENS unit can be recommended for the management of painful mononeuropathies. The TENS trial is safe and easy to perform, but in my experience the results have been generally unsatisfactory.

SUGGESTED READING

Fields HL. Pain syndromes in neurology. New York: Butterworth, 1990.

Max MB, Lynch SA, Muir J, et al. Effects of desipramine, amitriptyline, and fluoxetine on pain in diabetic neuropathy. N Engl J Med 1992; 326:1250–1256.
Portenoy RK, Foley KM, Inturrisi CE. The nature of opioid responsiveness and its implications for neuropathic pain: New hypotheses derived from studies of opioid infusions. Pain 1990; 43: 273.
Raja SN, Treede RD, Davis KD, Campbell JN. Systemic alpha-adrenergic blockade with phentolamine: A diagnostic test for sympathetically maintained pain. Anesthesiology 1991; 74:691.
Simone AD, Ochoa J. Early and late effects of prolonged topical capsaicin on cutaneous sensibility and neurogenic vasodilatation in humans. Pain 1991; 47:285.

COMPOUNDING PHARMACY

Professional Arts Pharmacy
1101 N Rolling Rd.
Baltimore, Maryland 21228
Telephone: (800) 832-9285

PATIENT RESOURCES

American Pain Society (APS)
1200 17th St. N.W., Suite 400
Washington, DC 20036
Telephone: (202) 296-9200

International Association for the Study of Pain (IASP)
909 NE 43rd St., Suite 306
Seattle, Washington 98105
Telephone: (206) 547-6409

PSYCHIATRIC DISEASE PRESENTING AS NEUROLOGIC DISEASE

CONVERSION DISORDER

MICHAEL J. KAMINSKY, M.D.
PHILLIP R. SLAVNEY, M.D.

Among the phenomena traditionally subsumed under the term *hysteria* none has been of greater interest to neurologists than conversion disorder, a behavior that suggests neurologic disease in the absence of a neurologic explanation. Patients whose symptoms simulate paralysis, blindness, ataxia, amnesia, seizures, or other neurologic dysfunctions are said to have conversion disorder if they are not consciously aware of their behavior. Such self-deceiving persons are to be distinguished from those who consciously intend to deceive others, for ultimate goals that are either obvious, as in malingering, or more obscure, as in factitious disorder. Although these distinctions are straightforward when diagnostic categories are being constructed, they may be difficult when patients are being assessed, for self-awareness is a continuum along which individuals may vary from time to time, depending on personality, circumstances, and the responses of others (including physicians) to behavior. What can be said about individuals in all three categories, however, is that the initial goal of their simulation is to be granted the *sick role,* a protected position from which other goals (e.g., interpersonal, financial) can be pursued. Given this common goal, many of the treatment principles outlined below for conversion disorder can also be applied to assessment of malingerers and to the care of patients with factitious disorder.

One other distinction should be noted at the outset. Hypochondriasis is the fear of having a disease, an anxiety that persists despite reassurance by physicians. The concept of hypochondriasis, therefore, depends on a state of mind (i.e., fear of disease) rather than on a behavior (e.g., simulation of dysfunction). Patients with conversion disorder may or may not have hypochondriacal preoccupations. When they do, they are anxious; when they do not, they seem less concerned about the potential significance of their complaints (*la belle indifférence*) than they do about the acceptance of those complaints as meriting the sick role.

DIAGNOSIS

Conversion disorder is suspected when there is a discrepancy between the patient's complaint and the physician's assessment. The simulation of dysfunction is often obvious if the patient is medically unsophisticated, though repeated examinations by careful physicians sometimes have the unintended effect of improving the imitation. Persons who have professional medical knowledge and lay people who have experience of certain disorders — either their own (as in pseudoseizures among epileptics) or someone close to them (as in pseudoparalyses among children caring for parents who have had cerebrovascular accidents) — may be capable of nearly perfect simulation.

When there is a discrepancy between the patient's complaint and the physician's assessment, more diagnostic weight should be given to signs than to symptoms, but it must be remembered that even certain "pathognomonic" signs of conversion disorder, such as sensory loss splitting the midline, can occur in patients rendered suggestible by delirium and other acute cerebral disorders.

The amobarbital interview may be helpful in the diagnosis (and treatment) of conversion disorder. During the disinhibited state produced by the drug, patients can be encouraged to abandon their apparent dysfunction and to reveal the circumstances under which it arose. While simulated motor and sensory loss is sometimes "cured" in this manner, amobarbital may not be useful when the complaint is intermittent, as in pseudoseizures.

The diagnostic approach we recommended is a modification of that proposed by Sir Francis Walshe. It has three criteria: (1) the absence of signs that require or tolerate neurologic diagnoses; (2) the presence of signs that are incongruous with neurologic diagnoses; and (3) evidence that the patient is simulating dysfunction in order to obtain the sick role. Unless the last criterion is met, there may be a tendency to regard any unexplained illness as hysterical, especially if the patient seems vague or dramatic in manner.

Symptoms suggesting conversion disorder are generally found in three settings: (1) associated with neurologic conditions; (2) associated with other psychiatric disorders; and (3) either singly in an acute form or associated with other medically unexplained symptoms in a chronic pattern of complaining to physicians.

Neurologic Disorders

Patients with neurologic disorders such as epilepsy, multiple sclerosis, and myasthenia gravis are entitled to the sick role and the benefits it confers. Under certain circumstances some of these patients simulate the manifestations of their neurologic condition because they have learned that being in the sick role helps them cope with interpersonal problems and other difficulties. It should also be noted that patients in the initial stages of a neurologic disorder that has an episodic course and subtle presentation are sometimes regarded as simulating dysfunctions when they are not. In these "false-positive" cases, a psychiatric history and continuing neurologic assessment help establish the correct diagnosis.

Other Psychiatric Disorders

Patients with other psychiatric conditions may consult neurologists for complaints that suggest conversion disorder because there is a discrepancy between symptoms and signs. These patients are not simulating illness; they are suffering it. Thus, for example, persons with anxiety disorders may report fatigue, dysphagia, impaired concentration, paresthesias, dizziness, or loss of consciousness; those with schizophrenia may experience somatic hallucinations of pain, heat, or tingling; and patients with depressive disorders can suffer from amnesia or psychomotor retardation. Such "false-positive" complaints do not occur as isolated phenomena, but as part of clinical syndromes whose other characteristic manifestations can be detected by psychiatric history and mental status examination.

Conversion Disorder and Somatization Disorder

When symptoms suggesting conversion disorder are not associated with other conditions, they present in two forms: conversion disorder per se and somatization disorder. In conversion disorder, single complaints may be provoked by sudden emotional distress, such as that experienced in combat, a natural disaster, or bereavement. Here, onset is usually acute and resolution may be rapid, even without formal treatment. When emotional distress is more gradual and lasts longer (as in troubled marriages), the simulation of dysfunction can persist until the patient's circumstances change. Histrionic traits of personality may or may not be present, and cultural factors sometimes encourage people to utilize the sick role as a means of dealing with interpersonal problems. Single conversion symptoms can occur at almost any age and seem to be equally frequent in men and women.

Multiple conversion symptoms can be seen in somatization disorder, a chronic illness consisting of otherwise unexplained complaints in a variety of organ systems. Somatization disorder typically begins before 30 years of age, is more commonly diagnosed in women, and seems to be prompted by histrionic and obsessional traits. Among the consequences of this illness are repeated hospitalization, excessive diagnostic procedures, and unnecessary surgery. When evaluating a single conversion symptom the physician should remember that it may be occurring in the context of somatization disorder. The diagnosis of somatization disorder rests on the review of systems, in which patients endorse many symptoms (and often do so in elaborate and mysterious detail).

TREATMENT

Patients for whom the diagnosis of conversion disorder is being considered should generally be referred to a psychiatrist for consultation. This can be an awkward moment, for it begins to redefine the patient's sick role from the neurologic to the psychiatric. Although an illness has been validated, it is a potentially stigmatizing one, and consultation may be refused.

Justifying Psychiatric Consultation

Refusal of consultation can often be avoided if it is clear that the reality of the patient's illness is not in question; only its cause. Some patients readily accept the view that, just as physical problems can affect emotional health, emotional problems can affect physical health, and that expert assessment of the latter possibility is needed if appropriate treatment is to be given. Other patients may be receptive to a more forthright approach and can be told that they have conversion disorder, which means that there is, indeed, something wrong, but that its ultimate cause is psychological, not physiologic; that the fundamental problem is not a lesion of the nervous system, but stressful circumstances that have yet to be detected. These justifications for psychiatric consultation may be welcomed by patients who have already wondered whether "pressure" is responsible for their illness. Still, many people with conversion disorder become angry or disappointed when psychiatric consultation is proposed. In these cases the referring physician may wish to express an interest in continuing to help the patient, with the understanding that consultation will be reconsidered if progress is not made.

When Consultation Is Refused

Although some patients who initially resist psychiatric consultation eventually agree to it, others continue to refuse. Patients in the latter group may be unwilling to give up the neurologic sick role because it has many psychological and practical advantages. For instance, as long as the problem is defined as physiologic, it is the physician who is obliged to correct it, not the patient.

In the face of continued refusal to accept consultation one approach that may be tried is "visit titration." The first goal of such treatment is protective, and regular appointments are made in order to prevent unnecessary hospitalizations, invasive diagnostic procedures, and iatrogenic addictions. Visits are brief and scheduled often enough ("titrated") so that the patient does not telephone between them. During each appointment an interim history is taken and an appropriate examination performed, but the focus of inquiry progressively shifts from the neurologic complaint to the patient's current situation and how he or she is coping with interpersonal, financial, and other stresses. This supportive, problem-solving technique, though indirect and time consuming, often accomplishes its eventual goal of symptom reduction or psychiatric consultation.

Some Principles of Psychiatric Treatment

When neurologic and psychiatric assessment lead to a diagnosis of conversion disorder, treatment directed to the patient's behavior can take several forms, one of which is based on the principles of control, confrontation, and change.

Control is often best obtained on a psychiatric ward, because it removes patients from the environment in which their behavior has been reinforced—if unwittingly—by family and friends. At first, control is external: staff discourage abnormal behaviors (e.g., using a wheelchair) and encourage normal ones (e.g., walking unassisted). In order to dispel any ambiguity about the nature of the complaint, unnecessary medications (e.g., anticonvulsants for patients who do not have epilepsy) are discontinued. Family members are educated about the nature of conversion disorder and, with the patient, begin to make changes in the circumstances that have initiated and sustained the behavior. As the patient comes to understand these matters, control becomes increasingly internal.

Confrontation involves telling patients that the problem is something they *do,* not something they *have,* and that they are responsible for their behavior. "Reacting to stress" is reinterpreted as "doing it for a reason." Although patients may previously have been unaware (or partly aware) of their motivations for seeking the sick role, those motivations are now clarified, and more appropriate problem-solving strategies are suggested.

The process of confrontation can be helped considerably if the neurologist, psychiatrist, and patient jointly review the results of the neurologic evaluation. This public analysis reduces the chance that patients will later misinterpret the neurologist's opinion when they are reminded that their illness is psychological, not physiologic, in origin. Giving patients material to read can also be useful, and the descriptions of conversion disorder and somatization disorder in the *Diagnostic and Statistical Manual of Mental Disorders* are quite suitable for this purpose. It is important that such reading be discussed with the psychiatrist, to avoid misunderstanding. Patients may be relieved to learn that their illness is a well-recognized one and are less likely to regard the diagnosis as merely an idiosyncratic judgment by a callous physician.

Confrontation is not condemnation, but sympathetic acknowledgment of the patient's situation: "This is the diagnosis and this is what it means. . . . People sometimes do things unawares. . . . Had they been aware, they might well have chosen another course of action." Confrontation provides an opportunity to do things differently, and, in our experience, many patients welcome it.

Once the nature of conversion disorder is understood, meaningful change is possible. Through the process of psychiatric assessment and psychotherapy, patients are helped to review their circumstances, vulnerabilities, and strengths. This aspect of treatment is very individualized. Although the opening focus of interpretation is generally the inappropriate use of the sick role, more personal themes soon emerge—the need for control, the fear of abandonment, the hope for reassurance, and the desire for attention. As the use of indirect means to accomplish hidden ends is revealed, patients become aware of their behavior and can decide to achieve their purposes in a more satisfactory manner.

Certain patients try to place the burden of change on the physician, as they have tried to place it on others: it is the physician who must persuade them of the diagnosis, make the connections that lead to insight, and establish relationships on a new footing. Such patients should be reminded that the final responsibility for change is theirs, but, in giving this message, physicians can be optimistic as well as realistic. Many people who inappropriately use the sick role do so because they cannot think of a better way to solve their problems; once they are shown that way, their response is most gratifying to those who help them.

SUGGESTED READING

Boffeli TJ, Guze SB. The simulation of neurologic disease. Psychiatr Clin North Am 1992; 15:301–310.

Kaminsky MJ, Slavney PR. Hysterical and obsessional features in patients with Briquet's syndrome (somatization disorder). Psychologic Med 1983; 13:111–120.

Kellner R. Somatization disorder. In: Treatments of psychiatric disorders: A task force report of the American Psychiatric Association. Vol. 3. Washington, DC: American Psychiatric Association, 1989: 2166–2171.

Merskey H. Conversion disorders. In: Treatments of psychiatric disorders: A task force report of the American Psychiatric Association. Vol. 3. Washington, DC: American Psychiatric Association, 1989: 2152–2159.

Slavney PR. Perspectives on "Hysteria." Baltimore: The Johns Hopkins University Press, 1990.

INDEX

Brain
  abscess of, 113-116
  arteriovenous malformation of, 189-193
  biopsy of, 138
  encephalitis and, 137-140
  encephalopathy and. *See* Encephalopathy
  hemorrhage of, 297
  neonatal, 27
Brain injury, 202-206
  neonatal, 97-100
  seizure and, 28, 44
Brain tumor
  in child, 215-220
  metastatic, 224-226
Brainstem
  glioma of, 217-218
  in Reye's syndrome, 325
  in unconscious patient, 4
Brevetoxins, 309
Bromocriptine
  for acromegaly, 233
  neuroleptic malignant syndrome and, 51
  for Parkinson's disease, 244
  for progressive supranuclear palsy, 251
  for prolactinoma, 232

C

Caffeine
  headache and, 92
  for orthostatic hypotension, 24
Calcium, polymyositis and, 394-395
Calcium channel blocker
  hypertensive encephalopathy and, 195
  ischemic stroke and, 172
  for migraine, 83
  subarachnoid hemorrhage and, 188
Calcium gluconate, for spider bite, 307
Caloric stimulation, 3
Canal, semicircular, 8-9
Cancer. *See* Tumor
Capillary malformation, 190
Capsaicin, 407-408
  for pain, 72
Carbamazepine
  complex partial seizures and, 61-63
  dystonia and, 263-264
  effectiveness of, 56
  encephalomyelitis and, 157
  Huntington's disease and, 248-249
  multiple sclerosis and, 161
  for pain, 405
  pharmacokinetics of, 58
  side effects of, 59
Carbidopa
  for neurodegenerative disease, 337
  for Parkinsonism, 50
Carboplatin, glioma and, 218
Carboxylase deficiency, 256, 340
Carcinoembryonic antigen, 229
Carcinoma. *See* Tumor
Carcinomatous meningitis, 228-230
Carcinomatous sensory neuropathy, 373
Cardiac syncope, 6-7
Cardioembolization, 174-179
  in pregnancy, 173
  transient ischemic attack caused by, 166, 168

Cardioinhibitory carotid sinus syncope, 6
Cardiomyopathy, in pregnancy, 173
Cardiovascular syncope, 5-7
Carnitine
  deficiency of, 401
  for Reye's syndrome, 325
Carnitine palmitoyl transferase deficiency, 400-401
Carotid endarterectomy, 168
Carotid sinus syncope, 5, 6
Carpal tunnel syndrome, 361-364
Catabolic state in Reye's syndrome, 324
Cataplexy, 17-18
Catapres
  for orthostatic hypotension, 23
  for Tourette's syndrome, 272
Cataract, 334
Catfish envenomation, 308
Cavernous arteriovenous malformation, 189-191
Cavus foot deformity, 375, 376
CCNU, neurotoxic effects of, 313
Cefotaxime
  for brain abscess, 115
  for Lyme disease, 130
  for meningitis, 111
Ceftazidime
  for brain abscess, 115
  for subdural empyema, 117
Ceftizoxime, for meningitis, 111
Ceftriaxone
  for brain abscess, 115
  Clostridium difficile and, 130
  for meningitis, 111
  for subdural empyema, 117
  for syphilis, 128
Cefuroxime axetil, 130
Central nervous system
  lymphoma of, 150-151, 239-241
  pain and, 73
  paraneoplastic syndromes of, 235-239
  Taenia solium infection of, 123-125
  tumors of. *See* Tumor
Cerebellar ataxia, hereditary, 254-261. *See also* Ataxia
Cerebellar degeneration
  paraneoplastic, 236, 237
  progressive, 258-260
Cerebellar dysfunction, chemotherapy causing, 314
Cerebellar glioma, 218
Cerebellar hematoma, 180-181
  management of, 182
Cerebral angiography, 199
Cerebral cysticercosis, 123-125
Cerebral edema
  ischemic stroke and, 172, 173
  Reye's syndrome and, 325
Cerebral hemorrhage
  dementia with, 297
  intracranial hematoma and, 179-185
Cerebral infarction, 177-178
Cerebral palsy, 78
Cerebral toxoplasmosis, 149
Cerebral vasculitis, 196-201
Cerebral venous occlusion, postpartum, 173
Cerebrospinal fluid
  brachial neuritis and, 354

  carcinomatous meningitis and, 229
  cerebellar hematoma and, 180-181
  chemotherapy toxicity and, 315-316
  cysticercosis and, 123, 125
  encephalitis and, 137
  HIV infection and, 151
  hydrocephalus and, 94-96
    posthemorrhagic, 98
  idiopathic intracranial hypertension and, 87
  infantile spasms and, 30
  inflammatory demyelinating polyradiculo-neuropathy and, 350
  Lyme disease and, 131
  lymphoma and, 240
  meningitis and, 110
  neonatal seizures and, 29
  paraneoplastic neurologic syndromes and, 236-237
  sarcoidosis and, 164
  syphilis and, 126-127, 128
  tuberculous meningitis and, 119
Cerebrotendinous xanthomatosis, 339-340
Cerebrovascular disease, 166-201
  arteriovenous malformations as, 189-193
  cardioembolic stroke as, 174-179
  dementia with, 296-297
  hypertensive encephalopathy as, 194-196
  intracranial hematoma as, 179-185
  ischemic stroke as, 169-174
  ruptured intracranial aneurysm as, 185-189
  transient ischemic attack as, 166-168
  vasculitis as, 196-201
Cerebrovascular syncope, 7
Ceroid lipofuscinosis, 339
Cervical dystonia, 266-270
Cervical spondylosis, 77-78
Cervicocephalic vasculitis, 196-197
Charcot-Marie-Tooth disease, 269-270, 374-375
Chelating agent, for hepatic porphyria, 317-318, 320-321
Chemotherapy, 221-222
  for brain metastases, 226
  for carcinomatous meningitis, 229-230
  for ependymoma, 219
  for glioma, 218, 221-222
  for lymphoma, 240-241
  for neuroectodermal tumor, 216-217
Chenodeoxycholic acid, 340
Cherry-red spot, 334
Chiari malformation, 102
Chickenpox, 135
Chickpea toxicity, 311
Child
  absence seizures in, 38-41
  ataxia in, 255, 258-260
  brain tumor in, 215-220
  cerebral cysticercosis in, 123-125
  febrile seizures in, 32-37
    recurrence of, 43
  headache in, 90-93
  neurodegenerative disease in, 334-341
Chloral hydrate
  for Alzheimer's disease, 284, 285
  for neurodegenerative disease, 337